Terminologia Anatomica

Terminologia Anatomica

International Anatomical Terminology

FCAT
Federative Committee on Anatomical Terminology

1998
Thieme Stuttgart · New York

Library of Congress Cataloging-in-Publication Data

Terminologia anatomica [Medienkombination] = International anatomival terimnology / Federative Committee on Anatomical Terminology. – Stuttgart : Thieme
Buch. 1998
CD-ROM. 1998

Typesetting by: ScreenArt GmbH & Co. KG,
D-72827 Wannweil, Germany

Printed in Germany by:
Druckhaus Thomas Müntzer,
D-99947 Bad Langensalza, Germany

ISBN 3-13-114361-4 (book) 1 2 3 4 5 6
ISBN 3-13-115251-6 (book and CD-ROM)

Preface

This book on anatomical terminology is the joint creation of the Federative Committee on Anatomical Terminology (FCAT) and the 56 Member Associations of the International Federation of Associations of Anatomists (IFAA). The IFAA is the only international body representing all aspects of anatomy and anatomical associations.

At the General Assembly of the Federative World Congress of Anatomy, held in Rio de Janeiro, Brazil, in August 1989, the FCAT was elected. Its objectives were defined thus:

"To present the official terminology of the anatomical sciences after consultation with all the members of the International Federation of Associations of Anatomists, thus ensuring a democratic input to the terminology."

Anatomical terminology is the foundation of medical terminology and it is important that doctors and scientists throughout the world use the same name for each structure.

The FCAT has met on several occasions since its inception:

- Nancy, France *11 September 1990*
- Toronto, Canada *4 July 1991*
- Nottingham, England *23 July 1992*
- Barcelona, Spain *21 July 1993*
- Utrecht, The Netherlands *6 to 8 April 1994*
- Lisbon, Portugal *21 to 30 July 1994*
- Southampton, England *14 to 17 Dec. 1994*
- Thessaloniki, Greece *23 to 27 September 1995*
- San Jose, Costa Rica *12 to 16 February 1996*
- Jena, Germany *25 to 26 March 1996*
- Fribourg, Switzerland *15 to 19 July 1996*
- New Orleans, USA *5 to 9 April 1997*
- São Paulo, Brazil *25 to 28 August 1997*
- Mainz, Germany *14 to 19 February 1998*

Early attempts to establish a working relationship with a previous terminology committee (the IANC) were unsuccessful and the FCAT has worked towards its objectives by reviewing and revising the Latin terminology, with the addition of a list of English terms in common usage. The FCAT has tried to avoid unnecessary change and has adopted many alternatives in common usage in order to encompass the variable way in which the terminology is used in different countries.

During 1996 a final draft of the terminology for macroscopic anatomy was sent to all the Member Associations of the IFAA for comment. The present work incorporates changes suggested by these Member Associations.

The FCAT is continuing work on histology, cytology, embryology, dental terminology and anthropology and hopes to present these works in published form soon. Future plans include a dictionary of anatomical terms, an illustrated terminology and electronic forms.

The terms are laid out in three columns, with each Latin term accompanied by a term in current usage in English-speaking countries. Alongside each pair is a unique identification number. The order in which the terms are set out follows the anatomy naturally through each system. Indentation and heading styles are used to indicate the relationship of one term to another. The book is completed by a comprehensive index of Latin and English terms and an index of eponyms that identifies the number of the appropriate non-eponymous term.

Only the Latin list of terms should be used as the basis for creating lists of equivalent terms in other languages. English equivalents are given in this list as English is spoken in many countries. It is not the basis for terminology in other languages.

The committee invites constructive comments from all quarters for consideration for future editions. Comments may be sent by postcard or Email to: leser.service@thieme.de.

Having been adopted by the IFAA this terminology supersedes all previous lists.

July 1998

Ian Whitmore
Chairman FCAT

Acknowledgements

Financial

During the period in which the Committee has worked on this terminology it has been fortunate to have the support of the societies and associations to which the individual members of the Committee belong. These organisations have helped with the travel costs and subsistence for meetings of the FCAT. The committee thanks them for their support.

In addition some meetings of the FCAT have been partially or totally sponsored by:

- Novartis Ltd, Switzerland
- ZLB Central Laboratory Blood Transfusion Service SRC, Switzerland
- Banco Real, Brazil
- American Association of Anatomists
- Anatomical Society of Great Britain and Ireland
- IFAA (International Federation of Anatomical Associations)
- Anatomische Gesellschaft
- Carl Zeiss Jena GmbH, Germany
- Dianova GmbH, Germany
- Freunde der Universität Mainz, Germany
- Georg Thieme Verlag, Germany
- Gustav Fischer Verlag, Germany
- Nederlandse Anatomen Vereniging
- Springer Verlag, Germany
- Universität Mainz, Germany
- Urban & Schwarzenberg Verlag für Medizin, Germany
- DFG, Germany

Meetings of the FCAT have been held in conjunction with and thus assisted by:

- International Symposia on Morphology at Nancy, France; Toronto, Canada; Barcelona, Spain; Thessaloniki, Greece; and San Jose, Costa Rica.
- Joint meetings of the Anatomical Society of Great Britain & Ireland, Anatomische Gesellschaft, and Nederlandse Anatomen Vereniging in Southampton, UK; Utrecht, Netherlands; and Jena, Germany.
- The meeting of the Anatomical Society of Great Britain and Ireland in Nottingham, UK.
- The IFAA congress held in Lisbon, Portugal.

Academic

The FCAT wishes to thank those individuals who assisted the Committee during its deliberations:

- Prof. B. Berkovitz
- Prof. L. Heimer
- Prof. C. K. Henkel
- Prof. T. P. Ma
- Dr. J. E. McNeal
- Prof. N. A. Moore
- Dr. R. P. Myers
- Prof. R. Nieuwenhuys
- Prof. G. Paxinos
- Prof. H. J. Ralston
- Prof. C. B. Saper
- Prof. J. E. Skandalakis
- Prof. L. W. Swanson
- Prof. H. B. M. Uylings
- Prof. J. Voogd

While the individuals acknowledged here gave valuable expert advice, the final terminology is the responsibility of the FCAT.

Members of the FCAT

Current members of FCAT are:

- Professor Ian Whitmore, Chairman, United Kingdom
- Professor Lutz Vollrath, Vice Chairman, Germany
- Professor Lee J. A. Di Dio, Secretary General, Brazil
- Professor Colin Wendell-Smith, Secretary, Australia
- Professor Georges Grignon, Secretary, France
- Professor David Brynmor Thomas, United Kingdom
- Professor Antoine Dhem, Belgium
- Professor Jan Drukker, The Netherlands
- Professor Raymond Gasser, United States of America
- Professor Jacques Gilloteaux, United States of America
- Professor Rolando Cruz Gutiérrez, Costa Rica
- Professor Duane E. Haines, United States of America
- Professor Lev L. Kolesnikov, Russia
- Professor Keith L. Moore, Canada
- Professor José Carlos Prates, Brazil
- Professor Alessandro Riva, Italy
- Professor Domingo Ruano-Gil, Spain
- Professor Haramichi Seguchi, Japan
- Professor Pierre Sprumont, Switzerland
- Professor Phillip V. Tobias, Republic of South Africa

Previous members were:

- Professor Giuseppe Balboni, Italy
- Professor Edward Klika, Czechoslovakia
- Professor George F. Martin, United States of America
- Professor Galina Satjukova, Russia
- Professor Kenjiro Yasuda, Japan

Contents

1 ...	**Anatomia generalis**	**General Anatomy**
1 ...	Nomina generalia	General terms
2 ...	Partes corporis humani	Parts of human body
3 ...	Plana, linea et regiones	Planes, lines and regions
7 ...	**Anatomia systemica**	**Systemic anatomy**
7 ...	**Ossa; Systema skeletale**	**Bones; Skeletal system**
7 ...	Nomina generalia	General terms
8 ...	Cranium	Cranium
9 ...	Ossa cranii	Bones of cranium
16 ...	Columna vertebralis	Vertebral column
17 ...	Skeleton thoracis	Thoracic skeleton
18 ...	Ossa membri superioris	Bones of upper limb
21 ...	Ossa membri inferioris	Bones of lower limb
25 ...	**Juncturae; Systema articulare**	**Joints; Articular system**
25 ...	Nomina generalia	General terms
26 ...	Juncturae cranii	Joints of skull
27 ...	Juncturae columnae vertebralis	Vertebral joints
28 ...	Juncturae thoracis	Thoracic joints
28 ...	Juncturae cinguli pelvici	Joints of pelvic girdle
28 ...	Juncturae membri superioris	Joints of upper limb
30 ...	Juncturae membri inferioris	Joints of lower limb
33 ...	**Musculi; Systema musculare**	**Muscles; Muscular system**
33 ...	Nomina generalia	General terms
34 ...	Musculi capitis	Muscles of head
35 ...	Musculi colli; Musculi cervicis	Muscles of neck
36 ...	Musculi dorsi	Muscles of back
37 ...	Musculi thoracis	Muscles of thorax
38 ...	Musculi abdominis	Muscles of abdomen
40 ...	Musculi membri superioris	Muscles of upper limb
42 ...	Musculi membri inferioris	Muscles of lower limb
44 ...	Vaginae tendinum et bursae	Tendon sheaths and bursae
47 ...	**Systema digestorium**	**Alimentary system**
47 ...	Os	Mouth
50 ...	Fauces	Fauces
50 ...	Pharynx	Pharynx
51 ...	Oesophagus	Oesophagus
51 ...	Gaster	Stomach
52 ...	Intestinum tenue	Small intestine
53 ...	Intestinum crassum	Large intestine
54 ...	Hepar	Liver
56 ...	Vesica biliaris; Vesica fellea	Gallbladder
56 ...	Pancreas	Pancreas

57 ...	**Systema respiratorium**	**Respiratory system**
57 ...	Nasus	Nose
58 ...	Larynx	Larynx
59 ...	Trachea	Trachea
59 ...	Bronchi	Bronchi
60 ...	Pulmones	Lungs
62 ...	**Cavitas thoracis; Cavitas thoracica**	**Thoracic cavity; Thorax**
63 ...	**Systema urinarium**	**Urinary system**
63 ...	Ren; Nephros	Kidney
64 ...	Ureter	Ureter
64 ...	Vesica urinaria	Urinary bladder
64 ...	Urethra feminina	Female urethra
64 ...	Urethra masculina	Male urethra
65 ...	**Systemata genitalia**	**Genital systems**
65 ...	Organa genitalia feminina interna	Female internal genitalia
66 ...	Organa genitalia feminina externa	Female external genitalia
67 ...	Organa genitalia masculina interna	Male internal genitalia
69 ...	Organa genitalia masculina externa	Male external genitalia
71 ...	Perineum	Perineum
72 ...	**Cavitas abdominis et pelvis**	**Abdominopelvic cavity**
74 ...	**Glandulae endocrinae**	**Endocrine glands**
75 ...	**Systema cardiovasculare**	**Cardiovascular system**
75 ...	Nomina generalia	General terms
75 ...	Cor	Heart
78 ...	Arteriae	Arteries
91 ...	Venae	Veins
99 ...	Trunci et ductus lymphatici	Lymphatic trunks and ducts
100 ...	**Systema lymphoideum**	**Lymphoid system**
100 ...	Organa lymphoidea primaria	Primary lymphoid organs
100 ...	Organa lymphoidea secundaria	Secondary lymphoid organs
101 ...	Nodi lymphoidei regionales	Regional lymph nodes
104 ...	**Systema nervosum**	**Nervous system**
104 ...	Nomina generalia	General terms
104 ...	Pars centralis; Systema nervosum centrale	Central nervous system
104 ...	Meninges	Meninges
105 ...	Medulla spinalis	Spinal cord
108 ...	Encephalon	Brain
108 ...	Myelencephalon; Medulla oblongata; Bulbus	Myelencephalon; Medulla oblongata; Bulb
112 ...	Pons	Pons
115 ...	Mesencephalon	Mesencephalon; Midbrain
118 ...	Cerebellum	Cerebellum
120 ...	Diencephalon	Diencephalon
124 ...	Telencephalon; Cerebrum	Telencephalon; Cerebrum
132 ...	Pars peripherica; Systema nervosum periphericum	Peripheral nervous system

133 ...	Nervi craniales	Cranial nerves
137 ...	Nervi spinales	Spinal nerves
141 ...	Divisio autonomica; Pars autonomica systematis nervosi peripherici	Autonomic division; Autonomic part of peripheral nervous system
141 ...	Pars sympathica	Sympathetic part
142 ...	Pars parasympathica	Parasympathetic part
142 ...	Plexus viscerales et ganglia visceralia	Peripheral autonomic plexuses and ganglia
144 ...	**Organa sensuum**	**Sense organs**
144 ...	Organum olfactorium; Organum olfactus	Olfactory organ
144 ...	Oculus et structurae pertinentes	Eye and related structures
148 ...	Auris	Ear
153 ...	Organum gustatorium; Organum gustus	Gustatory organ
154 ...	**Integumentum commune**	**The integument**
154 ...	Cutis	Skin
155 ...	Tela subcutanea; Hypodermis	Subcutaneous tissue

157 ... History of International Anatomical Terminology
163 ... Index of Eponyms
167 ... Index of Latin terms
227 ... Index of English terms

Anatomia generalis

General anatomy

	Nomina generalia	*General terms*
A01.0.00.001	Verticalis	Vertical
A01.0.00.002	Horizontalis	Horizontal
A01.0.00.003	Medianus	Median
A01.0.00.004	Coronalis	Coronal
A01.0.00.005	Sagittalis	Sagittal
A01.0.00.006	Dexter	Right
A01.0.00.007	Sinister	Left
A01.0.00.008	Intermedius	Intermediate
A01.0.00.009	Medialis	Medial
A01.0.00.010	Lateralis	Lateral
A01.0.00.011	Anterior	Anterior
A01.0.00.012	Posterior	Posterior
A01.0.00.013	Ventralis	Ventral
A01.0.00.014	Dorsalis	Dorsal
A01.0.00.015	Frontalis	Frontal
A01.0.00.016	Occipitalis	Occipital
A01.0.00.017	Superior	Superior
A01.0.00.018	Inferior	Inferior
A01.0.00.019	Cranialis	Cranial
A01.0.00.020	Caudalis	Caudal
A01.0.00.021	Rostralis	Rostral
A01.0.00.022	Apicalis	Apical
A01.0.00.023	Basalis	Basal
A01.0.00.024	Basilaris	Basilar
A01.0.00.025	Medius	Middle
A01.0.00.026	Transversus	Transverse
A01.0.00.027	Transversalis	Transverse
A01.0.00.028	Longitudinalis	Longitudinal
A01.0.00.029	Axialis	Axial
A01.0.00.030	Externus	External
A01.0.00.031	Internus	Internal
A01.0.00.032	Luminalis	Luminal
A01.0.00.033	Superficialis	Superficial
A01.0.00.034	Profundus	Deep
A01.0.00.035	Proximalis	Proximal
A01.0.00.036	Distalis	Distal
A01.0.00.037	Centralis	Central
A01.0.00.038	Periphericus; Peripheralis	Peripheral
A01.0.00.039	Radialis	Radial
A01.0.00.040	Ulnaris	Ulnar
A01.0.00.041	Fibularis; Peronealis	Fibular; Peroneal
A01.0.00.042	Tibialis	Tibial
A01.0.00.043	Palmaris; Volaris	Palmar; Volar
A01.0.00.044	Plantaris	Plantar
A01.0.00.045	Flexor	Flexor
A01.0.00.046	Extensor	Extensor

	Partes corporis humani	Parts of human body
A01.1.00.001	Caput	Head
A01.1.00.002	Sinciput	Forehead
A01.1.00.003	Occiput	Occiput
A01.1.00.004	Tempora	Temple
A01.1.00.005	Auris	Ear
A01.1.00.006	Facies	Face
A01.1.00.007	Oculus	Eye
A01.1.00.008	Bucca	Cheek
A01.1.00.009	Nasus	Nose
A01.1.00.010	Os	Mouth
A01.1.00.011	Mentum	Chin
A01.1.00.012	Collum; Cervix	Neck
A01.1.00.013	Truncus	Trunk
A01.1.00.014	Thorax	Thorax
A01.1.00.015	Pectus	Front of chest
A01.1.00.016	Abdomen	Abdomen
A01.1.00.017	Pelvis	Pelvis
A01.1.00.018	Dorsum	Back
A01.1.00.019	Membrum superius	Upper limb
A01.1.00.020	Cingulum pectorale; Cingulum membri superioris	Pectoral girdle; Shoulder girdle
A01.1.00.021	Axilla	Axilla
A01.1.00.022	Brachium	Arm
A01.1.00.023	Cubitus	Elbow
A01.1.00.024	Antebrachium	Forearm
A01.1.00.025	Manus	Hand
A01.1.00.026	Carpus	Wrist
A01.1.00.027	Metacarpus	Metacarpus
A01.1.00.028	Palma; Vola	Palm
A01.1.00.029	Dorsum manus	Dorsum of hand
A01.1.00.030	Digiti manus	Fingers including thumb
A01.1.00.031	Membrum inferius	Lower limb
A01.1.00.032	Cingulum pelvicum; Cingulum membri inferioris	Pelvic girdle
A01.1.00.033	Nates; Clunes	Buttocks
A01.1.00.034	Coxa	Hip
A01.1.00.035	Femur	Thigh
A01.1.00.036	Genu	Knee
A01.1.00.037	Poples	Posterior part of knee
A01.1.00.038	Crus	Leg
A01.1.00.039	Sura	Calf
A01.1.00.040	Pes	Foot
A01.1.00.041	Tarsus	Ankle
A01.1.00.042	Calx	Heel
A01.1.00.043	Metatarsus	Metatarsus
A01.1.00.044	Planta	Sole
A01.1.00.045	Dorsum pedis	Dorsum of foot
A01.1.00.046	Digiti pedis	Toes
A01.1.00.047	Cavitates	Cavities
A01.1.00.048	Cavitas cranii	Cranial cavity
A01.1.00.049	Cavitas thoracis	Thoracic cavity
A01.1.00.050	Cavitas abdominis et pelvis	Abdominopelvic cavity
A01.1.00.051	Cavitas abdominis	Abdominal cavity
A01.1.00.052	Cavitas pelvis	Pelvic cavity

* A01.2.00.000	**Plana, lineae et regiones**	**Planes, lines and regions**
A01.2.00.001	Plana frontalia; Plana coronalia	Frontal planes; Coronal planes
A01.2.00.002	Plana horizontalia	Horizontal planes
A01.2.00.003	Plana sagittalia	Sagittal planes
A01.2.00.004	Planum medianum	Median plane; Median sagittal plane
A01.2.00.005	Plana paramediana	Paramedian planes
A01.2.00.006	Plana transversalia	Transverse planes
A01.2.00.007	Planum transpyloricum	Transpyloric plane
A01.2.00.008	Planum subcostale	Subcostal plane
A01.2.00.009	Planum supracristale	Supracristal plane
A01.2.00.010	Planum intertuberculare	Intertubercular plane
A01.2.00.011	Planum interspinale	Interspinous plane
A01.2.00.012	Linea mediana anterior	Anterior median line
A01.2.00.013	Linea sternalis	Sternal line
A01.2.00.014	Linea parasternalis	Parasternal line
A01.2.00.015	Linea medioclavicularis	Midclavicular line
A01.2.00.016	Linea mammillaris	Mammillary line; Nipple line
A01.2.00.017	Linea axillaris anterior	Anterior axillary line
A01.2.00.018	Linea axillaris media	Midaxillary line
A01.2.00.019	Linea axillaris posterior	Posterior axillary line
A01.2.00.020	Linea scapularis	Scapular line
A01.2.00.021	Linea paravertebralis	Paravertebral line
A01.2.00.022	Linea mediana posterior	Posterior median line
A01.2.01.001	**Regiones capitis**	**Regions of head**
A01.2.01.002	Regio frontalis	Frontal region
A01.2.01.003	Regio parietalis	Parietal region
A01.2.01.004	Regio occipitalis	Occipital region
A01.2.01.005	Regio temporalis	Temporal region
A01.2.01.006	Regio auricularis	Auricular region
A01.2.01.007	Regio mastoidea	Mastoid region
A01.2.01.008	Regio facialis	Facial region
A01.2.01.009	Sulcus suprapalpebralis	Suprapalpebral sulcus
A01.2.01.010	Regio orbitalis	Orbital region
A01.2.01.011	Sulcus infrapalpebralis	Infrapalpebral sulcus
A01.2.01.012	Regio infraorbitalis	Infra-orbital region
A01.2.01.013	Regio buccalis	Buccal region
A01.2.01.014	Regio parotideomasseterica	Parotid region
A01.2.01.015	Regio zygomatica	Zygomatic region
A01.2.01.016	Regio nasalis	Nasal region
A01.2.01.017	Sulcus nasolabialis	Nasolabial sulcus
A01.2.01.018	Regio oralis	Oral region
A01.2.01.019	Sulcus mentolabialis	Mentolabial sulcus
A01.2.01.020	Regio mentalis	Mental region
A01.2.02.001	**Regiones cervicales**	**Regions of neck**
A01.2.02.002	Regio cervicalis anterior; Trigonum cervicale anterius; Trigonum colli anterius	Anterior cervical region; Anterior triangle
A01.2.02.003	Trigonum submandibulare	Submandibular triangle
A01.2.02.004	Trigonum caroticum	Carotid triangle
A01.2.02.005	Trigonum musculare; Trigonum omotracheale	Muscular triangle; Omotracheal triangle
A01.2.02.006	Trigonum submentale	Submental triangle
A01.2.02.007	Regio sternocleidomastoidea	Sternocleidomastoid region
A01.2.02.008	Fossa supraclavicularis minor	Lesser supraclavicular fossa
A01.2.02.009	Regio cervicalis lateralis; Trigonum cervicale posterius; Trigonum colli laterale	Lateral cervical region; Posterior triangle
A01.2.02.010	Trigonum omoclaviculare	Omoclavicular triangle; Subclavian triangle
A01.2.02.011	Fossa supraclavicularis major	Greater supraclavicular fossa

* **A01.2.00.000** *Regiones* The use of this term differs in practice. It may be restricted to areas of the surface of the body or be three dimensional.

A01.2.02.012	Regio cervicalis posterior; Regio colli posterior	Posterior cervical region
A01.2.03.001	**Regiones thoracicae anteriores et laterales**	**Anterior and lateral thoracic regions**
A01.2.03.002	Regio presternalis	Presternal region
A01.2.03.003	Fossa infraclavicularis	Infraclavicular fossa
A01.2.03.004	Trigonum clavipectorale; Trigonum deltopectorale	Clavipectoral triangle; Deltopectoral triangle
A01.2.03.005	Regio pectoralis	Pectoral region
* **A01.2.03.006**	Regio pectoralis lateralis	Lateral pectoral region
A01.2.03.007	Regio mammaria	Mammary region
A01.2.03.008	Regio inframammaria	Inframammary region
A01.2.03.009	Regio axillaris	Axillary region
A01.2.03.010	Fossa axillaris	Axillary fossa
A01.2.04.001	**Regiones abdominales**	**Abdominal regions**
A01.2.04.002	Hypochondrium; Regio hypochondriaca	Hypochondrium
A01.2.04.003	Epigastrium; Regio epigastrica; Fossa epigastrica	Epigastric region ; Epigastric fossa
A01.2.04.004	Latus; Regio lateralis	Flank; Lateral region
A01.2.04.005	Umbilicus; Regio umbilicalis	Umbilical region
A01.2.04.006	Inguen; Regio inguinalis	Groin; Inguinal region
A01.2.04.007	Hypogastrium; Regio pubica	Pubic region
A01.2.05.001	**Regiones dorsales; Regiones dorsi**	**Regions of back**
A01.2.05.002	Regio vertebralis	Vertebral region
A01.2.05.003	Regio sacralis	Sacral region
A01.2.05.004	(Foveola coccygea)	(Coccygeal foveola)
A01.2.05.005	Regio scapularis	Scapular region
* **A01.2.05.006**	Trigonum auscultationis	Auscultatory triangle; Triangle of auscultation
A01.2.05.007	Regio infrascapularis	Infrascapular region
A01.2.05.008	Regio lumbalis	Lumbar region
A01.2.05.009	(Trigonum lumbale inferius)	(Inferior lumbar triangle)
* **A01.2.05.010**	(Trigonum lumbale superius)	(Superior lumbar triangle)
A01.2.06.001	**Regio perinealis**	**Perineal region**
A01.2.06.002	Regio analis	Anal triangle
A01.2.06.003	Regio urogenitalis	Urogenital triangle
A01.2.07.001	**Regiones membri superioris**	**Regions of upper limb**
A01.2.07.002	Regio deltoidea	Deltoid region
A01.2.07.003	Regio brachialis	Brachial region
A01.2.07.004	Regio brachii anterior; Regio brachialis anterior	Anterior region of arm
A01.2.07.005	Sulcus bicipitalis lateralis; Sulcus bicipitalis radialis	Lateral bicipital groove
A01.2.07.006	Sulcus bicipitalis medialis; Sulcus bicipitalis ulnaris	Medial bicipital groove
A01.2.07.007	Regio brachii posterior; Regio brachialis posterior	Posterior region of arm
A01.2.07.008	Regio cubitalis	Cubital region
A01.2.07.009	Regio cubitalis anterior	Anterior region of elbow
A01.2.07.010	Fossa cubitalis	Cubital fossa
A01.2.07.011	Regio cubitalis posterior	Posterior region of elbow
A01.2.07.012	Regio antebrachialis	Antebrachial region
A01.2.07.013	Regio antebrachii anterior; Regio antebrachialis anterior	Anterior region of forearm

* **A01.2.03.006** *Regio pectoralis lateralis* The part of the pectoral region located between the anterior and posterior axillary lines.

* **A01.2.05.006** *Trigonum auscultationis* This triangle is formed by the lateral border of *m. trapezius*, the medial border of *m. rhomboideus major* and the superior border of *m. latissimus dorsi* with fascia over the seventh rib and adjacent intercostal spaces in its floor. With the upper limbs above the head, the triangles are at their largest and auscultation of the superior segments of the lower lobes of the lungs through them is facilitated. However, it has been said that the left triangle was so named because the drip of ingested fluids into the cardia of the stomach could be heard through it and timed in cases of oesophageal obstruction.

* **A01.2.05.010** *(Trigonum lumbale superius)* An inconstant triangle or rhombus through which abscesses may point or herniation occur. When present it is overlapped by *m. latissimus dorsi* and *m. obliquus externus abdominis* with *fascia thoracolumbalis* as its floor. It is bounded by the 12th rib and *m. serratus posterior inferior* superiorly, *m. erector spinae* medially and *m. obliquus internus abdominis* laterally.

A01.2.07.014	Regio antebrachii posterior; Regio antebrachialis posterior	Posterior region of forearm
A01.2.07.015	Margo radialis; Margo lateralis	Radial border; Lateral border
A01.2.07.016	Margo ulnaris; Margo medialis	Ulnar border; Medial border
A01.2.07.017	Regio manus	Hand region
A01.2.07.018	Regio carpalis	Carpal region
A01.2.07.019	Regio carpalis anterior	Anterior region of wrist
A01.2.07.020	Regio carpalis posterior	Posterior region of wrist
A01.2.07.021	Regio dorsalis manus	Dorsum of hand
A01.2.07.022	Palma; Vola; Regio palmaris	Palm; Palmar region
A01.2.07.023	Thenar; Eminentia thenaris	Thenar eminence
A01.2.07.024	Hypothenar; Eminentia hypothenaris	Hypothenar eminence
A01.2.07.025	Regio metacarpalis	Metacarpal region
A01.2.07.026	Digiti manus	Digits of hand; Fingers including thumb
A01.2.07.027	Pollex; Digitus primus [I]	Thumb
A01.2.07.028	Index; Digitus secundus [II]	Index finger
A01.2.07.029	Digitus medius; Digitus tertius [III]	Middle finger
A01.2.07.030	Digitus anularis; Digitus quartus [IV]	Ring finger
A01.2.07.031	Digitus minimus; Digitus quintus [V]	Little finger
A01.2.07.032	Facies palmares digitorum	Palmar surfaces of fingers
A01.2.07.033	Facies dorsales digitorum	Dorsal surfaces of fingers
A01.2.08.001	**Regiones membri inferioris**	**Regions of lower limb**
A01.2.08.002	Regio glutealis	Gluteal region
* A01.2.08.003	Crena analis; Crena ani; Crena intergluteali**s**	Intergluteal cleft; Natal cleft
A01.2.08.004	Sulcus glutealis	Gluteal fold
A01.2.08.005	Regio coxae	Hip region
A01.2.08.006	Regio femoris	Femoral region
A01.2.08.007	Regio femoris anterior	Anterior region of thigh
A01.2.08.008	Trigonum femoris	Femoral triangle
A01.2.08.009	Regio femoris posterior	Posterior region of thigh
A01.2.08.010	Regio genus	Knee region
A01.2.08.011	Regio genus anterior	Anterior region of knee
A01.2.08.012	Regio genus posterior	Posterior region of knee
A01.2.08.013	Fossa poplitea	Popliteal fossa
A01.2.08.014	Regio cruris	Leg region
A01.2.08.015	Regio cruris anterior	Anterior region of leg
A01.2.08.016	Regio cruris posterior	Posterior region of leg
A01.2.08.017	Regio surae	Sural region
A01.2.08.018	Regio talocruralis anterior	Anterior talocrural region; Anterior ankle region
A01.2.08.019	Regio talocruralis posterior	Posterior talocrural region; Posterior ankle region
A01.2.08.020	Regio retromalleolaris lateralis	Lateral retromalleolar region
A01.2.08.021	Regio retromalleolaris medialis	Medial retromalleolar region
A01.2.08.022	Regio pedis	Foot region
A01.2.08.023	Regio calcanea	Heel region
A01.2.08.024	Dorsum pedis; Regio dorsalis pedis	Dorsum of foot; Dorsal region of foot
A01.2.08.025	Planta; Regio plantaris	Sole; Plantar region
A01.2.08.026	Margo lateralis pedis; Margo fibularis pedis	Lateral border of foot; Fibular border of foot; Peroneal border of foot
A01.2.08.027	Margo medialis pedis; Margo tibialis pedis	Medial border of foot; Tibial border of foot
A01.2.08.028	Arcus pedis longitudinalis	Longitudinal arch of foot
A01.2.08.029	Pars lateralis	Lateral part
A01.2.08.030	Pars medialis	Medial part
A01.2.08.031	Arcus pedis transversus proximalis	Proximal transverse arch of foot
A01.2.08.032	Arcus pedis transversus distalis	Distal transverse arch of foot

* **A01.2.08.003** *Crena analis; crena ani; crena intergluteali*s The cleft between the buttocks, leading to the anus. Also called clunium, crena clunium, gluteal furrow, *intergluteal cleft*, rima ani, or rima clunium. Terms derived from *anus* and *gloutos* are preferred because those derived from *clunis* and *natis* may be confused with others from *cunnus* (vulva) and *natus* (birth).

A01.2.08.033	Regio tarsalis	Ankle region
A01.2.08.034	Regio metatarsalis	Metatarsal region
A01.2.08.035	Digiti pedis	Digits of foot; Toes
A01.2.08.036	Hallux; Digitus primus [I]	Great toe [I]
A01.2.08.037	Digitus secundus [II]	Second toe [II]
A01.2.08.038	Digitus tertius [III]	Third toe [III]
A01.2.08.039	Digitus quartus [IV]	Fourth toe [IV]
A01.2.08.040	Digitus minimus; Digitus quintus [V]	Little toe; Fifth toe [V]
A01.2.08.041	Facies plantares digitorum	Plantar surfaces of toes
A01.2.08.042	Facies dorsales digitorum	Dorsal surfaces of toes

Anatomia systemica | Systemic anatomy

A02.0.00.000 Ossa; Systema skeletale | Bones; skeletal system

	Nomina generalia	*General terms*
A02.0.00.001	Pars ossea	Bony part
A02.0.00.002	Substantia corticalis	Cortical bone
A02.0.00.003	Substantia compacta	Compact bone
A02.0.00.004	Substantia spongiosa; Substantia trabecularis	Spongy bone; Trabecular bone
A02.0.00.005	Pars cartilaginea	Cartilaginous part
A02.0.00.006	Pars membranacea	Membranous part
A02.0.00.007	Periosteum	Periosteum
A02.0.00.008	Perichondrium	Perichondrium
A02.0.00.009	Skeleton axiale	Axial skeleton
A02.0.00.010	Skeleton appendiculare	Appendicular skeleton
A02.0.00.011	Os longum	Long bone
A02.0.00.012	Os breve	Short bone
A02.0.00.013	Os planum	Flat bone
A02.0.00.014	Os irregulare	Irregular bone
A02.0.00.015	Os pneumaticum	Pneumatized bone
A02.0.00.016	Os sesamoideum	Sesamoid bone
A02.0.00.017	Diaphysis	Diaphysis
A02.0.00.018	Epiphysis	Epiphysis
A02.0.00.019	Cartilago epiphysialis	Epiphysial cartilage
A02.0.00.020	Lamina epiphysialis	Epiphysial plate; Growth plate
A02.0.00.021	Linea epiphysialis	Epiphysial line
A02.0.00.022	Metaphysis	Metaphysis
A02.0.00.023	Apophysis	Apophysis
A02.0.00.024	Tuber	Tuber; Tuberosity
A02.0.00.025	Tuberculum	Tubercle
A02.0.00.026	Tuberositas	Tuberosity
A02.0.00.027	Eminentia	Eminence
A02.0.00.028	Processus	Process
A02.0.00.029	Condylus	Condyle
A02.0.00.030	Epicondylus	Epicondyle
A02.0.00.031	Crista	Crest; Ridge
A02.0.00.032	Linea	Line
A02.0.00.033	Incisura	Notch
A02.0.00.034	Fossa	Fossa
A02.0.00.035	Sulcus	Groove
A02.0.00.036	Facies articularis	Articular surface
A02.0.00.037	Cavitas medullaris	Medullary cavity; Marrow cavity
* A02.0.00.038	Endosteum	Endosteum
A02.0.00.039	Medulla ossium flava	Yellow bone marrow
A02.0.00.040	Medulla ossium rubra	Red bone marrow
A02.0.00.041	Foramen nutricium	Nutrient foramen
A02.0.00.042	Canalis nutricius; Canalis nutriens	Nutrient canal
A02.0.00.043	Centrum ossificationis	Ossification centre▲
A02.0.00.044	Primarium	Primary
A02.0.00.045	Secundarium	Secondary

* **A02.0.00.038** *Endosteum* The incomplete layer of bone cells sometimes observed on the inner aspects of the bones constitutes the *endosteum* which is thus not a membrane like the *periosteum* but corresponds to the periosteal layer of the *dura mater.*

A02.1.00.001	Cranium	Cranium
A02.1.00.002	Norma facialis; Norma frontalis	Facial aspect; Frontal aspect
A02.1.00.003	Norma superior; Norma verticalis	Superior aspect; Vertical aspect
A02.1.00.004	Norma occipitalis	Occipital aspect
A02.1.00.005	Norma lateralis	Lateral aspect
A02.1.00.006	Norma inferior; Norma basalis	Inferior aspect
A02.1.00.007	Neurocranium	Neurocranium; Brain box
A02.1.00.008	Viscerocranium	Viscerocranium; Facial skeleton
A02.1.00.009	Chondrocranium	Chondrocranium
A02.1.00.010	Desmocranium	Desmocranium
A02.1.00.011	Pericranium; Periosteum externum cranii	Pericranium
A02.1.00.012	Cavitas cranii	Cranial cavity
A02.1.00.013	Frons	Forehead
A02.1.00.014	Occiput	Occiput
A02.1.00.015	Nasion	Nasion
A02.1.00.016	Bregma	Bregma
A02.1.00.017	Lambda	Lambda
A02.1.00.018	Inion	Inion
A02.1.00.019	Pterion	Pterion
A02.1.00.020	Asterion	Asterion
A02.1.00.021	Gonion	Gonion
A02.1.00.022	Fossa temporalis	Temporal fossa
A02.1.00.023	Arcus zygomaticus	Zygomatic arch
A02.1.00.024	Fossa infratemporalis	Infratemporal fossa
A02.1.00.025	Fossa pterygopalatina	Pterygopalatine fossa
A02.1.00.026	Fissura pterygomaxillaris	Pterygomaxillary fissure
A02.1.00.027	Fonticuli cranii	Fontanelles
A02.1.00.028	Fonticulus anterior	Anterior fontanelle
A02.1.00.029	Fonticulus posterior	Posterior fontanelle
A02.1.00.030	Fonticulus sphenoidalis; Fonticulus anterolateralis	Sphenoidal fontanelle
A02.1.00.031	Fonticulus mastoideus; Fonticulus posterolateralis	Mastoid fontanelle
A02.1.00.032	Calvaria	Calvaria
A02.1.00.033	Vertex	Vertex
A02.1.00.034	Lamina externa	External table
A02.1.00.035	Diploe	Diploe
A02.1.00.036	Canales diploici	Diploic canals
A02.1.00.037	Lamina interna	Internal table
A02.1.00.038	Sulcus sinus sagittalis superioris	Groove for superior sagittal sinus
A02.1.00.039	Foveolae granulares	Granular foveolae
A02.1.00.040	Impressiones gyrorum; Impressiones digitatae; Juga cerebralia	Impressions of cerebral gyri
A02.1.00.041	Sulci venosi	Venous grooves
A02.1.00.042	Sulci arteriosi	Arterial grooves
A02.1.00.043	(Os suturale)	(Sutural bone)
A02.1.00.044	Basis cranii	Cranial base; Basicranium
A02.1.00.045	Basis cranii interna	Internal surface of cranial base
A02.1.00.046	Fissura sphenopetrosa	Petrosphenoidal fissure; Sphenopetrosal fissure
A02.1.00.047	Fissura petrooccipitalis	Petro-occipital fissure
A02.1.00.048	Fossa cranii anterior	Anterior cranial fossa
A02.1.00.049	Fossa cranii media	Middle cranial fossa
A02.1.00.050	Fossa cranii posterior	Posterior cranial fossa
A02.1.00.051	Clivus	Clivus
A02.1.00.052	Sulcus sinus petrosi inferioris	Groove for inferior petrosal sinus
A02.1.00.053	Basis cranii externa	External surface of cranial base
A02.1.00.054	Foramen jugulare	Jugular foramen
A02.1.00.055	Foramen lacerum	Foramen lacerum

A02.1.00.056	Palatum osseum	Bony palate
A02.1.00.057	Canalis palatinus major	Greater palatine canal
A02.1.00.058	Foramen palatinum majus	Greater palatine foramen
A02.1.00.059	Foramina palatina minora	Lesser palatine foramina
A02.1.00.060	Fossa incisiva	Incisive fossa
A02.1.00.061	Canales incisivi	Incisive canals
A02.1.00.062	Foramina incisiva	Incisive foramina
A02.1.00.063	(Torus palatinus)	(Palatine torus)
A02.1.00.064	Canalis palatovaginalis	Palatovaginal canal
A02.1.00.065	Canalis vomerovaginalis	Vomerovaginal canal
A02.1.00.066	Canalis vomerorostralis	Vomerorostral canal
A02.1.00.067	Orbita	Orbit
A02.1.00.068	Cavitas orbitalis	Orbital cavity
A02.1.00.069	Aditus orbitalis	Orbital opening
A02.1.00.070	Margo orbitalis	Orbital margin
A02.1.00.071	Margo supraorbitalis	Supra-orbital margin
A02.1.00.072	Margo infraorbitalis	Infra-orbital margin
A02.1.00.073	Margo lateralis	Lateral margin
A02.1.00.074	Margo medialis	Medial margin
A02.1.00.075	Paries superior	Roof
A02.1.00.076	Paries inferior	Floor
A02.1.00.077	Paries lateralis	Lateral wall
A02.1.00.078	Paries medialis	Medial wall
A02.1.00.079	Foramen ethmoidale anterius	Anterior ethmoidal foramen
A02.1.00.080	Foramen ethmoidale posterius	Posterior ethmoidal foramen
A02.1.00.081	Sulcus lacrimalis	Lacrimal groove
A02.1.00.082	Fossa sacci lacrimalis	Fossa for lacrimal sac
A02.1.00.083	Fissura orbitalis superior	Superior orbital fissure
A02.1.00.084	Fissura orbitalis inferior	Inferior orbital fissure
A02.1.00.085	Canalis nasolacrimalis	Nasolacrimal canal
A02.1.00.086	Cavitas nasalis ossea	Bony nasal cavity
A02.1.00.087	Septum nasi osseum	Bony nasal septum
A02.1.00.088	Apertura piriformis	Piriform aperture
A02.1.00.089	Meatus nasi superior	Superior nasal meatus
A02.1.00.090	Meatus nasi medius	Middle nasal meatus
A02.1.00.091	Meatus nasi inferior	Inferior nasal meatus
A02.1.00.092	Ostium canalis nasolacrimalis	Opening of nasolacrimal canal
* A02.1.00.093	Meatus nasi communis	Common nasal meatus
A02.1.00.094	Recessus sphenoethmoidalis	Spheno-ethmoidal recess
A02.1.00.095	Meatus nasopharyngeus	Nasopharyngeal meatus
A02.1.00.096	Choana; Apertura nasalis posterior	Choana; Posterior nasal aperture
A02.1.00.097	Foramen sphenopalatinum	Sphenopalatine foramen

A02.1.01.001	Ossa cranii	Bones of cranium
A02.1.02.001	**Os parietale**	**Parietal bone**
A02.1.02.002	Facies interna	Internal surface
A02.1.02.003	Sulcus sinus sigmoidei	Groove for sigmoid sinus
A02.1.02.004	Sulcus sinus sagittalis superioris	Groove for superior sagittal sinus
A02.1.02.005	Sulcus arteriae meningeae mediae	Groove for middle meningeal artery
A02.1.02.006	Sulci arteriosi	Grooves for arteries
A02.1.02.007	Facies externa	External surface
A02.1.02.008	Linea temporalis superior	Superior temporal line
A02.1.02.009	Linea temporalis inferior	Inferior temporal line
A02.1.02.010	Tuber parietale; Eminentia parietalis	Parietal tuber; Parietal eminence
A02.1.02.011	Margo occipitalis	Occipital border
A02.1.02.012	Margo squamosus	Squamosal border

* **A02.1.00.093** *Meatus nasi communis* The common nasal meatus is the part of the nasal cavity between the conchae and the nasal septum.

A02.1.02.013	Margo sagittalis	Sagittal border
A02.1.02.014	Margo frontalis	Frontal border
A02.1.02.015	Angulus frontalis	Frontal angle
A02.1.02.016	Angulus occipitalis	Occipital angle
A02.1.02.017	Angulus sphenoidalis	Sphenoidal angle
A02.1.02.018	Angulus mastoideus	Mastoid angle
A02.1.02.019	Foramen parietale	Parietal foramen
A02.1.03.001	**Os frontale**	**Frontal bone**
A02.1.03.002	Squama frontalis	Squamous part
A02.1.03.003	Facies externa	External surface
A02.1.03.004	Tuber frontale; Eminentia frontalis	Frontal tuber; Frontal eminence
A02.1.03.005	Arcus superciliaris	Superciliary arch
A02.1.03.006	Glabella	Glabella
A02.1.03.007	(Sutura frontalis persistens; Sutura metopica)	(Frontal suture; Metopic suture)
A02.1.03.008	Margo supraorbitalis	Supra-orbital margin
A02.1.03.009	Incisura supraorbitalis/foramen supraorbitale	Supra-orbital notch/foramen
A02.1.03.010	Incisura frontalis/foramen frontale	Frontal notch/foramen
A02.1.03.011	Facies temporalis	Temporal surface
A02.1.03.012	Margo parietalis	Parietal margin
A02.1.03.013	Linea temporalis	Temporal line
A02.1.03.014	Processus zygomaticus	Zygomatic process
A02.1.03.015	Facies interna	Internal surface
A02.1.03.016	Crista frontalis	Frontal crest
A02.1.03.017	Sulcus sinus sagittalis superioris	Groove for superior sagittal sinus
A02.1.03.018	Foramen caecum	Foramen caecum▴
A02.1.03.019	Pars nasalis	Nasal part
A02.1.03.020	Spina nasalis	Nasal spine
A02.1.03.021	Margo nasalis	Nasal margin
A02.1.03.022	Pars orbitalis	Orbital part
A02.1.03.023	Facies orbitalis	Orbital surface
A02.1.03.024	(Spina trochlearis)	(Trochlear spine)
A02.1.03.025	Fovea trochlearis	Trochlear fovea
A02.1.03.026	Fossa glandulae lacrimalis	Fossa for lacrimal gland; Lacrimal fossa
A02.1.03.027	Margo sphenoidalis	Sphenoidal margin
A02.1.03.028	Incisura ethmoidalis	Ethmoidal notch
A02.1.03.029	Sinus frontalis	Frontal sinus
A02.1.03.030	Apertura sinus frontalis	Opening of frontal sinus
A02.1.03.031	Septum sinuum frontalium	Septum of frontal sinuses
A02.1.04.001	**Os occipitale**	**Occipital bone**
A02.1.04.002	Foramen magnum	Foramen magnum
A02.1.04.003	Basion	Basion
A02.1.04.004	Opisthion	Opisthion
A02.1.04.005	Pars basilaris	Basilar part
A02.1.04.006	Clivus	Clivus
A02.1.04.007	Tuberculum pharyngeum	Pharyngeal tubercle
A02.1.04.008	Sulcus sinus petrosi inferioris	Groove for inferior petrosal sinus
A02.1.04.009	Pars lateralis	Lateral part
A02.1.04.010	Squama occipitalis	Squamous part of occipital bone
A02.1.04.011	Margo mastoideus	Mastoid border
A02.1.04.012	Margo lambdoideus	Lambdoid border
A02.1.04.013	(Os interparietale)	(Interparietal bone)
A02.1.04.014	Condylus occipitalis	Occipital condyle
A02.1.04.015	Canalis condylaris	Condylar canal
A02.1.04.016	Canalis nervi hypoglossi	Hypoglossal canal
A02.1.04.017	Fossa condylaris	Condylar fossa
A02.1.04.018	Tuberculum jugulare	Jugular tubercle
A02.1.04.019	Incisura jugularis	Jugular notch

A02.1.04.020	Processus jugularis	Jugular process
A02.1.04.021	Processus intrajugularis	Intrajugular process
A02.1.04.022	Protuberantia occipitalis externa	External occipital protuberance
A02.1.04.023	(Crista occipitalis externa)	(External occipital crest)
A02.1.04.024	Linea nuchalis suprema	Highest nuchal line
A02.1.04.025	Linea nuchalis superior	Superior nuchal line
A02.1.04.026	Linea nuchalis inferior	Inferior nuchal line
A02.1.04.027	Planum occipitale	Occipital plane
A02.1.04.028	Eminentia cruciformis	Cruciform eminence
A02.1.04.029	Protuberantia occipitalis interna	Internal occipital protuberance
A02.1.04.030	(Crista occipitalis interna)	(Internal occipital crest)
A02.1.04.031	Sulcus sinus transversi	Groove for transverse sinus
A02.1.04.032	Sulcus sinus sigmoidei	Groove for sigmoid sinus
A02.1.04.033	Sulcus sinus occipitalis	Groove for occipital sinus
A02.1.04.034	Sulcus sinus marginalis	Groove for marginal sinus
A02.1.04.035	(Processus paramastoideus)	(Paramastoid process)
A02.1.04.036	Fossa cerebralis	Cerebral fossa
A02.1.04.037	Fossa cerebellaris	Cerebellar fossa
A02.1.05.001	**Os sphenoidale**	**Sphenoid; Sphenoidal bone**
A02.1.05.002	Corpus	Body
A02.1.05.003	Jugum sphenoidale	Jugum sphenoidale; Sphenoidal yoke
A02.1.05.004	Limbus sphenoidalis	Limbus of sphenoid
A02.1.05.005	Sulcus prechiasmaticus	Prechiasmatic sulcus
A02.1.05.006	Sella turcica	Sella turcica
A02.1.05.007	Tuberculum sellae	Tuberculum sellae
A02.1.05.008	(Processus clinoideus medius)	(Middle clinoid process)
A02.1.05.009	Fossa hypophysialis	Hypophysial fossa
A02.1.05.010	Dorsum sellae	Dorsum sellae
A02.1.05.011	Processus clinoideus posterior	Posterior clinoid process
A02.1.05.012	Sulcus caroticus	Carotid sulcus
A02.1.05.013	Lingula sphenoidalis	Sphenoidal lingula
A02.1.05.014	Crista sphenoidalis	Sphenoidal crest
A02.1.05.015	Rostrum sphenoidale	Sphenoidal rostrum
A02.1.05.016	Sinus sphenoidalis	Sphenoidal sinus
A02.1.05.017	Septum sinuum sphenoidalium	Septum of sphenoidal sinuses
A02.1.05.018	Apertura sinus sphenoidalis	Opening of sphenoidal sinus
A02.1.05.019	Concha sphenoidalis	Sphenoidal concha
A02.1.05.020	Ala minor	Lesser wing
A02.1.05.021	Canalis opticus	Optic canal
A02.1.05.022	Processus clinoideus anterior	Anterior clinoid process
A02.1.05.023	Fissura orbitalis superior	Superior orbital fissure
A02.1.05.024	Ala major	Greater wing
A02.1.05.025	Facies cerebralis	Cerebral surface
A02.1.05.026	Facies temporalis	Temporal surface
A02.1.05.027	Facies infratemporalis	Infratemporal surface
A02.1.05.028	Crista infratemporalis	Infratemporal crest
A02.1.05.029	Facies maxillaris	Maxillary surface
A02.1.05.030	Facies orbitalis	Orbital surface
A02.1.05.031	Margo zygomaticus	Zygomatic margin
A02.1.05.032	Margo frontalis	Frontal margin
A02.1.05.033	Margo parietalis	Parietal margin
A02.1.05.034	Margo squamosus	Squamosal margin
A02.1.05.035	Foramen rotundum	Foramen rotundum
A02.1.05.036	Foramen ovale	Foramen ovale
A02.1.05.037	(Foramen venosum)	(Sphenoidal emissary foramen)
A02.1.05.038	Foramen spinosum	Foramen spinosum
A02.1.05.039	(Foramen petrosum)	(Foramen petrosum)
A02.1.05.040	Spina ossis sphenoidalis	Spine of sphenoid bone

A02.1.05.041	Sulcus tubae auditivae; Sulcus tubae auditoriae	Sulcus of auditory tube
A02.1.05.042	Processus pterygoideus	Pterygoid process
A02.1.05.043	Lamina lateralis	Lateral plate
A02.1.05.044	Lamina medialis	Medial plate
A02.1.05.045	Incisura pterygoidea	Pterygoid notch
A02.1.05.046	Fossa pterygoidea	Pterygoid fossa
A02.1.05.047	Fossa scaphoidea	Scaphoid fossa
A02.1.05.048	Processus vaginalis	Vaginal process
A02.1.05.049	Sulcus palatovaginalis	Palatovaginal groove
A02.1.05.050	Sulcus vomerovaginalis	Vomerovaginal groove
A02.1.05.051	Hamulus pterygoideus	Pterygoid hamulus
A02.1.05.052	Sulcus hamuli pterygoidei	Groove of pterygoid hamulus
A02.1.05.053	Canalis pterygoideus	Pterygoid canal
A02.1.05.054	Processus pterygospinosus	Pterygospinous process
A02.1.06.001	**Os temporale**	**Temporal bone**
A02.1.06.002	Pars petrosa	Petrous part
A02.1.06.003	Margo occipitalis	Occipital margin
A02.1.06.004	Processus mastoideus	Mastoid process
A02.1.06.005	Incisura mastoidea	Mastoid notch
A02.1.06.006	Sulcus sinus sigmoidei	Groove for sigmoid sinus
A02.1.06.007	Sulcus arteriae occipitalis	Occipital groove
A02.1.06.008	Foramen mastoideum	Mastoid foramen
A02.1.06.009	Canalis nervi facialis	Facial canal
A02.1.06.010	Geniculum canalis nervi facialis	Geniculum of facial canal
A02.1.06.011	Canaliculus chordae tympani	Canaliculus for chorda tympani
A02.1.06.012	Apex partis petrosae	Apex of petrous part
A02.1.06.013	Canalis caroticus	Carotid canal
A02.1.06.014	Apertura externa canalis carotici	External opening of carotid canal
A02.1.06.015	Apertura interna canalis carotici	Internal opening of carotid canal
A02.1.06.016	Canaliculi caroticotympanici	Caroticotympanic canaliculi
A02.1.06.017	Canalis musculotubarius	Musculotubal canal
A02.1.06.018	Semicanalis musculi tensoris tympani	Canal for tensor tympani
A02.1.06.019	Semicanalis tubae auditivae; Semicanalis tubae auditoriae	Canal for auditory tube
A02.1.06.020	Septum canalis musculotubarii	Septum of musculotubal canal
A02.1.06.021	Facies anterior partis petrosae	Anterior surface of petrous part
A02.1.06.022	Tegmen tympani	Tegmen tympani
A02.1.06.023	Eminentia arcuata	Arcuate eminence
A02.1.06.024	Hiatus canalis nervi petrosi majoris	Hiatus for greater petrosal nerve
A02.1.06.025	Sulcus nervi petrosi majoris	Groove for greater petrosal nerve
A02.1.06.026	Hiatus canalis nervi petrosi minoris	Hiatus for lesser petrosal nerve
A02.1.06.027	Sulcus nervi petrosi minoris	Groove for lesser petrosal nerve
A02.1.06.028	Impressio trigeminalis	Trigeminal impression
A02.1.06.029	Margo superior partis petrosae	Superior border of petrous part
A02.1.06.030	Sulcus sinus petrosi superioris	Groove for superior petrosal sinus
A02.1.06.031	Facies posterior partis petrosae	Posterior surface of petrous part
A02.1.06.032	Porus acusticus internus	Internal acoustic opening
A02.1.06.033	Meatus acusticus internus	Internal acoustic meatus
A02.1.06.034	Fossa subarcuata	Subarcuate fossa
A02.1.06.035	Canaliculus vestibuli	Vestibular canaliculus
A02.1.06.036	Apertura canaliculi vestibuli	Opening of vestibular canaliculus
A02.1.06.037	Margo posterior partis petrosae	Posterior border of petrous part
A02.1.06.038	Sulcus sinus petrosi inferioris	Groove for inferior petrosal sinus
A02.1.06.039	Incisura jugularis	Jugular notch
A02.1.06.040	Facies inferior partis petrosae	Inferior surface of petrous part
A02.1.06.041	Fossa jugularis	Jugular fossa
A02.1.06.042	Canaliculus cochleae	Cochlear canaliculus
A02.1.06.043	Apertura canaliculi cochleae	Opening of cochlear canaliculus

A02.1.06.044	Canaliculus mastoideus	Mastoid canaliculus
A02.1.06.045	Incisura jugularis	Jugular notch
A02.1.06.046	Processus intrajugularis	Intrajugular process
A02.1.06.047	Processus styloideus	Styloid process
A02.1.06.048	Foramen stylomastoideum	Stylomastoid foramen
A02.1.06.049	Canaliculus tympanicus	Tympanic canaliculus
A02.1.06.050	Fossula petrosa	Petrosal fossula
A02.1.06.051	Cavitas tympani	Tympanic cavity
A02.1.06.052	Pars tympanica	Tympanic part
A02.1.06.053	Anulus tympanicus	Tympanic ring
A02.1.06.054	Porus acusticus externus	External acoustic opening
A02.1.06.055	Meatus acusticus externus	External acoustic meatus
A02.1.06.056	Spina tympanica major	Greater tympanic spine
A02.1.06.057	Spina tympanica minor	Lesser tympanic spine
A02.1.06.058	Sulcus tympanicus	Tympanic sulcus
A02.1.06.059	Incisura tympanica	Tympanic notch
A02.1.06.060	Vagina processus styloidei	Sheath of styloid process
A02.1.06.061	Pars squamosa	Squamous part
A02.1.06.062	Margo parietalis	Parietal border
A02.1.06.063	Incisura parietalis	Parietal notch
A02.1.06.064	Margo sphenoidalis	Sphenoidal margin
A02.1.06.065	Facies temporalis	Temporal surface
A02.1.06.066	Sulcus arteriae temporalis mediae	Groove for middle temporal artery
A02.1.06.067	Processus zygomaticus	Zygomatic process
A02.1.06.068	Crista supramastoidea	Supramastoid crest
A02.1.06.069	Foveola suprameatica; Foveola suprameatalis	Suprameatal triangle
A02.1.06.070	(Spina suprameatica; Spina suprameatalis)	(Suprameatal spine)
A02.1.06.071	Fossa mandibularis	Mandibular fossa
A02.1.06.072	Facies articularis	Articular surface
A02.1.06.073	Tuberculum articulare	Articular tubercle
A02.1.06.074	Fissura petrotympanica	Petrotympanic fissure
A02.1.06.075	Fissura petrosquamosa	Petrosquamous fissure
A02.1.06.076	Fissura tympanosquamosa	Tympanosquamous fissure
A02.1.06.077	Fissura tympanomastoidea	Tympanomastoid fissure
A02.1.06.078	Facies cerebralis	Cerebral surface
A02.1.07.001	**Os ethmoidale**	**Ethmoid; Ethmoidal bone**
A02.1.07.002	Lamina cribrosa	Cribriform plate
A02.1.07.003	Foramina cribrosa	Cribriform foramina
A02.1.07.004	Crista galli	Crista galli
A02.1.07.005	Ala cristae galli	Ala of crista galli
A02.1.07.006	Lamina perpendicularis	Perpendicular plate
A02.1.07.007	Labyrinthus ethmoidalis	Ethmoidal labyrinth
A02.1.07.008	Cellulae ethmoidales anteriores	Anterior ethmoidal cells
A02.1.07.009	Cellulae ethmoidales mediae	Middle ethmoidal cells
A02.1.07.010	Cellulae ethmoidales posteriores	Posterior ethmoidal cells
A02.1.07.011	Lamina orbitalis	Orbital plate
A02.1.07.012	Concha nasalis suprema	Supreme nasal concha
A02.1.07.013	Concha nasalis superior	Superior nasal concha
A02.1.07.014	Concha nasalis media	Middle nasal concha
A02.1.07.015	Bulla ethmoidalis	Ethmoidal bulla
A02.1.07.016	Processus uncinatus	Uncinate process
A02.1.07.017	Infundibulum ethmoidale	Ethmoidal infundibulum
A02.1.07.018	Hiatus semilunaris	Hiatus semilunaris
A02.1.08.001	**Concha nasalis inferior**	**Inferior nasal concha**
A02.1.08.002	Processus lacrimalis	Lacrimal process
A02.1.08.003	Processus maxillaris	Maxillary process
A02.1.08.004	Processus ethmoidalis	Ethmoidal process
A02.1.09.001	**Os lacrimale**	**Lacrimal bone**

A02.1.09.002	Crista lacrimalis posterior	Posterior lacrimal crest
A02.1.09.003	Sulcus lacrimalis	Lacrimal groove
A02.1.09.004	Hamulus lacrimalis	Lacrimal hamulus
A02.1.10.001	**Os nasale**	**Nasal bone**
A02.1.10.002	Sulcus ethmoidalis	Ethmoidal groove
A02.1.10.003	Foramina nasalia	Nasal foramina
A02.1.11.001	**Vomer**	**Vomer**
A02.1.11.002	Ala vomeris	Ala of vomer
A02.1.11.003	Sulcus vomeris	Vomerine groove
A02.1.11.004	Crista choanalis vomeris	Vomerine crest of choana
A02.1.11.005	Pars cuneiformis vomeris	Cuneiform part of vomer
A02.1.12.001	**Maxilla**	**Maxilla**
A02.1.12.002	Corpus maxillae	Body of maxilla
A02.1.12.003	Facies orbitalis	Orbital surface
A02.1.12.004	Canalis infraorbitalis	Infra-orbital canal
A02.1.12.005	Sulcus infraorbitalis	Infra-orbital groove
A02.1.12.006	Margo infraorbitalis	Infra-orbital margin
A02.1.12.007	Facies anterior	Anterior surface
A02.1.12.008	Foramen infraorbitale	Infra-orbital foramen
A02.1.12.009	Fossa canina	Canine fossa
A02.1.12.010	Incisura nasalis	Nasal notch
A02.1.12.011	Spina nasalis anterior	Anterior nasal spine
A02.1.12.012	Sutura zygomaticomaxillaris; Sutura infraorbitalis	Zygomaticomaxillary suture
A02.1.12.013	Facies infratemporalis	Infratemporal surface
A02.1.12.014	Foramina alveolaria	Alveolar foramina
A02.1.12.015	Canales alveolares	Alveolar canals
A02.1.12.016	Tuber maxillae; Eminentia maxillae	Maxillary tuberosity
A02.1.12.017	Facies nasalis	Nasal surface
A02.1.12.018	Sulcus lacrimalis	Lacrimal groove
A02.1.12.019	Crista conchalis	Conchal crest
A02.1.12.020	Margo lacrimalis	Lacrimal margin
A02.1.12.021	Hiatus maxillaris	Maxillary hiatus
A02.1.12.022	Sulcus palatinus major	Greater palatine groove
A02.1.12.023	Sinus maxillaris	Maxillary sinus
A02.1.12.024	Processus frontalis	Frontal process
A02.1.12.025	Crista lacrimalis anterior	Anterior lacrimal crest
A02.1.12.026	Incisura lacrimalis	Lacrimal notch
A02.1.12.027	Crista ethmoidalis	Ethmoidal crest
A02.1.12.028	Processus zygomaticus	Zygomatic process
A02.1.12.029	Processus palatinus	Palatine process
A02.1.12.030	Crista nasalis	Nasal crest
A02.1.12.031	(Os incisivum; Premaxilla)	(Incisive bone; Premaxilla)
A02.1.00.061	Canales incisivi	Incisive canals
A02.1.12.032	(Sutura incisiva)	(Incisive suture)
A02.1.12.033	Spinae palatinae	Palatine spines
A02.1.12.034	Sulci palatini	Palatine grooves
A02.1.12.035	Processus alveolaris	Alveolar process
A02.1.12.036	Arcus alveolaris	Alveolar arch
A02.1.12.037	Alveoli dentales	Dental alveoli
A02.1.12.038	Septa interalveolaria	Interalveolar septa
A02.1.12.039	Septa interradicularia	Interradicular septa
A02.1.12.040	Juga alveolaria	Alveolar yokes
A02.1.00.062	Foramina incisiva	Incisive foramina
A02.1.13.001	**Os palatinum**	**Palatine bone**
A02.1.13.002	Lamina perpendicularis	Perpendicular plate
A02.1.13.003	Facies nasalis	Nasal surface
A02.1.13.004	Facies maxillaris	Maxillary surface
A02.1.13.005	Incisura sphenopalatina	Sphenopalatine notch

A02.1.13.006	Sulcus palatinus major	Greater palatine groove
A02.1.13.007	Processus pyramidalis	Pyramidal process
A02.1.13.008	Canales palatini minores	Lesser palatine canals
A02.1.13.009	Crista conchalis	Conchal crest
A02.1.13.010	Crista ethmoidalis	Ethmoidal crest
A02.1.13.011	Processus orbitalis	Orbital process
A02.1.13.012	Processus sphenoidalis	Sphenoidal process
A02.1.13.013	Lamina horizontalis	Horizontal plate
A02.1.13.014	Facies nasalis	Nasal surface
A02.1.13.015	Facies palatina	Palatine surface
A02.1.13.016	Foramina palatina minora	Lesser palatine foramina
A02.1.13.017	Spina nasalis posterior	Posterior nasal spine
A02.1.13.018	Crista nasalis	Nasal crest
A02.1.13.019	Crista palatina	Palatine crest
A02.1.14.001	**Os zygomaticum**	**Zygomatic bone**
A02.1.14.002	Facies lateralis	Lateral surface
A02.1.14.003	Facies temporalis	Temporal surface
A02.1.14.004	Facies orbitalis	Orbital surface
A02.1.14.005	Processus temporalis	Temporal process
A02.1.14.006	Processus frontalis	Frontal process
A02.1.14.007	Tuberculum orbitale	Orbital tubercle
A02.1.14.008	(Tuberculum marginale)	(Marginal tubercle)
A02.1.14.009	Foramen zygomaticoorbitale	Zygomatico-orbital foramen
A02.1.14.010	Foramen zygomaticofaciale	Zygomaticofacial foramen
A02.1.14.011	Foramen zygomaticotemporale	Zygomaticotemporal foramen
A02.1.15.001	**Mandibula**	**Mandible**
A02.1.15.002	Corpus mandibulae	Body of mandible
A02.1.15.003	Basis mandibulae	Base of mandible
A02.1.15.004	(Symphysis mandibulae)	(Mandibular symphysis)
A02.1.15.005	Protuberantia mentalis	Mental protuberance
A02.1.15.006	Tuberculum mentale	Mental tubercle
A02.1.15.007	Foramen mentale	Mental foramen
A02.1.15.008	Linea obliqua	Oblique line
A02.1.15.009	Fossa digastrica	Digastric fossa
A02.1.15.010	Spina mentalis superior; Spina geni superior	Superior mental spine; Superior genial spine
A02.1.15.011	Spina mentalis inferior; Spina geni inferior	Inferior mental spine; Inferior genial spine
A02.1.15.012	Linea mylohyoidea	Mylohyoid line
A02.1.15.013	(Torus mandibularis)	(Mandibular torus)
A02.1.15.014	Fovea sublingualis	Sublingual fossa
A02.1.15.015	Fovea submandibularis	Submandibular fossa
A02.1.15.016	Pars alveolaris	Alveolar part
A02.1.15.017	Arcus alveolaris	Alveolar arch
A02.1.15.018	Alveoli dentales	Dental alveoli
A02.1.15.019	Septa interalveolaria	Interalveolar septa
A02.1.15.020	Septa interradicularia	Interradicular septa
A02.1.15.021	Juga alveolaria	Alveolar yokes
A02.1.15.022	Trigonum retromolare	Retromolar triangle
A02.1.15.023	Fossa retromolaris	Retromolar fossa
A02.1.15.024	Ramus mandibulae	Ramus of mandible
A02.1.15.025	Angulus mandibulae	Angle of mandible
A02.1.15.026	(Tuberositas masseterica)	(Masseteric tuberosity)
A02.1.15.027	(Tuberositas pterygoidea)	(Pterygoid tuberosity)
A02.1.15.028	Foramen mandibulae	Mandibular foramen
A02.1.15.029	Lingula mandibulae	Lingula
A02.1.15.030	Canalis mandibulae	Mandibular canal
A02.1.15.031	Sulcus mylohyoideus	Mylohyoid groove
A02.1.15.032	Processus coronoideus	Coronoid process
A02.1.15.033	Crista temporalis	Temporal crest
A02.1.15.034	Incisura mandibulae	Mandibular notch

A02.1.15.035	Processus condylaris	Condylar process
A02.1.15.036	Caput mandibulae; Condylus mandibulae	Head of mandible
A02.1.15.037	Collum mandibulae	Neck of mandible
A02.1.15.038	Fovea pterygoidea	Pterygoid fovea
A02.1.16.001	**Os hyoideum**	**Hyoid bone**
A02.1.16.002	Corpus ossis hyoidei	Body of hyoid bone
A02.1.16.003	Cornu minus	Lesser horn
A02.1.16.004	Cornu majus	Greater horn
A02.1.17.001	**Ossicula auditus; Ossicula auditoria** {vide paginam 149}	**Auditory ossicles** {see page 149}

A02.2.00.001	**Columna vertebralis**	**Vertebral column**
* **A02.2.00.002**	Curvatura primaria	Primary curvature
A02.2.00.003	Kyphosis thoracica	Thoracic kyphosis
A02.2.00.004	Kyphosis sacralis	Sacral kyphosis
* **A02.2.00.005**	Curvaturae secundariae	Secondary curvatures
A02.2.00.006	Lordosis cervicis; Lordosis colli	Cervical lordosis
A02.2.00.007	Lordosis lumbalis	Lumbar lordosis
A02.2.00.008	Scoliosis	Scoliosis
A02.2.00.009	Canalis vertebralis	Vertebral canal
A02.2.01.001	**Vertebra**	**Vertebra**
A02.2.01.002	Corpus vertebrae	Vertebral body
A02.2.01.003	Facies intervertebralis	Intervertebral surface
A02.2.01.004	Epiphysis anularis	Anular epiphysis
A02.2.01.005	Arcus vertebrae	Vertebral arch
A02.2.01.006	Pediculus arcus vertebrae	Pedicle
A02.2.01.007	Lamina arcus vertebrae	Lamina
A02.2.01.008	Foramen intervertebrale	Intervertebral foramen
A02.2.01.009	Incisura vertebralis superior	Superior vertebral notch
A02.2.01.010	Incisura vertebralis inferior	Inferior vertebral notch
A02.2.01.011	Foramen vertebrale	Vertebral foramen
A02.2.01.012	Processus spinosus	Spinous process
A02.2.01.013	Processus transversus	Transverse process
A02.2.01.014	Processus articularis superior; Zygapophysis superior	Superior articular process
A02.2.01.015	Facies articularis superior	Superior articular facet
A02.2.01.016	Processus articularis inferior; Zygapophysis inferior	Inferior articular process
A02.2.01.017	Facies articularis inferior	Inferior articular facet

A02.2.02.001	**Vertebrae cervicales [C I – C VII]**	**Cervical vertebrae [C I – C VII]**
A02.2.02.002	Uncus corporis; Processus uncinatus	Uncus of body; Uncinate process
A02.2.02.003	Foramen transversarium	Foramen transversarium
A02.2.02.004	Tuberculum anterius	Anterior tubercle
A02.2.02.005	Tuberculum caroticum	Carotid tubercle
A02.2.02.006	Tuberculum posterius	Posterior tubercle
A02.2.02.007	Sulcus nervi spinalis	Groove for spinal nerve
A02.2.02.101	**Atlas [C I]**	**Atlas [C I]**
A02.2.02.102	Massa lateralis atlantis	Lateral mass
A02.2.02.103	Facies articularis superior	Superior articular surface
A02.2.02.104	Facies articularis inferior	Inferior articular surface
A02.2.02.105	Arcus anterior atlantis	Anterior arch
A02.2.02.106	Fovea dentis	Facet for dens
A02.2.02.107	Tuberculum anterius	Anterior tubercle

* **A02.2.00.002** *Curvatura primaria* The primary curvature of the vertebral column is a result of the ventral flexion of the embryo and persists in the thoracic (*kyphosis thoracica*) and pelvic (*kyphosis sacralis*) regions.

* **A02.2.00.005** *Curvaturae secundariae* The secondary curvatures of the vertebral column (*lordosis cervicalis* and *lordosis lumbalis*) are dorsally concave and, being produced by fetal muscular action, are initially functional rather than structural.

A02.2.02.108	Arcus posterior atlantis	Posterior arch
A02.2.02.109	Sulcus arteriae vertebralis	Groove for vertebral artery
A02.2.02.110	(Canalis arteriae vertebralis)	(Canal for vertebral artery)
A02.2.02.111	Tuberculum posterius	Posterior tubercle
A02.2.02.201	**Axis [C II]**	**Axis [C II]**
A02.2.02.202	Dens axis	Dens
A02.2.02.203	Apex dentis	Apex
A02.2.02.204	Facies articularis anterior	Anterior articular facet
A02.2.02.205	Facies articularis posterior	Posterior articular facet
A02.2.02.301	**Vertebra prominens [C VII]**	**Vertebra prominens [C VII]**

A02.2.03.001	**Vertebrae thoracicae [T I – T XII]**	**Thoracic vertebrae [T I – T XII]**
A02.2.03.002	Fovea costalis superior	Superior costal facet
A02.2.03.003	Fovea costalis inferior	Inferior costal facet
A02.2.03.004	Fovea costalis processus transversi	Transverse costal facet
A02.2.03.005	Uncus corporis vertebrae thoracicae primae; Processus uncinatus vertebrae thoracicae primae	Uncus of body of first thoracic vertebra; Uncinate process of first thoracic vertebra

A02.2.04.001	**Vertebrae lumbales [L I – L V]**	**Lumbar vertebrae [L I – L V]**
A02.2.04.002	Processus accessorius	Accessory process
A02.2.04.003	Processus costiformis; Processus costalis	Costal process
A02.2.04.004	Processus mammillaris	Mammillary process

A02.2.05.001	**Os sacrum [vertebrae sacrales I – V]**	**Sacrum [sacral vertebrae I – V]**
A02.2.05.002	Basis ossis sacri	Base
A02.2.05.003	Promontorium	Promontory
A02.2.05.004	Ala ossis sacri	Ala; Wing
A02.2.05.005	Processus articularis superior	Superior articular process
A02.2.05.006	Pars lateralis	Lateral part
A02.2.05.007	Facies auricularis	Auricular surface
A02.2.05.008	Tuberositas ossis sacri	Sacral tuberosity
A02.2.05.009	Facies pelvica	Pelvic surface
A02.2.05.010	Lineae transversae	Transverse ridges
A02.2.05.011	Foramina intervertebralia	Intervertebral foramina
A02.2.05.012	Foramina sacralia anteriora	Anterior sacral foramina
A02.2.05.013	Facies dorsalis	Dorsal surface
A02.2.05.014	Crista sacralis mediana	Median sacral crest
A02.2.05.015	Foramina sacralia posteriora	Posterior sacral foramina
A02.2.05.016	Crista sacralis medialis	Intermediate sacral crest
A02.2.05.017	Crista sacralis lateralis	Lateral sacral crest
A02.2.05.018	Cornu sacrale	Sacral cornu; Sacral horn
A02.2.05.019	Canalis sacralis	Sacral canal
A02.2.05.020	Hiatus sacralis	Sacral hiatus
A02.2.05.021	Apex ossis sacri; Apex ossis sacralis	Apex

A02.2.06.001	**Os coccygis; Coccyx [vertebrae coccygeae I–IV]**	**Coccyx [coccygeal vertebrae I–IV]**
A02.2.06.002	Cornu coccygeum	Coccygeal cornu

A02.3.00.001	**Skeleton thoracis**	**Thoracic skeleton**
A02.3.01.001	**Costae [I–XII]**	**Ribs [I–XII]**
A02.3.01.002	Costae verae [I–VII]	True ribs [I–VII]
A02.3.01.003	Costae spuriae [VIII–XII]	False ribs [VIII–XII]
A02.3.01.004	Costae fluctuantes [XI–XII]	Floating ribs [XI–XII]
A02.3.01.005	Cartilago costalis	Costal cartilage
A02.3.02.001	**Costa**	**Rib**

	A02.3.02.002	Caput costae	Head
	A02.3.02.003	Facies articularis capitis costae	Articular facet
	A02.3.02.004	Crista capitis costae	Crest
	A02.3.02.005	Collum costae	Neck
	A02.3.02.006	Crista colli costae	Crest
	A02.3.02.007	Corpus costae	Body; Shaft
	A02.3.02.008	Tuberculum costae	Tubercle
	A02.3.02.009	Facies articularis tuberculi costae	Articular facet
	A02.3.02.010	Angulus costae	Angle
	A02.3.02.011	Sulcus costae	Costal groove
	A02.3.02.012	Crista costae	Crest
	A02.3.02.013	(Costa cervicalis; Costa colli)	(Cervical rib)
	A02.3.02.014	Costa prima [I]	First rib [I]
	A02.3.02.015	Tuberculum musculi scaleni anterioris	Scalene tubercle
	A02.3.02.016	Sulcus arteriae subclaviae	Groove for subclavian artery
	A02.3.02.017	Sulcus venae subclaviae	Groove for subclavian vein
	A02.3.02.018	Costa secunda [II]	Second rib [II]
	A02.3.02.019	Tuberositas musculi serrati anterioris	Tuberosity for serratus anterior
	A02.3.02.020	(Costa lumbalis)	(Lumbar rib)
	A02.3.03.001	**Sternum**	**Sternum**
	A02.3.03.002	Manubrium sterni	Manubrium of sternum
	A02.3.03.003	Incisura clavicularis	Clavicular notch
	A02.3.03.004	Incisura jugularis	Jugular notch; Suprasternal notch
	A02.3.03.005	Angulus sterni	Sternal angle
	A02.3.03.006	Corpus sterni	Body of sternum
	A02.3.03.007	Processus xiphoideus	Xiphoid process
	A02.3.03.008	Incisurae costales	Costal notches
	A02.3.03.009	(Ossa suprasternalia)	(Suprasternal bones)
	A02.2.03.001	**Vertebrae thoracicae [T I – T XII]**	**Thoracic vertebrae [T I – T XII]**
*	**A02.3.04.001**	**Cavea thoracis**	**Thoracic cage**
	A02.3.04.002	Cavitas thoracis	Thoracic cavity
*	**A02.3.04.003**	Apertura thoracis superior	Superior thoracic aperture; Thoracic inlet
*	**A02.3.04.004**	Apertura thoracis inferior	Inferior thoracic aperture; Thoracic outlet
	A02.3.04.005	Sulcus pulmonalis	Pulmonary groove
	A02.3.04.006	Arcus costalis	Costal margin; Costal arch
	A02.3.04.007	Spatium intercostale	Intercostal space
	A02.3.04.008	Angulus infrasternalis	Infrasternal angle; Subcostal angle

A02.4.00.001	**Ossa membri superioris**	**Bones of upper limb**
A02.4.00.002	**CINGULUM PECTORALE; CINGULUM MEMBRI SUPERIORIS**	**PECTORAL GIRDLE; SHOULDER GIRDLE**
A02.4.01.001	**Scapula**	**Scapula**
A02.4.01.002	Facies costalis; Facies anterior	Costal surface
A02.4.01.003	Fossa subscapularis	Subscapular fossa
A02.4.01.004	Facies posterior	Posterior surface
A02.4.01.005	Spina scapulae	Spine of scapula
A02.4.01.006	Tuberculum deltoideum	Deltoid tubercle
A02.4.01.007	Fossa supraspinata	Supraspinous fossa
A02.4.01.008	Fossa infraspinata	Infraspinous fossa
A02.4.01.009	Acromion	Acromion
A02.4.01.010	Facies articularis clavicularis	Clavicular facet
A02.4.01.011	Angulus acromii	Acromial angle
A02.4.01.012	Margo medialis	Medial border

* **A02.3.04.001** *Cavea thoracis* The term *compages thoracis* was introduced in the fourth edition of *Nomina Anatomica* as "a new term to denote the thoracic skeleton" (footnote 34, page A 28). However, it has not received wide acceptance and the appropriate term is *cavea* – a cage, rather than the previous *cavum* – a cavity.

* **A02.3.04.003 / A02.3.04.004** *Apertura thoracis superior/inferior* The terms "thoracic inlet" and "thoracic outlet" have been used differently by clinicians. Thus, the thoracic outlet syndrome refers to the thoracic inlet of this terminology.

A02.4.01.013	Margo lateralis	Lateral border
A02.4.01.014	Margo superior	Superior border
A02.4.01.015	Incisura scapulae	Suprascapular notch
A02.4.01.016	Angulus inferior	Inferior angle
A02.4.01.017	Angulus lateralis	Lateral angle
A02.4.01.018	Angulus superior	Superior angle
A02.4.01.019	Cavitas glenoidalis	Glenoid cavity
A02.4.01.020	Tuberculum supraglenoidale	Supraglenoid tubercle
A02.4.01.021	Tuberculum infraglenoidale	Infraglenoid tubercle
A02.4.01.022	Collum scapulae	Neck of scapula
A02.4.01.023	Processus coracoideus	Coracoid process
A02.4.02.001	**Clavicula**	**Clavicle**
A02.4.02.002	Extremitas sternalis	Sternal end
A02.4.02.003	Facies articularis sternalis	Sternal facet
A02.4.02.004	Impressio ligamenti costoclavicularis	Impression for costoclavicular ligament
A02.4.02.005	Corpus claviculae	Shaft of clavicle; Body of clavicle
A02.4.02.006	Sulcus musculi subclavii	Subclavian groove; Groove for subclavius
A02.4.02.007	Extremitas acromialis	Acromial end
A02.4.02.008	Facies articularis acromialis	Acromial facet
A02.4.02.009	Tuberositas ligamenti coracoclavicularis	Tuberosity for coracoclavicular ligament
A02.4.02.010	Tuberculum conoideum	Conoid tubercle
A02.4.02.011	Linea trapezoidea	Trapezoid line

A02.4.03.001	**PARS LIBERA MEMBRI SUPERIORIS**	**FREE PART OF UPPER LIMB**
A02.4.04.001	**Humerus**	**Humerus**
A02.4.04.002	Caput humeri	Head
A02.4.04.003	Collum anatomicum	Anatomical neck
A02.4.04.004	Collum chirurgicum	Surgical neck
A02.4.04.005	Tuberculum majus	Greater tubercle
A02.4.04.006	Tuberculum minus	Lesser tubercle
A02.4.04.007	Sulcus intertubercularis	Intertubercular sulcus; Bicipital groove
A02.4.04.008	Crista tuberculi majoris; Labium laterale	Crest of greater tubercle; Lateral lip
A02.4.04.009	Crista tuberculi minoris; Labium mediale	Crest of lesser tubercle; Medial lip
A02.4.04.010	Corpus humeri	Shaft of humerus; Body of humerus
A02.4.04.011	Facies anteromedialis	Anteromedial surface
A02.4.04.012	Facies anterolateralis	Anterolateral surface
A02.4.04.013	Facies posterior	Posterior surface
A02.4.04.014	Sulcus nervi radialis	Radial groove; Groove for radial nerve
A02.4.04.015	Margo medialis	Medial border
A02.4.04.016	Crista supraepicondylaris medialis; Crista supracondylaris medialis	Medial supraepicondylar ridge; Medial supracondylar ridge
A02.4.04.017	(Processus supracondylaris)	(Supracondylar process)
A02.4.04.018	Margo lateralis	Lateral margin
A02.4.04.019	Crista supraepicondylaris lateralis; Crista supracondylaris lateralis	Medial supraepicondylar ridge; Medial supracondylar ridge
A02.4.04.020	Tuberositas deltoidea	Deltoid tuberosity
A02.4.04.021	Condylus humeri	Condyle of humerus
A02.4.04.022	Capitulum humeri	Capitulum
A02.4.04.023	Trochlea humeri	Trochlea
A02.4.04.024	Fossa olecrani	Olecranon fossa
A02.4.04.025	Fossa coronoidea	Coronoid fossa
A02.4.04.026	Fossa radialis	Radial fossa
A02.4.04.027	Epicondylus medialis	Medial epicondyle
A02.4.04.028	Sulcus nervi ulnaris	Groove for ulnar nerve
A02.4.04.029	Epicondylus lateralis	Lateral epicondyle
A02.4.05.001	**Radius**	**Radius**
A02.4.05.002	Caput radii	Head
A02.4.05.003	Fovea articularis	Articular facet

A02.4.05.004	Circumferentia articularis	Articular circumference
A02.4.05.005	Collum radii	Neck
A02.4.05.006	Corpus radii	Shaft; Body
A02.4.05.007	Tuberositas radii	Radial tuberosity
A02.4.05.008	Facies anterior	Anterior surface
A02.4.05.009	Facies posterior	Posterior surface
A02.4.05.010	Facies lateralis	Lateral surface
A02.4.05.011	Tuberositas pronatoria	Pronator tuberosity
A02.4.05.012	Margo interosseus	Interosseous border
A02.4.05.013	Margo anterior	Anterior border
A02.4.05.014	Margo posterior	Posterior border
A02.4.05.015	Processus styloideus radii	Radial styloid process
A02.4.05.016	Crista suprastyloidea	Suprastyloid crest
A02.4.05.017	Tuberculum dorsale	Dorsal tubercle
A02.4.05.018	Sulci tendinum musculorum extensorum	Groove for extensor muscle tendons
A02.4.05.019	Incisura ulnaris	Ulnar notch
A02.4.05.020	Facies articularis carpalis	Carpal articular surface
A02.4.06.001	**Ulna**	**Ulna**
A02.4.06.002	Olecranon	Olecranon
A02.4.06.003	Processus coronoideus	Coronoid process
A02.4.06.004	Tuberositas ulnae	Tuberosity of ulna
A02.4.06.005	Incisura radialis	Radial notch
A02.4.06.006	Incisura trochlearis	Trochlear notch
A02.4.06.007	Corpus ulnae	Shaft; Body
A02.4.06.008	Facies anterior	Anterior surface
A02.4.06.009	Facies posterior	Posterior surface
A02.4.06.010	Facies medialis	Medial surface
A02.4.06.011	Margo interosseus	Interosseous border
A02.4.06.012	Margo anterior	Anterior border
A02.4.06.013	Margo posterior	Posterior border
A02.4.06.014	Crista musculi supinatoris	Supinator crest
A02.4.06.015	Caput ulnae	Head
A02.4.06.016	Circumferentia articularis	Articular circumference
A02.4.06.017	Processus styloideus ulnae	Ulnar styloid process

A02.4.07.001	**Ossa manus**	**Bones of hand**
A02.4.08.001	**Ossa carpi; Ossa carpalia**	**Carpal bones**
A02.4.08.002	(Os centrale)	(Os centrale)
A02.4.08.003	Os scaphoideum	Scaphoid
A02.4.08.004	Tuberculum ossis scaphoidei	Tubercle
A02.4.08.005	Os lunatum	Lunate
A02.4.08.006	Os triquetrum	Triquetrum
A02.4.08.007	Os pisiforme	Pisiform
A02.4.08.008	Os trapezium	Trapezium
A02.4.08.009	Tuberculum ossis trapezii	Tubercle
A02.4.08.010	Os trapezoideum	Trapezoid
A02.4.08.011	Os capitatum	Capitate
A02.4.08.012	Os hamatum	Hamate
A02.4.08.013	Hamulus ossis hamati	Hook of hamate
A02.4.08.014	Sulcus carpi	Carpal groove
A02.4.09.001	**Ossa metacarpi; Ossa metacarpalia [I–V]**	**Metacarpals [I–V]**
A02.4.09.002	Basis ossis metacarpi	Base
A02.4.09.003	Corpus ossis metacarpi	Shaft; Body
A02.4.09.004	Caput ossis metacarpi	Head
A02.4.09.005	Processus styloideus ossis metacarpi tertii [III]	Styloid process of third metacarpal [III]
A02.4.10.001	**Ossa digitorum; Phalanges**	**Phalanges**
A02.4.10.002	Phalanx proximalis	Proximal phalanx
A02.4.10.003	Phalanx media	Middle phalanx

A02.4.10.004	Phalanx distalis	Distal phalanx
A02.4.10.005	Tuberositas phalangis distalis	Tuberosity of distal phalanx
A02.4.10.006	Basis phalangis	Base of phalanx
A02.4.10.007	Corpus phalangis	Shaft of phalanx; Body of phalanx
A02.4.10.008	Caput phalangis	Head of phalanx
A02.4.10.009	Trochlea phalangis	Trochlea of phalanx
A02.4.11.001	**Ossa sesamoidea**	**Sesamoid bones**

A02.5.00.001	**Ossa membri inferioris**	**Bones of lower limb**
A02.5.00.002	**CINGULUM PELVICUM; CINGULUM MEMBRI INFERIORIS**	**PELVIC GIRDLE**
A02.2.05.001	**Os sacrum [vertebrae sacrales I–V]**	**Sacrum [sacral vertebrae I–V]**
A02.5.01.001	**Os coxae**	**Hip bone; Coxal bone; Pelvic bone**
A02.5.01.002	Acetabulum	Acetabulum
A02.5.01.003	Limbus acetabuli; Margo acetabuli	Acetabular margin
A02.5.01.004	Fossa acetabuli	Acetabular fossa
A02.5.01.005	Incisura acetabuli	Acetabular notch
A02.5.01.006	Facies lunata	Lunate surface
A02.5.01.007	Ramus ischiopubicus	Ischiopubic ramus
A02.5.01.008	Foramen obturatum	Obturator foramen
A02.5.01.009	Incisura ischiadica major	Greater sciatic notch
A02.5.01.101	**Os ilium; Ilium**	**Ilium**
A02.5.01.102	Corpus ossis ilii	Body of ilium
A02.5.01.103	Sulcus supraacetabularis	Supra-acetabular groove
A02.5.01.104	Ala ossis ilii	Ala of ilium; Wing of ilium
A02.5.01.105	Linea arcuata	Arcuate line
A02.5.01.106	Crista iliaca	Iliac crest
A02.5.01.107	Labium externum	Outer lip
A02.5.01.108	Tuberculum iliacum	Tuberculum of iliac crest
A02.5.01.109	Linea intermedia	Intermediate zone
A02.5.01.110	Labium internum	Inner lip
A02.5.01.111	Spina iliaca anterior superior	Anterior superior iliac spine
A02.5.01.112	Spina iliaca anterior inferior	Anterior inferior iliac spine
A02.5.01.113	Spina iliaca posterior superior	Posterior superior iliac spine
A02.5.01.114	Spina iliaca posterior inferior	Posterior inferior iliac spine
A02.5.01.115	Fossa iliaca	Iliac fossa
A02.5.01.116	Facies glutea	Gluteal surface
A02.5.01.117	Linea glutea anterior	Anterior gluteal line
A02.5.01.118	Linea glutea posterior	Posterior gluteal line
A02.5.01.119	Linea glutea inferior	Inferior gluteal line
A02.5.01.120	Facies sacropelvica	Sacropelvic surface
A02.5.01.121	Facies auricularis	Auricular surface
A02.5.01.122	Tuberositas iliaca	Iliac tuberosity
A02.5.01.201	**Os ischii; Ischium**	**Ischium**
A02.5.01.202	Corpus ossis ischii	Body
A02.5.01.203	Ramus ossis ischii	Ramus
A02.5.01.204	Tuber ischiadicum	Ischial tuberosity
A02.5.01.205	Spina ischiadica	Ischial spine
A02.5.01.206	Incisura ischiadica minor	Lesser sciatic notch
A02.5.01.301	**Os pubis; Pubis**	**Pubis**
A02.5.01.302	Corpus ossis pubis	Body
A02.5.01.303	Tuberculum pubicum	Pubic tubercle
A02.5.01.304	Facies symphysialis	Symphysial surface
A02.5.01.305	Crista pubica	Pubic crest
A02.5.01.306	Ramus superior ossis pubis	Superior pubic ramus
A02.5.01.307	Eminentia iliopubica	Iliopubic ramus
A02.5.01.308	Pecten ossis pubis	Pecten pubis; Pectineal line
A02.5.01.309	Crista obturatoria	Obturator crest

A02.5.01.310	Sulcus obturatorius	Obturator groove
A02.5.01.311	Tuberculum obturatorium anterius	Anterior obturator tubercle
A02.5.01.312	(Tuberculum obturatorium posterius)	(Posterior obturator tubercle)
A02.5.01.313	Ramus inferior ossis pubis	Inferior pubic ramus

A02.5.02.001	**Pelvis**	**Pelvis**
A02.5.02.002	Cavitas pelvis	Pelvic cavity
A02.5.02.003	Arcus pubicus	Pubic arch
A02.5.02.004	Angulus subpubicus	Subpubic angle
A02.5.02.005	Pelvis major	Greater pelvis; False pelvis
A02.5.02.006	Pelvis minor	Lesser pelvis; True pelvis
A02.5.02.007	Linea terminalis	Linea terminalis
A02.5.02.008	Apertura pelvis superior	Pelvic inlet
A02.5.02.009	Apertura pelvis inferior	Pelvic outlet
A02.5.02.010	Axis pelvis	Axis of pelvis
A02.5.02.011	Diameter transversa	Transverse diameter
A02.5.02.012	Diameter obliqua	Oblique diameter
A02.5.02.013	Conjugata anatomica	Anatomical conjugate
A02.5.02.014	Conjugata vera	True conjugate
A02.5.02.015	Conjugata diagonalis	Diagonal conjugate
A02.5.02.016	Conjugata recta	Straight conjugate
A02.5.02.017	Conjugata mediana	Median conjugate
A02.5.02.018	Conjugata externa	External conjugate
A02.5.02.019	Distantia interspinosa	Interspinous distance; Interspinous diameter
A02.5.02.020	Distantia intercristalis	Intercristal distance; Intercristal diameter
A02.5.02.021	Distantia intertrochanterica	Intertrochanteric distance; Intertrochanteric diameter
A02.5.02.022	Inclinatio pelvis	Pelvic inclination

A02.5.03.001	**PARS LIBERA MEMBRI INFERIORIS**	**FREE PART OF LOWER LIMB**
A02.5.04.001	**Femur; Os femoris**	**Femur; Thigh bone**
A02.5.04.002	Caput femoris	Head
A02.5.04.003	Fovea capitis femoris	Fovea for ligament of head
A02.5.04.004	Collum femoris	Neck
A02.5.04.005	Trochanter major	Greater trochanter
A02.5.04.006	Fossa trochanterica	Trochanteric fossa
A02.5.04.007	Trochanter minor	Lesser trochanter
A02.5.04.008	(Trochanter tertius)	(Third trochanter)
A02.5.04.009	Linea intertrochanterica	Intertrochanteric line
A02.5.04.010	Crista intertrochanterica	Intertrochanteric crest
A02.5.04.011	Tuberculum quadratum	Quadrate tubercle
A02.5.04.012	Corpus femoris	Shaft of femur; Body of femur
A02.5.04.013	Linea aspera	Linea aspera
A02.5.04.014	Labium laterale	Lateral lip
A02.5.04.015	Labium mediale	Medial lip
A02.5.04.016	Linea pectinea	Pectineal line; Spiral line
A02.5.04.017	Tuberositas glutea	Gluteal tuberosity
A02.5.04.018	Facies poplitea	Popliteal surface
A02.5.04.019	Linea supracondylaris medialis	Medial supracondylar line
A02.5.04.020	Linea supracondylaris lateralis	Lateral supracondylar line
A02.5.04.021	Condylus medialis	Medial condyle
A02.5.04.022	Epicondylus medialis	Medial epicondyle
A02.5.04.023	Tuberculum adductorium	Adductor tubercle
A02.5.04.024	Condylus lateralis	Lateral condyle
A02.5.04.025	Epicondylus lateralis	Lateral epicondyle
A02.5.04.026	Sulcus popliteus	Groove for popliteus
A02.5.04.027	Facies patellaris	Patellar surface
A02.5.04.028	Fossa intercondylaris	Intercondylar fossa

A02.5.04.029	Linea intercondylaris	Intercondylar line
A02.5.05.001	**Patella**	**Patella**
A02.5.05.002	Basis patellae	Base of patella
A02.5.05.003	Apex patellae	Apex of patella
A02.5.05.004	Facies articularis	Articular surface
A02.5.05.005	Facies anterior	Anterior surface
A02.5.06.001	**Tibia**	**Tibia**
A02.5.06.002	Facies articularis superior	Superior articular surface
A02.5.06.003	Condylus medialis	Medial condyle
A02.5.06.004	Condylus lateralis	Lateral condyle
A02.5.06.005	Facies articularis fibularis	Fibular articular facet
A02.5.06.006	Area intercondylaris anterior	Anterior intercondylar area
A02.5.06.007	Area intercondylaris posterior	Posterior intercondylar area
A02.5.06.008	Eminentia intercondylaris	Intercondylar eminence
A02.5.06.009	Tuberculum intercondylare mediale	Medial intercondylar tubercle
A02.5.06.010	Tuberculum intercondylare laterale	Lateral intercondylar tubercle
A02.5.06.011	Corpus tibiae	Shaft; Body
A02.5.06.012	Tuberositas tibiae	Tibial tuberosity
A02.5.06.013	Facies medialis	Medial surface
A02.5.06.014	Facies posterior	Posterior surface
A02.5.06.015	Linea musculi solei	Soleal line
A02.5.06.016	Facies lateralis	Lateral surface
A02.5.06.017	Margo anterior	Anterior border
A02.5.06.018	Margo medialis	Medial border
A02.5.06.019	Margo interosseus	Interosseous border
A02.5.06.020	Malleolus medialis	Medial malleolus
A02.5.06.021	Sulcus malleolaris	Malleolar groove
A02.5.06.022	Facies articularis malleoli medialis	Articular facet
A02.5.06.023	Incisura fibularis	Fibular notch
A02.5.06.024	Facies articularis inferior	Inferior articular surface
A02.5.07.001	**Fibula**	**Fibula**
A02.5.07.002	Caput fibulae	Head
A02.5.07.003	Facies articularis capitis fibulae	Articular facet
A02.5.07.004	Apex capitis fibulae	Apex of head
A02.5.07.005	Collum fibulae	Neck
A02.5.07.006	Corpus fibulae	Shaft; Body
A02.5.07.007	Facies lateralis	Lateral surface
A02.5.07.008	Facies medialis	Medial surface
A02.5.07.009	Facies posterior	Posterior surface
A02.5.07.010	Crista medialis	Medial crest
A02.5.07.011	Margo anterior	Anterior border
A02.5.07.012	Margo interosseus	Interosseous border
A02.5.07.013	Margo posterior	Posterior border
A02.5.07.014	Malleolus lateralis	Lateral malleolus
A02.5.07.015	Facies articularis malleoli lateralis	Articular facet
A02.5.07.016	Fossa malleoli lateralis	Malleolar fossa
A02.5.07.017	Sulcus malleolaris	Malleolar groove

A02.5.08.001	**Ossa pedis**	**Bones of foot**
A02.5.09.001	**Ossa tarsi; Ossa tarsalia**	**Tarsal bones**
A02.5.10.001	**Talus**	**Talus**
A02.5.10.002	Caput tali	Head
A02.5.10.003	Facies articularis navicularis	Navicular articular surface
A02.5.10.004	Facies articularis ligamenti calcaneonavicularis plantaris	Facet for plantar calcaneonavicular ligament
A02.5.10.005	Facies articularis partis calcaneonavicularis ligamenti bifurcati	Facet for calcaneonavicular part of bifurcate ligament
A02.5.10.006	Facies articularis calcanea anterior	Anterior facet for calcaneus

A02.5.10.007	Collum tali	Neck
A02.5.10.008	Facies articularis calcanea media	Middle facet for calcaneus
A02.5.10.009	Sulcus tali	Sulcus tali
A02.5.10.010	Corpus tali	Body
A02.5.10.011	Trochlea tali	Trochlea of talus
A02.5.10.012	Facies superior	Superior facet
A02.5.10.013	Facies malleolaris lateralis	Lateral malleolar facet
A02.5.10.014	Processus lateralis tali	Lateral process
A02.5.10.015	Facies malleolaris medialis	Medial malleolar facet
A02.5.10.016	Processus posterior tali	Posterior process
A02.5.10.017	Sulcus tendinis musculi flexoris hallucis longi	Groove for tendon of flexor hallucis longus
A02.5.10.018	Tuberculum laterale	Lateral tubercle
A02.5.10.019	Tuberculum mediale	Medial tubercle
A02.5.10.020	Facies articularis calcanea posterior	Posterior calcaneal articular facet
A02.5.10.021	(Os trigonum)	(Os trigonum)
A02.5.11.001	**Calcaneus**	**Calcaneus**
A02.5.11.002	Tuber calcanei	Calcaneal tuberosity
A02.5.11.003	Processus medialis tuberis calcanei	Medial process
A02.5.11.004	Processus lateralis tuberis calcanei	Lateral process
A02.5.11.005	Tuberculum calcanei	Calcaneal tubercle
A02.5.11.006	Sustentaculum tali	Sustentaculum tali; Talar shelf
A02.5.11.007	Sulcus tendinis musculi flexoris hallucis longi	Groove for tendon of flexor hallucis longus
A02.5.11.008	Sulcus calcanei	Calcaneal sulcus
A02.5.11.009	Sinus tarsi	Tarsal sinus
A02.5.11.010	Facies articularis talaris anterior	Anterior talar articular surface
A02.5.11.011	Facies articularis talaris media	Middle talar articular surface
A02.5.11.012	Facies articularis talaris posterior	Posterior talar articular surface
A02.5.11.013	Sulcus tendinis musculi fibularis longi; Sulcus tendinis musculi peronei longi	Groove for tendon of fibularis longus; Groove for tendon of peroneus longus
A02.5.11.014	Trochlea fibularis; Trochlea peronealis	Fibular trochlea; Peroneal trochlea; Peroneal tubercle
A02.5.11.015	Facies articularis cuboidea	Articular surface for cuboid
A02.5.12.001	**Os naviculare**	**Navicular**
A02.5.12.002	Tuberositas ossis navicularis	Tuberosity
A02.5.13.001	**Os cuneiforme mediale**	**Medial cuneiform**
A02.5.14.001	**Os cuneiforme intermedium**	**Intermediate cuneiform; Middle cuneiform**
A02.5.15.001	**Os cuneiforme laterale**	**Lateral cuneiform**
A02.5.16.001	**Os cuboideum**	**Cuboid**
A02.5.16.002	Sulcus tendinis musculi fibularis longi; Sulcus tendinis musculi peronei longi	Groove for tendon of fibularis longus; Groove for tendon of peroneus longus
A02.5.16.003	Tuberositas ossis cuboidei	Tuberosity
A02.5.16.004	Processus calcaneus	Calcaneal process
A02.5.17.001	**Ossa metatarsi; Ossa metatarsalia [I–V]**	**Metatarsals [I–V]**
A02.5.17.002	Basis ossis metatarsi	Base
A02.5.17.003	Corpus ossis metatarsi	Shaft; Body
A02.5.17.004	Caput ossis metatarsi	Head
A02.5.17.005	Tuberositas ossis metatarsi primi [I]	Tuberosity of first metatarsal bone [I]
A02.5.17.006	Tuberositas ossis metatarsi quinti [V]	Tuberosity of fifth metatarsal bone [V]
A02.5.18.001	**Ossa digitorum; Phalanges**	**Phalanges**
A02.5.18.002	Phalanx proximalis	Proximal phalanx
A02.5.18.003	Phalanx media	Middle phalanx
A02.5.18.004	Phalanx distalis	Distal phalanx
A02.5.18.005	Tuberositas phalangis distalis	Tuberosity of distal phalanx
A02.5.18.006	Basis phalangis	Base of phalanx
A02.5.18.007	Corpus phalangis	Shaft of phalanx; Body of phalanx
A02.5.18.008	Caput phalangis	Head of phalanx
A02.5.18.009	Trochlea phalangis	Trochlea of phalanx
A02.5.19.001	**Ossa sesamoidea**	**Sesamoid bones**

A03.0.00.000 Juncturae; Systema articulare — Joints; Articular system

	Nomina generalia	*General terms*
A03.0.00.001	Junctura	Joint
A03.0.00.002	Juncturae ossium	Bony joints
A03.0.00.003	Synarthrosis	Synarthrosis
A03.0.00.004	Junctura fibrosa	Fibrous joint
A03.0.00.005	Syndesmosis	Syndesmosis
A03.0.00.006	Gomphosis	Gomphosis; Socket
A03.0.00.007	Membrana interossea	Interosseous membrane
A03.0.00.008	Sutura	Suture
A03.0.00.009	Sutura plana	Plane suture
A03.0.00.010	Sutura squamosa	Squamous suture
A03.0.00.011	Sutura limbosa	Limbous suture
A03.0.00.012	Sutura serrata	Serrate suture
A03.0.00.013	Sutura denticulata	Denticulate suture
A03.0.00.014	Schindylesis	Schindylesis
A03.0.00.015	Junctura cartilaginea	Cartilaginous joint
A03.0.00.016	Synchondrosis	Synchondrosis
A03.0.00.017	Symphysis	Symphysis; Secondary cartilaginous joint
A03.0.00.018	Cartilago epiphysialis	Epiphysial cartilage; Primary cartilaginous joint
A03.0.00.019	Junctura ossea; Synostosis	Bony union; Synostosis
A03.0.00.020	Junctura synovialis; Articulatio; Diarthrosis	Synovial joint; Diarthrosis
A03.0.00.021	Facies articularis	Articular surface
A03.0.00.022	Cavitas articularis	Articular cavity
A03.0.00.023	Fossa articularis	Articular fossa
A03.0.00.024	(Caput articulare)	(Articular head)
A03.0.00.025	Labrum articulare	Labrum
A03.0.00.026	Capsula articularis	Joint capsule; Articular capsule
A03.0.00.027	Membrana fibrosa; Stratum fibrosum	Fibrous layer; Fibrous membrane
A03.0.00.028	Membrana synovialis; Stratum synoviale	Synovial membrane; Synovial layer
A03.0.00.029	Plicae synoviales	Synovial folds
A03.0.00.030	Villi synoviales	Synovial villi
A03.0.00.031	Synovia	Synovial fluid
A03.0.00.032	Discus articularis	Articular disc
A03.0.00.033	Meniscus articularis	Meniscus
A03.0.00.034	Ligamenta	Ligaments
A03.0.00.035	Ligg. intracapsularia	Intracapsular ligaments
A03.0.00.036	Ligg. capsularia	Capsular ligaments
A03.0.00.037	Ligg. extracapsularia	Extracapsular ligaments
A03.0.00.038	Recessus articularis	Articular recess
A03.0.00.039	Bursa synovialis	Synovial bursa
A03.0.00.040	Vagina synovialis	Synovial sheath
A03.0.00.041	Articulatio simplex	Simple joint
A03.0.00.042	Articulatio composita	Complex joint
A03.0.00.043	Articulatio plana	Plane joint
A03.0.00.044	Articulatio cylindrica	Cylindrical joint
A03.0.00.045	Articulatio trochoidea	Pivot joint
A03.0.00.046	Ginglymus	Hinge joint
A03.0.00.047	Articulatio bicondylaris	Bicondylar joint
A03.0.00.048	Articulatio sellaris	Saddle joint
A03.0.00.049	Articulatio ellipsoidea	Condylar joint; Ellipsoid joint
A03.0.00.050	Articulatio spheroidea; Enarthrosis	Ball and socket joint; Spheroidal joint
A03.0.00.051	Articulatio cotylica	Cotyloid joint
A03.0.00.052	Amphiarthrosis	Amphiarthrosis
A03.0.00.053	Abductio	Abduction
A03.0.00.054	Adductio	Adduction
A03.0.00.055	Rotatio externa; Exorotatio; Rotatio lateralis	Lateral rotation; External rotation

A03.0.00.056	Rotatio interna; Endorotatio; Rotatio medialis	Medial rotation; Internal rotation
A03.0.00.057	Circumductio	Circumduction
A03.0.00.058	Flexio	Flexion
A03.0.00.059	Extensio	Extension
A03.0.00.060	Pronatio	Pronation
A03.0.00.061	Supinatio	Supination
A03.0.00.062	Oppositio	Opposition
A03.0.00.063	Repositio	Reposition

A03.1.00.001	**Juncturae cranii**	**Joints of skull**
A03.1.00.002	**Juncturae fibrosae cranii**	**Cranial fibrous joints**
A03.1.01.001	**Syndesmoses cranii**	**Cranial syndesmoses**
A03.1.01.002	Lig. pterygospinale	Pterygospinous ligament
A03.1.01.003	Lig. stylohyoideum	Stylohyoid ligament
A03.1.02.001	**Suturae cranii**	**Cranial sutures**
A03.1.02.002	Sutura coronalis	Coronal suture
A03.1.02.003	Sutura sagittalis	Sagittal suture
A03.1.02.004	Sutura lambdoidea	Lambdoid suture
A03.1.02.005	Sutura occipitomastoidea	Occipitomastoid suture
A03.1.02.006	Sutura sphenofrontalis	Sphenofrontal suture
A03.1.02.007	Sutura sphenoethmoidalis	Spheno-ethmoidal suture
A03.1.02.008	Sutura sphenosquamosa	Sphenosquamous suture
A03.1.02.009	Sutura sphenoparietalis	Sphenoparietal suture
A03.1.02.010	Sutura squamosa	Squamous suture
A02.1.03.007	(Sutura frontalis persistens; Sutura metopica)	(Frontal suture; Metopic suture)
A03.1.02.011	Sutura parietomastoidea	Parietomastoid suture
A03.1.02.012	(Sutura squamomastoidea)	(Squamomastoid suture)
A03.1.02.013	Sutura frontonasalis	Frontonasal suture
A03.1.02.014	Sutura frontoethmoidalis	Fronto-ethmoidal suture
A03.1.02.015	Sutura frontomaxillaris	Frontomaxillary suture
A03.1.02.016	Sutura frontolacrimalis	Frontolacrimal suture
A03.1.02.017	Sutura frontozygomatica	Frontozygomatic suture
A03.1.02.018	Sutura zygomaticomaxillaris	Zygomaticomaxillary suture
A03.1.02.019	Sutura ethmoidomaxillaris	Ethmoidomaxillary suture
A03.1.02.020	Sutura ethmoidolacrimalis	Ethmoidolacrimal suture
A03.1.02.021	Sutura sphenovomeralis	Sphenovomerine suture
A03.1.02.022	Sutura sphenozygomatica	Sphenozygomatic suture
A03.1.02.023	Sutura sphenomaxillaris	Sphenomaxillary suture
A03.1.02.024	Sutura temporozygomatica	Temporozygomatic suture
A03.1.02.025	Sutura internasalis	Internasal suture
A03.1.02.026	Sutura nasomaxillaris	Nasomaxillary suture
A03.1.02.027	Sutura lacrimomaxillaris	Lacrimomaxillary suture
A03.1.02.028	Sutura lacrimoconchalis	Lacrimoconchal suture
A03.1.02.029	Sutura intermaxillaris	Intermaxillary suture
A03.1.02.030	Sutura palatomaxillaris	Palatomaxillary suture
A03.1.02.031	Sutura palatoethmoidalis	Palato-ethmoidal suture
A03.1.02.032	Sutura palatina mediana	Median palatine suture
A03.1.02.033	Sutura palatina transversa	Transverse palatine suture
A03.1.03.001	**Syndesmosis dentoalveolaris; Gomphosis**	**Dento-alveolar syndesmosis; Gomphosis**
A03.1.03.002	Periodontium	Periodontium; Periodontal membrane
A03.1.03.003	Gingiva	Gingiva
A03.1.03.004	Periodontium protectionis	Gum; Gingiva
A03.1.03.005	Periodontium insertionis	Inserting periodontium
A03.1.03.006	Desmodontium	Desmodentium; Periodontal fibre▲
A03.1.03.007	Cementum	Cement; Cementum
A03.1.03.008	Alveoli dentales	Dental alveoli

A03.1.04.001	**Juncturae cartilagineae cranii**	**Cranial cartilaginous joints**
A03.1.05.001	**Synchondroses cranii**	**Cranial synchondroses**
A03.1.05.002	Synchondrosis sphenooccipitalis	Spheno-occipital synchondrosis
A03.1.05.003	Synchondrosis sphenopetrosa	Sphenopetrosal synchondrosis
A03.1.05.004	Synchondrosis petrooccipitalis	Petro-occipital synchondrosis
A03.1.05.006	(Synchondrosis intraoccipitalis posterior)	(Posterior intra-occipital synchondrosis)
A03.1.05.007	(Synchondrosis intraoccipitalis anterior)	(Anterior intra-occipital synchondrosis)
A03.1.05.008	Synchondrosis sphenoethmoidalis	Spheno-ethmoidal synchondrosis

A03.1.06.001	**Articulationes cranii**	**Cranial synovial joints**
A03.1.07.001	**Articulatio temporomandibularis**	**Temporomandibular joint**
A03.1.07.002	Discus articularis	Articular disc
A03.1.07.003	Lig. laterale	Lateral ligament
A03.1.07.004	Lig. mediale	Medial ligament
A03.1.07.005	Membrana synovialis superior	Superior synovial membrane
A03.1.07.006	Membrana synovialis inferior	Inferior synovial membrane
A03.1.07.007	Lig. sphenomandibulare	Sphenomandibular ligament
A03.1.07.008	Lig. stylomandibulare	Stylomandibular ligament
A03.1.08.001	**Articulatio atlantooccipitalis**	**Atlanto-occipital joint**
A03.1.08.002	Membrana atlantooccipitalis anterior	Anterior atlanto-occipital membrane
A03.1.08.003	(Lig. atlantooccipitale anterius)	(Anterior atlanto-occipital ligament)
A03.1.08.004	Membrana atlantooccipitalis posterior	Posterior atlanto-occipital membrane
A03.1.08.005	Lig. atlantooccipitale laterale	Lateral atlanto-occipital ligament

A03.2.00.001	**Juncturae columnae vertebralis**	**Vertebral joints**
A03.2.01.001	**Syndesmoses columnae vertebralis**	**Syndesmoses of vertebral column**
A03.2.01.002	Ligg. interspinalia	Interspinous ligaments
A03.2.01.003	Ligg. flava	Ligamenta flava
A03.2.01.004	Ligg. intertransversaria	Intertransverse ligaments
A03.2.01.005	Lig. supraspinale	Supraspinous ligament
A03.2.01.006	Lig. nuchae	Ligamentum nuchae; Nuchal ligament
A03.2.01.007	Lig. longitudinale anterius	Anterior longitudinal ligament
A03.2.01.008	Lig. longitudinale posterius	Posterior longitudinal ligament
A03.2.01.009	Ligg. transversa	Transverse ligaments

A03.2.02.001	**Synchondroses columnae vertebralis**	**Synchondroses of vertebral column**
A03.2.02.002	Symphysis intervertebralis	Intervertebral joint
A03.2.02.003	Discus intervertebralis	Intervertebral disc
A03.2.02.004	Anulus fibrosus	Anulus fibrosus
A03.2.02.005	Nucleus pulposus	Nucleus pulposus

A03.2.03.001	**Articulationes columnae vertebralis**	**Vertebral synovial joints**
A03.2.04.001	**Articulatio atlantoaxialis mediana**	**Median atlanto-axial joint**
A03.2.04.002	Ligg. alaria	Alar ligaments
A03.2.04.003	Lig. apicis dentis	Apical ligament of dens
A03.2.04.004	Lig. cruciforme atlantis	Cruciate ligament of atlas
A03.2.04.005	Fasciculi longitudinales	Longitudinal bands
A03.2.04.006	Lig. transversum atlantis	Transverse ligament of atlas
A03.2.04.007	Membrana tectoria	Tectorial membrane
A03.2.05.001	**Articulatio atlantoaxialis lateralis**	**Lateral atlanto-axial joint**
A03.2.06.001	**Articulationes zygapophysiales**	**Zygapophysial joints**
A03.2.07.001	**Articulatio lumbosacralis**	**Lumbosacral joint**
A03.2.07.002	Lig. iliolumbale	Iliolumbar ligament
A03.2.08.001	**Articulatio sacrococcygea**	**Sacrococcygeal joint**
A03.2.08.002	Lig. sacrococcygeum posterius superficiale; Lig. sacrococcygeum dorsale superficiale	Superficial posterior sacrococcygeal ligament

A03.2.08.003	Lig. sacrococcygeum posterius profundum; Lig. sacrococcygeum dorsale profundum	Deep posterior sacrococcygeal ligament
A03.2.08.004	Lig. sacrococcygeum anterius; Lig. sacrococcygeum ventrale	Anterior sacrococcygeal ligament
A03.2.08.005	Lig. sacrococcygeum laterale	Lateral sacrococcygeal ligament

A03.3.00.001	**Juncturae thoracis**	**Thoracic joints**
A03.3.01.001	**Syndesmoses thoracis**	**Syndesmoses of thorax**
A03.3.01.002	Membrana intercostalis externa	External intercostal membrane
A03.3.01.003	Membrana intercostalis interna	Internal intercostal membrane

A03.3.02.001	**Synchondroses thoracis**	**Synchondroses of thorax**
A03.3.02.002	Synchondrosis costosternalis	Costosternal joint
A03.3.02.003	Synchondrosis costae primae	Synchondrosis of first rib
A03.3.02.004	Synchondroses sternales	Sternal synchondroses
A03.3.02.005	Symphysis xiphosternalis	Xiphisternal joint
A03.3.02.006	Symphysis manubriosternalis	Manubriosternal joint
A03.3.02.007	(Synchondrosis manubriosternalis)	(Manubriosternal synchondrosis)

A03.3.03.001	**Articulationes thoracis**	**Synovial joints of thorax**
A03.3.04.001	**Articulationes costovertebrales**	**Costovertebral joints**
A03.3.04.002	Articulatio capitis costae	Joint of head of rib
A03.3.04.003	Lig. capitis costae radiatum	Radiate ligament of head of rib
A03.3.04.004	Lig. capitis costae intraarticulare	Intra-articular ligament of head of rib
A03.3.04.005	Articulatio costotransversaria	Costotransverse joint
A03.3.04.006	Lig. costotransversarium	Costotransverse ligament
A03.3.04.007	Lig. costotransversarium superius	Superior costotransverse ligament
A03.3.04.008	Lig. costotransversarium laterale	Lateral costotransverse ligament
A03.3.04.009	Lig. lumbocostale	Lumbocostal ligament
A03.3.04.010	Foramen costotransversarium	Costotransverse foramen
A03.3.05.001	**Articulationes sternocostales**	**Sternocostal joints**
A03.3.05.002	Lig. sternocostale intraarticulare	Intra-articular sternocostal ligament
A03.3.05.003	Ligg. sternocostalia radiata	Radiate sternocostal ligaments
A03.3.05.004	Membrana sterni	Sternal membrane
A03.3.05.005	Ligg. costoxiphoidea	Costoxiphoid ligaments
A03.3.06.001	**Articulationes costochondrales**	**Costochondral joints**
A03.3.07.001	**Articulationes interchondrales**	**Interchondral joints**

A03.4.00.001	**Juncturae cinguli pelvici** (vide paginam 30)	**Joints of pelvic girdle** (see page 30)

A03.5.00.001	**Juncturae membri superioris**	**Joints of upper limb**
A03.5.00.002	**JUNCTURAE CINGULI PECTORALIS**	**JOINTS OF PECTORAL GIRDLE**
A03.5.01.001	**Syndesmoses cinguli pectoralis; Syndesmoses cinguli membri superioris**	**Syndesmoses of pectoral girdle; Syndesmoses of shoulder girdle**
A03.5.01.002	Lig. coracoacromiale	Coraco-acromial ligament
A03.5.01.003	Lig. transversum scapulae superius	Superior transverse scapular ligament
A03.5.01.004	(Lig. transversum scapulae inferius)	(Inferior transverse scapular ligament)

A03.5.02.001	**Articulationes cinguli pectoralis; Articulationes cinguli membri superioris**	**Synovial joints of pectoral girdle; Synovial joints of shoulder girdle**
A03.5.03.001	**Articulatio acromioclavicularis**	**Acromioclavicular joint**
A03.5.03.002	Lig. acromioclaviculare	Acromioclavicular ligament
A03.5.03.003	(Discus articularis)	(Articular disc)
A03.5.03.004	Lig. coracoclaviculare	Coracoclavicular ligament
A03.5.03.005	Lig. trapezoideum	Trapezoid ligament
A03.5.03.006	Lig. conoideum	Conoid ligament

A03.5.04.001	**Articulatio sternoclavicularis**	**Sternoclavicular joint**
A03.5.04.002	Discus articularis	Articular disc
A03.5.04.003	Lig. sternoclaviculare anterius	Anterior sternoclavicular ligament
A03.5.04.004	Lig. sternoclaviculare posterius	Posterior sternoclavicular ligament
A03.5.04.005	Lig. costoclaviculare	Costoclavicular ligament
A03.5.04.006	Lig. interclaviculare	Interclavicular ligament

A03.5.05.001	**JUNCTURAE MEMBRI SUPERIORIS LIBERI**	**JOINTS OF FREE UPPER LIMB**
A03.5.06.001	**Syndesmosis radioulnaris**	**Radio-ulnar syndesmosis**
A03.5.06.002	Membrana interossea antebrachii	Interosseous membrane of forearm
A03.5.06.003	Chorda obliqua	Oblique cord

A03.5.07.001	**Articulationes membri superioris liberi**	**Synovial joints of free upper limb**
A03.5.08.001	**Articulatio humeri; Articulatio glenohumeralis**	**Glenohumeral joint; Shoulder joint**
A03.5.08.002	Labrum glenoidale	Glenoid labrum
A03.5.08.003	Ligg. glenohumeralia	Glenohumeral ligaments
A03.5.08.004	Lig. coracohumerale	Coracohumeral ligament
A03.5.08.005	Lig. transversum humeri	Transverse humeral ligament
A03.5.09.001	**Articulatio cubiti**	**Elbow joint**
A03.5.09.002	Articulatio humeroulnaris	Humero-ulnar joint
A03.5.09.003	Articulatio humeroradialis	Humeroradial joint
A03.5.09.004	Articulatio radioulnaris proximalis	Proximal radio-ulnar joint
A03.5.09.005	Lig. collaterale ulnare	Ulnar collateral ligament
A03.5.09.006	Lig. collaterale radiale	Radial collateral ligament
A03.5.09.007	Lig. anulare radii	Anular ligament of radius
A03.5.09.008	Lig. quadratum	Quadrate ligament
A03.5.09.009	Recessus sacciformis	Sacciform recess
A03.5.10.001	**Articulatio radioulnaris distalis**	**Distal radio-ulnar joint**
A03.5.10.002	Discus articularis	Articular disc
A03.5.10.003	Recessus sacciformis	Sacciform recess
A03.5.11.001	**Articulationes manus**	**Joints of hand**
A03.5.11.002	Articulatio radiocarpalis	Wrist joint
A03.5.11.003	Lig. radiocarpale dorsale	Dorsal radiocarpal ligament
A03.5.11.004	Lig. radiocarpale palmare	Palmar radiocarpal ligament
A03.5.11.005	Lig. ulnocarpale dorsale	Dorsal ulnocarpal ligament
A03.5.11.006	Lig. ulnocarpale palmare	Palmar ulnocarpal ligament
A03.5.11.007	Lig. collaterale carpi ulnare	Ulnar collateral ligament of wrist joint
A03.5.11.008	Lig. collaterale carpi radiale	Radial collateral ligament of wrist joint
A03.5.11.101	Articulationes carpi; Articulationes intercarpales	Carpal joints; Intercarpal joints
A03.5.11.102	Articulatio mediocarpalis	Midcarpal joint
A03.5.11.103	Lig. carpi radiatum	Radiate carpal ligament
A03.5.11.104	Ligg. intercarpalia dorsalia	Dorsal intercarpal ligaments
A03.5.11.105	Ligg. intercarpalia palmaria	Palmar intercarpal ligaments
A03.5.11.106	Ligg. intercarpalia interossea	Interosseous intercarpal ligaments
A03.5.11.107	Articulatio ossis pisiformis	Pisiform joint
A03.5.11.108	Lig. pisohamatum	Pisohamate ligament
A03.5.11.109	Lig. pisometacarpale	Pisometacarpal ligament
A03.5.11.201	Canalis carpi	Carpal tunnel
A03.5.11.202	Canalis ulnaris	Ulnar canal
A03.5.11.301	Articulationes carpometacarpales	Carpometacarpal joints
A03.5.11.302	Ligg. carpometacarpalia dorsalia	Dorsal carpometacarpal ligaments
A03.5.11.303	Ligg. carpometacarpalia palmaria	Palmar carpometacarpal ligaments
A03.5.11.304	Articulatio carpometacarpalis pollicis	Carpometacarpal joint of thumb
A03.5.11.401	Articulationes intermetacarpales	Intermetacarpal joints
A03.5.11.402	Ligg. metacarpalia dorsalia	Dorsal metacarpal ligaments
A03.5.11.403	Ligg. metacarpalia palmaria	Palmar metacarpal ligaments
A03.5.11.404	Ligg. metacarpalia interossea	Interosseous metacarpal ligaments

A03.5.11.405	Spatia interossea metacarpi	Interosseous metacarpal spaces
A03.5.11.501	Articulationes metacarpophalangeae	Metacarpophalangeal joints
A03.5.11.502	Ligg. collateralia	Collateral ligaments
A03.5.11.503	Ligg. palmaria	Palmar ligaments
A03.5.11.504	Lig. metacarpale transversum profundum	Deep transverse metacarpal ligament
A03.5.11.601	Articulationes interphalangeae manus	Interphalangeal joints of hand
A03.5.11.602	Ligg. collateralia	Collateral ligaments
A03.5.11.603	Ligg. palmaria	Palmar ligaments

A03.6.00.001	**Juncturae membri inferioris**	**Joints of lower limb**
A03.4.00.001	**JUNCTURAE CINGULI PELVICI**	**JOINTS OF PELVIC GIRDLE**
A03.6.01.001	**Syndesmoses cinguli pelvici**	**Syndesmoses of pelvic girdle**
A03.6.01.002	Membrana obturatoria	Obturator membrane
A03.6.01.003	Canalis obturatorius	Obturator canal
A03.6.02.001	**Symphysis pubica**	**Pubic symphysis**
A03.6.02.002	Discus interpubicus; Fibrocartilago interpubica	Interpubic disc; Interpubic fibrocartilage
A03.6.02.003	Lig. pubicum superius	Superior pubic ligament
A03.6.02.004	Lig. pubicum inferius	Inferior pubic ligament
A03.6.03.001	**Articulatio sacroiliaca**	**Sacro-iliac joint**
A03.6.03.002	Lig. sacroiliacum anterius	Anterior sacro-iliac ligament
A03.6.03.003	Lig. sacroiliacum interosseum	Interosseous sacro-iliac ligament
A03.6.03.004	Lig. sacroiliacum posterius	Posterior sacro-iliac ligament
A03.6.03.005	Lig. sacrotuberale	Sacrotuberous ligament
A03.6.03.006	Processus falciformis	Falciform process
A03.6.03.007	Lig. sacrospinale	Sacrospinous ligament
A03.6.03.008	Foramen ischiadicum majus	Greater sciatic foramen
A03.6.03.009	Foramen ischiadicum minus	Lesser sciatic foramen

A03.6.04.001	**JUNCTURAE MEMBRI INFERIORIS LIBERI**	**JOINTS OF FREE LOWER LIMB**
A03.6.05.001	**Syndesmosis tibiofibularis**	**Tibiofibular syndesmosis; Inferior tibiofibular joint**
A03.6.05.002	Membrana interossea cruris	Interosseous membrane of leg
A03.6.05.003	Lig. tibiofibulare anterius	Anterior tibiofibular ligament
A03.6.05.004	Lig. tibiofibulare posterius	Posterior tibiofibular ligament

A03.6.06.001	**Articulationes membri inferioris liberi**	**Synovial joints of free lower limb**
A03.6.07.001	**Articulatio coxae; Articulatio coxofemoralis**	**Hip joint**
A03.6.07.002	Zona orbicularis	Zona orbicularis
A03.6.07.003	Lig. iliofemorale	Iliofemoral ligament
A03.6.07.004	Pars transversa	Transverse part
A03.6.07.005	Pars descendens	Descending part
A03.6.07.006	Lig. ischiofemorale	Ischiofemoral ligament
A03.6.07.007	Lig. pubofemorale	Pubofemoral ligament
A03.6.07.008	Labrum acetabuli	Acetabular labrum
A03.6.07.009	Lig. transversum acetabuli	Transverse acetabular ligament
A03.6.07.010	Lig. capitis femoris	Ligament of head of femur
A03.6.08.001	**Articulatio genus**	**Knee joint**
A03.6.08.002	Meniscus lateralis	Lateral meniscus
A03.6.08.003	Lig. meniscofemorale anterius	Anterior meniscofemoral ligament
A03.6.08.004	Lig. meniscofemorale posterius	Posterior meniscofemoral ligament
A03.6.08.005	Meniscus medialis	Medial meniscus
A03.6.08.006	Lig. transversum genus	Transverse ligament of knee
A03.6.08.007	Lig. cruciatum anterius	Anterior cruciate ligament
A03.6.08.008	Lig. cruciatum posterius	Posterior cruciate ligament
A03.6.08.009	Plica synovialis infrapatellaris	Infrapatellar synovial fold
A03.6.08.010	Plicae alares	Alar folds
A03.6.08.011	Lig. collaterale fibulare	Fibular collateral ligament

A03.6.08.012	Lig. collaterale tibiale	Tibial collateral ligament
A03.6.08.013	Lig. popliteum obliquum	Oblique popliteal ligament
A03.6.08.014	Lig. popliteum arcuatum	Arcuate popliteal ligament
A03.6.08.015	Lig. patellae	Patellar ligament
A03.6.08.016	Retinaculum patellae mediale	Medial patellar retinaculum
A03.6.08.017	Retinaculum patellae laterale	Lateral patellar retinaculum
A03.6.08.018	Corpus adiposum infrapatellare	Infrapatellar fat pad
A03.6.09.001	**Articulatio tibiofibularis**	**Tibiofibular joint; Superior tibiofibular joint**
A03.6.09.002	Lig. capitis fibulae anterius	Anterior ligament of fibular head
A03.6.09.003	Lig. capitis fibulae posterius	Posterior ligament of fibular head
A03.6.10.001	**Articulationes pedis**	**Joints of foot**
A03.6.10.002	Articulatio talocruralis	Ankle joint
A03.6.10.003	Lig. collaterale mediale; Lig. deltoideum	Medial ligament; Deltoid ligament
A03.6.10.004	Pars tibionavicularis	Tibionavicular part
A03.6.10.005	Pars tibiocalcanea	Tibiocalcaneal part
A03.6.10.006	Pars tibiotalaris anterior	Anterior tibiotalar part
A03.6.10.007	Pars tibiotalaris posterior	Posterior tibiotalar part
A03.6.10.008	Lig. collaterale laterale	Lateral ligament
A03.6.10.009	Lig. talofibulare anterius	Anterior talofibular ligament
A03.6.10.010	Lig. talofibulare posterius	Posterior talofibular ligament
A03.6.10.011	Lig. calcaneofibulare	Calcaneofibular ligament
A03.6.10.101	Articulatio subtalaris; Articulatio talocalcanea	Subtalar joint; Talocalcaneal joint
A03.6.10.102	Lig. talocalcaneum laterale	Lateral talocalcaneal ligament
A03.6.10.103	Lig. talocalcaneum mediale	Medial talocalcaneal ligament
A03.6.10.104	Lig. talocalcaneum posterius	Posterior talocalcaneal ligament
A03.6.10.201	Articulatio tarsi transversa	Transverse tarsal joint
A03.6.10.202	Articulatio talocalcaneonavicularis	Talocalcaneonavicular joint
A03.6.10.203	Lig. calcaneonaviculare plantare	Plantar calcaneonavicular ligament; Spring ligament
A03.6.10.204	Articulatio calcaneocuboidea	Calcaneocuboid joint
A03.6.10.301	Articulatio cuneonavicularis	Cuneonavicular joint
A03.6.10.401	Articulationes intercuneiformes	Intercuneiform joints
A03.6.10.501	Ligamenta tarsi	Tarsal ligaments
A03.6.10.502	Ligg. tarsi interossea	Tarsal interosseous ligaments
A03.6.10.503	Lig. talocalcaneum interosseum	Talocalcaneal interosseous ligament
A03.6.10.504	Lig. cuneocuboideum interosseum	Cuneocuboid interosseous ligament
A03.6.10.505	Ligg. intercuneiformia interossea	Intercuneiform interosseous ligaments
A03.6.10.506	Ligg. tarsi dorsalia	Dorsal tarsal ligaments
A03.6.10.507	Lig. talonaviculare	Talonavicular ligament
A03.6.10.508	Ligg. intercuneiformia dorsalia	Dorsal intercuneiform ligament
A03.6.10.509	Lig. cuneocuboideum dorsale	Dorsal cuneocuboid ligament
A03.6.10.510	Lig. cuboideonaviculare dorsale	Dorsal cuboideonavicular ligament
A03.6.10.511	Lig. bifurcatum	Bifurcate ligament
A03.6.10.512	Lig. calcaneonaviculare	Calcaneonavicular ligament
A03.6.10.513	Lig. calcaneocuboideum	Calcaneocuboid ligament
A03.6.10.514	Ligg. cuneonavicularia dorsalia	Dorsal cuneonavicular ligament
A03.6.10.515	Lig. calcaneocuboideum dorsale	Dorsal calcaneocuboid ligament
A03.6.10.516	Ligg. tarsi plantaria	Plantar tarsal ligaments
A03.6.10.517	Lig. plantare longum	Long plantar ligament
A03.6.10.518	Lig. calcaneocuboideum plantare	Plantar calcaneocuboid ligament; Short plantar ligament
A03.6.10.203	Lig. calcaneonaviculare plantare	Plantar calcaneonavicular ligament; Spring ligament
A03.6.10.519	Ligg. cuneonavicularia plantaria	Plantar cuneonavicular ligaments
A03.6.10.520	Lig. cuboideonaviculare plantare	Plantar cuboideonavicular ligament
A03.6.10.521	Ligg. intercuneiformia plantaria	Plantar intercuneiform ligaments
A03.6.10.522	Lig. cuneocuboideum plantare	Plantar cuneocuboid ligament
A03.6.10.601	Articulationes tarsometatarsales	Tarsometatarsal joints
A03.6.10.602	Ligg. tarsometatarsalia dorsalia	Dorsal tarsometatarsal ligaments

A03.6.10.603	Ligg. tarsometatarsalia plantaria	Plantar tarsometatarsal ligaments
A03.6.10.604	Ligg. cuneometatarsalia interossea	Cuneometatarsal interosseous ligaments
A03.6.10.701	Articulationes intermetatarsales	Intermetatarsal joints
A03.6.10.702	Ligg. metatarsalia interossea	Metatarsal interosseous ligaments
A03.6.10.703	Ligg. metatarsalia dorsalia	Dorsal metatarsal ligaments
A03.6.10.704	Ligg. metatarsalia plantaria	Plantar metatarsal ligaments
A03.6.10.705	Spatia interossea metatarsi	Intermetatarsal spaces
A03.6.10.801	Articulationes metatarsophalangeae	Metatarsophalangeal joints
A03.6.10.802	Ligg. collateralia	Collateral ligaments
A03.6.10.803	Ligg. plantaria	Plantar ligaments
A03.6.10.804	Lig. metatarsale transversum profundum	Deep transverse metatarsal ligament
A03.6.10.901	Articulationes interphalangeae pedis	Interphalangeal joints of foot
A03.6.10.902	Ligg. collateralia	Collateral ligaments
A03.6.10.903	Ligg. plantaria	Plantar ligaments

A04.0.00.000	**Musculi; Systema musculare**	**Muscles; Muscular system**
	Nomina generalia	*General terms*
A04.0.00.001	Caput	Head
A04.0.00.002	Venter	Belly
* **A04.0.00.003**	Insertio	Attachment
A04.0.00.004	Punctum fixum	Fixed end
A04.0.00.005	Punctum mobile	Mobile end
A04.0.00.006	M. fusiformis	Fusiform muscle
A04.0.00.007	M. planus	Flat muscle
A04.0.00.008	M. rectus	Straight muscle
A04.0.00.009	M. triangularis	Triangular muscle
A04.0.00.010	M. quadratus	Quadrate muscle
A04.0.00.011	M. biventer	Two-bellied muscle
A04.0.00.012	M. biceps	Two-headed muscle
A04.0.00.013	M. triceps	Three-headed muscle
A04.0.00.014	M. quadriceps	Four-headed muscle
A04.0.00.015	M. semipennatus; M. unipennatus	Semipennate muscle; Unipennate muscle
A04.0.00.016	M. pennatus; M. bipennatus	Pennate muscle; Bipennate muscle
A04.0.00.017	M. multipennatus	Multipennate muscle
A04.0.00.018	M. orbicularis	Orbicular muscle
A04.0.00.019	M. cutaneus	Cutaneous muscle
A04.0.00.020	M. abductor	Abductor muscle
A04.0.00.021	M. adductor	Adductor muscle
A04.0.00.022	M. rotator	Rotator muscle
A04.0.00.023	M. flexor	Flexor muscle
A04.0.00.024	M. extensor	Extensor muscle
A04.0.00.025	M. pronator	Pronator muscle
A04.0.00.026	M. supinator	Supinator muscle
A04.0.00.027	M. opponens	Opponens muscle
A04.0.00.028	M. sphincter	Sphincter muscle
A04.0.00.029	M. dilatator	Dilator muscle
A04.0.00.030	Compartimentum	Compartment
* **A04.0.00.031**	Fascia	Fascia
A04.0.00.032	Fascia capitis et colli	Fascia of head and neck
A04.0.00.033	Fascia trunci	Fascia of trunk
* **A04.0.00.034**	Fascia parietalis	Parietal fascia
* **A04.0.00.035**	Fascia extraserosalis	Extraserosal fascia
* **A04.0.00.036**	Fascia visceralis	Visceral fascia

* **A04.0.00.003** *Insertio* The Latin word *insertio* means attachment. The terms insertion and origo/origin have not been used as they change with function.

* **A04.0.00.031** *Fascia* As the term is used here, *fascia* consists of sheaths, sheets or other dissectible connective tissue aggregations. Most form from condensations of mesenchyme as organs or cavities grow within them (condensation fasciae); some are left behind as organs move (migration fasciae); others are formed as serosal surfaces fuse (fusion fasciae). The list appearing under *fascia* includes all categories for which the use of the term is recommended. It thus includes not only the sheaths of muscles but also the investments of viscera and dissectible structures related to them. Nevertheless, for convenience and reference, the complete list is entered under *Muscles*. Not all of the structures which have been regarded (by some) as *fascia* are included. The fifth (1983) edition of *Nomina Anatomica* introduced the terms, *fascia superficialis* and *fascia profunda*. These are not recommended for use as generic terms in an unqualified way. In English, the view was that the connective tissue between the skin and muscle fascia was also a fascia and was called *fascia superficialis*, in contradistinction to the fascia of muscles, viscera and related structures that was called *fascia profunda*. However, the terms were anglocentric and have not been taken up in other languages. Thus, in the interests of international understanding, the recommended terms are now *tela subcutanea* – subcutaneous tissue, *fascia musculorum* and *fascia visceralis*. The problem was that *fascia superficialis* in English described the whole of the *tela subcutanea*, in Italian it excluded the *panniculus adiposus*, in French it excluded both the *panniculus adiposus* and the *textus connectivus laxus* beneath the *stratum membranosum*, whereas in German it described the superficial layer of the *fascia musculorum* and thus excluded the *panniculus adiposus*, the *stratum membranosum* and the *textus connectivus laxus*. Perhaps the most frequent use of the term *fascia* no longer recommended was for parts of the *tela subcutanea* of the anterior abdominal wall (Camper's fascia, now *panniculus adiposus abdominis*; Scarpa's fascia, now *stratum membranosum abdominis*), of the penis (Colles' fascia, now *stratum membranosum penis*) and of the perineum (Colles' fascia, now *stratum membranosum perinei*).

* **A04.0.00.034 / A04.0.00.035 / A04.0.00.036** *Fascia parietalis/fascia extraserosalis/fascia visceralis* *Fascia parietalis* is a generic term for the fascia which lies outside the parietal layer of a serosa (pericardium, peritoneum, pleura or *tunica vaginalis testis*) and lines the wall of a body cavity. *Fascia parietalis* may be or may not be a separate layer from the *fascia investiens profunda* outside it and/or the *tela subserosa parietalis* inside it. *Fascia visceralis* is a generic term for the fascia which lies immediately outside the visceral layer of the serosae together with that which immediately surrounds the viscera. *Fascia visceralis* may or may not be a separate layer from the *tela subserosa visceralis*. *Fascia extraserosalis* is a generic term of exclusion for any other fascia which lies inside the *fascia parietalis* and outside the *fascia visceralis*. The most obvious *fascia extraserosalis* is in the pelvis where it forms ligaments, such as the cardinal ligament of the uterus.

A04.0.00.037	Fasciae membrorum	Fascia of limbs
A04.0.00.038	Fasciae musculorum	Fascia of muscles
A04.0.00.039	Fascia investiens	Investing layer
A04.0.00.040	Fascia propria musculi	Fascia of individual muscle; Muscle sheath
A04.0.00.041	Epimysium	Epimysium
A04.0.00.042	Perimysium	Perimysium
A04.0.00.043	Endomysium	Endomysium
A04.0.00.044	Tendo	Tendon
A04.0.00.045	Tendo intermedius	Intermediate tendon
A04.0.00.046	Intersectio tendinea	Tendinous intersection
A04.0.00.047	Aponeurosis	Aponeurosis
A04.0.00.048	Arcus tendineus	Tendinous arch
A04.0.00.049	Trochlea muscularis	Muscular trochlea
A03.0.00.039	Bursa synovialis	Synovial bursa
A03.0.00.040	Vagina synovialis	Synovial sheath

A04.1.00.001	**Musculi capitis**	**Muscles of head**
A04.1.01.001	**Musculi externi bulbi oculi** {vide paginam 147}	**Extra-ocular muscles** {see page 147}
A04.1.02.001	**Musculi ossiculorum auditus** {vide paginam 150}	**Muscles of auditory ossicles** {see page 150}
A04.1.03.001	**Musculi faciei**	**Facial muscles**
A04.1.03.002	M. epicranius	Epicranius
A04.1.03.003	M. occipitofrontalis	Occipitofrontalis
A04.1.03.004	Venter frontalis	Frontal belly
A04.1.03.005	Venter occipitalis	Occipital belly
A04.1.03.006	M. temporoparietalis	Temporoparietalis
A04.1.03.007	Galea aponeurotica; Aponeurosis epicranialis	Epicranial aponeurosis
A04.1.03.008	M. procerus	Procerus
A04.1.03.009	M. nasalis	Nasalis
A04.1.03.010	Pars transversa	Transverse part
A04.1.03.011	Pars alaris	Alar part
A04.1.03.012	M. depressor septi nasi	Depressor septi nasi
A04.1.03.013	M. orbicularis oculi	Orbicularis oculi
A04.1.03.014	Pars palpebralis	Palpebral part
A04.1.03.015	Fasciculus ciliaris	Ciliary bundle
* **A04.1.03.016**	Pars profunda	Deep part
A04.1.03.017	Pars orbitalis	Orbital part
A04.1.03.018	M. corrugator supercilii	Corrugator supercilii
A04.1.03.019	M. depressor supercilii	Depressor supercilii
A04.1.03.020	M. auricularis anterior	Auricularis anterior
A04.1.03.021	M. auricularis superior	Auricularis superior
A04.1.03.022	M. auricularis posterior	Auricularis posterior
A04.1.03.023	M. orbicularis oris	Orbicularis oris
A04.1.03.024	Pars marginalis	Marginal part
A04.1.03.025	Pars labialis	Labial part
A04.1.03.026	M. depressor anguli oris	Depressor anguli oris
A04.1.03.027	M. transversus menti	Transversus menti
A04.1.03.028	M. risorius	Risorius
A04.1.03.029	M. zygomaticus major	Zygomaticus major
A04.1.03.030	M. zygomaticus minor	Zygomaticus minor
A04.1.03.031	M. levator labii superioris	Levator labii superioris
A04.1.03.032	M. levator labii superioris alaeque nasi	Levator labii superioris alaeque nasi
A04.1.03.033	M. depressor labii inferioris	Depressor labii inferioris
A04.1.03.034	M. levator anguli oris	Levator anguli oris
A04.1.03.035	Modiolus anguli oris	Modiolus

* **A04.1.03.016** *Pars profunda* Previously known as the *pars lacrimalis*, this is the deep part of the *pars palpebralis*. Jones L. T. 1960. "The Anatomy of the Lower Eyelid." *Am J Ophthalmol* 49: 29–36.

A04.1.03.036	M. buccinator	Buccinator
A04.1.03.037	M. mentalis	Mentalis
A04.1.04.001	**Musculi masticatorii**	**Masticatory muscles**
A04.1.04.002	M. masseter	Masseter
A04.1.04.003	Pars superficialis	Superficial part
A04.1.04.004	Pars profunda	Deep part
A04.1.04.005	M. temporalis	Temporalis; Temporal muscle
A04.1.04.006	M. pterygoideus lateralis	Lateral pterygoid
A04.1.04.007	Caput superius	Upper head; Superior head
A04.1.04.008	Caput inferius	Lower head; Inferior head
A04.1.04.009	M. pterygoideus medialis	Medial pterygoid
A04.1.04.010	Fascia buccopharyngea	Buccopharyngeal fascia
A04.1.04.011	Fascia masseterica	Masseteric fascia
A04.1.04.012	Fascia parotidea	Parotid fascia
A04.1.04.013	Fascia temporalis	Temporal fascia
A04.1.04.014	Lamina superficialis	Superficial layer
A04.1.04.015	Lamina profunda	Deep layer
A04.1.05.001	**Musculi linguae** {vide paginam 49}	**Muscles of tongue** {see page 49}
A04.1.06.001	**Musculi palati mollis et faucium** {vide paginam 50}	**Muscles of soft palate and fauces** {see page 50}

A04.2.00.001	Musculi colli; Musculi cervicis	Muscles of neck
A04.2.01.001	Platysma	Platysma
A04.2.01.002	M. longus colli; M. longus cervicis	Longus colli
A04.2.01.003	M. longus capitis	Longus capitis
A04.2.01.004	M. scalenus anterior	Scalenus anterior; Anterior scalene
A04.2.01.005	M. scalenus medius	Scalenus medius; Middle scalene
A04.2.01.006	M. scalenus posterior	Scalenus posterior; Posterior scalene
A04.2.01.007	(M. scalenus minimus)	(Scalenus minimus)
A04.2.01.008	M. sternocleidomastoideus	Sternocleidomastoid
A04.2.02.001	**Musculi suboccipitales**	**Suboccipital muscles**
A04.2.02.002	M. rectus capitis anterior	Rectus capitis anterior
A04.2.02.003	M. rectus capitis lateralis	Rectus capitis lateralis
A04.2.02.004	M. rectus capitis posterior major	Rectus capitis posterior major
A04.2.02.005	M. rectus capitis posterior minor	Rectus capitis posterior minor
A04.2.02.006	M. obliquus capitis superior	Obliquus capitis superior
A04.2.02.007	M. obliquus capitis inferior	Obliquus capitis inferior
A04.2.03.001	**Musculi suprahyoidei**	**Suprahyoid muscles**
A04.2.03.002	M. digastricus	Digastric
A04.2.03.003	Venter anterior	Anterior belly
A04.2.03.004	Venter posterior	Posterior belly
A04.2.03.005	M. stylohyoideus	Stylohyoid
A04.2.03.006	M. mylohyoideus	Mylohyoid
A04.2.03.007	M. geniohyoideus	Geniohyoid
A04.2.04.001	**Musculi infrahyoidei**	**Infrahyoid muscles**
A04.2.04.002	M. sternohyoideus	Sternohyoid
A04.2.04.003	M. omohyoideus	Omohyoid
A04.2.04.004	Venter superior	Superior belly
A04.2.04.005	Venter inferior	Inferior belly
A04.2.04.006	M. sternothyroideus	Sternothyroid
A04.2.04.007	M. thyrohyoideus	Thyrohyoid
A04.2.04.008	(M. levator glandulae thyroideae)	(Levator glandulae thyroideae)
A04.2.05.001	**Fascia cervicalis; Fascia colli**	**Cervical fascia**
A04.2.05.002	Lamina superficialis	Investing layer; Superficial layer
A04.2.05.003	Spatium suprasternale	Suprasternal space
A04.2.05.004	Lamina pretrachealis	Pretracheal layer

*	A04.2.05.005	Lig. suspensorium glandulae thyroideae	Suspensory ligament of thyroid gland
	A04.2.05.006	Lamina prevertebralis	Prevertebral layer
	A04.2.05.007	Vagina carotica	Carotid sheath
	A04.2.06.001	**Musculi pharyngis {vide paginam 51}**	**Pharyngeal muscles {see page 51}**
	A04.2.07.001	**Musculi laryngis {vide paginam 59}**	**Laryngeal muscles {see page 59}**

	A04.3.00.001	**Musculi dorsi**	**Muscles of back**
	A04.3.01.001	M. trapezius	Trapezius
	A04.3.01.002	Pars descendens	Descending part; Superior part
	A04.3.01.003	Pars transversa	Transverse part; Middle part
	A04.3.01.004	Pars ascendens	Ascending part; Inferior part
	A04.3.01.005	(M. transversus nuchae)	(Transversus nuchae)
	A04.3.01.006	M. latissimus dorsi	Latissimus dorsi
	A04.3.01.007	M. rhomboideus major	Rhomboid major
	A04.3.01.008	M. rhomboideus minor	Rhomboid minor
	A04.3.01.009	M. levator scapulae	Levator scapulae
	A04.3.01.010	M. serratus posterior inferior	Serratus posterior inferior
	A04.3.01.011	M. serratus posterior superior	Serratus posterior superior
	A04.3.01.012	Mm. intertransversarii anteriores cervicis; Mm. intertransversarii anteriores colli	Anterior cervical intertransversarii
	A04.3.01.013	Mm. intertransversarii posteriores laterales cervicis; Mm. intertransversarii posteriores laterales colli	Lateral posterior cervical intertransversarii
	A04.3.01.014	Mm. intertransversarii laterales lumborum	Intertransversarii laterales lumborum
	A04.3.01.015	Partes dorsales	Dorsal parts
	A04.3.01.016	Partes ventrales	Ventral parts
	A04.3.01.017	Fascia nuchae	Nuchal fascia

*	**A04.3.02.001**	**Musculi dorsi proprii**	**Musles of back proper**
	A04.3.02.002	**Musculus erector spinae**	**Erector spinae**
	A04.3.02.003	Aponeurosis m. erectoris spinae	Erector spinae aponeurosis
	A04.3.02.004	Septum intermusculare	Intermuscular septum
	A04.3.02.005	M. iliocostalis	Iliocostalis
	A04.3.02.006	M. iliocostalis lumborum	Iliocostalis lumborum
	A04.3.02.007	Pars lumbalis; Divisio lateralis m. erectoris spinae lumborum	Lumbar part; Lateral division of lumbar erector spinae
	A04.3.02.008	Pars thoracica	Thoracic part
	A04.3.02.009	M. iliocostalis cervicis; M. iliocostalis colli	Iliocostalis cervicis
	A04.3.02.010	M. longissimus	Longissimus
	A04.3.02.011	M. longissimus thoracis	Longissimus thoracis
	A04.3.02.012	Pars lumbalis; Divisio medialis m. erectoris spinae lumborum	Lumbar part; Medial division of lumbar erector spinae
	A04.3.02.013	M. longissimus cervicis; M. longissimus colli	Longissimus cervicis
	A04.3.02.014	M. longissimus capitis	Longissimus capitis
	A04.3.02.015	M. spinalis	Spinalis
	A04.3.02.016	M. spinalis thoracis	Spinalis thoracis
	A04.3.02.017	M. spinalis cervicis; M. spinalis colli	Spinalis cervicis
*	A04.3.02.018	M. spinalis capitis	Spinalis capitis
	A04.3.02.101	**Musculi spinotransversales**	**Spinotransversales**
	A04.3.02.102	M. splenius	Splenius

* **A04.2.05.005** *Lig. suspensorium glandulae thyroideae* The thyroid gland is suspended from the thyroid and cricoid cartilages and from the trachea by thickenings of the pretracheal fascia. Loré J. M. Jr 1983. "Practical Anatomical Considerations in Thyroid Surgery." *Arch J Otolaryngol* 109: 568–574. The name *lig. supensorium glandulae thyroideae* was formerly limited to the thickenings attaching the lobes of the thyroid gland to the sides of the cricoid cartilage.

* **A04.3.02.001** *Musculi dorsi proprii* The muscles under this heading, being epaxial muscles, are supplied by *rami posteriores* and may be regarded as the only true back muscles. In this sense the *mm. intertransversarii anteriores, mm. posteriores laterales cervicis*, and *mm. intertransversarii laterales lumborum*, being hypaxial muscles and homologues of *mm. levatores costarum* and being supplied by *rami anteriores* are not true back muscles.

* **A04.3.02.018** *M. spinalis capitis* Generally considered to be the most medial part of *m. semispinalis capitis*, this muscle may be a separate entity. Martin A. 1994. "Spinalis Capitis, or an Accessory Paraspinous Muscle." *J Anat* 185: 195–198.

A04.3.02.103	M. splenius capitis	Splenius capitis
A04.3.02.104	M. splenius cervicis; M. splenius colli	Splenius cervicis
A04.3.02.201	**Musculi transversospinales**	**Transversospinales**
* A04.3.02.202	Mm. multifidi	Multifidus
A04.3.02.203	M. multifidus lumborum	Multifidus lumborum
A04.3.02.204	M. multifidus thoracis	Multifidus thoracis
A04.3.02.205	M. multifidus cervicis; M. multifidus colli	Multifidus cervicis
A04.3.02.206	M. semispinalis	Semispinalis
A04.3.02.207	M. semispinalis thoracis	Semispinalis thoracis
A04.3.02.208	M. semispinalis cervicis; M. semispinalis colli	Semispinalis cervicis
A04.3.02.209	M. semispinalis capitis	Semispinalis capitis
A04.3.02.210	Mm. rotatores	Rotatores
A04.3.02.211	(Mm. rotatores lumborum)	(Rotatores lumborum)
A04.3.02.212	Mm. rotatores thoracis	Rotatores thoracis
A04.3.02.213	Mm. rotatores cervicis; Mm. rotatores colli	Rotatores cervicis
A04.3.02.301	**Musculi interspinales**	**Interspinales**
A04.3.02.302	Mm. interspinales lumborum	Interspinales lumborum
A04.3.02.303	Mm. interspinales thoracis	Interspinales thoracis
A04.3.02.304	Mm. interspinales cervicis; Mm. interspinales colli	Interspinales cervicis
A04.3.02.401	**Musculi intertransversarii**	**Intertransversarii**
A04.3.02.402	Mm. intertransversarii mediales lumborum	Medial lumbar intertransversarii
A04.3.02.403	Mm. intertransversarii thoracis	Thoracic intertransversarii
A04.3.02.404	Mm. intertransversarii posteriores mediales cervicis; Mm. intertransversarii posteriores mediales colli	Medial posterior cervical intertransversarii
A04.3.02.501	**Fascia thoracolumbalis**	**Thoracolumbar fascia**
A04.3.02.502	Lamina posterior; Lamina superficialis	Posterior layer
A04.3.02.503	Lamina media	Middle layer
A04.3.02.504	Lamina anterior; Lamina profunda; Fascia musculi quadrati lumborum	Anterior layer; Quadratus lumborum fascia

A04.4.00.001	Musculi thoracis	Muscles of thorax
A04.4.01.001	(M. sternalis)	(Sternalis)
A04.4.01.002	M. pectoralis major	Pectoralis major
A04.4.01.003	Pars clavicularis	Clavicular head
A04.4.01.004	Pars sternocostalis	Sternocostal head
A04.4.01.005	Pars abdominalis	Abdominal part
A04.4.01.006	M. pectoralis minor	Pectoralis minor
A04.4.01.007	M. subclavius	Subclavius
A04.4.01.008	M. serratus anterior	Serratus anterior
A04.4.01.009	Mm. levatores costarum	Levatores costarum
A04.4.01.010	Mm. levatores costarum longi	Levatores costarum longi
A04.4.01.011	Mm. levatores costarum breves	Levatores costarum breves
A04.4.01.012	Mm. intercostales externi	External intercostal muscle
A03.3.01.002	Membrana intercostalis externa	External intercostal membrane
A04.4.01.013	Mm. intercostales interni	Internal intercostal muscle
A03.3.01.003	Membrana intercostalis interna	Internal intercostal membrane
A04.4.01.014	Mm. intercostales intimi	Innermost intercostal muscle
A04.4.01.015	Mm. subcostales	Subcostales
A04.4.01.016	M. transversus thoracis	Transversus thoracis
A04.4.01.017	Fascia pectoralis	Pectoral fascia
A04.4.01.018	Fascia clavipectoralis	Clavipectoral fascia
A04.4.01.019	Fascia thoracica	Thoracic fascia
A04.4.01.020	Fascia endothoracica; Fascia parietalis thoracis	Endothoracic fascia; Parietal fascia of thorax

* **A04.3.02.202** *Mm. multifidi* Although listed under *musculi transversospinales* for conventional reasons, *m. multifidus* consists of a series of overlapping unisegmentally innervated spinotransverse muscles. Macintosh J. E. et al. 1986. "The Morphology of the Human Lumbar Multifidus." *Clin Biochem* 1: 196–204.

A04.4.02.001	**Diaphragma**	**Diaphragm**
A04.4.02.002	Pars lumbalis diaphragmatis	Lumbar part
A04.4.02.003	Crus dextrum	Right crus
A04.4.02.004	Crus sinistrum	Left crus
A04.4.02.005	Lig. arcuatum medianum	Median arcuate ligament
A04.4.02.006	Lig. arcuatum mediale	Medial arcuate ligament
A04.4.02.007	Lig. arcuatum laterale	Lateral arcuate ligament
A04.4.02.008	Pars costalis diaphragmatis	Costal part
A04.4.02.009	Pars sternalis diaphragmatis	Sternal part
A04.4.02.010	Hiatus aorticus	Aortic hiatus
A04.4.02.011	Hiatus oesophageus	Oesophageal hiatus▲
A04.4.02.012	Lig. phrenicooesophagealis	Phrenico-oesophageal ligament▲
A04.4.02.013	Centrum tendineum	Central tendon
A04.4.02.014	Foramen venae cavae	Caval opening
A04.4.02.015	Trigonum sternocostale	Sternocostal triangle
A04.4.02.016	Trigonum lumbocostale	Lumbocostal triangle
A04.4.02.017	Fascia diaphragmatica	Diaphragmatic fascia

A04.5.00.001	**Musculi abdominis**	**Muscles of abdomen**
A04.5.01.001	M. rectus abdominis	Rectus abdominis
A04.5.01.002	Intersectiones tendineae	Tendinous intersections
A04.5.01.003	Vagina musculi recti abdominis	Rectus sheath
A04.5.01.004	Lamina anterior	Anterior layer
A04.5.01.005	Lamina posterior	Posterior layer
A04.5.01.006	Linea arcuata	Arcuate line
A04.5.01.007	M. pyramidalis	Pyramidalis
A04.5.01.008	M. obliquus externus abdominis	External oblique
A04.5.01.009	Lig. inguinale; Arcus inguinalis	Inguinal ligament
A04.5.01.010	Lig. lacunare	Lacunar ligament
A04.5.01.011	Lig. pectineum	Pectineal ligament
A04.5.01.012	Lig. reflexum	Reflected ligament
A04.5.01.013	Anulus inguinalis superficialis	Superficial inguinal ring
A04.5.01.014	Crus mediale	Medial crus
A04.5.01.015	Crus laterale	Lateral crus
A04.5.01.016	Fibrae intercrurales	Intercrural fibres▲
A04.5.01.017	M. obliquus internus abdominis	Internal oblique
A04.5.01.018	M. cremaster ♂	Cremaster ♂
A04.5.01.019	M. transversus abdominis	Transversus abdominis; Transverse abdominal
A04.5.01.020	Falx inguinalis; Tendo conjunctivus	Inguinal falx; Conjoint tendon
A04.5.01.021	Anulus inguinalis profundus	Deep inguinal ring
A04.5.01.022	Linea alba	Linea alba
A04.5.01.023	Anulus umbilicalis	Umbilical ring
A04.5.01.024	Adminiculum lineae albae	Posterior attachment of linea alba
A04.5.01.025	Linea semilunaris	Linea semilunaris
A04.5.01.026	Canalis inguinalis	Inguinal canal
A04.5.01.027	M. quadratus lumborum	Quadratus lumborum
* A04.5.02.001	**Fascia abdominis**	**Abdominal fascia**
A04.5.02.002	Fascia abdominis visceralis	Visceral abdominal fascia
A04.5.02.003	Fascia propria organi	Fascia of individual organ
A04.5.02.004	Fascia extraperitonealis	Extraperitoneal fascia
A04.5.02.005	Lig. extraperitoneale	Extraperitoneal ligament
* A04.5.02.006	Fascia abdominis parietalis; Fascia endoabdominalis	Parietal abdominal fascia; Endo-abdominal fascia

* **A04.5.02.001** *Fascia abdominis* The list is from within outwards and for completeness and reference includes terms for all items which have previously been regarded as part of *fascia abdominis*. It thus includes a number for which the term *fascia* is no longer recommended (see footnote to A04.0.00.031 and also to A04.0.00.034/5/6).

* **A04.5.02.006** *Fascia endoabdominalis* These terms are sometimes used generically to include not only parietal fascia but also extraperitoneal fascia and visceral fascia in the abdomen and pelvis.

A04.5.02.003	Fascia propria organi	Fascia of individual organ
A04.5.02.007	Fascia iliopsoas; Fascia iliaca	Iliopsoas fascia; Fascia iliaca
A04.5.02.008	Pars psoatica	Psoas fascia
A04.5.02.009	Pars iliaca	Iliac fascia
A04.5.02.010	Arcus iliopectineus	Iliopectineal arch
A04.5.02.011	Fascia transversalis	Transversalis fascia
A04.5.02.012	Lig. interfoveolare	Interfoveolar ligament
A04.5.02.013	Tractus iliopubicus	Iliopubic tract
* A04.5.02.014	Fascia umbilicalis	Umbilical fascia
A04.5.02.015	Fascia investiens abdominis	Investing abdominal fascia
A04.5.02.016	Fascia investiens profunda	Deep investing fascia
A04.5.02.017	Fasciae investientes intermediae	Intermediate investing fascia
A04.5.02.018	Fascia investiens superficialis	Superficial investing fascia
A04.5.02.019	Lig. suspensorium clitoridis ♀	Suspensory ligament of clitoris ♀
A04.5.02.019	Lig. suspensorium penis ♂	Suspensory ligament of penis ♂
A04.5.02.020	Textus connectivus laxus	Loose connective tissue
A04.5.02.021	Tela subcutanea abdominis	Subcutaneous tissue of abdomen
A04.5.02.022	Stratum membranosum	Membranous layer
A04.5.02.023	Lig. fundiforme clitoridis ♀	Fundiform ligament of clitoris ♀
A04.5.02.023	Lig. fundiforme penis ♂	Fundiform ligament of penis ♂
A04.5.02.024	Panniculus adiposus	Fatty layer
A04.5.03.001	**Fascia pelvis; Fascia pelvica**	**Pelvic fascia**
A04.5.03.002	Fascia pelvis visceralis	Visceral pelvic fascia
A04.5.03.003	Fascia propria organi	Fascia of individual organ
A04.5.03.004	Fascia rectoprostatica; Septum rectovesicale ♂	Rectoprostatic fascia; Rectovesical septum ♂
A04.5.03.004	Fascia rectovaginalis; Septum rectovaginale ♀	Rectovaginal fascia; Rectovaginal septum ♀
A04.5.03.005	Fascia extraperitonealis	Extraperitoneal fascia
A04.5.03.006	Lig. extraperitoneale	Extraperitoneal ligament
* A04.5.03.007	Fascia pelvis parietalis; Fascia endopelvina	Parietal pelvic fascia; Endopelvic fascia
A04.5.03.008	Fascia propria organi	Fascia of individual organ
A04.5.03.009	Fascia obturatoria	Obturator fascia
A04.5.03.010	Arcus tendineus fasciae pelvis	Tendinous arch of pelvic fascia
A04.5.03.011	Fascia musculi piriformis	Piriformis fascia
A04.5.03.012	Fascia superior diaphragmatis pelvis	Superior fascia of pelvic diaphragm
A04.5.03.013	Lig. pubovesicale; Lig. mediale puboprostaticum ♂	Pubovesical ligament; Medial puboprostatic ligament ♂
A04.5.03.013	Lig. mediale pubovesicale ♀	Medial pubovesical ligament ♀
A04.5.03.014	M. pubovesicalis	Pubovesicalis
A04.5.03.015	Lig. puboprostaticum; Lig. laterale puboprostaticum ♂	Puboprostatic ligament; Lateral puboprostatic ligament ♂
A04.5.03.015	Lig. laterale pubovesicale ♀	Lateral pubovesical ligament ♀
A04.5.03.016	Lig. laterale vesicae	Lateral ligament of bladder
A04.5.03.017	M. rectovesicalis	Rectovesicalis
A04.5.03.018	Fascia presacralis	Presacral fascia
A04.5.03.019	Fascia rectosacralis	Rectosacral fascia
A04.5.03.020	Fascia inferior diaphragmatis pelvis	Inferior fascia of pelvic diaphragm
A04.5.04.001	**Diaphragma pelvis**	**Pelvic diaphragm; Pelvic floor**
A04.5.03.012	Fascia superior diaphragmatis pelvis	Superior fascia of pelvic diaphragm
A04.5.03.020	Fascia inferior diaphragmatis pelvis	Inferior fascia of pelvic diaphragm
A04.5.04.002	M. levator ani	Levator ani
A04.5.04.003	M. pubococcygeus	Pubococcygeus
A04.5.04.004	M. puboperinealis	Puboperinealis
A04.5.04.005	M. puboprostaticus; M. levator prostatae ♂	Puboprostaticus; Levator prostatae ♂
A04.5.04.005	M. pubovaginalis ♀	Pubovaginalis ♀
A04.5.04.006	M. puboanalis	Pubo-analis

* **A04.5.02.014** *Fascia umbilicalis* A thickening in *fascia transversalis* behind the umbilicus. Orda R., Nathan H. 1973. "Surgical Anatomy of the Umbilical Structures." *Int Surg* 58: 458–464.
* **A04.5.03.007** *Fascia endopelvina* These terms are sometimes used generically to include not only parietal fascia but also extraperitoneal fascia and visceral fascia in the abdomen and pelvis.

A04.5.04.007	M. puborectalis	Puborectalis
A04.5.04.008	M. iliococcygeus	Iliococcygeus
A04.5.04.009	(Arcus tendineus musculi levatoris ani)	(Tendinous arch of levator ani)
A04.5.04.010	Hiatus urogenitalis	Urogenital hiatus
A04.5.04.011	M. ischiococcygeus; M. coccygeus	Ischiococcygeus; Coccygeus
A04.5.04.012	M. sphincter ani externus	External anal sphincter
A04.5.04.013	Pars subcutanea	Subcutaneous part
A04.5.04.014	Pars superficialis	Superficial part
A04.5.04.015	Pars profunda	Deep part
* A04.5.04.016	Corpus anococcygeum; Lig. anococcygeum	Anococcygeal body; Anococcygeal ligament
A04.5.04.017	Tendo musculi pubococcygei	Pubococcygeal tendon
A04.5.04.018	Raphe musculi iliococcygei	Iliococcygeal raphe
A04.5.04.019	Insertio partis superficialis musculi sphincteris ani externi	Attachment of superficial external anal sphincter
A04.5.05.001	**Mm. perinei** {vide paginam 71}	**Perineal muscles** {see page 71}

A04.6.00.001	Musculi membri superioris	Muscles of upper limb
A04.6.01.001	**Compartimenta**	**Compartments**
A04.6.01.002	Compartimentum brachii anterius; Compartimentum brachii flexorum	Anterior compartment of arm; Flexor compartment of arm
A04.6.01.003	Compartimentum brachii posterius; Compartimentum brachii extensorum	Posterior compartment of arm; Extensor compartment of arm
A04.6.01.004	Compartimentum antebrachii anterius; Compartimentum antebrachii flexorum	Anterior compartment of forearm; Flexor compartment of forearm
A04.6.01.005	Pars superficialis	Superficial part
A04.6.01.006	Pars profunda	Deep part
A04.6.01.007	Compartimentum antebrachii posterius; Compartimentum antebrachii extensorum	Posterior compartment of forearm; Extensor compartment of forearm
A04.6.01.008	Pars lateralis; Pars radialis	Lateral part; Radial part
A04.6.02.001	**Musculi**	**Muscles**
A04.6.02.002	M. deltoideus	Deltoid
A04.6.02.003	Pars clavicularis	Clavicular part
A04.6.02.004	Pars acromialis	Acromial part
A04.6.02.005	Pars spinalis	Spinal part
A04.6.02.006	M. supraspinatus	Supraspinatus
A04.6.02.007	Fascia supraspinata	Supraspinous fascia
A04.6.02.008	M. infraspinatus	Infraspinatus
A04.6.02.009	Fascia infraspinata	Infraspinous fascia
A04.6.02.010	M. teres minor	Teres minor
A04.6.02.011	M. teres major	Teres major
A04.6.02.012	M. subscapularis	Subscapularis
A04.6.02.013	M. biceps brachii	Biceps brachii
A04.6.02.014	Caput longum	Long head
A04.6.02.015	Caput breve	Short head
A04.6.02.016	Aponeurosis musculi bicipitis brachii; Aponeurosis bicipitalis; Lacertus fibrosus	Bicipital aponeurosis
A04.6.02.017	M. coracobrachialis	Coracobrachialis
A04.6.02.018	M. brachialis	Brachialis
A04.6.02.019	M. triceps brachii	Triceps brachii
A04.6.02.020	Caput longum	Long head
A04.6.02.021	Caput laterale	Lateral head
A04.6.02.022	Caput mediale; Caput profundum	Medial head; Deep head
A04.6.02.023	M. anconeus	Anconeus
A04.6.02.024	M. articularis cubiti	Articularis cubiti
A04.6.02.025	M. pronator teres	Pronator teres
A04.6.02.026	Caput humerale	Humeral head

* **A04.5.04.016** *Corpus anococcygeum* The term *corpus*, rather than *ligamentum*, has been used here because it is a stratified nonligamentous structure in which fleshy muscle attachments underlie a tendon.

A04.6.02.027	Caput ulnare	Ulnar head
A04.6.02.028	M. flexor carpi radialis	Flexor carpi radialis
A04.6.02.029	M. palmaris longus	Palmaris longus
A04.6.02.030	M. flexor carpi ulnaris	Flexor carpi ulnaris
A04.6.02.031	Caput humerale	Humeral head
A04.6.02.032	Caput ulnare	Ulnar head
A04.6.02.033	M. flexor digitorum superficialis	Flexor digitorum superficialis
A04.6.02.034	Caput humeroulnare	Humero-ulnar head
A04.6.02.035	Caput radiale	Radial head
A04.6.02.036	M. flexor digitorum profundus	Flexor digitorum profundus
A04.6.02.037	M. flexor pollicis longus	Flexor pollicis longus
A04.6.02.038	M. pronator quadratus	Pronator quadratus
A04.6.02.039	M. brachioradialis	Brachioradialis
A04.6.02.040	M. extensor carpi radialis longus	Extensor carpi radialis longus
A04.6.02.041	M. extensor carpi radialis brevis	Extensor carpi radialis brevis
A04.6.02.042	M. extensor digitorum	Extensor digitorum
A04.6.02.043	Connexus intertendinei	Intertendinous connections
A04.6.02.044	M. extensor digiti minimi	Extensor digiti minimi
A04.6.02.045	M. extensor carpi ulnaris	Extensor carpi ulnaris
A04.6.02.046	Caput humerale	Humeral head
A04.6.02.047	Caput ulnare	Ulnar head
A04.6.02.048	M. supinator	Supinator
A04.6.02.049	M. abductor pollicis longus	Abductor pollicis longus
A04.6.02.050	M. extensor pollicis brevis	Extensor pollicis brevis
A04.6.02.051	M. extensor pollicis longus	Extensor pollicis longus
A04.6.02.052	M. extensor indicis	Extensor indicis
A04.6.02.053	M. palmaris brevis	Palmaris brevis
A04.6.02.054	M. abductor pollicis brevis	Abductor pollicis brevis
A04.6.02.055	M. flexor pollicis brevis	Flexor pollicis brevis
A04.6.02.056	Caput superficiale	Superficial head
A04.6.02.057	Caput profundum	Deep head
A04.6.02.058	M. opponens pollicis	Opponens pollicis
A04.6.02.059	M. adductor pollicis	Adductor pollicis
A04.6.02.060	Caput obliquum	Oblique head
A04.6.02.061	Caput transversum	Transverse head
A04.6.02.062	M. abductor digiti minimi	Abductor digiti minimi
A04.6.02.063	M. flexor digiti minimi brevis	Flexor digiti minimi brevis
A04.6.02.064	M. opponens digiti minimi	Opponens digiti minimi
A04.6.02.065	Mm. lumbricales	Lumbricals
A04.6.02.066	Mm. interossei dorsales	Dorsal interossei
A04.6.02.067	Mm. interossei palmares	Palmar interossei
A04.6.03.001	**Fasciae**	**Fascia**
A04.6.03.002	Fascia axillaris	Axillary fascia
A04.6.03.003	Lig. suspensorium axillae	Suspensory ligament of axilla
A04.6.03.004	Fascia deltoidea	Deltoid fascia
A04.6.03.005	Fascia brachii	Brachial fascia
A04.6.03.006	Septum intermusculare brachii mediale	Medial intermuscular septum of arm
A04.6.03.007	Septum intermusculare brachii laterale	Lateral intermuscular septum of arm
A04.6.03.008	Fascia antebrachii	Antebrachial fascia
A04.6.03.009	Fascia dorsalis manus	Dorsal fascia of hand
A04.6.03.010	Retinaculum musculorum extensorum	Extensor retinaculum
A04.6.03.011	Lig. metacarpale transversum superficiale	Superficial transverse metacarpal ligament
A04.6.03.012	Aponeurosis palmaris	Palmar aponeurosis
A04.6.03.013	Retinaculum musculorum flexorum	Flexor retinaculum
A04.6.03.014	Chiasma tendinum	Tendinous chiasm

A04.7.00.001	Musculi membri inferioris	Muscles of lower limb
A04.7.01.001	**Compartimenta**	**Compartments**
A04.7.01.002	Compartimentum femoris anterius; Compartimentum femoris extensorum	Anterior compartment of thigh; Extensor compartment of thigh
A04.7.01.003	Compartimentum femoris posterius; Compartimentum femoris flexorum	Posterior compartment of thigh; Flexor compartment of thigh
A04.7.01.004	Compartimentum femoris mediale; Compartimentum femoris adductorum	Medial compartment of thigh; Adductor compartment of thigh
A04.7.01.005	Compartimentum cruris anterius; Compartimentum cruris extensorum	Anterior compartment of leg; Extensor compartment of leg
A04.7.01.006	Compartimentum cruris posterius; Compartimentum cruris flexorum	Posterior compartment of leg; Flexor compartment of leg
A04.7.01.007	Pars superficialis; Pars gastrocnemialis; Pars tricipitalis	Superficial part
A04.7.01.008	Pars profunda; Pars solealis	Deep part
A04.7.01.009	Compartimentum cruris laterale; Compartimentum cruris fibularium; Compartimentum cruris peroneorum	Lateral compartment of leg; Fibular compartment of leg; Peroneal compartment of leg
A04.7.02.001	**Musculi**	**Muscles**
A04.7.02.002	M. iliopsoas	Iliopsoas
A04.7.02.003	M. iliacus	Iliacus
A04.7.02.004	M. psoas major	Psoas major
A04.7.02.005	(M. psoas minor)	(Psoas minor)
A04.7.02.006	M. gluteus maximus	Gluteus maximus
A04.7.02.007	M. gluteus medius	Gluteus medius
A04.7.02.008	M. gluteus minimus	Gluteus minimus
A04.7.02.009	Aponeurosis glutea	Gluteal aponeurosis
A04.7.02.010	M. tensor fasciae latae	Tensor fasciae latae; Tensor of fascia lata
A04.7.02.011	M. piriformis	Piriformis
A04.7.02.012	M. obturatorius internus	Obturator internus
A04.7.02.013	M. gemellus superior	Gemellus superior; Superior gemellus
A04.7.02.014	M. gemellus inferior	Gemellus inferior; Inferior gemellus
A04.7.02.015	M. quadratus femoris	Quadratus femoris
A04.7.02.016	M. sartorius	Sartorius
A04.7.02.017	M. quadriceps femoris	Quadriceps femoris
A04.7.02.018	M. rectus femoris	Rectus femoris
A04.7.02.019	Caput rectum	Straight head
A04.7.02.020	Caput reflexum	Reflected head
A04.7.02.021	M. vastus lateralis	Vastus lateralis
A04.7.02.022	M. vastus intermedius	Vastus intermedius
A04.7.02.023	M. vastus medialis	Vastus medialis
A04.7.02.024	M. articularis genus	Articularis genus; Articular muscle of knee
A04.7.02.025	M. pectineus	Pectineus
A04.7.02.026	M. adductor longus	Adductor longus
A04.7.02.027	M. adductor brevis	Adductor brevis
A04.7.02.028	M. adductor magnus	Adductor magnus
A04.7.02.029	M. adductor minimus	Adductor minimus
A04.7.02.030	M. gracilis	Gracilis
A04.7.02.031	M. obturatorius externus	Obturator externus
A04.7.02.032	M. biceps femoris	Biceps femoris
A04.7.02.033	Caput longum	Long head
A04.7.02.034	Caput breve	Short head
A04.7.02.035	M. semitendinosus	Semitendinosus
A04.7.02.036	M. semimembranosus	Semimembranosus
A04.7.02.037	M. tibialis anterior	Tibialis anterior
A04.7.02.038	M. extensor digitorum longus	Extensor digitorum longus
A04.7.02.039	M. fibularis tertius; M. peroneus tertius	Fibularis tertius; Peroneus tertius
A04.7.02.040	M. extensor hallucis longus	Extensor hallucis longus
A04.7.02.041	M. fibularis longus; M. peroneus longus	Fibularis longus; Peroneus longus
A04.7.02.042	M. fibularis brevis; M. peroneus brevis	Fibularis brevis; Peroneus brevis

A04.7.02.043	M. triceps surae	Triceps surae
A04.7.02.044	M. gastrocnemius	Gastrocnemius
A04.7.02.045	Caput laterale	Lateral head
A04.7.02.046	Caput mediale	Medial head
A04.7.02.047	M. soleus	Soleus
A04.7.02.048	Tendo calcaneus	Calcaneal tendon
A04.7.02.049	M. plantaris	Plantaris
A04.7.02.050	M. popliteus	Popliteus
A04.7.02.051	M. tibialis posterior	Tibialis posterior
A04.7.02.052	M. flexor digitorum longus	Flexor digitorum longus
A04.7.02.053	M. flexor hallucis longus	Flexor hallucis longus
A04.7.02.054	M. extensor hallucis brevis	Extensor hallucis brevis
A04.7.02.055	M. extensor digitorum brevis	Extensor digitorum brevis
A04.7.02.056	M. abductor hallucis	Abductor hallucis
A04.7.02.057	M. flexor hallucis brevis	Flexor hallucis brevis
A04.7.02.058	Caput mediale	Medial head
A04.7.02.059	Caput laterale	Lateral head
A04.7.02.060	M. adductor hallucis	Adductor hallucis
A04.7.02.061	Caput obliquum	Oblique head
A04.7.02.062	Caput transversum	Transverse head
A04.7.02.063	M. abductor digiti minimi	Abductor digiti minimi
A04.7.02.064	(M. abductor metatarsi quinti)	(Abductor of fifth metatarsal)
A04.7.02.065	(M. opponens digiti minimi)	(Opponens digiti minimi)
A04.7.02.066	M. flexor digiti minimi brevis	Flexor digiti minimi brevis
A04.7.02.067	M. flexor digitorum brevis	Flexor digitorum brevis
A04.7.02.068	M. quadratus plantae; M. flexor accessorius	Quadratus plantae; Flexor accessorius
A04.7.02.069	Mm. lumbricales	Lumbricals
A04.7.02.070	Mm. interossei dorsales	Dorsal interossei
A04.7.02.071	Mm. interossei plantares	Plantar interossei
A04.7.03.001	**Fasciae**	**Fascia**
A04.7.03.002	Fascia lata	Fascia lata
A04.7.03.003	Tractus iliotibialis	Iliotibial tract
A04.7.03.004	Septum intermusculare femoris laterale	Lateral femoral intermuscular septum
A04.7.03.005	Septum intermusculare femoris mediale	Medial femoral intermuscular septum
A04.7.03.006	Canalis adductorius	Adductor canal
A04.7.03.007	Septum intermusculare vastoadductorium	Anteromedial intermuscular septum; Subsartorial fascia
A04.7.03.008	Hiatus adductorius	Adductor hiatus
A04.7.03.009	Fascia iliaca	Iliac fascia
A04.7.03.010	Lacuna musculorum	Muscular space
A04.5.02.010	Arcus iliopectineus	Iliopectineal arch
A04.7.03.011	Lacuna vasorum	Vascular space
A04.7.03.012	Canalis femoralis	Femoral canal
A04.7.03.013	Trigonum femorale	Femoral triangle
A04.7.03.014	Anulus femoralis	Femoral ring
A04.7.03.015	Septum femorale	Femoral septum
A04.7.03.016	Hiatus saphenus	Saphenous opening
A04.7.03.017	Margo falciformis; Margo arcuatus	Falciform margin
A04.7.03.018	Cornu superius; Crus superius	Superior horn
A04.7.03.019	Cornu inferius; Crus inferius	Inferior horn
A04.7.03.020	Fascia cribrosa	Cribriform fascia
A04.7.03.021	Fascia cruris	Deep fascia of leg
A04.7.03.022	Septum intermusculare cruris anterius	Anterior intermuscular septum of leg
A04.7.03.023	Septum intermusculare cruris posterius	Posterior intermuscular septum of leg
A04.7.03.024	Arcus tendineus musculi solei	Tendinous arch of soleus
A04.7.03.025	Retinaculum musculorum extensorum superius	Superior extensor retinaculum
A04.7.03.026	Retinaculum musculorum flexorum	Flexor retinaculum
A04.7.03.027	Retinaculum musculorum extensorum inferius	Inferior extensor retinaculum

A04.7.03.028	Retinaculum musculorum fibularium superius; Retinaculum musculorum peroneorum superius	Superior fibular retinaculum; Superior peroneal retinaculum
A04.7.03.029	Retinaculum musculorum fibularium inferius; Retinaculum musculorum peroneorum inferius	Inferior fibular retinaculum; Inferior peroneal retinaculum
A04.7.03.030	Fascia dorsalis pedis	Dorsal fascia of foot
A04.7.03.031	Aponeurosis plantaris	Plantar aponeurosis
A04.7.03.032	Fasciculi transversi	Transverse fascicles
A04.7.03.033	Lig. metatarsale transversum superficiale	Superficial transverse metatarsal ligament

A04.8.00.001	Vaginae tendinum et bursae	Tendon sheaths and bursae
	Nomina generalia	*General terms*
A04.8.01.001	Bursa subcutanea	Subcutaneous bursa
A04.8.01.002	Bursa submuscularis	Submuscular bursa
A04.8.01.003	Bursa subfascialis	Subfascial bursa
A04.8.01.004	Bursa subtendinea	Subtendinous bursa
A04.8.01.005	Vagina tendinis	Tendon sheath
A04.8.01.006	Stratum fibrosum; Vagina fibrosa	Fibrous sheath
A04.8.01.007	Stratum synoviale;vagina synovialis	Synovial sheath
A04.8.01.008	Mesotendineum	Mesotendon
A04.8.02.001	**Bursae colli**	**Bursae of neck**
A04.8.02.002	Bursa musculi tensoris veli palatini	Bursa of tensor veli palatini
A04.8.02.003	Bursa subcutanea prominentiae laryngeae	Subcutaneous bursa of laryngeal prominence
A04.8.02.004	Bursa infrahyoidea	Infrahyoid bursa
A04.8.02.005	Bursa retrohyoidea	Retrohyoid bursa
A04.8.03.001	**Bursae membri superioris**	**Bursae of upper limb**
A04.8.03.002	Bursa subtendinea musculi trapezii	Subtendinous bursa of trapezius
A04.8.03.003	(Bursa subcutanea acromialis)	(Subcutaneous acromial bursa)
A04.8.03.004	Bursa subacromialis	Subacromial bursa
A04.8.03.005	Bursa subdeltoidea	Subdeltoid bursa
A04.8.03.006	(Bursa musculi coracobrachialis)	(Coracobrachial bursa)
A04.8.03.007	Bursa subtendinea musculi infraspinati	Subtendinous bursa of infraspinatus
A04.8.03.008	Bursa subtendinea musculi subscapularis	Subtendinous bursa of subscapularis
A04.8.03.009	Bursa subtendinea musculi teretis majoris	Subtendinous bursa of teres major
A04.8.03.010	Bursa subtendinea musculi latissimi dorsi	Subtendinous bursa of latissimus dorsi
A04.8.03.011	Bursa subcutanea olecrani	Subcutaneous olecranon bursa
A04.8.03.012	(Bursa intratendinea olecrani)	(Intratendinous olecranon bursa)
A04.8.03.013	Bursa subtendinea musculi tricipitis brachii	Subtendinous bursa of triceps brachii
A04.8.03.014	Bursa bicipitoradialis	Bicipitoradial bursa
A04.8.03.015	(Bursa cubitalis interossea)	(Interosseous cubital bursa)
A04.8.04.001	**Vaginae tendinum membri superioris**	**Tendinous sheaths of upper limb**
A04.8.04.002	Vagina tendinis intertubercularis	Intertubercular tendon sheath
A04.8.04.003	Vaginae tendinum carpales	Carpal tendinous sheaths
A04.8.04.004	Vaginae tendinum carpales palmares	Palmar carpal tendinous sheaths
A04.8.04.005	Vagina tendinis musculi flexoris pollicis longi	Tendinous sheath of flexor pollicis longus
A04.8.04.006	Vagina tendinis musculi flexoris carpi radialis	Tendinous sheath of flexor carpi radialis
A04.8.04.007	Vagina communis tendinum musculorum flexorum	Common flexor sheath
A04.8.04.008	Vaginae tendinum carpales dorsales	Dorsal carpal tendinous sheaths
A04.8.04.009	Vagina tendinum musculorum abductoris longi et extensoris pollicis brevis	Tendinous sheath of abductor longus and extensor pollicis brevis
A04.8.04.010	Vagina tendinum musculorum extensorum carpi radialium	Tendinous sheath of extensores carpi radiales
A04.8.04.011	Vagina tendinis musculi extensoris pollicis longi	Tendinous sheath of extensor pollicis longus
A04.8.04.012	Vagina tendinum musculorum extensoris digitorum et extensoris indicis	Tendinous sheath of extensor digitorum and extensor indicis

A04.8.04.013	Vagina tendinis musculi extensoris digiti minimi brevis	Tendinous sheath of extensor digiti minimi brevis
A04.8.04.014	Vagina tendinis musculi extensoris carpi ulnaris	Tendinous sheath of extensor carpi ulnaris
A04.8.04.015	Vaginae fibrosae digitorum manus	Fibrous sheaths of digits of hand
A04.8.04.016	Pars anularis vaginae fibrosae	Anular part of fibrous sheath
A04.8.04.017	Pars cruciformis vaginae fibrosae	Cruciform part of fibrous sheath
A04.8.04.018	Vaginae synoviales digitorum manus	Synovial sheaths of digits of hand
A04.8.04.019	Vincula tendinum	Vincula tendinum
A04.8.04.020	Vinculum longum	Vinculum longum
A04.8.04.021	Vinculum breve	Vinculum breve
A04.8.05.001	**Bursae membri inferioris**	**Bursae of lower limb**
A04.8.05.002	Bursa subcutanea trochanterica	Subcutaneous trochanteric bursa
A04.8.05.003	Bursa trochanterica musculi glutei maximi	Trochanteric bursa of gluteus maximus
A04.8.05.004	Bursae trochantericae musculi glutei medii	Trochanteric bursae of gluteus medius
A04.8.05.005	Bursa trochanterica musculi glutei minimi	Trochanteric bursa of gluteus minimus
A04.8.05.006	Bursa musculi piriformis	Bursa of piriformis
A04.8.05.007	Bursa ischiadica musculi obturatorii interni	Sciatic bursa of obturator internus
A04.8.05.008	Bursa subtendinea musculi obturatorii interni	Subtendinous bursa of obturator internus
A04.8.05.009	Bursae intermusculares musculorum gluteorum	Intermuscular gluteal bursae
A04.8.05.010	Bursa ischiadica musculi glutei maximi	Sciatic bursa of gluteus maximus
A04.8.05.011	(Bursa iliopectinea)	(Iliopectineal bursa)
A04.8.05.012	Bursa subtendinea iliaca	Subtendinous bursa of iliacus
A04.8.05.013	Bursa musculi bicipitis femoris superior	Superior bursa of biceps femoris
A04.8.05.014	Bursa subcutanea prepatellaris	Subcutaneous prepatellar bursa
A04.8.05.015	(Bursa subfascialis prepatellaris)	(Subfascial prepatellar bursa)
A04.8.05.016	(Bursa subtendinea prepatellaris)	(Subtendinous prepatellar bursa)
A04.8.05.017	Bursa suprapatellaris	Suprapatellar bursa
A04.8.05.018	Bursa subcutanea infrapatellaris	Subcutaneous infrapatellar bursa
A04.8.05.019	Bursa infrapatellaris profunda	Deep infrapatellar bursa
A04.8.05.020	Bursa subcutanea tuberositatis tibiae	Subcutaneous bursa of tuberosity of tibia
A04.8.05.021	Bursae subtendineae musculi sartorii	Subtendinous bursa of sartorius
A04.8.05.022	Bursa anserina	Anserine bursa
A04.8.05.023	Bursa subtendinea musculi bicipitis femoris inferior	Inferior subtendinous bursa of biceps femoris
A04.8.05.024	Recessus subpopliteus	Subpopliteal recess
A04.8.05.025	Bursa subtendinea musculi gastrocnemii lateralis	Lateral subtendinous bursa of gastrocnemius
A04.8.05.026	Bursa subtendinea musculi gastrocnemii medialis	Medial subtendinous bursa of gastrocnemius
A04.8.05.027	Bursa musculi semimembranosi	Semimembranosus bursa
A04.8.05.028	Bursa subcutanea malleoli lateralis	Subcutaneous bursa of lateral malleolus
A04.8.05.029	Bursa subcutanea malleoli medialis	Subcutaneous bursa of medial malleolus
A04.8.05.030	Bursa subtendinea musculi tibialis anterioris	Subtendinous bursa of tibialis anterior
A04.8.05.031	Bursa subcutanea calcanea	Subcutaneous calcaneal bursa
A04.8.05.032	Bursa tendinis calcanei	Bursa of tendo calcaneus; Bursa of calcaneal tendon; Retrocalcaneal bursa
A04.8.06.001	**Vaginae tendinum membri inferioris**	**Tendinous sheaths of lower limb**
A04.8.06.002	Vaginae tendinum tarsales anteriores	Anterior tarsal tendinous sheaths
A04.8.06.003	Vagina tendinis musculi tibialis anterioris	Tendinous sheath of tibialis anterior
A04.8.06.004	Vagina tendinis musculi extensoris hallucis longi	Tendinous sheath of extensor hallucis longus
A04.8.06.005	Vagina tendinum musculi extensoris digitorum longi	Tendinous sheath of extensor digitorum longus
A04.8.06.006	Vaginae tendinum tarsales tibiales	Tibial tarsal tendinous sheaths
A04.8.06.007	Vagina tendinum musculi flexoris digitorum longi	Tendinous sheath of flexor digitorum longus
A04.8.06.008	Vagina tendinis musculi tibialis posterioris	Tendinous sheath of tibialis posterior

A04.8.06.009	Vagina tendinis musculi flexoris hallucis longi	Tendinous sheath of flexor hallucis longus
A04.8.06.010	Vaginae tendinum tarsales fibulares	Fibular tarsal tendinous sheaths
A04.8.06.011	Vagina communis tendinum musculorum fibularium; Vagina communis tendinum musculorum peroneorum	Common tendinous sheath of fibulares; Common tendinous sheath of peronei
A04.8.06.012	Vagina plantaris tendinis musculi fibularis longi; Vagina plantaris tendinis musculi peronei longi	Plantar tendinous sheath of fibularis longus; Plantar tendinous sheath of peroneus longus
A04.8.06.013	Vagina tendinum digitorum pedis	Tendinous sheaths of toes
A04.8.06.014	Vaginae fibrosae digitorum pedis	Fibrous sheaths of toes
A04.8.06.015	Pars anularis vaginae fibrosae	Anular part
A04.8.06.016	Pars cruciformis vaginae fibrosae	Cruciform part
A04.8.06.017	Vaginae synoviales digitorum pedis	Synovial sheaths of toes
A04.8.06.018	Vincula tendinum	Vincula tendinum

A05.0.00.000	**Systema digestorium**	**Alimentary system**
A05.1.00.001	**Os**	**Mouth**
A05.1.01.001	**Cavitas oris**	**Oral cavity**
A05.1.01.002	Tunica mucosa oris	Mucous membrane of mouth
A05.1.01.003	**Vestibulum oris**	**Oral vestibule**
A05.1.01.004	Rima oris	Oral fissure; Oral opening
A05.1.01.005	Labia oris	Lips
A05.1.01.006	Labium superius	Upper lip
A05.1.01.007	Philtrum	Philtrum
A05.1.01.008	Tuberculum	Tubercle
A05.1.01.009	Labium inferius	Lower lip
A05.1.01.010	Frenulum labii superioris	Frenulum of upper lip
A05.1.01.011	Frenulum labii inferioris	Frenulum of lower lip
A05.1.01.012	Commissura labiorum	Labial commissure
A05.1.01.013	Angulus oris	Angle of mouth
A05.1.01.014	Bucca	Cheek
A05.1.01.015	Corpus adiposum buccae	Buccal fat pad
* **A05.1.01.016**	Organum juxtaorale	Juxta-oral organ
A05.1.01.017	Papilla ductus parotidei	Papilla of parotid duct
A05.1.01.101	**Cavitas oris propria**	**Oral cavity proper**
A05.1.01.102	Palatum	Palate
A05.1.01.103	Palatum durum	Hard palate
A05.1.01.104	Palatum molle;velum palatinum	Soft palate
A05.1.01.105	Raphe palati	Palatine raphe
A05.1.01.106	Plicae palatinae transversae; Rugae palatinae	Transverse palatine folds; Palatine rugae
A05.1.01.107	Papilla incisiva	Incisive papilla
A05.1.01.108	Gingiva	Gingiva; Gum
A05.1.01.109	Margo gingivalis	Gingival margin
A05.1.01.110	Papilla gingivalis; Papilla interdentalis	Gingival papilla; Interdental papilla
A05.1.01.111	Sulcus gingivalis	Gingival sulcus; Gingival groove
A05.1.01.112	Caruncula sublingualis	Sublingual caruncle
A05.1.01.113	Plica sublingualis	Sublingual fold

A05.1.02.001	**Glandulae oris**	**Glands of mouth**
A05.1.02.002	**Glandulae salivariae majores**	**Major salivary glands**
A05.1.02.003	Glandula parotidea	Parotid gland
A05.1.02.004	Pars superficialis	Superficial part
A05.1.02.005	Pars profunda	Deep part
A05.1.02.006	Glandula parotidea accessoria	Accessory parotid gland
A05.1.02.007	Ductus parotideus	Parotid duct
A05.1.02.008	Glandula sublingualis	Sublingual gland
A05.1.02.009	Ductus sublingualis major	Major sublingual duct
A05.1.02.010	Ductus sublinguales minores	Minor sublingual ducts
A05.1.02.011	Glandula submandibularis	Submandibular gland
A05.1.02.012	Ductus submandibularis	Submandibular duct
A05.1.02.013	**Glandulae salivariae minores**	**Minor salivary glands**
A05.1.02.014	Glandulae labiales	Labial glands
A05.1.02.015	Glandulae buccales	Buccal glands
A05.1.02.016	Glandulae molares	Molar glands
A05.1.02.017	Glandulae palatinae	Palatine glands
A05.1.02.018	Glandulae linguales	Lingual glands

* **A05.1.01.016** *Organum juxtaorale* For a detailed description of this mechanoreceptive secretory organ, see: Zenker W. 1982. "Juxtaoral Organ (Chievitz' Organ). Morphology and Clinical Aspects." Baltimore, Munich: Urban & Schwarzenberg.

A05.1.03.001	**Dentes**	**Teeth**
A05.1.03.002	Arcus dentalis maxillaris; Arcus dentalis superior	Maxillary dental arcade; Upper dental arcade
A05.1.03.003	Arcus dentalis mandibularis; Arcus dentalis inferior	Mandibular dental arcade; Lower dental arcade
A05.1.03.004	Dens incisivus	Incisor tooth
A05.1.03.005	Dens caninus	Canine tooth
A05.1.03.006	Dens premolaris	Premolar tooth
A05.1.03.007	Dens molaris	Molar tooth
A05.1.03.008	Dens molaris tertius; Dens serotinus	Third molar tooth; Wisdom tooth
A05.1.03.009	Corona dentis	Crown
A05.1.03.010	Cuspis dentis	Cusp; Cuspid
A05.1.03.011	Apex cuspidis	Apex of cusp
A05.1.03.012	Cuspis accessoria	Accessory cusp
A05.1.03.013	Tuberculum dentis	Tubercle
A05.1.03.014	Crista transversalis	Transverse ridge
A05.1.03.015	Crista triangularis	Triangular ridge
A05.1.03.016	Crista obliqua	Oblique ridge
A05.1.03.017	Fissura occlusalis	Occlusal fissure
A05.1.03.018	Fossa occlusalis	Occlusal fossa
A05.1.03.019	Cuspis buccalis	Buccal cusp
A05.1.03.020	Cuspis palatinalis	Palatal cusp
A05.1.03.021	Cuspis lingualis	Lingual cusp
A05.1.03.022	Cuspis mesiobuccalis	Mesiobuccal cusp
A05.1.03.023	Cuspis mesiopalatalis	Mesiopalatal cusp
A05.1.03.024	Cuspis mesiolingualis	Mesiolingual cusp
A05.1.03.025	Cuspis distobuccalis	Distobuccal cusp
A05.1.03.026	Cuspis distopalatinalis	Distopalatal cusp
A05.1.03.027	Cuspis distolingualis	Distolingual cusp
A05.1.03.028	Cuspis distalis	Distal cusp; Hypoconulid
A05.1.03.029	Corona clinica	Clinical crown
A05.1.03.030	Cervix dentis	Neck; Cervix
A05.1.03.031	Radix dentis	Root
A05.1.03.032	Apex radicis dentis	Root apex
A05.1.03.033	Radix clinica	Clinical root
A05.1.03.034	Facies occlusalis	Occlusal surface
A05.1.03.035	Facies vestibularis	Vestibular surface
A05.1.03.036	Facies buccalis	Buccal surface
A05.1.03.037	Facies labialis	Labial surface
A05.1.03.038	Facies lingualis	Lingual surface
A05.1.03.039	Facies palatinalis	Palatal surface
A05.1.03.040	Facies mesialis	Mesial surface
A05.1.03.041	Facies distalis	Distal surface
A05.1.03.042	Facies approximalis	Approximal surface; Interproximal surface
A05.1.03.043	Area contingens	Contact zone
A05.1.03.044	Cingulum	Cingulum
A05.1.03.045	Crista marginalis	Marginal ridge
A05.1.03.046	Margo incisalis	Incisal margin
A05.1.03.047	Cavitas dentis; Cavitas pulparis	Pulp cavity
A05.1.03.048	Cavitas coronae	Pulp cavity of crown
A05.1.03.049	Canalis radicis dentis	Root canal; Pulp canal
A05.1.03.050	Foramen apicis dentis	Apical foramen
A05.1.03.051	Pulpa dentis	Dental pulp
A05.1.03.052	Pulpa coronalis	Crown pulp
A05.1.03.053	Pulpa radicularis	Root pulp
A05.1.03.054	Papilla dentis	Dental papilla
A05.1.03.055	Dentinum	Dentine
A05.1.03.056	Enamelum	Enamel
A05.1.03.057	Cementum	Cement

A05.1.03.058	Periodontium	Periodontium
A05.1.03.059	Mammillae	Mammelons
A05.1.03.060	Stria canina; Sulcus caninus	Canine groove
A05.1.03.061	Fossa canina	Canine fossa
A05.1.03.062	Fovea mesialis	Mesial fovea
A05.1.03.063	Fovea distalis	Distal fovea
A05.1.03.064	Radix buccalis	Buccal root
A05.1.03.065	Radix palatinalis	Palatal root
A05.1.03.066	Radix mesialis	Mesial root
A05.1.03.067	Radix distalis	Distal root
A05.1.03.068	Radix mesiobuccalis	Mesiobuccal root
A05.1.03.069	Radix mesiolingualis	Mesiolingual root
A05.1.03.070	Radix accessoria	Accessory root
A05.1.03.071	(Tuberculum anomale)	(Anomalous tubercle)
A05.1.03.072	Cuspis paramolaris; Tuberculum paramolare	Paramolar cusp; Paramolar tubercle
A05.1.03.073	Tuberculum molare	Molar tubercle
A05.1.03.074	Alveolus dentalis	Tooth socket
A05.1.03.075	Curvea occlusalis	Occlusal curves
A05.1.03.076	Dentes decidui	Deciduous teeth
A05.1.03.077	Dentes permanentes	Permanent teeth
A05.1.03.078	(Diastema)	(Diastema)

A05.1.04.001	**Lingua**	**Tongue**
A05.1.04.002	Corpus linguae	Body of tongue
A05.1.04.003	Radix linguae	Root of tongue
A05.1.04.004	Dorsum linguae	Dorsum of tongue
A05.1.04.005	Pars anterior; Pars presulcalis	Anterior part; Presulcal part
A05.1.04.006	Pars posterior; Pars postsulcalis	Posterior part; Postsulcal part
A05.1.04.007	Facies inferior linguae	Inferior surface of tongue
A05.1.04.008	Plica fimbriata	Fimbriated fold
A05.1.04.009	Margo linguae	Margin of tongue
A05.1.04.010	Apex linguae	Apex of tongue; Tip of tongue
A05.1.04.011	Tunica mucosa linguae	Mucous membrane of tongue
A05.1.04.012	Frenulum linguae	Frenulum of tongue
A05.1.04.013	Papillae linguales	Papillae of tongue; Lingual papillae
A05.1.04.014	Papillae filiformes	Filiform papillae
A05.1.04.015	Papillae fungiformes	Fungiform papillae
A05.1.04.016	Papillae vallatae	Vallate papillae
A05.1.04.017	Papillae foliatae	Foliate papillae
A05.1.04.018	Sulcus medianus linguae	Midline groove of tongue; Median sulcus of tongue
A05.1.04.019	Sulcus terminalis linguae	Terminal sulcus of tongue
A05.1.04.020	Foramen caecum linguae	Foramen caecum of tongue▲
A05.1.04.021	(Ductus thyroglossalis)	(Thyroglossal duct)
A05.1.04.022	Tonsilla lingualis	Lingual tonsil
A05.1.04.023	Noduli lymphoidei	Lymphoid nodules
A05.1.04.024	Septum linguae	Lingual septum
A05.1.04.025	Aponeurosis linguae	Lingual aponeurosis
A04.1.05.001	**Musculi linguae**	**Muscles of tongue**
A05.1.04.101	M. genioglossus	Genioglossus
A05.1.04.102	M. hyoglossus	Hyoglossus
A05.1.04.103	M. chondroglossus	Chondroglossus
A05.1.04.104	M. ceratoglossus	Ceratoglossus
A05.1.04.105	M. styloglossus	Styloglossus
A05.1.04.106	M. longitudinalis superior	Superior longitudinal muscle
A05.1.04.107	M. longitudinalis inferior	Inferior longitudinal muscle
A05.1.04.108	M. transversus linguae	Transverse muscle
A05.1.04.109	M. verticalis linguae	Vertical muscle
A05.1.04.110	M. palatoglossus	Palatoglossus

A05.2.01.001	**FAUCES**	**FAUCES**
A05.2.01.002	Isthmus faucium	Isthmus of fauces; Oropharyngeal isthmus
A05.2.01.003	Palatum molle; Velum palatinum	Soft palate
A05.2.01.004	Uvula palatina	Uvula
A05.2.01.005	Arcus palatoglossus; Plica anterior faucium	Palatoglossal arch; Anterior pillar of fauces
A05.2.01.006	(Plica triangularis)	(Triangular fold)
A05.2.01.007	Arcus palatopharyngeus; Plica posterior faucium	Palatopharyngeal arch; Posterior pillar of fauces
A05.2.01.008	(Plica semilunaris)	(Semilunar fold)
A05.2.01.009	Fossa tonsillaris; Sinus tonsillaris	Tonsillar sinus; Tonsillar fossa; Tonsillar bed
A05.2.01.010	Fossa supratonsillaris	Supratonsillar fossa
A05.2.01.011	Tonsilla palatina	Palatine tonsil
A05.2.01.012	Capsula tonsillae	Tonsillar capsule
* A05.2.01.013	(Fissura tonsillaris; Fissura intratonsillaris)	(Tonsillar cleft; Intratonsillar cleft)
A05.2.01.014	Fossulae tonsillae	Tonsillar pits
A05.2.01.015	Cryptae tonsillae	Tonsillar crypts
A04.1.06.001	**Musculi palati mollis et faucium**	**Muscles of soft palate and fauces**
A05.2.01.101	Aponeurosis palatina	Palatine aponeurosis
A05.2.01.102	M. levator veli palatini	Levator veli palatini
A05.2.01.103	M. tensor veli palatini	Tensor veli palatini
A05.2.01.104	M. uvulae	Musculus uvulae
A05.1.04.110	M. palatoglossus	Palatoglossus
A05.2.01.105	M. palatopharyngeus	Palatopharyngeus
A05.2.01.106	Fasciculus anterior	Anterior fascicle
A05.2.01.107	Fasciculus posterior; M. sphincter palatopharyngeus	Posterior fascicle; Palatopharyngeal sphincter

A05.3.01.001	**PHARYNX**	**PHARYNX**
A05.3.01.002	**Cavitas pharyngis**	**Cavity of pharynx**
A05.3.01.003	**Pars nasalis pharyngis**	**Nasopharynx**
A05.3.01.004	Fornix pharyngis	Vault of pharynx
A05.3.01.005	Hypophysis pharyngealis	Pharyngeal hypophysis
A05.3.01.006	Tonsilla pharyngealis	Pharyngeal tonsil
A05.3.01.007	Fossulae tonsillae	Tonsillar pits
A05.3.01.008	Cryptae tonsillae	Tonsillar crypts
A05.3.01.009	Noduli lymphoidei pharyngeales	Pharyngeal lymphoid nodules
A05.3.01.010	(Bursa pharyngealis)	(Pharyngeal bursa)
A05.3.01.011	Ostium pharyngeum tubae auditivae; Ostium pharyngeum tubae auditoriae	Pharyngeal opening of auditory tube
A05.3.01.012	Torus tubarius	Torus tubarius
A05.3.01.013	Plica salpingopharyngea	Salpingopharyngeal fold
A05.3.01.014	Plica salpingopalatina	Salpingopalatine fold
A05.3.01.015	Torus levatorius	Torus levatorius
A05.3.01.016	Tonsilla tubaria	Tubal tonsil
A05.3.01.017	Recessus pharyngeus	Pharyngeal recess
A05.3.01.018	Crista palatopharyngea	Palatopharyngeal ridge
A05.3.01.019	**Pars oralis pharyngis**	**Oropharynx**
A05.3.01.020	Vallecula epiglottica	Epiglottic vallecula
A05.3.01.021	Plica glossoepiglottica mediana	Median glosso-epiglottic fold
A05.3.01.022	Plica glossoepiglottica lateralis	Lateral glosso-epiglottic fold
A05.3.01.023	**Pars laryngea pharyngis**	**Laryngopharynx; Hypopharynx**
A05.3.01.024	Recessus piriformis	Piriform fossa; Piriform recess
A05.3.01.025	Plica nervi laryngei superioris	Fold of superior laryngeal nerve
A05.3.01.026	Constrictio pharyngooesophagealis	Pharyngo-oesophageal constriction▲
A05.3.01.027	Fascia pharyngobasilaris	Pharyngobasilar fascia

* **A05.2.01.013** (*Fissura tonsillaris; fissura intratonsillaris*) A deep cleft in the palatine tonsil which curves parallel to the convex dorsum of the tongue and retrogresses during childhood and puberty. It is not situated above the tonsil and thus the term *fossa supratonsillaris*, if used in this way, is a misnomer. The term properly refers only to that part of the tonsillar fossa lying above the palatine tonsil.

A05.3.01.028	Tela submucosa	Submucosa
A05.3.01.029	Tunica mucosa	Mucosa; Mucous membrane
A05.3.01.030	Glandulae pharyngeales	Pharyngeal glands
A04.2.06.001	**Musculi pharyngis; Tunica muscularis pharyngis**	**Pharyngeal muscles; Muscle layer of pharynx**
A05.3.01.101	Raphe pharyngis	Pharyngeal raphe
A05.3.01.102	Raphe pterygomandibularis	Pterygomandibular raphe
A05.3.01.103	M. constrictor pharyngis superior	Superior constrictor
A05.3.01.104	Pars pterygopharyngea	Pterygopharyngeal part
A05.3.01.105	Pars buccopharyngea	Buccopharyngeal part
A05.3.01.106	Pars mylopharyngea	Mylopharyngeal part
A05.3.01.107	Pars glossopharyngea	Glossopharyngeal part
A05.3.01.108	M. constrictor pharyngis medius	Middle constrictor
A05.3.01.109	Pars chondropharyngea	Chondropharyngeal part
A05.3.01.110	Pars ceratopharyngea	Ceratopharyngeal part
A05.3.01.111	M. constrictor pharyngis inferior	Inferior constrictor
A05.3.01.112	Pars thyropharyngea; M. thyropharyngeus	Thyropharyngeal part; Thyropharyngeus
A05.3.01.113	Pars cricopharyngea; M. cricopharyngeus	Cricopharyngeal part; Cricopharyngeus
A05.3.01.114	M. stylopharyngeus	Stylopharyngeus
A05.3.01.115	M. salpingopharyngeus	Salpingopharyngeus
A05.2.01.105	M. palatopharyngeus	Palatopharyngeus
A05.3.01.116	Fascia buccopharyngealis	Buccopharyngeal fascia
A05.3.01.117	Spatium peripharyngeum	Peripharyngeal space
A05.3.01.118	Spatium retropharyngeum	Retropharyngeal space
A05.3.01.119	Spatium lateropharyngeum; Spatium pharyngeum laterale; Spatium parapharyngeum	Parapharyngeal space; Lateral pharyngeal space

A05.4.01.001	OESOPHAGUS	OESOPHAGUS▲
A05.4.01.002	Pars cervicalis; Pars colli	Cervical part
A05.4.01.003	Pars thoracica	Thoracic part
A05.4.01.004	Constrictio partis thoracicae; Constrictio bronchoaortica	Thoracic constriction; Broncho-aortic constriction
A05.4.01.005	Constrictio phrenica; Constrictio diaphragmatica	Diaphragmatic constriction
A05.4.01.006	Pars abdominalis	Abdominal part
A05.4.01.007	Tunica serosa	Serosa; Serous coat
A05.4.01.008	Tela subserosa	Subserosa; Subserous layer
A05.4.01.009	Tunica adventitia	Adventitia
A05.4.01.010	Tunica muscularis	Muscular layer; Muscular coat
A05.4.01.011	Tendo cricooesophageus	Crico-oesophageal tendon▲
A05.4.01.012	M. bronchooesophageus	Broncho-oesophageus▲
A05.4.01.013	M. pleurooesophageus	Pleuro-oesophageus▲
A05.4.01.014	Tela submucosa	Submucosa
A05.4.01.015	Tunica mucosa	Mucosa; Mucous membrane
A05.4.01.016	Lamina muscularis mucosae	Muscularis mucosae
A05.4.01.017	Glandulae oesophageae	Oesophageal glands▲

A05.5.01.001	GASTER	STOMACH
A05.5.01.002	Paries anterior	Anterior wall
A05.5.01.003	Paries posterior	Posterior wall
A05.5.01.004	Curvatura major	Greater curvature
A05.5.01.005	Curvatura minor	Lesser curvature
A05.5.01.006	Incisura angularis	Angular incisure
A05.5.01.007	Cardia; Pars cardiaca	Cardia; Cardial part
A05.5.01.008	Ostium cardiacum	Cardial orifice
A05.5.01.009	Fundus gastricus	Fundus of stomach
A05.5.01.010	Fornix gastricus	Fornix of stomach

A05.5.01.011	Incisura cardialis	Cardial notch
A05.5.01.012	Corpus gastricum	Body of stomach
A05.5.01.013	Canalis gastricus	Gastric canal
A05.5.01.014	Pars pylorica	Pyloric part
A05.5.01.015	Antrum pyloricum	Pyloric antrum
A05.5.01.016	Canalis pyloricus	Pyloric canal
A05.5.01.017	Pylorus	Pylorus
A05.5.01.018	Ostium pyloricum	Pyloric orifice
A05.5.01.019	Tunica serosa	Serosa; Serous coat
A05.5.01.020	Tela subserosa	Subserosa; Subserous layer
A05.5.01.021	Tunica muscularis	Muscular layer; Muscular coat
A05.5.01.022	Stratum longitudinale	Longitudinal layer
A05.5.01.023	Stratum circulare	Circular layer
A05.5.01.024	M. sphincter pyloricus	Pyloric sphincter
A05.5.01.025	Fibrae obliquae	Oblique fibres▲
A05.5.01.026	Tela submucosa	Submucosa
A05.5.01.027	Tunica mucosa	Mucosa; Mucous membrane
A05.5.01.028	Plicae gastricae	Gastric folds; Gastric rugae
A05.5.01.029	Lamina muscularis mucosae	Muscularis mucosae
A05.5.01.030	Areae gastricae	Gastric areas
A05.5.01.031	Plicae villosae	Villous folds
A05.5.01.032	Foveolae gastricae	Gastric pits
A05.5.01.033	Glandulae gastricae	Gastric glands

A05.6.01.001	**Intestinum tenue**	**Small intestine**
A05.6.01.002	Tunica serosa	Serosa; Serous coat
A05.6.01.003	Tela subserosa	Subserosa; Subserous layer
A05.6.01.004	Tunica muscularis	Muscular layer; Muscular coat
* A05.6.01.005	Stratum longitudinale; Stratum helicoidale longi gradus	Longitudinal layer; Long pitch helicoidal layer
* A05.6.01.006	Stratum circulare; Stratum helicoidale brevis gradus	Circular layer; Short pitch helicoidal layer
A05.6.01.007	Plicae circulares	Circular folds
A05.6.01.008	Tela submucosa	Submucosa
A05.6.01.009	Tunica mucosa	Mucosa; Mucous membrane
A05.6.01.010	Lamina muscularis mucosae	Muscularis mucosae
A05.6.01.011	Villi intestinales	Intestinal villi
A05.6.01.012	Glandulae intestinales	Intestinal glands
A05.6.01.013	Noduli lymphoidei solitarii	Solitary lymphoid nodules
A05.6.01.014	Noduli lymphoidei aggregati	Aggregated lymphoid nodules

A05.6.02.001	**DUODENUM**	**DUODENUM**
A05.6.02.002	Pars superior	Superior part
A05.6.02.003	Ampulla; Bulbus	Ampulla; Duodenal cap
A05.6.02.004	Flexura duodeni superior	Superior duodenal flexure
A05.6.02.005	Pars descendens	Descending part
A05.6.02.006	Flexura duodeni inferior	Inferior duodenal flexure
A05.6.02.007	Pars horizontalis; Pars inferior	Inferior part; Horizontal part; Transverse part
A05.6.02.008	Pars ascendens	Ascending part
A05.6.02.009	Flexura duodenojejunalis	Duodenojejunal flexure
A05.6.02.010	Pars tecta duodeni	Hidden part of duodenum
A05.6.02.011	M. suspensorius duodeni; Lig. suspensorium duodeni	Suspensory muscle of duodenum; Suspensory ligament of duodenum
A05.6.02.012	Pars phrenicocoeliaca	Phrenicocoeliac part▲
A05.6.02.013	Pars coeliacoduodenalis	Coeliacoduodenal part▲

* **A05.6.01.005 / A05.6.01.006** *Stratum helicoidale longi gradus/stratum helicoidale brevis gradus* These new terms recognize that the disposition of the fibres in the muscular layers of the wall of the small intestine is not truly longitudinal or circular but helicoidal with a long pitch and a short pitch respectively. Carey E. J. 1921. "Studies on the Structure and Function of the Small Intestine." *Anat Rec* 21: 189–216.

A05.6.02.014	Plica longitudinalis duodeni	Longitudinal fold of duodenum
A05.6.02.015	Papilla duodeni major	Major duodenal papilla
A05.6.02.016	Papilla duodeni minor	Minor duodenal papilla
A05.6.02.017	Glandulae duodenales	Duodenal glands

A05.6.03.001	**JEJUNUM**	**JEJUNUM**

A05.6.04.001	**ILEUM**	**ILEUM**
A05.6.04.002	Pars terminalis	Terminal ileum
A05.6.04.003	(Diverticulum ilei)	(Ileal diverticulum)

A05.7.01.001	**Intestinum crassum**	**Large intestine**
A05.7.01.002	Tunica serosa	Serosa; Serous coat
A05.7.01.003	Tela subserosa	Subserosa; Subserous layer
A05.7.01.004	Tunica muscularis	Muscular layer; Muscular coat
A05.7.01.005	Tela submucosa	Submucosa
A05.7.01.006	Tunica mucosa	Mucosa; Mucous membrane
A05.7.01.007	Lamina muscularis mucosae	Muscularis mucosae
A05.7.01.008	Glandulae intestinales	Intestinal glands

A05.7.02.001	**CAECUM**	**CAECUM**▲
A05.7.02.002	Papilla ilealis	Ileal papilla
* A05.7.02.003	Ostium ileale	Ileal orifice; Orifice of ileal papilla
A05.7.02.004	Frenulum ostii ilealis	Frenulum of ileal orifice
A05.7.02.005	Labrum ileocolicum; Labrum superius	Ileocolic lip; Superior lip
A05.7.02.006	Labrum ileocaecale; Labrum inferius	Ileocaecal lip; Inferior lip
A05.7.02.007	Appendix vermiformis	Appendix; Vermiform appendix
A05.7.02.008	Ostium appendicis vermiformis	Orifice of vermiform appendix
A05.7.02.009	Noduli lymphoidei aggregati	Aggregated lymphoid nodules
A05.7.02.010	(Fascia precaecocolica)	(Precaecocolic fascia)▲

A05.7.03.001	**COLON**	**COLON**
A05.7.03.002	Colon ascendens	Ascending colon
A05.7.03.003	Flexura coli dextra; Flexura coli hepatica	Right colic flexure; Hepatic flexure
A05.7.03.004	Colon transversum	Transverse colon
A05.7.03.005	Flexura coli sinistra; Flexura coli splenica	Left colic flexure; Splenic flexure
A05.7.03.006	Colon descendens	Descending colon
A05.7.03.007	Colon sigmoideum	Sigmoid colon
A05.7.03.008	Plicae semilunares coli	Semilunar folds of colon
A05.7.03.009	Haustra coli	Haustra of colon
A05.7.03.010	Appendices omentales; Appendices adiposae coli; Appendices epiploicae	Omental appendices; Fatty appendices of colon
A05.7.03.011	Tunica muscularis	Muscular layer; Muscular coat
A05.7.03.012	Stratum longitudinale	Longitudinal layer
A05.7.03.013	Taeniae coli	Taeniae coli▲
A05.7.03.014	Taenia mesocolica	Mesocolic taenia▲
A05.7.03.015	Taenia omentalis	Omental taenia▲
A05.7.03.016	Taenia libera	Free taenia▲
A05.7.03.017	Stratum circulare	Circular layer

A05.7.04.001	**RECTUM**	**RECTUM**
A05.7.04.002	Flexura sacralis	Sacral flexure
A05.7.04.003	Flexurae laterales	Lateral flexures

* **A05.7.02.003** *Ostium ileale* The ileal orifice is found at the apex of the *papilla ilealis*. While the orifice may have lips which meet at the frenula, it is no longer appropriate to describe these structures as constituting an ileocaecal valve, the mechanism for closure of the orifice lying in the terminal ileum. Rosenberg J. C. and DiDio L. J. A. 1969. "In Vivo Appearance and Function of the Termination of the Ileum as Observed Directly Through a Caecostomy." *Am J Gastroenterol* 52: 411–419.

A05.7.04.004	Flexura superodextra lateralis; Flexura superior lateralis	Superodextral lateral flexure; Superior lateral flexure
A05.7.04.005	Flexura intermediosinistra lateralis; Flexura intermedia lateralis	Intermediosinistral lateral flexure; Intermediate lateral flexure
A05.7.04.006	Flexura inferodextra lateralis; Flexura inferior lateralis	Inferodextral lateral flexure; Inferior lateral flexure
A05.7.04.007	Plicae transversae recti	Transverse folds of rectum
A05.7.04.008	Ampulla recti	Rectal ampulla
A05.7.04.009	Tunica muscularis	Muscular layer; Muscular coat
A05.7.04.010	Stratum longitudinale	Longitudinal layer
A05.7.04.011	M. rectococcygeus	Rectococcygeus
A05.7.04.012	Mm. anorectoperineales; Mm. rectourethrales	Anorectoperineal muscles; Recto-urethral muscles
A05.7.04.013	M. rectoperinealis; M. rectourethralis superior	Rectoperinealis; Recto-urethralis superior
A05.7.04.014	M. anoperinealis; M. rectourethralis inferior	Anoperinealis; Recto-urethralis inferior
A04.5.03.017	M. rectovesicalis	Rectovesicalis
A05.7.04.015	Stratum circulare	Circular layer
A05.7.04.016	Lig. recti laterale	Lateral ligament of rectum; Rectal stalk

A05.7.05.001	**CANALIS ANALIS**	**ANAL CANAL**
A05.7.05.002	Flexura anorectalis; Flexura perinealis	Anorectal flexure; Perineal flexure
A05.7.05.003	Junctio anorectalis	Anorectal junction
A05.7.05.004	Columnae anales	Anal columns
A05.7.05.005	Valvulae anales	Anal valves
A05.7.05.006	Sinus anales	Anal sinuses
A05.7.05.007	Zona transitionalis analis	Anal transition zone
A05.7.05.008	Linea anocutanea	Anocutaneous line
A05.7.05.009	Linea pectinata	Pectinate line
A05.7.05.010	Pecten analis	Anal pecten
A05.7.05.011	M. sphincter ani internus	Internal anal sphincter
A05.7.05.012	Sulcus intersphinctericus	Intersphincteric groove
A04.5.04.012	M. sphincter ani externus	External anal sphincter
A04.5.04.015	Pars profunda	Deep part
A04.5.04.014	Pars superficialis	Superficial part
A04.5.04.013	Pars subcutanea	Subcutaneous part
A05.7.05.013	Anus	Anus

A05.8.01.001	**Hepar**	**Liver**
A05.8.01.002	Facies diaphragmatica	Diaphragmatic surface
A05.8.01.003	Pars superior	Superior part
A05.8.01.004	Impressio cardiaca	Cardiac impression
A05.8.01.005	Pars anterior	Anterior part
A05.8.01.006	Pars dextra	Right part
A05.8.01.007	Pars posterior	Posterior part
A05.8.01.008	Area nuda	Bare area
A05.8.01.009	Sulcus venae cavae	Groove for vena cava
A05.8.01.010	Fissura ligamenti venosi	Fissure for ligamentum venosum
A05.8.01.011	Lig. venosum	Ligamentum venosum
A05.8.01.012	Facies visceralis	Visceral surface
A05.8.01.013	Fossa vesicae biliaris; Fossa vesicae felleae	Fossa for gallbladder
A05.8.01.014	Fissura ligamenti teretis	Fissure for ligamentum teres; Fissure for round ligament
A05.8.01.015	Lig. teres hepatis	Round ligament of the liver
A05.8.01.016	Porta hepatis	Porta hepatis
A05.8.01.017	Tuber omentale	Omental tuberosity
A05.8.01.018	Impressio oesophageale	Oesophageal impression▲
A05.8.01.019	Impressio gastrica	Gastric impression

A05.8.01.020	Impressio duodenalis	Duodenal impression
A05.8.01.021	Impressio colica	Colic impression
A05.8.01.022	Impressio renalis	Renal impression
A05.8.01.023	Impressio suprarenalis	Suprarenal impression
A05.8.01.024	Margo inferior	Inferior border
A05.8.01.025	Incisura ligamenti teretis	Notch for ligamentum teres
* A05.8.01.026	Lobus hepatis dexter	Right lobe of liver
* A05.8.01.027	Lobus hepatis sinister	Left lobe of liver
A05.8.01.028	Appendix fibrosa hepatis	Fibrous appendix of liver
* A05.8.01.029	Lobus quadratus	Quadrate lobe
A05.8.01.030	Lobus caudatus	Caudate lobe
A05.8.01.031	Processus papillaris	Papillary process
A05.8.01.032	Processus caudatus	Caudate process
A05.8.01.033	**Segmentatio hepatis: lobi, partes, divisiones et segmenta**	**Hepatic segmentation: lobes, parts, divisions and segments**
A05.8.01.034	Fissura umbilicalis	Umbilical fissure
A05.8.01.035	Fissura portalis principalis	Main portal fissure
A05.8.01.036	Fissura portalis dextra	Right portal fissure
A05.8.01.037	Pars hepatis sinistra	Left liver; Left part of liver
A05.8.01.038	Divisio lateralis sinistra	Left lateral division
A05.8.01.039	Segmentum posterius laterale sinistrum; Segmentum II	Left posterior lateral segment; Segment II
A05.8.01.040	Segmentum anterius laterale sinistrum; Segmentum III	Left anterior lateral segment; Segment III
A05.8.01.041	Divisio medialis sinistra	Left medial division
A05.8.01.042	Segmentum mediale sinistrum; Segmentum IV	Left medial segment; Segment IV
A05.8.01.043	Pars posterior hepatis; Lobus caudatus	Posterior liver; Posterior part of liver; Caudate lobe
A05.8.01.044	Segmentum posterius; Lobus caudatus; Segmentum I	Posterior segment; Caudate lobe; Segment I
A05.8.01.045	Pars hepatis dextra	Right liver; Right part of liver
A05.8.01.046	Divisio medialis dextra	Right medial division
A05.8.01.047	Segmentum anterius mediale dextrum; Segmentum V	Anterior medial segment; Segment V
A05.8.01.048	Segmentum posterius mediale dextrum; Segmentum VIII	Posterior medial segment; Segment VIII
A05.8.01.049	Divisio lateralis dextra	Right lateral division
A05.8.01.050	Segmentum anterius laterale dextrum; Segmentum VI	Anterior lateral segment; Segment VI
A05.8.01.051	Segmentum posterius laterale dextrum; Segmentum VII	Posterior lateral segment; Segment VII
A05.8.01.052	Tunica serosa	Serosa; Serous coat
A05.8.01.053	Tela subserosa	Subserosa; Subserous layer
A05.8.01.054	Tunica fibrosa	Fibrous capsule
A05.8.01.055	Capsula fibrosa perivascularis	Perivascular fibrous capsule
A05.8.01.056	Lobuli hepatis	Lobules of liver
A05.8.01.057	Aa. interlobulares	Interlobular arteries
A05.8.01.058	Vv. interlobulares	Interlobular veins
A05.8.01.059	Vv. centrales	Central veins

A05.8.01.026 / A05.8.01.027 / A05.8.01.029 *Lobi hepatis* These are the traditional right, left and quadrate lobes that were based on external appearance and are not functional entities. For this reason and because *lobus* has been used in different ways by different groups and nationalities, the traditional terms are expected to become redundant. The new terms under A05.8.01.033 accommodate the different usages. Van Damme J.-P. J. 1993. "Behavioral Anatomy of the Abdominal Arteries." *Surg Clin North Am* 73: 699–725.

A05.8.01.033 *Segmentatio hepatis: lobi, partes, divisiones et segmenta* These are the developmental, functional and surgically separable units of the liver and are based on the distribution of the *v. portae hepatis, aa. hepaticae* and *ductus hepatici.* The segments are numbered according to Couinaud (1957): the *segmentum posterius*, which corresponds to the *lobus caudatus*, is numbered as I and the remainder II–VIII clockwise from the left beginning with the *segmentum posterius laterale sinistrum*. The *divisio lateralis sinistra* (II & III) is separated from the *divisio medialis sinistra* (IV) and the *pars posterior hepatis* (I) by the *fissura umbilicalis*. The *pars hepatis sinistra* and the *pars hepatis dextra* are separated by an oblique plane, *fissura portalis principalis*, that runs anteriorly from a line between the long axis of the *fossa vesicae biliaris* and the middle of the *vena cava inferior* as it lies in contact with the liver posteriorly and transects the *lobus quadratus*. The *divisio medialis dextra* (V & VIII) is separated from the *divisio lateralis dextra* (VI & VII) by the *fissura portalis dextra*. Couinaud C. 1957. *Le foie – Etudes Anatomiques et Chirurgicales*. Paris: Masson.

A05.8.01.060	Ductus biliferi interlobulares	Interlobular bile ducts
A05.8.01.061	**Ductus hepaticus communis**	**Common hepatic duct**
A05.8.01.062	Ductus hepaticus dexter	Right hepatic duct
A05.8.01.063	R. anterior	Anterior branch
A05.8.01.064	R. posterior	Posterior branch
A05.8.01.065	Ductus hepaticus sinister	Left hepatic duct
A05.8.01.066	R. lateralis	Lateral branch
A05.8.01.067	R. medialis	Medial branch
A05.8.01.068	Ductus lobi caudati dexter	Right duct of caudate lobe
A05.8.01.069	Ductus lobi caudati sinister	Left duct of caudate lobe

A05.8.02.001	Vesica biliaris; Vesica fellea	Gallbladder
A05.8.02.002	Fundus vesicae biliaris; Fundus vesicae felleae	Fundus of gallbladder
A05.8.02.003	Infundibulum vesicae biliaris; Infundibulum vesicae felleae	Infundibulum of gallbladder
A05.8.02.004	Corpus vesicae biliaris; Corpus vesicae felleae	Body of gallbladder
A05.8.02.005	Collum vesicae biliaris; Collum vesicae felleae	Neck of gallbladder
A05.8.02.006	Tunica serosa	Serosa; Serous coat
A05.8.02.007	Tela subserosa	Subserosa; Subserous layer
A05.8.02.008	Tunica muscularis	Muscular layer; Muscular coat
A05.8.02.009	Tunica mucosa	Mucosa; Mucous membrane
A05.8.02.010	Plicae mucosae; Rugae	Mucosal folds; Rugae
A05.8.02.011	**Ductus cysticus**	**Cystic duct**
A05.8.02.012	Plica spiralis	Spiral fold
A05.8.02.013	**Ductus choledochus; Ductus biliaris**	**Bile duct**
A05.8.02.014	M. sphincter ductus choledochi; M. sphincter ductus biliaris	Sphincter of bile duct
A05.8.02.015	M. sphincter superior	Superior sphincter
A05.8.02.016	M. sphincter inferior	Inferior sphincter
A05.8.02.017	Ampulla hepatopancreatica; Ampulla biliaropancreatica	Hepatopancreatic ampulla; Biliaropancreatic ampulla
A05.8.02.018	M. sphincter ampullae	Sphincter of ampulla
A05.8.02.019	Glandulae ductus choledochi; Glandulae ductus biliaris	Glands of bile duct

A05.9.01.001	Pancreas	Pancreas
A05.9.01.002	Caput pancreatis	Head of pancreas
A05.9.01.003	Processus uncinatus	Uncinate process
A05.9.01.004	Incisura pancreatis	Pancreatic notch
A05.9.01.005	Collum pancreatis	Neck of pancreas
A05.9.01.006	Corpus pancreatis	Body of pancreas
A05.9.01.007	Facies anterosuperior	Anterosuperior surface
A05.9.01.008	Facies posterior	Posterior surface
A05.9.01.009	Facies anteroinferior	Antero-inferior surface
A05.9.01.010	Margo superior	Superior border
A05.9.01.011	Margo anterior	Anterior border
A05.9.01.012	Margo inferior	Inferior border
A05.9.01.013	Tuber omentale	Omental eminence
A05.9.01.014	Cauda pancreatis	Tail of pancreas
A05.9.01.015	Ductus pancreaticus	Pancreatic duct
A05.9.01.016	M. sphincter ductus pancreatici	Sphincter of pancreatic duct
A05.9.01.017	Ductus pancreaticus accessorius	Accessory pancreatic duct
A05.9.01.018	(Pancreas accessorium)	(Accessory pancreas)
A05.9.01.019	Insulae pancreaticae	Pancreatic islets

A06.0.00.000	**Systema respiratorium**	**Respiratory system**
A06.1.01.001	**NASUS**	**NOSE**
A06.1.01.002	Radix nasi	Root of nose
A06.1.01.003	Dorsum nasi	Dorsum of nose
A06.1.01.004	Apex nasi	Apex of nose; Tip of nose
A06.1.01.005	Ala nasi	Ala of nose
A06.1.01.006	Cartilagines nasi	Nasal cartilages
A06.1.01.007	Cartilago alaris major	Major alar cartilage
A06.1.01.008	Crus mediale	Medial crus
A06.1.01.009	Pars mobilis septi nasi	Mobile part of nasal septum
A06.1.01.010	Crus laterale	Lateral crus
A06.1.01.011	Cartilagines alares minores	Minor alar cartilages
A06.1.01.012	Cartilagines nasi accessoriae	Accessory nasal cartilages
A06.1.01.013	Cartilago septi nasi	Septal nasal cartilage
A06.1.01.014	Processus lateralis	Lateral process
A06.1.01.015	Processus posterior; Processus sphenoidalis	Posterior process; Sphenoid process
A06.1.01.016	Cartilago vomeronasalis	Vomeronasal cartilage
A06.1.02.001	**Cavitas nasi**	**Nasal cavity**
A06.1.02.002	Nares	Nares; Nostrils
A06.1.02.003	Choanae	Choanae; Posterior nasal apertures
A06.1.02.004	Septum nasi	Nasal septum
A06.1.02.005	Pars membranacea	Membranous part
A06.1.02.006	Pars cartilaginea	Cartilaginous part
A06.1.02.007	Pars ossea	Bony part
A06.1.02.008	Organum vomeronasale	Vomeronasal organ
A06.1.02.009	Vestibulum nasi	Nasal vestibule
A06.1.02.010	Limen nasi	Limen nasi
A06.1.02.011	Sulcus olfactorius	Olfactory groove
A06.1.02.012	Concha nasi suprema	Highest nasal concha
A06.1.02.013	Concha nasi superior	Superior nasal concha
A06.1.02.014	Concha nasi media	Middle nasal concha
A06.1.02.015	Concha nasi inferior	Inferior nasal concha
A06.1.02.016	Plexus cavernosus conchae	Cavernous plexus of conchae
A06.1.02.017	Tunica mucosa	Mucosa; Mucous membrane
A06.1.02.018	Pars respiratoria	Respiratory region
A06.1.02.019	Pars olfactoria	Olfactory region
A06.1.02.020	Glandulae nasales	Nasal glands
A06.1.02.021	Agger nasi	Agger nasi
A06.1.02.022	Recessus sphenoethmoidalis	Spheno-ethmoidal recess
A06.1.02.023	Meatus nasi superior	Superior nasal meatus
A06.1.02.024	Meatus nasi medius	Middle nasal meatus
A06.1.02.025	Atrium meatus medii	Atrium of middle meatus
A06.1.02.026	Bulla ethmoidalis	Ethmoidal bulla
A06.1.02.027	Infundibulum ethmoidale	Ethmoidal infundibulum
A06.1.02.028	Hiatus semilunaris	Semilunar hiatus
A06.1.02.029	Meatus nasi inferior	Inferior nasal meatus
A06.1.02.030	Apertura ductus nasolacrimalis	Opening of nasolacrimal duct
A06.1.02.031	Meatus nasi communis	Common nasal meatus
A06.1.02.032	Meatus nasopharyngeus	Nasopharyngeal meatus
A06.1.02.033	(Ductus incisivus)	(Incisive duct)
A06.1.03.001	**Sinus paranasales**	**Paranasal sinuses**
A06.1.03.002	Sinus maxillaris	Maxillary sinus
A06.1.03.003	Sinus sphenoidalis	Sphenoidal sinus
A06.1.03.004	Sinus frontalis	Frontal sinus
A06.1.03.005	Cellulae ethmoidales	Ethmoidal cells
A06.1.03.006	Cellulae ethmoidales anteriores	Anterior ethmoidal cells

A06.1.02.031 *Meatus nasi communis* The common nasal meatus is the part of the nasal cavity between the conchae and the nasal septum.

A06.1.03.007	Cellulae ethmoidales mediae	Middle ethmoidal cells
A06.1.03.008	Cellulae ethmoidales posteriores	Posterior ethmoidal cells

A06.2.01.001	LARYNX	LARYNX
A06.2.02.001	**Cartilagines et articulationes laryngis**	**Laryngeal cartilages and joints**
A06.2.02.002	**Cartilago thyroidea**	**Thyroid cartilage**
A06.2.02.003	Prominentia laryngea	Laryngeal prominence
A06.2.02.004	Lamina dextra/sinistra	Right/left lamina
A06.2.02.005	Incisura thyroidea superior	Superior thyroid notch
A06.2.02.006	Incisura thyroidea inferior	Inferior thyroid notch
A06.2.02.007	Tuberculum thyroideum superius	Superior thyroid tubercle
A06.2.02.008	Tuberculum thyroideum inferius	Inferior thyroid tubercle
A06.2.02.009	Linea obliqua	Oblique line
A06.2.02.010	Cornu superius	Superior horn
A06.2.02.011	Cornu inferius	Inferior horn
A06.2.02.012	(Foramen thyroideum)	(Thyroid foramen)
A06.2.02.013	Membrana thyrohyoidea	Thyrohyoid membrane
A06.2.02.014	Lig. thyrohyoideum medianum	Median thyrohyoid ligament
A06.2.02.015	Bursa retrohyoidea	Retrohyoid bursa
A06.2.02.016	Bursa infrahyoidea	Infrahyoid bursa
A06.2.02.017	Lig. thyrohyoideum laterale	Lateral thyrohyoid ligament
A06.2.02.018	Cartilago triticea	Triticeal cartilage
A06.2.03.001	**Cartilago cricoidea**	**Cricoid cartilage**
A06.2.03.002	Arcus cartilaginis cricoideae	Arch of cricoid cartilage
A06.2.03.003	Lamina cartilaginis cricoideae	Lamina of cricoid cartilage
A06.2.03.004	Facies articularis arytenoidea	Arytenoid articular surface
A06.2.03.005	Facies articularis thyroidea	Thyroid articular surface
A06.2.03.006	**Articulatio cricothyroidea**	**Cricothyroid joint**
A06.2.03.007	Capsula articularis cricothyroidea	Capsule of cricothyroid joint
A06.2.03.008	Lig. ceratocricoideum	Ceratocricoid ligament
A06.2.03.009	Lig. cricothyroideum medianum	Median cricothyroid ligament
A06.2.03.010	Lig. cricotracheale	Cricotracheal ligament
A06.2.04.001	**Cartilago arytenoidea**	**Arytenoid cartilage**
A06.2.04.002	Facies articularis	Articular surface
A06.2.04.003	Basis cartilaginis arytenoideae	Base of arytenoid cartilage
A06.2.04.004	Facies anterolateralis	Anterolateral surface
A06.2.04.005	Processus vocalis	Vocal process
A06.2.04.006	Crista arcuata	Arcuate crest
A06.2.04.007	Colliculus	Colliculus
A06.2.04.008	Fovea oblonga	Oblong fovea
A06.2.04.009	Fovea triangularis	Triangular fovea
A06.2.04.010	Facies medialis	Medial surface
A06.2.04.011	Facies posterior	Posterior surface
A06.2.04.012	Apex cartilaginis arytenoideae	Apex of arytenoid cartilage
A06.2.04.013	Processus muscularis	Muscular process
A06.2.04.014	**Articulatio cricoarytenoidea**	**Crico-arytenoid joint**
A06.2.04.015	Capsula articularis cricoarytenoidea	Capsule of crico-arytenoid joint
A06.2.04.016	Lig. cricoarytenoideum	Crico-arytenoid ligament
A06.2.04.017	Lig. cricopharyngeum	Cricopharyngeal ligament
A06.2.04.018	(Cartilago sesamoidea)	(Sesamoid cartilage)
A06.2.05.001	**Cartilago corniculata**	**Corniculate cartilage**
A06.2.05.002	Tuberculum corniculatum	Corniculate tubercle
A06.2.06.001	**Cartilago cuneiformis**	**Cuneiform cartilage**
A06.2.06.002	Tuberculum cuneiforme	Cuneiform tubercle
A06.2.07.001	**Epiglottis**	**Epiglottis**
A06.2.07.002	Cartilago epiglottica	Epiglottic cartilage
A06.2.07.003	Petiolus epiglottidis	Stalk of epiglottis
A06.2.07.004	Tuberculum epiglotticum	Epiglottic tubercle

A06.2.07.005	Lig. thyroepiglotticum	Thyro-epiglottic ligament
A06.2.07.006	Lig. hyoepiglotticum	Hyo-epiglottic ligament
A06.2.07.007	Corpus adiposum preepiglotticum	Pre-epiglottic fat body
A04.2.07.001	**Musculi laryngis**	**Laryngeal muscles**
A06.2.08.001	M. cricothyroideus	Cricothyroid
A06.2.08.002	Pars recta	Straight part
A06.2.08.003	Pars obliqua	Oblique part
A06.2.08.004	M. cricoarytenoideus posterior	Posterior crico-arytenoid
A06.2.08.005	(M. ceratocricoideus)	(Ceratocricoid)
A06.2.08.006	M. cricoarytenoideus lateralis	Lateral crico-arytenoid
A06.2.08.007	M. vocalis	Vocalis
A06.2.08.008	M. thyroarytenoideus	Thyro-arytenoid
A06.2.08.009	Pars thyroepiglottica	Thyro-epiglottic part
A06.2.08.010	M. arytenoideus obliquus	Oblique arytenoid
A06.2.08.011	Pars aryepiglottica	Ary-epiglottic part
A06.2.08.012	M. arytenoideus transversus	Transverse arytenoid
A06.2.09.001	**Cavitas laryngis**	**Laryngeal cavity**
A06.2.09.002	Aditus laryngis	Laryngeal inlet
A06.2.09.003	Plica aryepiglottica	Ary-epiglottic fold
A06.2.09.004	Tuberculum corniculatum	Corniculate tubercle
A06.2.09.005	Tuberculum cuneiforme	Cuneiform tubercle
A06.2.09.006	Incisura interarytenoidea	Interarytenoid notch
A06.2.09.007	Vestibulum laryngis	Laryngeal vestibule
A06.2.09.008	Plica vestibularis	Vestibular fold
A06.2.09.009	Rima vestibuli	Rima vestibuli
A06.2.09.010	Ventriculus laryngis	Laryngeal ventricle
A06.2.09.011	Sacculus laryngis	Laryngeal saccule
A06.2.09.012	Glottis	Glottis
A06.2.09.013	Plica vocalis	Vocal fold
A06.2.09.014	Rima glottidis; Rima vocalis	Rima glottidis
A06.2.09.015	Pars intermembranacea	Intermembranous part
A06.2.09.016	Pars intercartilaginea	Intercartilaginous part
A06.2.09.017	Plica interarytenoidea	Interarytenoid fold
A06.2.09.018	Cavitas infraglottica	Infraglottic cavity
A06.2.09.019	Tunica mucosa	Mucosa; Mucous membrane
A06.2.09.020	Glandulae laryngeales	Laryngeal glands
A06.2.09.021	Membrana fibroelastica laryngis	Fibro-elastic membrane of larynx
A06.2.09.022	Membrana quadrangularis	Quadrangular membrane
A06.2.09.023	Lig. vestibulare	Vestibular ligament
A06.2.09.024	Conus elasticus	Conus elasticus; Cricovocal membrane
A06.2.09.025	Lig. vocale	Vocal ligament

A06.3.01.001	TRACHEA	TRACHEA
A06.3.01.002	Pars cervicalis; Pars colli	Cervical part
A06.3.01.003	Pars thoracica	Thoracic part
A06.3.01.004	Cartilagines tracheales	Tracheal cartilages
A06.3.01.005	M. trachealis	Trachealis
A06.3.01.006	Ligg. anularia; Ligg. trachealia	Anular ligaments
A06.3.01.007	Paries membranaceus	Membranous wall
A06.3.01.008	Bifurcatio tracheae	Tracheal bifurcation
A06.3.01.009	Carina tracheae	Carina of trachea
A06.3.01.010	Tunica mucosa	Mucosa; Mucous membrane
A06.3.01.011	Glandulae tracheales	Tracheal glands

A06.4.01.001	BRONCHI	BRONCHI
A06.4.01.002	Arbor bronchialis	Bronchial tree
A06.4.01.003	Bronchus principalis dexter	Right main bronchus
A06.4.01.004	Bronchus principalis sinister	Left main bronchus

A06.4.02.001	**Bronchi lobares et segmentales**	**Lobar and segmental bronchi**
A06.4.02.002	Bronchus lobaris superior dexter	Right superior lobar bronchus
A06.4.02.003	Bronchus segmentalis apicalis [B I]	Apical segmental bronchus [B I]
A06.4.02.004	Bronchus segmentalis posterior [B II]	Posterior segmental bronchus [B II]
A06.4.02.005	Bronchus segmentalis anterior [B III]	Anterior segmental bronchus [B III]
A06.4.02.006	Bronchus lobaris medius	Middle lobar bronchus
A06.4.02.007	Bronchus segmentalis lateralis [B IV]	Lateral segmental bronchus [B IV]
A06.4.02.008	Bronchus segmentalis medialis [B V]	Medial segmental bronchus [B V]
A06.4.02.009	Bronchus lobaris inferior dexter	Right inferior lobar bronchus
A06.4.02.010	Bronchus segmentalis superior [B VI]	Superior segmental bronchus [B VI]
A06.4.02.011	Bronchus segmentalis basalis medialis; Bronchus cardiacus [B VII]	Medial basal segmental bronchus [B VII]
A06.4.02.012	Bronchus segmentalis basalis anterior [B VIII]	Anterior basal segmental bronchus [B VIII]
A06.4.02.013	Bronchus segmentalis basalis lateralis [B IX]	Lateral basal segmental bronchus [B IX]
A06.4.02.014	Bronchus segmentalis basalis posterior [B X]	Posterior basal segmental bronchus [B X]
A06.4.02.015	Bronchus lobaris superior sinister	Left superior lobar bronchus
A06.4.02.016	Bronchus segmentalis apicoposterior [B I+II]	Apicoposterior segmental bronchus [B I+II]
A06.4.02.017	Bronchus segmentalis anterior [B III]	Anterior segmental bronchus [B III]
A06.4.02.018	Bronchus lingularis superior [B IV]	Superior lingular bronchus [B IV]
A06.4.02.019	Bronchus lingularis inferior [B V]	Inferior lingular bronchus [B V]
A06.4.02.020	Bronchus lobaris inferior sinister	Left inferior lobar bronchus
A06.4.02.021	Bronchus segmentalis superior [B VI]	Superior segmental bronchus [B VI]
A06.4.02.022	Bronchus segmentalis basalis medialis; Bronchus cardiacus [B VII]	Medial basal segmental bronchus [B VII]
A06.4.02.023	Bronchus segmentalis basalis anterior [B VIII]	Anterior basal segmental bronchus [B VIII]
A06.4.02.024	Bronchus segmentalis basalis lateralis [B IX]	Lateral basal segmental bronchus [B IX]
A06.4.02.025	Bronchus segmentalis basalis posterior [B X]	Posterior basal segmental bronchus [B X]
A06.4.02.026	Bronchi intrasegmentales	Intrasegmental bronchi
A06.4.02.027	Tunica fibromusculocartilaginea	Fibromusculocartilaginous layer
A06.4.02.028	Tela submucosa	Submucosa
A06.4.02.029	Tunica mucosa	Mucosa; Mucous membrane
A06.4.02.030	Glandulae bronchiales	Bronchial glands

A06.5.01.001	**PULMONES**	**LUNGS**
A06.5.01.002	Pulmo dexter	Left lung
A06.5.01.003	Pulmo sinister	Right lung
A06.5.01.004	Basis pulmonis	Base of lung
A06.5.01.005	Apex pulmonis	Apex of lung
A06.5.01.006	Facies costalis	Costal surface
A06.5.01.007	Pars vertebralis	Vertebral part
A06.5.01.008	Facies mediastinalis	Mediastinal surface
A06.5.01.009	Impressio cardiaca	Cardiac impression
A06.5.01.010	Facies diaphragmatica	Diaphragmatic surface
A06.5.01.011	Facies interlobaris	Interlobar surface
A06.5.01.012	Margo anterior	Anterior border
A06.5.01.013	Incisura cardiaca pulmonis sinistri	Cardiac notch of left lung
A06.5.01.014	Margo inferior	Inferior border
A06.5.01.015	Hilum pulmonis	Hilum of lung
A06.5.01.016	Radix pulmonis	Root of lung
A06.5.01.017	Lobus superior	Superior lobe; Upper lobe
A06.5.01.018	Lingula pulmonis sinistri	Lingula of left lung
A06.5.01.019	Lobus medius pulmonis dextri	Middle lobe of right lung
A06.5.01.020	Lobus inferior	Inferior lobe; Lower lobe
A06.5.01.021	Fissura obliqua	Oblique fissure
A06.5.01.022	Fissura horizontalis pulmonis dextri	Horizontal fissure of right lung
A06.5.01.023	Vasa sanguinea intrapulmonalia	Intrapulmonary blood vessels
A06.5.02.001	**Segmenta bronchopulmonalia**	**Bronchopulmonary segments**
A06.5.02.002	Pulmo dexter, lobus superior	Right lung, superior lobe

A06.5.02.003	Segmentum apicale [S I]	Apical segment [S I]
A06.5.02.004	Segmentum posterius [S II]	Posterior segment [S II]
A06.5.02.005	Segmentum anterius [S III]	Anterior segment [S III]
A06.5.02.006	Pulmo dexter, lobus medius	Right lung, middle lobe
A06.5.02.007	Segmentum laterale [S IV]	Lateral segment [S IV]
A06.5.02.008	Segmentum mediale [S V]	Medial segment [S V]
A06.5.02.009	Pulmo dexter, lobus inferior	Right lung, inferior lobe
A06.5.02.010	Segmentum superius [S VI]	Superior segment [S VI]
A06.5.02.011	Segmentum basale mediale; Segmentum cardiacum [S VII]	Medial basal segment [S VII]
A06.5.02.012	Segmentum basale anterius [S VIII]	Anterior basal segment [S VIII]
A06.5.02.013	Segmentum basale laterale [S IX]	Lateral basal segment [S IX]
A06.5.02.014	Segmentum basale posterius [S X]	Posterior basal segment [S X]
A06.5.02.015	Pulmo sinister, lobus superior	Left lung, superior lobe
A06.5.02.016	Segmentum apicoposterius [S I+II]	Apicoposterior segment [S I+II]
A06.5.02.017	Segmentum anterius [S III]	Anterior segment [S III]
A06.5.02.018	Segmentum lingulare superius [S IV]	Superior lingular segment [S IV]
A06.5.02.019	Segmentum lingulare inferius [S V]	Inferior lingular segment [S V]
A06.5.02.020	Pulmo sinister, lobus inferior	Left lung, inferior lobe
A06.5.02.021	Segmentum superius [S VI]	Superior segment [S VI]
A06.5.02.022	Segmentum basale mediale; Segmentum cardiacum [S VII]	Medial basal segment [S VII]
A06.5.02.023	Segmentum basale anterius [S VIII]	Anterior basal segment [S VIII]
A06.5.02.024	Segmentum basale laterale [S IX]	Lateral basal segment [S IX]
A06.5.02.025	Segmentum basale posterius [S X]	Posterior basal segment [S X]
A06.5.02.026	Bronchioli	Bronchioles
A06.5.02.027	Lobulus	Lobule

A02.3.04.002	**Cavitas thoracis; Cavitas thoracica**	**Thoracic cavity; Thorax**
A07.1.01.001	**Cavitas pleuralis**	**Pleural cavity**
A07.1.02.001	**Pleura**	**Pleura**
A07.1.02.002	Pleura visceralis; Pleura pulmonalis	Visceral pleura; Pulmonary pleura
A07.1.02.003	Tunica serosa	Serosa; Serous coat
A07.1.02.004	Tela subserosa	Subserosa; Subserous layer
A07.1.02.005	Pleura parietalis	Parietal pleura
A07.1.02.006	Cupula pleurae	Cervical pleura; Dome of pleura; Pleural cupula
A07.1.02.007	Pars costalis	Costal part
A07.1.02.008	Pars diaphragmatica	Diaphragmatic part
A07.1.02.009	Pars mediastinalis	Mediastinal part
A07.1.02.010	Tunica serosa	Serosa; Serous coat
A07.1.02.011	Tela subserosa	Subserosa; Subserous layer
A07.1.02.012	Recessus pleurales	Pleural recesses
A07.1.02.013	Recessus costodiaphragmaticus	Costodiaphragmatic recess
A07.1.02.014	Recessus costomediastinalis	Costomediastinal recess
A07.1.02.015	Recessus phrenicomediastinalis	Phrenicomediastinal recess
A07.1.02.016	Recessus vertebromediastinalis	Vertebromediastinal recess
A07.1.02.017	Lig. pulmonale	Pulmonary ligament
A04.4.01.020	Fascia endothoracica; Fascia parietalis thoracis	Endothoracic fascia; Parietal fascia of thorax
A07.1.02.018	Membrana suprapleuralis	Suprapleural membrane
A07.1.02.019	Fascia phrenicopleuralis	Phrenicopleural fascia
A07.1.02.101	**Mediastinum**	**Mediastinum**
A07.1.02.102	Mediastinum superius	Superior mediastinum
A07.1.02.103	Mediastinum inferius	Inferior mediastinum
A07.1.02.104	Mediastinum anterius	Anterior mediastinum
A07.1.02.105	Mediastinum medium	Middle mediastinum
A07.1.02.106	Mediastinum posterius	Posterior mediastinum
A07.1.03.001	**Cavitas pericardiaca** (vide paginam 77)	**Pericardial cavity** (see page 77)

A08.0.00.000 Systema urinarium — Urinary system

A08.1.01.001	REN; NEPHROS	KIDNEY
A08.1.01.002	Margo lateralis	Lateral border
A08.1.01.003	Margo medialis	Medial border
A08.1.01.004	Hilum renale	Hilum of kidney
A08.1.01.005	Sinus renalis	Renal sinus
A08.1.01.006	Facies anterior	Anterior surface
A08.1.01.007	Facies posterior	Posterior surface
A08.1.01.008	Extremitas superior; Polus superior	Superior pole; Superior extremity
A08.1.01.009	Extremitas inferior; Polus inferior	Inferior pole; Inferior extremity
A08.1.01.010	Fascia renalis	Renal fascia
A08.1.01.011	Corpus adiposum pararenale	Paranephric fat; Pararenal fat body
A08.1.01.012	Capsula adiposa	Perinephric fat; Perirenal fat capsule
A08.1.01.013	Capsula fibrosa	Fibrous capsule
A08.1.01.014	Lobi renales	Kidney lobes
* A08.1.01.015	Cortex renalis	Renal cortex
A08.1.01.016	Labyrinthus corticis	Cortical labyrinth
A08.1.01.017	Cortex corticis	Cortex corticis
A08.1.01.018	Radii medullares	Medullary rays
A08.1.01.019	Columnae renales	Renal columns
* A08.1.01.020	Medulla renalis	Renal medulla
A08.1.01.021	Zona externa	Outer zone
A08.1.01.022	Stria externa	Outer stripe
A08.1.01.023	Stria interna	Inner stripe
A08.1.01.024	Fasciculi vasculares	Vascular bundles
A08.1.01.025	Regio interfascicularis	Interbundle region
A08.1.01.026	Zona interna	Inner zone
A08.1.01.027	Papilla renalis	Renal papilla
A08.1.01.028	Crista renalis	Renal crest
A08.1.01.029	Pyramides renales	Renal pyramids
A08.1.01.030	Area cribrosa	Cribriform area
A08.1.01.031	Foramina papillaria	Openings of papillary ducts
A08.1.02.001	**Segmenta renalia**	**Renal segments**
A08.1.02.002	Segmentum superius	Superior segment
A08.1.02.003	Segmentum anterius superius	Anterior superior segment
A08.1.02.004	Segmentum anterius inferius	Anterior inferior segment
A08.1.02.005	Segmentum inferius	Inferior segment
A08.1.02.006	Segmentum posterius	Posterior segment
* A08.1.03.001	**Arteriae intrarenales**	**Intrarenal arteries**
A08.1.03.002	Aa. interlobares	Interlobar arteries
A08.1.03.003	Aa. arcuatae	Arcuate arteries
A08.1.03.004	Aa. corticales radiatae; Aa. interlobulares	Cortical radiate arteries; Interlobular arteries
A08.1.03.005	Arteriola glomerularis afferens	Afferent glomerular arteriole
A08.1.03.006	Arteriola glomerularis efferens	Efferent glomerular arteriole
A08.1.03.007	Aa. perforantes radiatae	Perforating radiate arteries
A08.1.03.008	Arteriolae rectae; Vasa recta	Vasa recta; Straight arterioles
A08.1.03.009	Rr. capsulares	Capsular branches
* A08.1.04.001	**Venae intrarenales**	**Intrarenal veins**
A08.1.04.002	Vv. interlobares	Interlobar veins
A08.1.04.003	Vv. arcuatae	Arcuate veins
A08.1.04.004	Vv. corticales radiatae; Vv. interlobulares	Cortical radiate veins; Interlobular veins
A08.1.04.005	Venulae rectae	Venulae rectae; Straight venules
A08.1.04.006	Vv. stellatae	Stellate veins

* **A08.1.01.015 / A08.1.01.020** *Cortex/medulla renalis* The subdivisions of the renal cortex and the renal medulla follow the recommendations given by The Renal Commission of the International Union of Physiological Sciences (IUPS) 1988. "A Standard Nomenclature for Structures of the Kidney" *Am J Physiol* 254: F1–8, *Pflugers Arch* 411: 113–120, *Kidney Int* 33: 1–7 and *Anat Embryol* (Berlin) 178: N1–8.

* **A08.1.03.001 / A08.1.04.001** *Arteriae/venae intrarenales* For further details regarding the nomenclature of renal blood vessels, see the publications mentioned above in A07.1.01.015.

A08.1.05.001	**Pelvis renalis**	**Renal pelvis**
A08.1.05.002	Typus dendriticus	Branching type
A08.1.05.003	Calices renales majores	Major calices
A08.1.05.004	Calyx superior	Superior calyx
A08.1.05.005	Calyx medius	Middle calyx
A08.1.05.006	Calyx inferior	Inferior calyx
A08.1.05.007	Calices renales minores	Minor calices
A08.1.05.008	(Typus ampullaris)	(Ampullary type)
A08.1.05.009	Tunica adventitia	Adventitia
A08.1.05.010	Tunica muscularis	Muscular layer; Muscular coat
A08.1.05.011	Tunica mucosa	Mucosa; Mucous membrane

A08.2.01.001	URETER	URETER
A08.2.01.002	Pars abdominalis	Abdominal part
A08.2.01.003	Pars pelvica	Pelvic part
A08.2.01.004	Pars intramuralis	Intramural part
A08.2.01.005	Tunica adventitia	Adventitia
A08.2.01.006	Tunica muscularis	Muscular layer; Muscular coat
A08.2.01.007	Tunica mucosa	Mucosa; Mucous membrane

A08.3.01.001	VESICA URINARIA	URINARY BLADDER
A08.3.01.002	Apex vesicae	Apex of bladder
A08.3.01.003	Corpus vesicae	Body of bladder
A08.3.01.004	Fundus vesicae	Fundus of bladder
A08.3.01.005	Cervix vesicae; Collum vesicae	Neck of bladder
A08.3.01.006	Uvula vesicae	Uvula of bladder
A08.3.01.007	Lig. umbilicale medianum	Median umbilical ligament
A08.3.01.008	Tunica serosa	Serosa; Serous coat
A08.3.01.009	Tela subserosa	Subserosa; Subserous layer
A08.3.01.010	Tunica muscularis	Muscular layer; Muscular coat
A08.3.01.011	Mm. trigoni vesicae	Trigonal muscles
A08.3.01.012	M. trigoni vesicae superficialis	Superficial trigone
A08.3.01.013	M. trigoni vesicae profundus	Deep trigone
A08.3.01.014	M. detrusor vesicae	Detrusor
A08.3.01.015	Pars nonstratificata	Unstratified part
A08.3.01.016	Pars cervicis vesicae; Pars colli vesicae	Bladder neck part
A08.3.01.017	Stratum externum longitudinale	External longitudinal layer
A08.3.01.018	Stratum circulare	Circular layer
A08.3.01.019	Stratum internum longitudinale	Internal longitudinal layer
A08.3.01.020	M. pubovesicalis	Pubovesicalis
A04.5.03.017	M. rectovesicalis	Rectovesicalis
A08.3.01.021	M. vesicoprostaticus ♂	Vesicoprostaticus ♂
A08.3.01.021	M. vesicovaginalis ♀	Vesicovaginalis ♀
A08.3.01.022	Tela submucosa	Submucosa
A08.3.01.023	Tunica mucosa	Mucosa; Mucous membrane
A08.3.01.024	Trigonum vesicae	Trigone of bladder
A08.3.01.025	Plica interureterica	Interureteric crest
A08.3.01.026	Ostium ureteris	Ureteric orifice
* A08.3.01.027	Ostium urethrae internum	Internal urethral orifice

A08.4.01.001	**Urethra feminina** (vide paginam 67)	**Female urethra** (see page 67)

A08.5.01.001	**Urethra masculina** (vide paginam 70)	**Male urethra** (see page 70)

* **A08.3.01.027** *Ostium urethrae internum* This term describes the opening of the urethra from the bladder. However, superimposed lateral cystograms and voiding cystourethrograms show that the ostium in the bladder that is filling differs from the ostium in the bladder that is voiding. The bladder around the *ostium urethrae accipiens* usually forms a flat disc or baseplate, the *pars intramuralis urethrae* (bladder neck) is closed and the urethra is at its longest. With the onset of voiding the baseplate becomes progressively funnel-shaped and the bladder neck opens and becomes incorporated into the funnel so that the bladder appears to descend and the urethra to shorten. The *ostium urethrae internum evacuans* then lies some 20% closer to the *ostium urethrae externum* in the female, and at the *basis prostatae* in the male.

A09.0.00.000	**Systemata genitalia**	**Genital systems**
A09.0.00.001	Systema genitale femininum	Female genital system
A09.0.00.002	Systema genitale masculinum	Male genital system

A09.1.00.001	**Organa genitalia feminina interna**	**Female internal genitalia**
A09.1.01.001	OVARIUM	OVARY
A09.1.01.002	Hilum ovarii	Hilum of ovary
A09.1.01.003	Facies medialis	Medial surface
A09.1.01.004	Facies lateralis	Lateral surface
A09.1.01.005	Margo liber	Free border
A09.1.01.006	Margo mesovaricus	Mesovarian border
A09.1.01.007	Extremitas tubaria	Tubal extremity
A09.1.01.008	Extremitas uterina	Uterine extremity
A09.1.01.009	Tunica albuginea	Tunica albuginea
A09.1.01.010	Stroma ovarii	Ovarian stroma
A09.1.01.011	Cortex ovarii	Ovarian cortex
A09.1.01.012	Medulla ovarii	Ovarian medulla
A09.1.01.013	Folliculi ovarici vesiculosi	Vesicular ovarian follicle
A09.1.01.014	Corpus rubrum	Corpus rubrum
A09.1.01.015	Corpus luteum	Corpus luteum
A09.1.01.016	Corpus albicans	Corpus albicans
A09.1.01.017	Lig. ovarii proprium; Lig. uteroovaricum	Ligament of ovary
A09.1.01.018	Lig. suspensorium ovarii	Suspensory ligament of ovary; Infundibulopelvic ligament

A09.1.02.001	TUBA UTERINA; SALPINX	UTERINE TUBE
A09.1.02.002	Ostium abdominale tubae uterinae	Abdominal ostium
A09.1.02.003	Infundibulum tubae uterinae	Infundibulum
A09.1.02.004	Fimbriae tubae uterinae	Fimbriae
A09.1.02.005	Fimbria ovarica	Ovarian fimbria
A09.1.02.006	Ampulla tubae uterinae	Ampulla
A09.1.02.007	Isthmus tubae uterinae	Isthmus
A09.1.02.008	Pars uterina	Uterine part; Intramural part
A09.1.02.009	Ostium uterinum tubae uterinae	Uterine ostium
A09.1.02.010	Tunica serosa	Serosa; Serous coat
A09.1.02.011	Tela subserosa	Subserosa; Subserous layer
A09.1.02.012	Tunica muscularis	Muscular layer; Muscular coat
A09.1.02.013	Tunica mucosa	Mucosa; Mucous membrane
A09.1.02.014	Plicae tubariae	Folds of uterine tube

A09.1.03.001	UTERUS	UTERUS
A09.1.03.002	Fundus uteri	Fundus of uterus
A09.1.03.003	Corpus uteri	Body of uterus
A09.1.03.004	Cornu uteri	Uterine horn
A09.1.03.005	Margo uteri	Border of uterus
A09.1.03.006	Facies intestinalis; Facies posterior	Intestinal surface; Posterior surface
A09.1.03.007	Cavitas uteri	Uterine cavity
A09.1.03.008	Facies vesicalis; Facies anterior	Vesical surface; Anterior surface
A09.1.03.009	Ostium anatomicum uteri internum	Anatomical internal os
A09.1.03.010	Cervix uteri	Cervix of uterus
A09.1.03.011	Portio supravaginalis cervicis	Supravaginal part
A09.1.03.012	Isthmus uteri	Isthmus of uterus
* A09.1.03.013	Ostium histologicum uteri internum	Histological internal os

* **A09.1.03.013** *Ostium histologicum uteri internum* The histological internal os is the lower limit of the *isthmus uteri* and can be recognized with the unaided eye: above endometrium is present that undergoes menstrual changes; below cervical mucosa is present that does not. Frankl O. 1933. "On the Physiology and Pathology of the Isthmus Uteri." *J Obstet Gynecol Br Commonw.* 40: 397–422.

A09.1.03.014	Portio vaginalis cervicis	Vaginal part
A09.1.03.015	Ostium uteri	External os of uterus
A09.1.03.016	Labium anterius	Anterior lip
A09.1.03.017	Labium posterius	Posterior lip
A09.1.03.018	Canalis cervicis uteri	Cervical canal
A09.1.03.019	Plicae palmatae	Palmate folds
A09.1.03.020	Glandulae cervicales	Cervical glands
A09.1.03.021	Parametrium	Parametrium
A09.1.03.022	Paracervix	Paracervix
A09.1.03.023	Tunica serosa; Perimetrium	Serosa; Serous coat; Perimetrium
A09.1.03.024	Tela subserosa	Subserosa; Subserous layer
A09.1.03.025	Tunica muscularis; Myometrium	Myometrium
A09.1.03.026	M. rectouterinus	Recto-uterinus
A09.1.03.027	Tunica mucosa; Endometrium	Endometrium
A09.1.03.028	Glandulae uterinae	Uterine glands
A09.1.03.029	Lig. teres uteri	Round ligament of uterus
A09.1.03.030	Lig. pubocervicale	Pubocervical ligament
A09.1.03.031	Lig. cardinale; Lig. transversum cervicis	Cardinal ligament; Transverse cervical ligament
A09.1.03.032	Lig. rectouterinum	Uterosacral ligament; Recto-uterine ligament

A09.1.04.001	**VAGINA**	**VAGINA**
A09.1.04.002	Fornix vaginae	Vaginal fornix
A09.1.04.003	Pars anterior	Anterior part
A09.1.04.004	Pars posterior	Posterior part
A09.1.04.005	Pars lateralis	Lateral part
A09.1.04.006	Paries anterior	Anterior wall
A09.1.04.007	Paries posterior	Posterior wall
A09.1.04.008	Hymen	Hymen
A09.1.04.009	Carunculae hymenales	Carunculae hymenales; Hymenal caruncles
A09.1.04.010	Tunica muscularis	Muscular layer; Muscular coat
A09.1.04.011	Tunica mucosa	Mucosa; Mucous membrane
A09.1.04.012	Rugae vaginales	Vaginal rugae
A09.1.04.013	Columnae rugarum	Vaginal columns
A09.1.04.014	Columna rugarum anterior	Anterior vaginal column
A09.1.04.015	Columna rugarum posterior	Posterior vaginal column
A09.1.04.016	Carina urethralis vaginae	Urethral carina of vagina
A09.1.04.017	Tunica spongiosa	Spongy layer

A09.1.05.001	**Epoophoron**	**Epoophoron**
A09.1.05.002	Ductus longitudinalis	Longitudinal duct
A09.1.05.003	Ductuli transversi	Transverse ductules
A09.1.05.004	Appendices vesiculosae	Vesicular appendices
A09.1.06.001	**Paroophoron**	**Paroophoron**
A09.1.06.002	(Ductus deferens vestigialis)	(Vestige of ductus deferens)

A09.2.00.001	**Organa genitalia feminina externa**	**Female external genitalia**
A09.2.01.001	**PUDENDUM FEMININUM; VULVA**	**PUDENDUM; VULVA**
A09.2.01.002	Mons pubis	Mons pubis
A09.2.01.003	Labium majus pudendi	Labium majus
A09.2.01.004	Commissura labiorum anterior	Anterior commissure
A09.2.01.005	Commissura labiorum posterior	Posterior commissure
A09.2.01.006	Rima pudendi	Pudendal cleft
A09.2.01.007	Labium minus pudendi	Labium minus
A09.2.01.008	Frenulum labiorum pudendi	Frenulum of labia minora; Fourchette
A09.2.01.009	Preputium clitoridis	Prepuce of clitoris
A09.2.01.010	Frenulum clitoridis	Frenulum of clitoris
A09.2.01.012	Vestibulum vaginae	Vestibule
A09.2.01.012	Fossa vestibuli vaginae	Vestibular fossa

A09.2.01.013	Bulbus vestibuli	Bulb of vestibule
A09.2.01.014	Commissura bulborum	Commissure of bulbs
A09.2.01.015	Ostium vaginae	Vaginal orifice
A09.2.01.016	Glandula vestibularis major	Greater vestibular gland
A09.2.01.017	Glandulae vestibulares minores	Lesser vestibular glands
A09.2.02.001	**Clitoris**	**Clitoris**
A09.2.02.002	Crus clitoridis	Crus of clitoris
A09.2.02.003	Corpus clitoridis	Body of clitoris
A09.2.02.004	Glans clitoridis	Glans of clitoris
A09.2.02.005	Corpus cavernosum clitoridis	Corpus cavernosum of clitoris
A09.2.02.006	Septum corporum cavernosorum	Septum of corpora cavernosa
A09.2.02.007	Fascia clitoridis	Fascia of clitoris
A04.5.02.019	Lig. suspensorium clitoridis	Suspensory ligament of clitoris
A04.5.02.023	Lig. fundiforme clitoridis	Fundiform ligament of clitoris
A08.4.01.001	**Urethra feminina**	**Female urethra**
* A08.3.01.028	Ostium urethrae internum	Internal urethral orifice; Internal urinary meatus
A09.2.03.001	Ostium urethrae internum accipiens	Filling internal urethral orifice
A09.2.03.002	Ostium urethrae internum evacuans	Voiding internal urethral orifice
A09.2.03.003	Pars intramuralis	Intramural part
A09.2.03.004	Crista urethralis	Urethral crest
A09.2.03.005	Ostium urethrae externum	External urethral orifice
A09.2.03.006	M. sphincter urethrae externus	External urethral sphincter
A09.2.03.007	Tunica muscularis	Muscular layer; Muscular coat
A09.2.03.008	Stratum circulare	Circular layer
A09.2.03.009	Sphincter urethrae internus	Internal urethral sphincter
A09.2.03.010	Stratum longitudinale	Longitudinal layer
A09.2.03.011	Tunica spongiosa	Spongy layer
A09.2.03.012	Tunica mucosa	Mucosa; Mucous membrane
A09.2.03.013	Glandulae urethrales	Urethral glands
A09.2.03.014	Lacunae urethrales	Urethral lacunae
A09.2.03.015	(Ductus paraurethrales)	(Para-urethral ducts)

A09.3.00.001	**Organa genitalia masculina interna**	**Male internal genitalia**
A09.3.01.001	**TESTIS; ORCHIS**	**TESTIS**
A09.3.01.002	Extremitas superior; Polus superior	Upper pole; Superior pole
A09.3.01.003	Extremitas inferior; Polus inferior	Lower pole; Inferior pole
A09.3.01.004	Facies lateralis	Lateral surface
A09.3.01.005	Facies medialis	Medial surface
A09.3.01.006	Margo anterior	Anterior border
A09.3.01.007	Margo posterior	Posterior border
A09.3.01.008	Tunica vaginalis testis	Tunica vaginalis
A09.3.01.009	Lamina parietalis	Parietal layer
A09.3.01.010	Lamina visceralis	Visceral layer
A09.3.01.011	Lig. epididymidis superius	Superior ligament of epididymis
A09.3.01.012	Lig. epididymidis inferius	Inferior ligament of epididymis
A09.3.01.013	Sinus epididymidis	Sinus of epididymis
A09.3.01.014	Tunica serosa	Serosa; Serous coat
A09.3.01.015	Tela subserosa	Subserosa; Subserous layer
A09.3.01.016	Tunica albuginea	Tunica albuginea
A09.3.01.017	Tunica vasculosa	Vascular layer
A09.3.01.018	Mediastinum testis	Mediastinum of testis
A09.3.01.019	Septula testis	Septa testis
A09.3.01.020	Lobuli testis	Lobules of testis

* **A08.3.01.028** *Ostium urethrae internum* This term describes the opening of the urethra from the bladder. However, superimposed lateral cystograms and voiding cystourethrograms show that the ostium in the bladder that is filling differs from the ostium in the bladder that is voiding. The bladder around the *ostium urethrae accipiens* usually forms a flat disc or baseplate, the *pars intramuralis urethrae* (bladder neck) is closed and the urethra is at its longest. With the onset of voiding the baseplate becomes progressively funnel-shaped and the bladder neck opens and becomes incorporated into the funnel so that the bladder appears to descend and the urethra to shorten. The *ostium urethrae internum evacuans* then lies some 20% closer to the *ostium urethrae externum* in the female, and at the *basis prostatae* in the male.

A09.3.01.021	Parenchyma testis	Parenchyma of testis
A09.3.01.022	Tubuli seminiferi contorti	Seminiferous tubules; Convoluted seminiferous tubules
A09.3.01.023	Tubuli seminiferi recti	Straight tubules
A09.3.01.024	Rete testis	Rete testis
A09.3.01.025	Ductuli efferentes testis	Efferent ductules

A09.3.02.001	**EPIDIDYMIS**	**EPIDIDYMIS**
A09.3.02.002	Caput epididymidis	Head of epididymis
A09.3.02.003	Lobuli epididymidis; Coni epididymidis	Lobules of epididymis; Conical lobules of epidiymis
A09.3.02.004	Corpus epididymidis	Body of epididymis
A09.3.02.005	Cauda epididymidis	Tail of epididymis
A09.3.02.006	Ductus epididymidis	Duct of epididymis
A09.3.02.007	Ductuli aberrantes	Aberrant ductules
A09.3.02.008	(Ductulus aberrans superior)	(Superior aberrant ductule)
A09.3.02.009	(Ductulus aberrans inferior)	(Inferior aberrant ductule)
A09.3.02.010	Appendix testis	Appendix of testis
A09.3.02.011	(Appendix epididymidis)	(Appendix of epididymis)

A09.3.03.001	**(PARADIDYMIS)**	**(PARADIDYMIS)**

A09.3.04.001	**FUNICULUS SPERMATICUS**	**SPERMATIC CORD**
A09.3.04.002	Fascia spermatica externa	External spermatic fascia
A09.3.04.003	M. cremaster	Cremaster
A09.3.04.004	Fascia cremasterica	Cremasteric fascia
A09.3.04.005	Fascia spermatica interna	Internal spermatic fascia
A09.3.04.006	(Vestigium processus vaginalis)	(Vestige of processus vaginalis)

A09.3.05.001	**DUCTUS DEFERENS**	**DUCTUS DEFERENS; VAS DEFERENS**
A09.3.05.002	Pars scrotalis	Scrotal part
A09.3.05.003	Pars funicularis	Funicular part
A09.3.05.004	Pars inguinalis	Inguinal part
A09.3.05.005	Pars pelvica	Pelvic part
A09.3.05.006	Ampulla ductus deferentis	Ampulla of ductus deferens
A09.3.05.007	Diverticula ampullae	Diverticula of ampulla
A09.3.05.008	Tunica adventitia	Adventitia
A09.3.05.009	Tunica muscularis	Muscular layer; Muscular coat
A09.3.05.010	Tunica mucosa	Mucosa; Mucous membrane

* **A09.3.06.001**	**GLANDULA VESICULOSA; GLANDULA SEMINALIS; VESICULA SEMINALIS**	**SEMINAL GLAND; SEMINAL VESICLE**
A09.3.06.002	Tunica adventitia	Adventitia
A09.3.06.003	Tunica muscularis	Muscular layer; Muscular coat
A09.3.06.004	Tunica mucosa	Mucosa; Mucous membrane
A09.3.06.005	Ductus excretorius	Excretory duct

A09.3.07.001	**Ductus ejaculatorius**	**Ejaculatory duct**

* **A09.3.08.001**	**PROSTATA**	**PROSTATE**
A09.3.08.002	Basis prostatae	Base of prostate
A09.3.08.003	Pars proximalis	Proximal part
A09.3.08.004	Zona glandularum periurethralium	Peri-urethral gland zone
A09.3.08.005	Pars distalis	Distal part

* **A09.3.06.001** *Glandula vesiculosa* This term should be used instead of *vesicula seminalis* because the organ is not a reservoir for semen, but a gland secreting a substantial part of seminal plasma.
* **A09.3.08.001** *Prostata* The term *glandula prostatica* has been omitted because the prostate is more than its glandular part which comprises only about two-thirds of the tissue inside the prostatic capsule.

A09.3.08.006	Apex prostatae	Apex of prostate
A09.3.08.007	Facies anterior	Anterior surface
A09.3.08.008	Facies posterior	Posterior surface
A09.3.08.009	Facies inferolateralis	Inferolateral surface
A09.3.08.010	Lobi prostatae dexter et sinister	Right and left lobes of prostate
* A09.3.08.011	Lobulus inferoposterior	Inferoposterior lobule
* A09.3.08.012	Lobulus inferolateralis	Inferolateral lobule
* A09.3.08.013	Lobulus superomedialis	Superomedial lobule
* A09.3.08.014	Lobulus anteromedialis	Anteromedial lobule
A09.3.08.015	(Lobus medius)	(Middle lobe)
A09.3.08.016	Isthmus prostatae; Commissura prostatae	Isthmus of prostate; Commissure of prostate
A09.3.08.017	Capsula prostatica	Capsule of prostate
A09.3.08.018	Parenchyma	Parenchyma
A09.3.08.019	Ductuli prostatici	Prostatic ducts
A09.3.08.020	Substantia muscularis	Muscular tissue
A04.5.04.005	M. puboprostaticus	Puboprostaticus
A08.3.01.021	M. vesicoprostaticus	Vesicoprostaticus
* A09.3.08.021	Area trapezoidea	Trapezoid area

A09.3.09.001	**GLANDULA BULBOURETHRALIS**	**BULBO-URETHRAL GLAND**
A09.3.09.002	Ductus glandulae bulbourethralis	Duct of bulbo-urethral gland

A09.4.00.001	**Organa genitalia masculina externa**	**Male external genitalia**
A09.4.01.001	**PENIS**	**PENIS**
A09.4.01.002	Radix penis	Root of penis
A09.4.01.003	Corpus penis	Body of penis
A09.4.01.004	Crus penis	Crus of penis
A09.4.01.005	Dorsum penis	Dorsum of penis
A09.4.01.006	Facies urethralis	Urethral surface
A09.4.01.007	Glans penis	Glans penis
A09.4.01.008	Corona glandis	Corona of glans
A09.4.01.009	Septum glandis	Septum of glans
A09.4.01.010	Collum glandis	Neck of glans
A09.4.01.011	Preputium penis	Prepuce; Foreskin
A09.4.01.012	Frenulum preputii	Frenulum
A09.4.01.013	Raphe penis	Raphe of penis
A09.4.01.014	Corpus cavernosum penis	Corpus cavernosum penis
A09.4.01.015	Corpus spongiosum penis	Corpus spongiosum penis
A09.4.01.016	Bulbus penis	Bulb of penis
A09.4.01.017	Tunica albuginea corporum cavernosorum	Tunica albuginea of corpora cavernosa
A09.4.01.018	Tunica albuginea corporis spongiosi	Tunica albuginea of corpus spongiosum
A09.4.01.019	Septum penis	Septum penis
A09.4.01.020	Trabeculae corporum cavernosorum	Trabeculae of corpora cavernosa
A09.4.01.021	Trabeculae corporis spongiosi	Trabeculae of corpus spongiosum
A09.4.01.022	Cavernae corporum cavernosorum	Cavernous spaces of corpora cavernosa
A09.4.01.023	Cavernae corporis spongiosi	Cavernous spaces of corpus spongiosum
A09.4.01.024	Aa. helicinae	Helicine arteries
A09.4.01.025	Vv. cavernosae	Cavernous veins
A09.4.01.026	Fascia penis	Fascia of penis
A04.5.02.019	Lig. suspensorium penis	Suspensory ligament of penis

* **A09.3.08.011 / A09.3.08.012 / A09.3.08.013 / A09.3.08.014** *Lobuli prostatae* Within each lobe of the prostate, four lobules are defined by the arrangement of ducts and connective tissue and may be distinguished with the unaided eye. The combined inferoposterior/inferolateral lobules, the superomedial lobules and the anteromedial lobules correspond to the histological entities of McNeal [1988. *Am J Surg Pathol* 12: 619–633], and widely called after his usage, peripheral, central and transition zones respectively. A technique for the gross dissection of the inferoposterior, inferolateral and combined superomedial/anteromedial lobules was described by Tisell and Salander [1975. *Scand J Urol Nephrol* 9: 185–191 1975]. The inferoposterior and inferolateral lobules, together with the commissure, form a hollow cone within which the superomedial lobes surround the ejaculatory ducts and the anteromedial lobes flank the proximal urethra.

* **A09.3.08.021** *Area trapezoidea* A hyperechoic area found distal to the prostate, bounded superiorly by the *m. rectoperinealis* applied to the prostate, anteriorly by the *pars intermedia urethrae*, inferiorly by the *m. anoperinealis* and posteriorly by the anorectal flexure.

A09.4.01.027	Tela subcutanea penis	Subcutaneous tissue of penis
A04.5.02.023	Lig. fundiforme penis	Fundiform ligament of penis
A09.4.01.028	Glandulae preputiales	Preputial glands

A08.5.01.001	**URETHRA MASCULINA**	**MALE URETHRA**
* **A08.3.01.027**	Ostium urethrae internum	Internal urethral orifice; Internal urinary meatus
A09.4.02.001	Ostium urethrae internum accipiens	Filling internal urethral orifice
A09.4.02.002	Ostium urethrae internum evacuans	Emptying internal urethral orifice
A09.4.02.003	Pars intramuralis; Pars preprostatica	Intramural part; Preprostatic part
A09.4.02.004	Pars prostatica	Prostatic urethra
A09.4.02.005	Pars proximalis	Proximal part
A09.4.02.006	Pars distalis	Distal part
A09.4.02.007	Crista urethralis	Urethral crest
A09.4.02.008	Colliculus seminalis	Seminal colliculus
A09.4.02.009	Utriculus prostaticus	Prostatic utricle
A09.4.02.010	Sinus prostaticus	Prostatic sinus
A09.4.02.011	Tunica muscularis	Muscular layer; Muscular coat
A09.4.02.012	Stratum circulare	Circular layer
A09.4.02.013	M. sphincter urethrae internus; M. sphincter supracollicularis	Internal urethral sphincter; Supracollicular sphincter; Preprostatic sphincter
A09.4.02.014	Stratum longitudinale	Longitudinal layer
A09.4.02.015	Tunica mucosa	Mucosa; Mucous membrane
A09.4.02.016	M. sphincter urethrae externus	External urethral sphincter
* **A09.4.02.017**	Pars intermedia; Pars membranacea	Intermediate part of urethra; Membranous urethra
A09.4.02.018	Tunica muscularis	Muscular layer; Muscular coat
A09.4.02.019	Stratum longitudinale	Longitudinal layer
A09.4.02.020	Tunica mucosa	Mucosa; Mucous membrane
A09.4.02.021	Pars spongiosa	Spongy urethra
A09.4.02.022	Fossa navicularis urethrae	Navicular fossa
A09.4.02.023	(Valvula fossae navicularis)	(Valve of navicular fossa)
A09.4.02.024	Lacunae urethrales	Urethral lacunae
A09.4.02.025	Glandulae urethrales	Urethral glands
A09.4.02.026	Ductus paraurethrales	Para-urethral ducts
A09.4.02.027	Tunica muscularis	Muscular layer; Muscular coat
A09.4.02.028	Stratum longitudinale	Longitudinal layer
A09.4.02.029	Tunica mucosa	Mucosa; Mucous membrane
A09.4.02.030	Ostium urethrae externum	External urethral orifice; External urinary meatus

A09.4.03.001	**SCROTUM**	**SCROTUM**
A09.4.03.002	Raphe scroti	Raphe of scrotum
A09.4.03.003	Tunica dartos	Dartos fascia; Superficial fascia of scrotum
A09.4.03.004	Septum scroti	Septum of scrotum
A09.4.03.005	M. dartos	Dartos muscle

* **A08.3.01.028** *Ostium urethrae internum* This term describes the opening of the urethra from the bladder. However, superimposed lateral cystograms and voiding cystourethrograms show that the ostium in the bladder that is filling differs from the ostium in the bladder that is voiding. The bladder around the *ostium urethrae accipiens* usually forms a flat disc or baseplate, the *pars intramuralis urethrae* (bladder neck) is closed and the urethra is at its longest. With the onset of voiding the baseplate becomes progressively funnel-shaped and the bladder neck opens and becomes incorporated into the funnel so that the bladder appears to descend and the urethra to shorten. The *ostium urethrae internum evacuans* then lies some 20% closer to the *ostium urethrae externum* in the female, and at the *basis prostatae* in the male.

* **A09.4.02.017** *Pars intermedia* With the abandonment of the term urogenital diaphragm, pars membranacea has become a misnomer, it being the part between the *pars prostatica urethrae* and the *pars spongiosa urethrae* and not just the part passing through the *membrana perinealis*. The isthmus urethrae extends between the *membrana perinealis* and the distal end of the *colliculus seminalis* that may be 0–1 cm above the apex of the prostate. Myers R. P. 1991. "Male Urethral Sphincteric Anatomy and Radical Prostatectomy." *Urol Clin North Am* 18: 211–227

* **A09.5.00.001**	**Perineum**	**Perineum**
A09.2.00.001	**Organa genitalia feminina externa** {vide paginam 66}	**Female external genitalia** {see page 66}
A09.4.00.001	**Organa genitalia masculina externa** {vide paginam 69}	**Male external genitalia** {see page 69}
A09.5.00.002	Raphe perinei	Perineal raphe
A04.5.05.001	Mm. perinei	Perineal muscles
A09.5.00.003	M. regionis analis	Muscle of anal triangle
A04.5.04.012	M. sphincter ani externus	External anal sphincter
A09.5.00.004	Mm. regionis urogenitalis	Muscles of urogenital triangle
* **A09.5.00.005**	Corpus perineale; Centrum perinei	Perineal body
* **A04.5.04.016**	Corpus anococcygeum; Lig. anococcygeum	Anococcygeal body; Anococcygeal ligament
A09.5.00.006	Tela subcutanea perinei	Subcutaneous tissue of perineum
A09.5.00.007	Stratum membranosum	Membranous layer
* **A09.5.01.001**	**Saccus subcutaneus perinei**	**Subcutaneous perineal pouch**
* **A09.5.02.001**	**Compartimentum superficiale perinei; Spatium superficiale perinei**	**Superficial perineal pouch; Superficial perineal compartment; Superficial perineal space**
A09.5.02.002	Fascia perinei; Fascia investiens perinei superficialis	Perineal fascia; Superficial investing fascia of perineum; Deep perineal fascia
A09.5.02.003	M. transversus perinei superficialis	Superficial transverse perineal muscle
A09.5.02.004	M. ischiocavernosus	Ischiocavernosus
A09.5.02.005	M. bulbospongiosus	Bulbospongiosus
* **A09.5.03.001**	**Saccus profundus perinei; Spatium profundum perinei**	**Deep perineal pouch; Deep perineal space**
A09.5.03.002	Membrana perinei	Perineal membrane
* **A09.5.03.003**	Lig. transversum perinei ♂	Transverse perineal ligament ♂
* **A09.5.03.004**	M. transversus perinei profundus ♂	Deep transverse perineal muscle ♂
A09.4.02.016	M. sphincter urethrae externus ♂	External urethral sphincter ♂
A09.2.03.006	M. sphincter urethrae externus ♀	External urethral sphincter ♀
* **A09.5.03.005**	M. compressor urethrae ♀	Compressor urethrae ♀
* **A09.5.03.006**	M. sphincter urethrovaginalis ♀	Sphincter urethrovaginalis ♀
A09.5.04.001	**Fossa ischioanalis**	**Ischio-anal fossa**
A09.5.04.002	Corpus adiposum fossae ischioanalis	Fat body of ischio-anal fossa
A09.5.04.003	Canalis pudendalis	Pudendal canal

* **A09.5.00.001** *Perineum* This term, like the term *fascia*, has been used in different ways in different languages and circumstances. In its most restricted sense, and in obstetrics, it has equated with perineal body; in an intermediate sense it has included only superficial structures within anal and urogenital triangles; in its widest sense, as used here, it includes all structures within those triangles, extending deeply as far as the inferior fascia of the pelvic diaphragm that separates it from pelvic cavity.

* **A09.5.00.005** *Corpus perineale* Tendineum has been omitted from the alternative *centrum perinei*: the perineal body is fibromuscular rather than tendinous and quite unlike the *centrum tendineum* of the diaphragm.

* **A04.5.04.016** *Corpus anococcygeum* The term *corpus*, rather than *ligamentum*, has been used here because it is a stratified nonligamentous structure in which fleshy muscle attachments underlie a tendon.

* **A09.5.01.001 / A09.5.02.001 / A09.5.03.001** *Saccus subcutaneus perinei/compartimentum superficiale perinei/recessus profundus perinei* The subcutaneous perineal pouch is a potential space between the membranous layer of perineal subcutaneous tissue and the superficial layer of the investing fascia of perineal muscles. Extravasations or collections in the subcutaneous pouch may track, deep to the membranous layer of subcutaneous tissue, into the anterior abdominal wall, along the clitoris/penis and/or into the labia or scrotum. The superficial pouch is a fully enclosed compartment, being bounded below by the perineal fascia (the superficial layer of the investing fascia of the superficial perineal muscles) and above by the perineal membrane. The deep perineal pouch, on the other hand, is not an enclosed compartment but is open above. This and the deep urogenital muscles are bounded below by the perineal membrane but extend up into the pelvis rendering the old terms *diaphragma urogenitalis* and *fascia diaphragmatis urogenitale inferior* misnomers. Oelrich T. M. 1980. "The Urethral Sphincter in the Male." *Am J Anat* 158: 229–264; Oelrich T. M. 1983. "The Striated Urogenital Sphincter in the Female." *Anat Rec* 205: 223–232; Roberts W. H., Habenicht J., Krishingner G. 1954. "The Pelvic and Perineal Fasciae and their Neural and Vascular Relationships." *Anat Rec* 149: 707–720.

* **A09.5.03.003** *Lig. transversum perinei* There is no transverse perineal ligament as such in the female. Milley P. S., Nichols D. H. 1971. "The Relationship Between the Pubourethral Ligament and the Urogenital Diaphragm in the Human Female." *Anat Rec* 170: 281–284.

* **A09.5.03.004 / A09.5.03.005 / A09.5.03.006** *M. transversus perinei profundus ♂/m. compressor urethrae ♀/m. sphincter urethrovaginalis ♀* The male symbol appears after *m. transversus perinei profundus* because in the female this muscle is represented only by smooth muscle. The female muscles are a part of the urogenital sphincter described by Oelrich T. M. 1983. "The Striated Urogenital Sphincter in the Human Female." *Anat Rec* 205: 223–232.

A10.1.00.000	**Cavitas abdominis et pelvis**	**Abdominopelvic cavity**
A10.1.00.001	Cavitas abdominis; Cavitas abdominalis	Abdominal cavity
A10.1.00.002	Cavitas pelvis; Cavitas pelvina	Pelvic cavity

A10.1.01.001	**Spatium extraperitoneale**	**Extraperitoneal space**
A10.1.01.002	Spatium retroperitoneale	Retroperitoneal space
A10.1.01.003	Spatium retropubicum	Retropubic space
A10.1.01.004	Spatium retroinguinale	Retro-inguinal space

A10.1.02.001	**Cavitas peritonealis**	**Peritoneal cavity**

A10.1.02.002	**Peritoneum**	**Peritoneum**
A10.1.02.003	Tunica serosa	Serosa; Serous coat
A10.1.02.004	Tela subserosa	Subserosa; Subserous layer
A10.1.02.005	Peritoneum parietale	Parietal peritoneum
A10.1.02.006	Peritoneum viscerale	Visceral peritoneum
A10.1.02.007	**Mesenterium**	**Mesentery**
A10.1.02.008	Radix mesenterii	Root of mesentery
A10.1.02.009	**Mesocolon**	**Mesocolon**
A10.1.02.010	Mesocolon transversum	Transverse mesocolon
A10.1.02.011	(Mesocolon ascendens)	(Ascending mesocolon)
A10.1.02.012	(Mesocolon descendens)	(Descending mesocolon)
A10.1.02.013	Mesocolon sigmoideum	Sigmoid mesocolon
A10.1.02.014	Mesoappendix	Meso-appendix
A10.1.02.101	**Omentum minus**	**Lesser omentum**
A10.1.02.102	Lig. hepatophrenicum	Hepatophrenic ligament
A10.1.02.103	Lig. hepatoesophageale	Hepato-oesophageal ligament▲
A10.1.02.104	Lig. hepatogastricum	Hepatogastric ligament
A10.1.02.105	Lig. hepatoduodenale	Hepatoduodenal ligament
A10.1.02.106	(Lig. hepatocolicum)	(Hepatocolic ligament)
A10.1.02.201	**Omentum majus**	**Greater omentum**
A10.1.02.202	Lig. gastrophrenicum	Gastrophrenic ligament
A10.1.02.203	Lig. gastrosplenicum; Lig. gastrolienale	Gastrosplenic ligament
A10.1.02.204	Plica presplenica	Presplenic fold
A10.1.02.205	(Lig. gastrocolicum)	(Gastrocolic ligament)
A10.1.02.206	Lig. phrenicosplenicum	Phrenicosplenic ligament
A10.1.02.207	Lig. splenorenale; Lig. lienorenale	Splenorenal ligament; Lienorenal ligament
A10.1.02.208	Lig. pancreaticosplenicum	Pancreaticosplenic ligament
A10.1.02.209	Lig. pancreaticocolicum	Pancreaticocolic ligament
A10.1.02.210	Lig. splenocolicum	Splenocolic ligament
A10.1.02.211	Lig. phrenicocolicum	Phrenicocolic ligament
A10.1.02.301	**Ligamenta hepatis**	**Peritoneal attachments of liver**
A10.1.02.302	Lig. coronarium	Coronary ligament
A10.1.02.303	Lig. falciforme	Falciform ligament
A10.1.02.304	Lig. triangulare dextrum	Right triangular ligament
A10.1.02.305	Lig. triangulare sinistrum	Left triangular ligament
A10.1.02.306	Lig. hepatorenale	Hepatorenal ligament
A10.1.02.401	**Recessus, fossae et plicae**	**Recesses, fossae and folds**
A10.1.02.402	Bursa omentalis	Omental bursa; Lesser sac
A10.1.02.403	Foramen omentale; Foramen epiploicum	Omental foramen; Epiploic foramen
A10.1.02.404	Vestibulum	Vestibule
A10.1.02.405	Recessus superior	Superior recess
A10.1.02.406	Recessus inferior	Inferior recess
A10.1.02.407	Recessus splenicus; Recessus lienalis	Splenic recess
A10.1.02.408	Plica gastropancreatica	Gastropancreatic fold
A10.1.02.409	Plica hepatopancreatica	Hepatopancreatic fold

A10.1.02.410	Plica duodenalis superior; Plica duodenojejunalis	Superior duodenal fold; Duodenojejunal fold
A10.1.02.411	Recessus duodenalis superior	Superior duodenal fossa
A10.1.02.412	Plica duodenalis inferior; Plica duodenomesocolica	Inferior duodenal fold; Duodenomesocolic fold
A10.1.02.413	Recessus duodenalis inferior	Inferior duodenal fossa
A10.1.02.414	(Plica paraduodenalis)	(Paraduodenal fold)
A10.1.02.415	(Recessus paraduodenalis)	(Paraduodenal recess)
A10.1.02.416	(Recessus retroduodenalis)	(Retroduodenal recess)
A10.1.02.417	Recessus intersigmoideus	Intersigmoid recess
A10.1.02.418	Recessus ileocaecalis superior	Superior ileocaecal recess▲
A10.1.02.419	Plica caecalis vascularis	Vascular fold of caecum▲
A10.1.02.420	Recessus ileocaecalis inferior	Inferior ileocaecal recess▲
A10.1.02.421	Plica ileocaecalis	Ileocaecal fold▲
A10.1.02.422	Recessus retrocaecalis	Retrocaecal recess▲
A10.1.02.423	Plicae caecales	Caecal folds▲
A10.1.02.424	Sulci paracolici	Paracolic gutters
A10.1.02.425	Recessus subphrenicus	Subphrenic space
A10.1.02.426	Recessus subhepaticus	Subhepatic space
A10.1.02.427	Recessus hepatorenalis	Hepatorenal recess
A10.1.02.428	Trigonum cystohepaticum	Cystohepatic triangle
A10.1.02.429	Plica umbilicalis mediana	Median umbilical fold
A10.1.02.430	Fossa supravesicalis	Supravesical fossa
A10.1.02.431	Plica umbilicalis medialis	Medial umbilical fold
A10.1.02.432	Fossa inguinalis medialis	Medial inguinal fossa
A10.1.02.433	Trigonum inguinale	Inguinal triangle
A10.1.02.434	Plica umbilicalis lateralis; Plica epigastrica	Lateral umbilical fold; Epigastric fold
A10.1.02.435	Fossa inguinalis lateralis	Lateral inguinal fossa
A10.1.02.501	**Peritoneum urogenitale**	**Urogenital peritoneum**
A10.1.02.502	Fossa paravesicalis	Paravesical fossa
A10.1.02.503	Plica vesicalis transversa	Transverse vesical fold
A10.1.02.504	Excavatio vesicouterina ♀	Vesico-uterine pouch ♀
A10.1.02.505	Lig. latum uteri ♀	Broad ligament of uterus ♀
A10.1.02.506	Mesometrium ♀	Mesometrium ♀
A10.1.02.507	Mesosalpinx ♀	Mesosalpinx ♀
A10.1.02.508	Mesovarium ♀	Mesovarium ♀
* **A10.1.02.509**	Trigonum parietale laterale pelvis ♀	Pelvic lateral wall triangle ♀
A10.1.02.510	Fossa ovarica ♀	Ovarian fossa ♀
A09.1.01.018	Lig. suspensorium ovarii ♀	Suspensory ligament of ovary; Infundibulopelvic ligament ♀
A10.1.02.511	Plica rectouterina ♀	Recto-uterine fold ♀
A10.1.02.512	Excavatio rectouterina ♀	Recto-uterine pouch ♀
A10.1.02.513	Excavatio rectovesicalis ♂	Recto-vesical pouch ♂
A10.1.02.514	Fossa pararectalis	Pararectal fossa

* **A10.1.02.509** *Trigonum parietale laterale pelvis* Laparoscopists enter pelvic extraperitoneal tissue planes through this triangle which is bounded anteriorly by *lig. teres*, laterally by *a. iliacus externus* and medially by *lig. suspensorium ovarii*.

A11.0.00.000 Glandulae endocrinae — Endocrine glands

A11.1.00.001	**Hypophysis; Glandula pituitaria**	**Pituitary gland**
A11.1.00.002	Adenohypophysis; Lobus anterior	Adenohypophysis; Anterior lobe
A11.1.00.003	Pars tuberalis	Pars tuberalis
A11.1.00.004	Pars intermedia	Pars intermedia
A11.1.00.005	Pars distalis	Pars distalis; Pars anterior
A11.1.00.006	Neurohypophysis; Lobus posterior	Neurohypophysis; Posterior lobe
A11.1.00.007	Infundibulum	Infundibulum
A11.1.00.008	Lobus nervosus; Pars nervosa	Neural lobe; Pars nervosa

* **A11.2.00.001**	**Glandula pinealis; Corpus pineale**	**Pineal gland; Pineal body**

A11.3.00.001	**Glandula thyroidea**	**Thyroid gland**
A11.3.00.002	Lobus	Lobe
A11.3.00.003	Isthmus glandulae thyroideae	Isthmus
A11.3.00.004	(Lobus pyramidalis)	(Pyramidal lobe)
A11.3.00.005	Glandulae thyroideae accessoriae	Accessory thyroid glands
A11.3.00.006	Capsula fibrosa	Fibrous capsule
A11.3.00.007	Stroma	Stroma
A11.3.00.008	Parenchyma	Parenchyma
A11.3.00.009	Lobuli	Lobules

A11.4.00.001	**Glandula parathyroidea**	**Parathyroid gland**
A11.4.00.002	Glandula parathyroidea superior	Superior parathyroid gland
A11.4.00.003	Glandula parathyroidea inferior	Inferior parathyroid gland
A11.4.00.004	Glandulae parathyroideae accessoriae	Accessory parathyroid glands

A11.5.00.001	**Glandula suprarenalis**	**Suprarenal gland; Adrenal gland**
A11.5.00.002	Facies anterior	Anterior surface
A11.5.00.003	Facies posterior	Posterior surface
A11.5.00.004	Facies renalis	Renal surface
A11.5.00.005	Margo superior	Superior border
A11.5.00.006	Margo medialis	Medial border
A11.5.00.007	Cortex	Cortex
A11.5.00.008	Medulla	Medulla
A11.5.00.009	Hilum	Hilum
A11.5.00.010	V. centralis	Central vein
A11.5.00.011	Glandulae suprarenales accessoriae	Accessory suprarenal glands

A05.9.01.019	**Insulae pancreaticae**	**Pancreatic islets**

* **A11.2.00.001** *Glandula pinealis* This is known under many different names, e.g. *epiphysis cerebri, corpus pineale, organum pineale, glandula pinealis, conarium*, commonly used English terms being pineal gland, pineal body, or simply pineal. The term *glandula pinealis* is preferred, because the endocrine function of the pineal gland has been established beyond any doubt.

A12.0.00.000 Systema cardiovasculare — Cardiovascular system

	Nomina generalia	*General terms*
A12.0.00.001	Vas sanguineum	Blood vessel
* **A12.0.00.002**	Anastomosis arteriolovenularis; Anastomosis arteriovenosa	Arteriolovenular anastomosis; Arteriovenous anastomosis
A12.0.00.003	Arteria	Artery
A12.0.00.004	A. nutricia; A. nutriens	Nutrient artery
A12.0.00.005	Arteriola	Arteriole
A12.0.00.006	Circulus arteriosus	Arterial circle
A12.0.00.007	Circulus vasculosus	Vascular circle
A12.0.00.008	Cisterna	Cistern
A12.0.00.009	Haema; Sanguis	Blood
A12.0.00.010	Plexus vasculosus	Vascular plexus
A12.0.00.011	Plexus venosus	Venous plexus
A12.0.00.012	Rete arteriosum	Arterial plexus
A12.0.00.013	Rete mirabile	Rete mirabile
A12.0.00.014	Rete vasculosum articulare	Articular vascular plexus
A12.0.00.015	Rete venosum	Venous plexus
A12.0.00.016	Sinus venosus	Sinus venosus
A12.0.00.017	Tunica externa	Tunica externa
A12.0.00.018	Tunica intima	Tunica intima
A12.0.00.019	Tunica media	Tunica media
A12.0.00.020	Valva	Valve
A12.0.00.021	Valvula	Cusp
A12.0.00.022	Cuspis	Cusp
A12.0.00.023	Valvula venosa	Venous valve
A12.0.00.024	Vas anastomoticum	Anastomotic vessel
A12.0.00.025	Vas capillare	Capillary
A12.0.00.026	Vas collaterale	Collateral vessel
A12.0.00.027	Vas sinusoideum	Sinusoid
A12.0.00.028	Vasa vasorum	Vasa vasorum
A12.0.00.029	Vasa nervorum	Vessels of nerves
A12.0.00.030	Vena	Vein
A12.0.00.031	V. comitans	Vena comitans
A12.0.00.032	V. cutanea	Cutaneous vein
A12.0.00.033	V. emissaria	Emissary vein
A12.0.00.034	V. nutricia; V. nutriens	Nutrient vein
A12.0.00.035	V. profunda	Deep vein
A12.0.00.036	V. superficialis	Superficial vein
A12.0.00.037	Venula	Venule
A12.0.00.038	Vas lymphaticum	Lymphatic vessel
A12.0.00.039	Vas lymphaticum superficiale	Superficial lymph vessel
A12.0.00.040	Vas lymphaticum profundum	Deep lymph vessel
A12.0.00.041	Plexus lymphaticus	Lymphatic plexus
A12.0.00.042	Valvula lymphatica	Lymphatic valvule
A12.0.00.043	Lympha	Lymph
A12.0.00.044	Vas lymphocapillare	Lymphatic capillary
A12.0.00.045	Rete lymphocapillare	Lymphatic rete

A12.1.00.001	**Cor**	**Heart**
A12.1.00.002	Basis cordis	Base of heart
A12.1.00.003	Facies sternocostalis; Facies anterior	Anterior surface; Sternocostal surface
A12.1.00.004	Facies diaphragmatica; Facies inferior	Diaphragmatic surface; Inferior surface
A12.1.00.005	Facies pulmonalis dextra/sinistra	Right/left pulmonary surface

* **A12.0.00.002** *Anastomosis arteriolovenularis* Although the term *anastomosis arteriovenosa* is widely used, for the sake of correctness *anastomosis arteriolovenularis* is the preferred term, since the structure in question does not link an artery and a vein, but an arteriole and a venule.

A12.1.00.006	Margo dexter	Right border
A12.1.00.007	Apex cordis	Apex of heart
A12.1.00.008	Incisura apicis cordis	Notch of cardiac apex
A12.1.00.009	Sulcus interventricularis anterior	Anterior interventricular sulcus
A12.1.00.010	Sulcus interventricularis posterior	Posterior interventricular sulcus
A12.1.00.011	Sulcus coronarius	Coronary sulcus
A12.1.00.012	Ventriculus cordis dexter/sinister	Right/left ventricle
A12.1.00.013	Septum interventriculare	Interventricular septum
A12.1.00.014	Pars muscularis	Muscular part
A12.1.00.015	Pars membranacea	Membranous part
A12.1.00.016	Septum atrioventriculare	Atrioventricular septum
A12.1.00.017	Atrium cordis dextrum/sinistrum	Right/ left atrium
A12.1.00.018	Auricula atrii	Auricle
A12.1.00.019	Septum interatriale	Interatrial septum
A12.1.00.020	Trabeculae carneae	Trabeculae carneae
A12.1.00.021	Vortex cordis	Vortex of heart
A12.1.00.022	Mm. papillares	Papillary muscles
A12.1.00.023	Chordae tendineae	Chordae tendineae; Tendinous cords
A12.1.00.024	Chordae tendineae falsae; Chordae tendineae spuriae	False chordae tendineae
A12.1.00.025	Trigonum fibrosum dextrum	Right fibrous trigone
A12.1.00.026	Trigonum fibrosum sinistrum	Left fibrous trigone
A12.1.00.027	Anulus fibrosus dexter/sinister	Right/left fibrous ring
A12.1.00.028	Tendo infundibuli	Tendon of infundibulum
A12.1.00.029	Tendo valvulae venae cavae inferioris	Tendon of valve of inferior vena cava
A12.1.00.030	Trigonum nodi sinuatrialis	Triangle of sinu-atrial node

A12.1.01.001	**Atrium dextrum**	**Right atrium**
A12.1.01.002	Auricula dextra	Right auricle
A12.1.01.003	Crista terminalis	Crista terminalis
A12.1.01.004	Foramina venarum minimarum	Openings of smallest cardiac veins
A12.1.01.005	Fossa ovalis	Fossa ovalis; Oval fossa
A12.1.01.006	Limbus fossae ovalis	Limbus fossae ovalis; Border of oval fossa
A12.1.01.007	(Foramen ovale cordis)	(Foramen ovale)
A12.1.01.008	Mm. pectinati	Musculi pectinati; Pectinate muscles
A12.1.01.009	Ostium sinus coronarii	Opening of coronary sinus
A12.1.01.010	Ostium venae cavae inferioris	Opening of inferior vena cava
A12.1.01.011	Ostium venae cavae superioris	Opening of superior vena cava
A12.1.01.012	Sinus venarum cavarum	Sinus of venae cavae
A12.1.01.013	Sulcus terminalis cordis	Sulcus terminalis cordis
A12.1.01.014	Tuberculum intervenosum	Intervenous tubercle
A12.1.01.015	Valvula venae cavae inferioris	Valve of inferior vena cava
A12.1.01.016	Valvula sinus coronarii	Valve of coronary sinus

A12.1.02.001	**Ventriculus dexter**	**Right ventricle**
A12.1.02.002	Ostium atrioventriculare dextrum	Right atrioventricular orifice
A12.1.02.003	Valva atrioventricularis dextra; Valva tricuspidalis	Tricuspid valve; Right atrioventricular valve
A12.1.02.004	Cuspis anterior	Anterior cusp
A12.1.02.005	Cuspis posterior	Posterior cusp
A12.1.02.006	Cuspis septalis	Septal cusp
A12.1.02.007	Crista supraventricularis	Supraventricular crest
A12.1.02.008	Conus arteriosus	Conus arteriosus; Infundibulum
A12.1.02.009	Ostium trunci pulmonalis	Opening of pulmonary trunk
A12.1.02.010	Valva trunci pulmonalis	Pulmonary valve

* A12.1.02.011	Valvula semilunaris dextra	Right semilunar cusp
* A12.1.02.012	Valvula semilunaris sinistra	Left semilunar cusp
* A12.1.02.013	Valvula semilunaris anterior	Anterior semilunar cusp
A12.1.02.014	Noduli valvularum semilunarium	Nodules of semilunar cusps
A12.1.02.015	Lunulae valvularum semilunarium	Lunules of semilunar cusps
A12.1.02.016	Commissurae valvularum semilunarium	Commissures of semilunar cusps
A12.1.02.017	M. papillaris anterior	Anterior papillary muscle
A12.1.02.018	M. papillaris posterior	Posterior papillary muscle
A12.1.02.019	M. papillaris septalis	Septal papillary muscle
A12.1.02.020	Trabecula septomarginalis	Septomarginal trabecula; Moderator band
A12.1.02.021	Trabeculae carneae	Trabeculae carneae

A12.1.03.001	**Atrium sinistrum**	**Left atrium**
A12.1.03.002	Auricula sinistra	Left auricle
A12.1.03.003	Mm. pectinati	Musculi pectinati; Pectinate muscles
A12.1.03.004	Ostia venarum pulmonalium	Openings of pulmonary veins
A12.1.03.005	Valvula foraminis ovalis	Valve of foramen ovale

A12.1.04.001	**Ventriculus sinister**	**Left ventricle**
A12.1.04.002	Ostium atrioventriculare sinistrum	Left atrioventricular orifice
A12.1.04.003	Valva atrioventricularis sinistra; Valva mitralis	Mitral valve; Left atrioventricular valve
A12.1.04.004	Cuspis anterior	Anterior cusp
A12.1.04.005	Cuspis posterior	Posterior cusp
* A12.1.04.006	Cuspides commissurales	Commissural cusps
A12.1.04.007	M. papillaris anterior	Anterior papillary muscle
A12.1.04.008	M. papillaris posterior	Posterior papillary muscle
A12.1.04.009	Vestibulum aortae	Aortic vestibule
A12.1.04.010	Ostium aortae	Aortic orifice
A12.1.04.011	Trabeculae carneae	Trabeculae carneae
A12.1.04.012	Valva aortae	Aortic valve
* A12.1.04.013	Valvula semilunaris dextra; Valvula coronaria dextra	Right semilunar cusp; Right coronary cusp
* A12.1.04.014	Valvula semilunaris sinistra; Valvula coronaria sinistra	Left semilunar cusp; Left coronary cusp
* A12.1.04.015	Valvula semilunaris posterior; Valvula non coronaria	Posterior semilunar cusp; Noncoronary cusp
A12.1.04.016	Noduli valvularum semilunarium	Nodules of semilunar cusps
A12.1.04.017	Lunulae valvularum semilunarium	Lunules of semilunar cusps
A12.1.04.018	Commissurae valvularum semilunarium	Commissures of semilunar cusps
A12.1.05.001	**Endocardium**	**Endocardium**
A12.1.06.001	**Myocardium**	**Myocardium**
A12.1.06.002	Complexus stimulans cordis; Systema conducente cordis	Conducting system of heart
A12.1.06.003	Nodus sinuatrialis	Sinu-atrial node
A12.1.06.004	Nodus atrioventricularis	Atrioventricular node
A12.1.06.005	Fasciculus atrioventricularis	Atrioventricular bundle
A12.1.06.006	Crus dextrum	Right bundle
A12.1.06.007	Crus sinistrum	Left bundle
A12.1.06.008	Rr. subendocardiales	Subendocardial branches
A07.1.03.001	**Cavitas pericardiaca**	**Pericardial cavity**
A12.1.07.001	Sinus transversus pericardii	Transverse pericardial sinus

* **A12.1.02.011 / A12.1.02.012 / A12.1.02.013** *Valvulae semilunares trunci pulmonalis* For didactic reasons the cusps of the pulmonary valve are named from their positions in fetal anatomy. In the adult, due to rotation in development, their positions become right anterior, posterior and left anterior respectively.

* **A12.1.04.006** *Cuspides commissurales* Small accessory cusps are almost always found between the two major cusps of the *valva atrioventricularis sinistra.*

* **A12.1.04.013 / A12.1.04.014 / A12.1.04.015** *Valvulae semilunares aortae* For didactic reasons the cusps of the aortic valve are named from their positions in fetal anatomy and from the origins of the coronary arteries. In the adult, due to rotation in development, their positions become anterior, left posterior and right posterior respectively.

A12.1.07.002	Sinus obliquus pericardii	Oblique pericardial sinus
A12.1.08.001	**Pericardium**	**Pericardium**
A12.1.08.002	Pericardium fibrosum	Fibrous pericardium
A12.1.08.003	Ligg. sternopericardiaca	Sternopericardial ligaments
* A12.1.08.004	Membrana bronchopericardiaca	Bronchopericardial membrane
A12.1.08.005	Pericardium serosum	Serous pericardium
A12.1.08.006	Lamina parietalis	Parietal layer
A12.1.08.007	Lamina visceralis; Epicardium	Visceral layer; Epicardium
A12.1.08.008	Tunica serosa	Serosa; Serous coat
A12.1.08.009	Tela subserosa	Subserosa; Subserous layer
A12.1.08.010	Plica venae cavae sinistrae	Fold of left vena cava

A12.2.00.001	**Arteriae**	**Arteries**
A12.2.01.001	**TRUNCUS PULMONALIS**	**PULMONARY TRUNK**
A12.2.01.002	Sinus trunci pulmonalis	Sinus of pulmonary trunk
A12.2.01.003	Crista supravalvularis	Supravalvular ridge
A12.2.01.004	Bifurcatio trunci pulmonalis	Bifurcation of pulmonary trunk

A12.2.01.101	**Arteria pulmonalis dextra**	**Right pulmonary artery**
A12.2.01.102	Aa. lobares superiores	Superior lobar arteries
A12.2.01.103	A. segmentalis apicalis	Apical segmental artery
A12.2.01.104	A. segmentalis anterior	Anterior segmental artery
A12.2.01.105	R. ascendens	Ascending branch
A12.2.01.106	R. descendens	Descending branch
A12.2.01.107	A. segmentalis posterior	Posterior segmental artery
A12.2.01.108	R. ascendens	Ascending branch
A12.2.01.109	R. descendens	Descending branch
A12.2.01.110	A. lobaris media	Middle lobar artery
A12.2.01.111	A. segmentalis medialis	Medial segmental artery
A12.2.01.112	A. segmentalis lateralis	Lateral segmental artery
A12.2.01.113	Aa. lobares inferiores	Inferior lobar arteries
A12.2.01.114	A. segmentalis superior	Superior segmental artery
A12.2.01.115	Pars basalis	Basal part
A12.2.01.116	A. segmentalis basalis anterior	Anterior basal segmental artery
A12.2.01.117	A. segmentalis basalis lateralis	Lateral basal segmental artery
A12.2.01.118	A. segmentalis basalis medialis	Medial basal segmental artery
A12.2.01.119	A. segmentalis basalis posterior	Posterior basal segmental artery

A12.2.01.201	**Arteria pulmonalis sinistra**	**Left pulmonary artery**
A12.2.01.202	Lig. arteriosum (Ductus arteriosus)	Ligamentum arteriosum (Ductus arteriosus)
A12.2.01.203	Aa. lobares superiores	Superior lobar arteries
A12.2.01.204	A. segmentalis apicalis	Apical segmental artery
A12.2.01.205	A. segmentalis anterior	Anterior segmental artery
A12.2.01.206	R. ascendens	Ascending branch
A12.2.01.207	R. descendens	Descending branch
A12.2.01.208	A. segmentalis posterior	Posterior segmental artery
A12.2.01.209	R. ascendens	Ascending branch
A12.2.01.210	R. descendens	Descending branch
A12.2.01.211	A. lingularis	Lingular artery

* **A12.1.08.004** *Membrana bronchopericardiaca* A connective tissue membrane consisting mainly of collagenous fibres that extends from the anterior surface of the tracheal bifurcation via the dorsal wall of the pericardium to the diaphragm. Three fibre directions can be discerned. Vertical fibres run in the direction just mentioned. Transverse fibres run from the pericardium into the lung where they join the adventitia of the large pulmonary veins. Oblique fibres extend from the two main bronchi diagonally over the pericardium into the opposite pulmonal ligaments. The membrane is the borderline between the middle and the posterior mediastinum, together with the tracheal bifurcation. Its function is to stabilize the tracheal bifurcation and that of the main bronchi, in relation to the dorsal aspect of the pericardium and the pulmonary hilus, during movements relating to respiration, the larynx, and the head. *Benninghoff Anatomie*. 1994. Edited by Drenckhahn D. and Zenker W. Vol. 1, p. 557. München-Wien-Baltimore: Urban & Schwarzenberg. Rauber/Kopsch. 1987. *Anatomie des Menschen*. Edited by Leonhardt H. Vol. 2, p. 159. "Innere Organe." Stuttgart, New York: Georg Thieme.

A12.2.01.212	A. lingularis inferior	Inferior lingular artery
A12.2.01.213	A. lingularis superior	Superior lingular artery
A12.2.01.214	Aa. lobares inferiores	Inferior lobar arteries
A12.2.01.215	A. segmentalis superior	Superior segmental artery
A12.2.01.216	Pars basalis	Basal part
A12.2.01.217	A. segmentalis basalis anterior	Anterior basal segmental artery
A12.2.01.218	A. segmentalis basalis lateralis	Lateral basal segmental artery
A12.2.01.219	A. segmentalis basalis medialis	Medial basal segmental artery
A12.2.01.220	A. segmentalis basalis posterior	Posterior basal segmental artery

A12.2.02.001	**AORTA**	**AORTA**
A12.2.03.001	**Pars ascendens aortae; Aorta ascendens**	**Ascending aorta**
A12.2.03.002	Sinus aortae	Aortic sinus
A12.2.03.003	Crista supravalvularis	Supravalvular ridge
A12.2.03.004	Bulbus aortae	Aortic bulb
A12.2.03.101	**Arteria coronaria dextra**	**Right coronary artery**
A12.2.03.102	Rr. atrioventriculares	Atrioventricular branches
A12.2.03.103	R. coni arteriosi	Conus branch
A12.2.03.104	R. nodi sinuatrialis	Sinu-atrial nodal branch
A12.2.03.105	Rr. atriales	Atrial branches
A12.2.03.106	R. marginalis dexter	Right marginal branch
A12.2.03.107	R. atrialis intermedius	Intermediate atrial branch
A12.2.03.108	R. interventricularis posterior	Posterior interventricular branch
A12.2.03.109	Rr. interventriculares septales	Interventricular septal branches
A12.2.03.110	R. nodi atrioventricularis	Atrioventricular nodal branch
A12.2.03.111	(R. posterolateralis dexter)	(Right posterolateral branch)
A12.2.03.201	**Arteria coronaria sinistra**	**Left coronary artery**
A12.2.03.202	R. interventricularis anterior	Anterior interventricular branch
A12.2.03.203	R. coni arteriosi	Conus branch
A12.2.03.204	R. lateralis	Lateral branch
A12.2.03.205	Rr. interventriculares septales	Interventricular septal branches
A12.2.03.206	R. circumflexus	Circumflex branch
A12.2.03.207	R. atrialis anastomoticus	Atrial anastomotic branch
A12.2.03.208	Rr. atrioventriculares	Atrioventricular branches
A12.2.03.209	R. marginalis sinister	Left marginal artery
A12.2.03.210	R. atrialis intermedius	Intermediate atrial branch
A12.2.03.211	R. posterior ventriculi sinistri	Posterior left ventricular branch
A12.2.03.212	(R. nodi sinuatrialis)	(Sinu-atrial nodal branch)
A12.2.03.213	(R. nodi atrioventricularis)	(Atrioventricular nodal branch)
A12.2.03.214	Rr. atriales	Atrial branches

A12.2.04.001	**Arcus aortae**	**Arch of aorta; Aortic arch**
A12.2.04.002	(Isthmus aortae)	(Aortic isthmus)
A12.2.04.003	Corpora paraaortica; Glomera aortica	Para-aortic bodies; Aortic glomera

A12.2.04.004	**Truncus brachiocephalicus**	**Brachiocephalic trunk**
A12.2.04.005	(A. thyroidea ima)	(Thyroid ima artery)

A12.2.04.006	**Arteria carotis communis**	**Common carotid artery**
A12.2.04.007	Glomus caroticum	Carotid body
A12.2.04.008	Sinus caroticus	Carotid sinus
A12.2.04.009	Bifurcatio carotidis	Carotid bifurcation

A12.2.05.001	**Arteria carotis externa**	**External carotid artery**
A12.2.05.002	**A. thyroidea superior**	**Superior thyroid artery**
A12.2.05.003	R. infrahyoideus	Infrahyoid branch

A12.2.05.004	R. sternocleidomastoideus	Sternocleidomastoid branch
A12.2.05.005	A. laryngea superior	Superior laryngeal artery
A12.2.05.006	R. cricothyroideus	Cricothyroid branch
A12.2.05.007	R. glandularis anterior	Anterior glandular branch
A12.2.05.008	R. glandularis posterior	Posterior glandular branch
A12.2.05.009	R. glandularis lateralis	Lateral glandular branch
A12.2.05.010	**Arteria pharyngea ascendens**	**Ascending pharyngeal artery**
A12.2.05.011	A. meningea posterior	Posterior meningeal artery
A12.2.05.012	Rr. pharyngeales	Pharyngeal branches
A12.2.05.013	A. tympanica inferior	Inferior tympanic artery
A12.2.05.014	**(Truncus linguofacialis)**	**(Linguofacial trunk)**
A12.2.05.015	**Arteria lingualis**	**Lingual artery**
A12.2.05.016	R. suprahyoideus	Suprahyoid branch
A12.2.05.017	Rr. dorsales linguae	Dorsal lingual branches
A12.2.05.018	A. sublingualis	Sublingual artery
A12.2.05.019	A. profunda linguae	Deep lingual artery
A12.2.05.020	**Arteria facialis**	**Facial artery**
A12.2.05.021	A. palatina ascendens	Ascending palatine artery
A12.2.05.022	R. tonsillaris	Tonsillar branch
A12.2.05.023	A. submentalis	Submental artery
A12.2.05.024	Rr. glandulares	Glandular branches
A12.2.05.025	A. labialis inferior	Inferior labial branch
A12.2.05.026	A. labialis superior	Superior labial branch
A12.2.05.027	R. septi nasi	Nasal septal branch
A12.2.05.028	R. lateralis nasi	Lateral nasal branch
A12.2.05.029	A. angularis	Angular artery
A12.2.05.030	**Arteria occipitalis**	**Occipital artery**
A12.2.05.031	R. mastoideus	Mastoid branch
A12.2.05.032	R. auricularis	Auricular branch
A12.2.05.033	Rr. sternocleidomastoidei	Sternocleidomastoid branches
A12.2.05.034	Rr. occipitales	Occipital branches
A12.2.05.035	(R. meningeus)	(Meningeal branch)
A12.2.05.036	R. descendens	Descending branch
A12.2.05.037	**Arteria auricularis posterior**	**Posterior auricular artery**
A12.2.05.038	A. stylomastoidea	Stylomastoid artery
A12.2.05.039	A. tympanica posterior	Posterior tympanic artery
A12.2.05.040	Rr. mastoidei	Mastoid branch
A12.2.05.041	(R. stapedius)	(Stapedial branch)
A12.2.05.042	R. auricularis	Auricular branch
A12.2.05.043	R. occipitalis	Occipital branch
A12.2.05.044	R. parotideus	Parotid branch
A12.2.05.045	**Arteria temporalis superficialis**	**Superficial temporal artery**
A12.2.05.046	R. parotideus	Parotid branch
A12.2.05.047	A. transversa faciei	Transverse facial artery
A12.2.05.048	Rr. auriculares anteriores	Anterior auricular branches
A12.2.05.049	A. zygomaticoorbitalis	Zygomatico-orbital artery
A12.2.05.050	A. temporalis media	Middle temporal artery
A12.2.05.051	R. frontalis	Frontal branch
A12.2.05.052	R. parietalis	Parietal branch
A12.2.05.053	**Arteria maxillaris**	**Maxillary artery**
A12.2.05.054	A. auricularis profunda	Deep auricular artery
A12.2.05.055	A. tympanica anterior	Anterior tympanic artery
A12.2.05.056	A. alveolaris inferior	Inferior alveolar artery
A12.2.05.057	Rr. dentales	Dental branches
A12.2.05.058	Rr. peridentales	Peridental branches
A12.2.05.059	R. mentalis	Mental branch
A12.2.05.060	R. mylohyoideus	Mylohyoid branch
A12.2.05.061	A. meningea media	Middle meningeal artery
A12.2.05.062	R. accessorius	Accessory branch

A12.2.05.063	R. frontalis	Frontal branch
A12.2.05.064	R. orbitalis	Orbital branch
A12.2.05.065	R. parietalis	Parietal branch
A12.2.05.066	R. petrosus	Petrosal branch
A12.2.05.067	A. tympanica superior	Superior tympanic artery
A12.2.05.068	R. anastomoticus cum a. lacrimali	Anastomotic branch with lacrimal artery
A12.2.05.069	A. pterygomeningea	Pterygomeningeal artery
A12.2.05.070	A. masseterica	Masseteric artery
A12.2.05.071	A. temporalis profunda anterior	Anterior deep temporal artery
A12.2.05.072	A. temporalis profunda posterior	Posterior deep temporal artery
A12.2.05.073	Rr. pterygoidei	Pterygoid branches
A12.2.05.074	A. buccalis	Buccal artery
A12.2.05.075	A. alveolaris superior posterior	Posterior superior alveolar artery
A12.2.05.076	Rr. dentales	Dental branches
A12.2.05.077	Rr. peridentales	Peridental branches
A12.2.05.078	A. infraorbitalis	Infra-orbital artery
A12.2.05.079	Aa. alveolares superiores anteriores	Anterior superior alveolar arteries
A12.2.05.080	Rr. dentales	Dental branches
A12.2.05.081	Rr. peridentales	Peridental branches
A12.2.05.082	A. canalis pterygoidei	Artery of pterygoid canal
A12.2.05.083	R. pharyngeus	Pharyngeal branch
A12.2.05.084	A. palatina descendens	Descending palatine artery
A12.2.05.085	A. palatina major	Greater palatine artery
A12.2.05.086	Aa. palatinae minores	Lesser palatine arteries
A12.2.05.087	R. pharyngeus	Pharyngeal branch
A12.2.05.088	A. sphenopalatina	Sphenopalatine artery
A12.2.05.089	Aa. nasales posteriores laterales	Posterior lateral nasal arteries
A12.2.05.090	Rr. septales posteriores	Posterior septal branches

A12.2.06.001	**Arteria carotis interna**	**Internal carotid artery**
A12.2.06.002	**Pars cervicalis**	**Cervical part**
A12.2.06.003	Sinus caroticus	Carotid sinus
A12.2.06.004	**Pars petrosa**	**Petrous part**
A12.2.06.005	Aa. caroticotympanicae	Caroticotympanic arteries
A12.2.06.006	A. canalis pterygoidei	Artery of pterygoid canal
A12.2.06.007	**Pars cavernosa**	**Cavernous part**
A12.2.06.008	R. basalis tentorii	Tentorial basal branch
A12.2.06.009	R. marginalis tentorii	Tentorial marginal branch
A12.2.06.010	R. meningeus	Meningeal branch
A12.2.06.011	R. sinus cavernosi	Cavernous branch
A12.2.06.012	A. hypophysialis inferior	Inferior hypophysial artery
A12.2.06.013	Rr. ganglionares trigeminales	Branches to trigeminal ganglion
A12.2.06.014	Rr. nervorum	Branches to nerves
A12.2.06.015	**Pars cerebralis**	**Cerebral part**
A12.2.06.016	A. ophthalmica	Ophthalmic artery
A12.2.06.017	A. hypophysialis superior	Superior hypophysial artery
A12.2.06.018	A. communicans posterior	Posterior communicating artery
A12.2.06.019	A. choroidea anterior	Anterior choroidal artery
A12.2.06.020	A. uncalis	Uncal artery
A12.2.06.021	Rr. clivales	Clivus branches
A12.2.06.022	R. meningeus	Meningeal branch
A12.2.06.023	**Siphon caroticum**	**Carotid syphon**
A12.2.06.016	**Arteria ophthalmica**	**Ophthalmic artery**
A12.2.06.024	A. centralis retinae	Central retinal artery
A12.2.06.025	Pars extraocularis	Extraocular part
A12.2.06.026	Pars intraocularis	Intraocular part
A12.2.06.027	A. lacrimalis	Lacrimal artery

A12.2.06.028	R. anastomoticus cum a. meningea media	Anastomotic branch with middle meningeal artery
A12.2.06.029	Aa. palpebrales laterales	Lateral palpebral arteries
A12.2.06.030	R. meningeus recurrens	Recurrent meningeal branch
A12.2.06.031	Aa. ciliares posteriores breves	Short posterior ciliary arteries
A12.2.06.032	Aa. ciliares posteriores longae	Long posterior ciliary arteries
A12.2.06.033	Aa. musculares	Muscular arteries
A12.2.06.034	Aa. ciliares anteriores	Anterior ciliary arteries
A12.2.06.035	Aa. conjunctivales anteriores	Anterior conjunctival arteries
A12.2.06.036	Aa. episclerales	Episcleral arteries
A12.2.06.037	A. supraorbitalis	Supra-orbital artery
A12.2.06.038	R. diploicus	Diploic branch
A12.2.06.039	A. ethmoidalis anterior	Anterior ethmoidal artery
A12.2.06.040	R. meningeus anterior	Anterior meningeal branch
A12.2.06.041	Rr. septales anteriores	Anterior septal branches
A12.2.06.042	Rr. nasales anteriores laterales	Anterior lateral nasal branches
A12.2.06.043	A. ethmoidalis posterior	Posterior ethmoidal artery
A12.2.06.044	Aa. palpebrales mediales	Medial palpebral arteries
A12.2.06.045	Aa. conjunctivales posteriores	Posterior conjunctival arteries
A12.2.06.046	Arcus palpebralis inferior	Inferior palpebral arch
A12.2.06.047	Arcus palpebralis superior	Superior palpebral arch
A12.2.06.048	A. supratrochlearis	Supratrochlear artery
A12.2.06.049	A. dorsalis nasi	Dorsal nasal artery; External nasal artery

A12.2.07.001	**Arteriae encephali**	**Arteries of brain**
A12.2.06.019	**A. choroidea anterior**	**Anterior choroidal artery**
A12.2.07.002	Rr. choroidei ventriculi lateralis	Choroidal branches to lateral ventricle
A12.2.07.003	(Rr. choroidei ventriculi tertii)	(Choroidal branches to third ventricle)
A12.2.07.004	Rr. substantiae perforatae anterioris	Branches to anterior perforated substance
A12.2.07.005	Rr. chiasmatici	Branches to optic chiasm; Branches to optic chiasma
A12.2.07.006	Rr. tractus optici	Branches to optic tract
A12.2.07.007	Rr. corporis geniculati lateralis	Branches to lateral geniculate body
A12.2.07.008	Rr. genus capsulae internae	Branches to internal capsule, genu
A12.2.07.009	Rr. cruris posterioris capsulae internae	Branches to internal capsule, posterior limb
A12.2.07.010	Rr. partis retrolentiformis capsulae internae	Branches to internal capsule, retrolentiform limb
A12.2.07.011	Rr. globi pallidi	Branches to globus pallidus
A12.2.07.012	Rr. caudae nuclei caudati	Branches to tail of caudate nucleus
A12.2.07.013	Rr. hippocampi	Branches to hippocampus
A12.2.07.014	(Rr. uncales)	(Branches to uncus)
A12.2.07.015	Rr. corporis amygdaloidei	Branches to amygdaloid body
A12.2.07.016	(Rr. tuberis cinerei)	(Branches to tuber cinereum)
A12.2.07.017	(Rr. nucleorum hypothalami)	(Branches to hypothalamic nuclei)
A12.2.07.018	Rr. nucleorum thalami	Branches to thalamic nuclei
A12.2.07.019	Rr. substantiae nigrae	Branches to substantia nigra
A12.2.07.020	Rr. nuclei rubri	Branches to red nucleus
A12.2.07.021	Rr. cruris cerebri	Branches to crus cerebri
A12.2.07.022	**Arteria cerebri anterior**	**Anterior cerebral artery**
A12.2.07.023	Pars precommunicalis; Segmentum A1	Precommunicating part; A1 segment
A12.2.07.024	Aa. centrales anteromediales	Anteromedial central arteries
A12.2.07.025	Aa. striatae mediales proximales	Proximal medial striate arteries
A12.2.07.026	A. supraoptica	Supraoptic artery
A12.2.07.027	Aa. perforantes anteriores	Anterior perforating arteries
A12.2.07.028	Aa. preopticae	Preoptic arteries
A12.2.07.029	A. communicans anterior	Anterior communicating artery
A12.2.07.024	Aa. centrales anteromediales	Anteromedial central arteries
A12.2.07.030	A. suprachiasmatica	Suprachiasmatic artery
A12.2.07.031	A. commissuralis mediana	Median commissural artery

A12.2.07.032	A. callosa mediana	Median callosal artery
A12.2.07.033	Pars postcommunicalis; Segmentum A2	Postcommunicating part; A2 segment
A12.2.07.034	A. striata medialis distalis	Distal medial striate artery
A12.2.07.035	A. frontobasalis medialis; A. orbitofrontalis medialis	Medial frontobasal artery; Medial orbitofrontal artery
A12.2.07.036	A. polaris frontalis	Polar frontal artery
A12.2.07.037	A. callosomarginalis	Callosomarginal artery
A12.2.07.038	R. frontalis anteromedialis	Anteromedial frontal branch
A12.2.07.039	R. frontalis intermediomedialis	Intermediomedial frontal branch
A12.2.07.040	R. frontalis posteromedialis	Posteromedial frontal branch
A12.2.07.041	R. cingularis	Cingular branch
A12.2.07.042	Rr. paracentrales	Paracentral branches
A12.2.07.043	A. pericallosa	Pericallosal artery
A12.2.07.042	(Rr. paracentrales)	(Paracentral branches)
A12.2.07.044	Rr. precuneales	Precuneal branches
A12.2.07.045	Rr. parietooccipitales	Parieto-occipital branches
A12.2.07.046	**Arteria cerebri media**	**Middle cerebral artery**
A12.2.07.047	Pars sphenoidalis; Pars horizontalis; Segmentum M1	Sphenoid part; Horizontal part; M1 segment
A12.2.07.048	Aa. centrales anterolaterales	Anterolateral central arteries; Lenticulostriate arteries
A12.2.07.049	Rr. proximales laterales striati	Proximal lateral striate branches
A12.2.07.050	Rr. distales laterales striati	Distal lateral striate branches
A12.2.06.020	(A. uncalis)	(Uncal artery)
A12.2.07.051	A. polaris temporalis	Polar temporal artery
A12.2.07.052	A. temporalis anterior	Anterior temporal artery
A12.2.07.053	Pars insularis; Segmentum M2	Insular part; M2 segment
A12.2.07.054	Aa. insulares	Insular arteries
A12.2.07.055	Rr. terminales inferiores; Rr. corticales inferiores; Segmentum M2	Inferior terminal branches; Inferior cortical branches; M2 segment
A12.2.07.056	R. temporalis anterior	Anterior temporal branch
A12.2.07.057	R. temporalis medius	Middle temporal branch
A12.2.07.058	R. temporalis posterior	Posterior temporal branch
A12.2.07.059	R. temporooccipitalis	Temporo-occipital branch
A12.2.07.060	R. gyri angularis	Branch to angular gyrus
A12.2.07.061	Rr. terminales superiores; Rr. corticales superiores; Segmentum M2	Superior terminal branches; Superior cortical branches; M2 segment
A12.2.07.062	A. frontobasalis lateralis; A. orbitofrontalis lateralis	Lateral frontobasal artery; Lateral orbitofrontal artery
A12.2.07.063	A. prefrontalis	Prefrontal artery
A12.2.07.064	A. sulci precentralis	Artery of precentral sulcus
A12.2.07.065	A. sulci centralis	Artery of central sulcus
A12.2.07.066	A. sulci postcentralis	Artery of postcentral sulcus
A12.2.07.067	A. parietalis anterior	Anterior parietal artery
A12.2.07.068	A. parietalis posterior	Posterior parietal artery
A12.2.06.018	**Arteria communicans posterior**	**Posterior communicating artery**
A12.2.07.069	Aa. centrales posteromediales	Posteromedial central arteries
A12.2.07.070	Rr. anteriores	Anterior branches
A12.2.07.071	Rr. posteriores	Posterior branches
A12.2.07.072	R. chiasmaticus	Chiasmatic branch
A12.2.07.073	Aa. tuberis cinerei	Artery of tuber cinereum
A12.2.07.074	Rr. mediales	Medial branches
A12.2.07.075	Rr. laterales	Lateral branches
A12.2.07.076	A. thalamotuberalis	Thalamotuberal artery; Premammillary artery
A12.2.07.077	R. hypothalamicus	Hypothalamic branch
A12.2.07.078	Aa. mammillares	Mammillary arteries
A12.2.07.079	R. nervi oculomotorii	Branch to oculomotor nerve
A12.2.07.080	**Circulus arteriosus cerebri**	**Cerebral arterial circle**
A12.2.06.001	A. carotis interna	Internal carotid artery
A12.2.07.022	A. cerebri anterior	Anterior cerebral artery

A12.2.07.029	A. communicans anterior	Anterior communicating artery
A12.2.07.046	A. cerebri media	Middle cerebral artery
A12.2.06.018	A. communicans posterior	Posterior communicating artery
A12.2.07.081	A. basilaris	Basilar artery
A12.2.07.082	A. cerebri posterior	Posterior cerebral artery
A12.2.07.082	**Arteria cerebri posterior**	**Posterior cerebral artery**
A12.2.07.083	Pars precommunicalis; Segmentum P1	Precommunicating part; P1 segment
A12.2.07.084	Aa. centrales posteromediales	Posteromedial central arteries; Paramedian arteries
A12.2.07.085	Aa. circumferentiales breves	Short circumferential arteries
A12.2.07.086	A. thalami perforans	Thalamoperforating artery
A12.2.07.087	A. collicularis; A. quadrigeminalis	Collicular artery; Quadrigeminal artery
A12.2.07.088	Pars postcommunicalis; Segmentum P2	Postcommunicating part; P2 segment
A12.2.07.089	Aa. centrales posterolaterales	Posterolateral central arteries
A12.2.07.090	A. thalamogeniculata	Thalamogeniculate artery
A12.2.07.091	Rr. choroidei posteriores mediales	Posterior medial choroidal branches
A12.2.07.092	Rr. choroidei posteriores laterales	Posterior lateral choroidal branches
A12.2.07.093	Rr. pedunculares	Peduncular branches
A12.2.07.094	A. occipitalis lateralis; Segmentum P3	Lateral occipital artery; P3 segment
A12.2.07.095	Rr. temporales anteriores	Anterior temporal branches
A12.2.07.096	Rr. temporales intermedii; Rr. temporales medii	Intermediate temporal branches; Middle temporal branches
A12.2.07.097	Rr. temporales posteriores	Posterior temporal branches
A12.2.07.098	A. occipitalis medialis; Segmentum P4	Medial occipital artery; P4 segment
A12.2.07.099	R. corporis callosi dorsalis	Dorsal branch to corpus callosum
A12.2.07.100	R. parietalis	Parietal branch
A12.2.07.101	R. parietooccipitalis	Parieto-occipital branch
A12.2.07.102	R. calcarinus	Calcarine branch
A12.2.07.103	R. occipitotemporalis	Occipitotemporal branch

A12.2.08.001	**Arteria subclavia**	**Subclavian artery**
A12.2.08.002	**Arteria vertebralis**	**Vertebral artery**
A12.2.08.003	Pars prevertebralis	Prevertebral part
A12.2.08.004	Pars transversaria; Pars cervicalis	Cervical part
A12.2.08.005	Rr. spinales	Spinal branches
A12.2.08.006	Rr. radiculares	Radicular branches
A12.2.08.007	A. medullaris segmentalis	Segmental medullary artery
A12.2.08.008	Rr. musculares	Muscular branches
A12.2.08.009	Pars atlantica	Atlantic part
A12.2.08.010	Pars intracranialis	Intracranial part
A12.2.08.011	Rr. meningei	Meningeal branches
A12.2.08.012	A. inferior posterior cerebelli	Posterior inferior cerebellar artery
A12.2.08.013	A. spinalis posterior	Posterior spinal artery
A12.2.08.014	R. tonsillae cerebelli	Cerebellar tonsillar branch
A12.2.08.015	R. choroideus ventriculi quarti	Choroidal branch to fourth ventricle
A12.2.08.016	A. spinalis anterior	Anterior spinal artery
A12.2.08.017	Rr. medullares mediales	Medial medullary branches
A12.2.08.018	Rr. medullares laterales	Lateral medullary branches
A12.2.07.081	**Arteria basilaris**	**Basilar artery**
A12.2.08.019	A. inferior anterior cerebelli	Anterior inferior cerebellar artery
A12.2.08.020	A. labyrinthi	Labyrinthine artery
A12.2.08.021	Aa. pontis	Pontine arteries
A12.2.08.022	Rr. mediales	Medial branches; Paramedian pontine branches
A12.2.08.023	Rr. laterales	Lateral branches; Circumferential pontine branches
A12.2.08.024	Aa. mesencephalicae	Mesencephalic arteries
A12.2.08.025	A. superior cerebelli	Superior cerebellar artery

A12.2.08.026	R. medialis	Medial branch; Medial superior cerebellar artery
A12.2.08.027	A. vermis superior	Superior vermian branch
A12.2.08.028	R. lateralis	Lateral branch; Lateral superior cerebellar artery
A12.2.07.082	A. cerebri posterior	Posterior cerebral artery
A12.2.08.029	**Arteria thoracica interna**	**Internal thoracic artery**
A12.2.08.030	Rr. mediastinales	Mediastinal branches
A12.2.08.031	Rr. thymici	Thymic branches
A12.2.08.032	(Rr. bronchiales)	(Bronchial branches)
A12.2.08.033	(Rr. tracheales)	(Tracheal branches)
A12.2.08.034	A. pericardiacophrenica	Pericardiacophrenic artery
A12.2.08.035	Rr. sternales	Sternal branches
A12.2.08.036	Rr. perforantes	Perforating branches
A12.2.08.037	Rr. mammarii mediales	Medial mammary branches
A12.2.08.038	(R. costalis lateralis)	(Lateral costal branch)
A12.2.08.039	Rr. intercostales anteriores	Anterior intercostal branches
A12.2.08.040	A. musculophrenica	Musculophrenic artery
A12.2.08.041	A. epigastrica superior	Superior epigastric artery
A12.2.08.042	**Truncus thyrocervicalis**	**Thyrocervical trunk**
A12.2.08.043	A. thyroidea inferior	Inferior thyroid artery
A12.2.08.044	A. laryngea inferior	Inferior laryngeal artery
A12.2.08.045	Rr. glandulares	Glandular branches
A12.2.08.046	Rr. pharyngeales	Pharyngeal branches
A12.2.08.047	Rr. oesophageales	Oesophageal branches▲
A12.2.08.048	Rr. tracheales	Tracheal branches
A12.2.08.049	A. cervicalis ascendens	Ascending cervical artery
A12.2.08.050	Rr. spinales	Spinal branches
A12.2.08.051	A. suprascapularis	Suprascapular artery
A12.2.08.052	R. acromialis	Acromial branch
A12.2.08.053	A. transversa colli; A. transversa cervicis	Transverse cervical artery
A12.2.08.054	R. superficialis	Superficial cervical artery
A12.2.08.055	R. ascendens	Ascending branch
A12.2.08.056	R. descendens	Descending branch
A12.2.08.057	R. profundus; A. dorsalis scapulae	Deep branch; Dorsal scapular artery
A12.2.08.058	(A. dorsalis scapulae)	(Dorsal scapular artery)
A12.2.08.059	**Truncus costocervicalis**	**Costocervical trunk**
A12.2.08.060	A. cervicalis profunda	Deep cervical artery
A12.2.08.061	A. intercostalis suprema	Supreme intercostal artery
A12.2.08.062	A. intercostalis posterior prima	First posterior intercostal artery
A12.2.08.063	A. intercostalis posterior secunda	Second posterior intercostal artery
A12.2.08.064	Rr. dorsales	Dorsal branches
A12.2.08.065	Rr. spinales	Spinal branches

A12.2.09.001	ARTERIAE MEMBRI SUPERIORIS	ARTERIES OF UPPER LIMB
A12.2.09.002	**Arteria axillaris**	**Axillary artery**
A12.2.09.003	Rr. subscapulares	Subscapular branches
A12.2.09.004	A. thoracica superior	Superior thoracic artery
A12.2.09.005	A. thoracoacromialis	Thoraco-acromial artery
A12.2.09.006	R. acromialis	Acromial branch
A12.2.09.007	Rete acromiale	Acromial anastomosis
A12.2.09.008	R. clavicularis	Clavicular branch
A12.2.09.009	R. deltoideus	Deltoid branch
A12.2.09.010	Rr. pectorales	Pectoral branches
A12.2.09.011	A. thoracica lateralis	Lateral thoracic artery
A12.2.09.012	Rr. mammarii laterales	Lateral mammary branches
A12.2.09.013	A. subscapularis	Subscapular artery
A12.2.09.014	A. thoracodorsalis	Thoracodorsal artery

A12.2.09.015	A. circumflexa scapulae	Circumflex scapular artery
A12.2.09.016	A. circumflexa humeri anterior	Anterior circumflex humeral artery
A12.2.09.017	A. circumflexa humeri posterior	Posterior circumflex humeral artery
A12.2.09.018	**Arteria brachialis**	**Brachial artery**
A12.2.09.019	(A. brachialis superficialis)	(Superficial brachial artery)
A12.2.09.020	A. profunda brachii	Profunda brachii artery; Deep artery of arm
A12.2.09.021	Aa. nutriciae humeri; Aa. nutrientes humeri	Humeral nutrient arteries
A12.2.09.022	R. deltoideus	Deltoid branch
A12.2.09.023	A. collateralis media	Medial collateral artery
A12.2.09.024	A. collateralis radialis	Radial collateral artery
A12.2.09.025	A. collateralis ulnaris superior	Superior ulnar collateral artery
A12.2.09.026	A. collateralis ulnaris inferior	Inferior ulnar collateral artery
A12.2.09.027	**Arteria radialis**	**Radial artery**
A12.2.09.028	A. recurrens radialis	Radial recurrent artery
A12.2.09.029	A. nutricia radii; A. nutriens radii	Nutrient artery of radius
A12.2.09.030	R. carpalis palmaris	Palmar carpal branch
A12.2.09.031	R. palmaris superficialis	Superficial palmar branch
A12.2.09.032	R. carpalis dorsalis	Dorsal carpal branch
A12.2.09.033	Rete carpale dorsale	Dorsal carpal arch
A12.2.09.034	Aa. metacarpales dorsales	Dorsal metacarpal arteries
A12.2.09.035	Aa. digitales dorsales	Dorsal digital arteries
A12.2.09.036	A. princeps pollicis	Princeps pollicis artery
A12.2.09.037	A. radialis indicis	Radialis indicis artery
A12.2.09.038	Arcus palmaris profundus	Deep palmar arch
A12.2.09.039	Aa. metacarpales palmares	Palmar metacarpal arteries
A12.2.09.040	Rr. perforantes	Perforating branches
A12.2.09.041	**Arteria ulnaris**	**Ulnar artery**
A12.2.09.042	A. recurrens ulnaris	Ulnar recurrent artery
A12.2.09.043	R. anterior	Anterior branch
A12.2.09.044	R. posterior	Posterior branch
A12.2.09.045	Rete articulare cubiti	Cubital anastomosis
A12.2.09.046	A. nutricia ulnae; A. nutriens ulnae	Nutrient artery of ulna
A12.2.09.047	A. interossea communis	Common interosseous artery
A12.2.09.048	A. interossea anterior	Anterior interosseous artery
A12.2.09.049	A. comitans nervi mediani	Median artery
A12.2.09.050	A. interossea posterior	Posterior interosseous artery
A12.2.09.051	R. perforans	Perforating branch
A12.2.09.052	A. interossea recurrens	Recurrent interosseous artery
A12.2.09.053	R. carpalis dorsalis	Dorsal carpal branch
A12.2.09.054	R. carpalis palmaris	Palmar carpal branch
A12.2.09.055	R. palmaris profundus	Deep palmar branch
A12.2.09.056	Arcus palmaris superficialis	Superficial palmar arch
A12.2.09.057	Aa. digitales palmares communes	Common palmar digital arteries
A12.2.09.058	Aa. digitales palmares propriae	Proper palmar digital arteries

A12.2.10.001	**Pars descendens aortae; Aorta descendens**	**Descending aorta**

A12.2.11.001	**Pars thoracica aortae; Aorta thoracica**	**Thoracic aorta**
A12.2.11.002	Rr. bronchiales	Bronchial branches
A12.2.11.003	Rr. oesophageales	Oesophageal branches▲
A12.2.11.004	Rr. pericardiaci	Pericardial branches
A12.2.11.005	Rr. mediastinales	Mediastinal branches
A12.2.11.006	Aa. phrenicae superiores	Superior phrenic arteries
A12.2.11.007	Aa. intercostales posteriores	Posterior intercostal arteries
A12.2.11.008	R. dorsalis	Dorsal branch
A12.2.11.009	R. cutaneus medialis	Medial cutaneous branch
A12.2.11.010	R. cutaneus lateralis	Lateral cutaneous branch

* A12.2.11.011	Rr. spinales	Spinal branches
A12.2.11.012	R. postcentralis	Postcentral branch
A12.2.11.013	R. prelaminaris	Prelaminar branch
A12.2.11.014	A. radicularis posterior	Posterior radicular artery
A12.2.11.015	A. radicularis anterior	Anterior radicular artery
A12.2.11.016	A. medullaris segmentalis	Segmental medullary artery
A12.2.11.017	R. collateralis	Collateral branch
A12.2.11.018	R. cutaneus lateralis	Lateral cutaneous branch
A12.2.11.019	Rr. mammarii laterales	Lateral mammary branches
A12.2.11.020	A. subcostalis	Subcostal artery
A12.2.11.021	R. dorsalis	Dorsal branch
A12.2.11.022	R. spinalis	Spinal branch

A12.2.12.001	**Pars abdominalis aortae; Aorta abdominalis**	**Abdominal aorta**
A12.2.12.002	**A. phrenica inferior**	**Inferior phrenic artery**
A12.2.12.003	Aa. suprarenales superiores	Superior suprarenal arteries
A12.2.12.004	**Aa. lumbales**	**Lumbar arteries**
A12.2.12.005	R. dorsalis	Dorsal branch
A12.2.12.006	R. spinalis	Spinal branch
A12.2.12.007	A. medullaris segmentalis	Segmental medullary artery
A12.2.12.008	**A. sacralis mediana**	**Median sacral artery**
A12.2.12.009	Aa. lumbales imae	Arteriae lumbales imae
A12.2.12.010	Rr. sacrales laterales	Lateral sacral branches
A12.2.12.011	Glomus coccygeum	Coccygeal body
A12.2.12.012	**Truncus coeliacus**	**Coeliac trunk**▲
A12.2.12.013	A. gastrica sinistra	Left gastric artery
A12.2.12.014	Rr. oesophageales	Oesophageal branches▲
A12.2.12.015	A. hepatica communis	Common hepatic artery
A12.2.12.016	A. gastroduodenalis	Gastroduodenal artery
A12.2.12.017	(A. supraduodenalis)	(Supraduodenal artery)
A12.2.12.018	A. pancreaticoduodenalis superior posterior	Posterior superior pancreaticoduodenal artery
A12.2.12.019	Rr. pancreatici	Pancreatic branches
A12.2.12.020	Rr. duodenales	Duodenal branches
A12.2.12.021	Aa. retroduodenales	Retroduodenal arteries
A12.2.12.022	A. gastroomentalis dextra	Right gastro-omental artery; Right gastro-epiploic artery
A12.2.12.023	Rr. gastrici	Gastric branches
A12.2.12.024	Rr. omentales	Omental branches
A12.2.12.025	A. pancreaticoduodenalis superior anterior	Anterior superior pancreaticoduodenal artery
A12.2.12.026	Rr. pancreatici	Pancreatic branches
A12.2.12.027	Rr. duodenales	Duodenal branches
A12.2.12.028	A. gastrica dextra	Right gastric artery
A12.2.12.029	A. hepatica propria	Hepatic artery proper
A12.2.12.030	R. dexter	Right branch
A12.2.12.031	A. cystica	Cystic artery
A12.2.12.032	A. lobi caudati	Artery of caudate lobe
A12.2.12.033	A. segmenti anterioris	Anterior segmental artery
A12.2.12.034	A. segmenti posterioris	Posterior segmental artery
A12.2.12.035	R. sinister	Left branch
A12.2.12.036	A. lobi caudati	Artery of caudate lobe
A12.2.12.037	A. segmenti medialis	Medial segmental artery
A12.2.12.038	A. segmenti lateralis	Lateral segmental artery

A12.2.11.011 *Rr. spinales* The branches of the *ramus dorsalis* of an *arteria intercostalis posterior* that enter an intervertebral foramen include one that tracks behind the *corpus vertebrae (ramus postcentralis)*, one that tracks in front of the *lamina arcus vertebrae (ramus prelaminaris)*, one to the anterior root of the spinal nerve (*arteria radicularis anterior*), one to the posterior root of the spinal nerve (*arteria radicularis posterior*), and one that anastomoses with the anterior spinal artery (*arteria medullaris segmentalis*).

A12.2.12.039	R. intermedius	Intermediate branch
A12.2.12.040	A. splenica; A. lienalis	Splenic artery
A12.2.12.041	Rr. pancreatici	Pancreatic branches
A12.2.12.042	A. pancreatica dorsalis	Dorsal pancreatic artery
A12.2.12.043	A. pancreatica inferior	Inferior pancreatic artery
A12.2.12.044	A. prepancreatica	Prepancreatic artery
A12.2.12.045	A. pancreatica magna	Greater pancreatic artery
A12.2.12.046	A. caudae pancreatis	Artery to tail of pancreas
A12.2.12.047	A. gastroomentalis sinistra	Left gastro-omental artery; Left gastro-epiploic artery
A12.2.12.048	Rr. gastrici	Gastric branches
A12.2.12.049	Rr. omentales	Omental branches
A12.2.12.050	Aa. gastricae breves	Short gastric arteries
A12.2.12.051	Rr. splenici; Rr. lienales	Splenic branches
A12.2.12.052	A. gastrica posterior	Posterior gastric artery
A12.2.12.053	**Arteria mesenterica superior**	**Superior mesenteric artery**
A12.2.12.054	A. pancreaticoduodenalis inferior	Inferior pancreaticoduodenal artery
A12.2.12.055	R. anterior	Anterior branch
A12.2.12.056	R. posterior	Posterior branch
A12.2.12.057	Aa. jejunales	Jejunal arteries
A12.2.12.058	Aa. ileales	Ileal arteries
A12.2.12.059	A. ileocolica	Ileocolic artery
A12.2.12.060	A. caecalis anterior	Anterior caecal artery▲
A12.2.12.061	A. caecalis posterior	Posterior caecal artery▲
A12.2.12.062	A. appendicularis	Appendicular artery
A12.2.12.063	R. ilealis	Ileal branch
A12.2.12.064	R. colicus	Colic branch
A12.2.12.065	A. colica dextra	Right colic artery
A12.2.12.066	A. flexurae dextrae	Right flexural artery
A12.2.12.067	A. colica media	Middle colic artery
A12.2.12.068	A. marginalis coli; A. juxtacolica; Arcus marginalis coli	Marginal artery; Juxtacolic artery; Marginal arcade
A12.2.12.069	**A. mesenterica inferior**	**Inferior mesenteric artery**
A12.2.12.070	A. ascendens	Ascending artery
A12.2.12.071	A. colica sinistra	Left colic artery
A12.2.12.072	Aa. sigmoideae	Sigmoid arteries
A12.2.12.073	A. rectalis superior	Superior rectal artery
A12.2.12.074	**A. suprarenalis media**	**Middle suprarenal artery**
A12.2.12.075	**A. renalis**	**Renal artery**
A12.2.12.076	Rr. capsulares	Capsular branches
A12.2.12.077	A. suprarenalis inferior	Inferior suprarenal artery
A12.2.12.078	R. anterior	Anterior branch
A12.2.12.079	A. segmenti superioris	Superior segmental artery
A12.2.12.080	A. segmenti anterioris superioris	Anterior superior segmental artery
A12.2.12.081	A. segmenti anterioris inferioris	Anterior inferior segmental artery
A12.2.12.082	A. segmenti inferioris	Inferior segmental artery
A12.2.12.083	R. posterior	Posterior branch
A12.2.12.084	A. segmenti posterioris	Posterior segmental artery
A12.2.12.085	Rr. ureterici	Ureteric branches
* A08.1.03.001	Aa. intrarenales	Intrarenal arteries
A12.2.12.086	**A. ovarica** ♀	**Ovarian artery** ♀
A12.2.12.087	Rr. ureterici ♀	Ureteric branches ♀
A12.2.12.088	Rr. tubarii ♀	Tubal branches ♀
A12.2.12.086	**A. testicularis** ♂	**Testicular artery** ♂
A12.2.12.087	Rr. ureterici ♂	Ureteric branches ♂
A12.2.12.088	Rr. epididymales ♂	Epididymal branches ♂

* **A08.1.03.001** *Arteriae/venae intrarenales* For further details regarding the nomenclature of renal blood vessels, see the publications mentioned above in A08.1.01.015.

A12.2.13.001	**Bifurcatio aortae**	**Aortic bifurcation**
A12.2.14.001	**Arteria iliaca communis**	**Common iliac artery**
A12.2.15.001	**Arteria iliaca interna**	**Internal iliac artery**
A12.2.15.002	**A. iliolumbalis**	**Iliolumbar artery**
A12.2.15.003	R. lumbalis	Lumbar branch
A12.2.15.004	R. spinalis	Spinal branch
A12.2.15.005	R. iliacus	Iliacus branch
A12.2.15.006	**Aa. sacrales laterales**	**Lateral sacral arteries**
A12.2.15.007	Rr. spinales	Spinal branches
A12.2.15.008	**A. obturatoria**	**Obturator artery**
A12.2.15.009	R. pubicus	Pubic branch
A12.2.15.010	R. acetabularis	Acetabular branch
A12.2.15.011	R. anterior	Anterior branch
A12.2.15.012	R. posterior	Posterior branch
A12.2.15.013	**A. glutea superior**	**Superior gluteal artery**
A12.2.15.014	R. superficialis	Superficial branch
A12.2.15.015	R. profundus	Deep branch
A12.2.15.016	R. superior	Superior branch
A12.2.15.017	R. inferior	Inferior branch
A12.2.15.018	**A. glutea inferior**	**Inferior gluteal artery**
A12.2.15.019	A. comitans nervi ischiadici	Artery to sciatic nerve
A12.2.15.020	**A. umbilicalis**	**Umbilical artery**
A12.2.15.021	Pars patens	Patent part
A12.2.15.022	A. ductus deferentis ♂	Artery to ductus deferens; Artery to vas deferens ♂
A12.2.15.023	Rr. ureterici	Ureteric branches
A12.2.15.024	Aa. vesicales superiores	Superior vesical arteries
A12.2.15.025	Pars occlusa	Occluded part
A12.2.15.026	Chorda a. umbilicalis	Cord of umbilical artery
A12.2.15.027	**A. vesicalis inferior**	**Inferior vesical artery**
A12.2.15.028	Rr. prostatici ♂	Prostatic branches ♂
A12.2.15.029	**A. uterina** ♀	**Uterine artery** ♀
A12.2.15.030	Rr. helicini ♀	Helicine branches ♀
A12.2.15.031	Rr. vaginales ♀	Vaginal branches ♀
A12.2.15.032	(A. azygos vaginae) ♀	(Azygos artery of vagina) ♀
A12.2.15.033	R. ovaricus ♀	Ovarian branches ♀
A12.2.15.034	R. tubarius ♀	Tubal branch ♀
A12.2.15.035	**A. vaginalis** ♀	**Vaginal artery** ♀
A12.2.15.036	**A. rectalis media**	**Middle rectal artery**
A12.2.15.037	Rr. vaginales ♀	Vaginal branches ♀
A12.2.15.037	Rr. prostatici ♂	Prostatic branches♂
A12.2.15.038	**A. pudenda interna**	**Internal pudendal artery**
A12.2.15.039	A. rectalis inferior	Inferior rectal artery
A12.2.15.040	A. perinealis	Perineal artery
A12.2.15.041	Rr. labiales posteriores ♀	Posterior labial branches ♀
A12.2.15.041	Rr. scrotales posteriores ♂	Posterior scrotal branches ♂
A12.2.15.042	A. urethralis	Urethral artery
A12.2.15.043	A. bulbi vestibuli ♀	Artery of bulb of vestibule ♀
A12.2.15.043	A. bulbi penis ♂	Artery of bulb of penis ♂
A12.2.15.044	A. dorsalis clitoridis ♀	Dorsal artery of clitoris ♀
A12.2.15.044	A. dorsalis penis ♂	Dorsal artery of penis ♂
A12.2.15.045	A. profunda clitoridis ♀	Deep artery of clitoris ♀
A12.2.15.045	A. profunda penis ♂	Deep artery of penis ♂
A12.2.15.046	Aa. perforantes penis ♂	Perforating arteries of penis ♂

A12.2.16.001	ARTERIAE MEMBRI INFERIORIS	ARTERIES OF LOWER LIMB
A12.2.16.002	**Arteria iliaca externa**	**External iliac artery**
A12.2.16.003	A. epigastrica inferior	Inferior epigastric artery
A12.2.16.004	R. pubicus	Pubic branch
A12.2.16.005	R. obturatorius	Obturator branch
A12.2.16.006	(A. obturatoria accessoria)	(Accessory obturator artery)
A12.2.16.007	A. cremasterica ♂	Cremasteric artery ♂
A12.2.16.007	A. ligamenti teretis uteri ♀	Artery of round ligament of uterus ♀
A12.2.16.008	A. circumflexa ilium profunda	Deep circumflex iliac artery
A12.2.16.009	R. ascendens	Ascending branch
A12.2.16.010	**Arteria femoralis**	**Femoral artery**
A12.2.16.011	A. epigastrica superficialis	Superficial epigastric artery
A12.2.16.012	A. circumflexa ilium superficialis	Superficial circumflex iliac artery
A12.2.16.013	A. pudenda externa superficialis	Superficial external pudendal artery
A12.2.16.014	A. pudenda externa profunda	Deep external pudendal artery
A12.2.16.015	Rr. labiales anteriores ♀	Anterior labial branches ♀
A12.2.16.015	Rr. scrotales anteriores ♂	Anterior scrotal branches ♂
A12.2.16.016	Rr. inguinales	Inguinal branches
A12.2.16.017	A. descendens genus	Descending genicular artery
A12.2.16.018	R. saphenus	Saphenous branch
A12.2.16.019	Rr. articulares	Articular branches
A12.2.16.020	**Arteria profunda femoris**	**Deep artery of thigh**
A12.2.16.021	A. circumflexa femoris medialis	Medial circumflex femoral artery
A12.2.16.022	R. superficialis	Superficial branch
A12.2.16.023	R. profundus	Deep branch
A12.2.16.024	R. acetabularis	Acetabular branch
A12.2.16.025	R. ascendens	Ascending branch
A12.2.16.026	R. descendens	Descending branch
A12.2.16.027	A. circumflexa femoris lateralis	Lateral circumflex femoral artery
A12.2.16.028	R. ascendens	Ascending branch
A12.2.16.029	R. descendens	Descending branch
A12.2.16.030	R. transversus	Transverse branch
A12.2.16.031	Aa. perforantes	Perforating arteries
A12.2.16.032	Aa. nutriciae femoris; Aa. nutrientes femoris	Femoral nutrient arteries
A12.2.16.033	**Arteria poplitea**	**Popliteal artery**
A12.2.16.034	A. superior lateralis genus	Superior lateral genicular artery
A12.2.16.035	A. superior medialis genus	Superior medial genicular artery
A12.2.16.036	A. media genus	Middle genicular artery
A12.2.16.037	Aa. surales	Sural arteries
A12.2.16.038	A. inferior lateralis genus	Inferior lateral genicular artery
A12.2.16.039	A. inferior medialis genus	Inferior medial genicular artery
A12.2.16.040	Rete articulare genus	Genicular anastomosis
A12.2.16.041	Rete patellare	Patellar anastomosis
A12.2.16.042	**Arteria tibialis anterior**	**Anterior tibial artery**
A12.2.16.043	A. recurrens tibialis anterior	Anterior tibial recurrent artery
A12.2.16.044	(A. recurrens tibialis posterior)	(Posterior tibial recurrent artery)
A12.2.16.045	A. malleolaris anterior lateralis	Anterior lateral malleolar artery
A12.2.16.046	A. malleolaris anterior medialis	Anterior medial malleolar artery
A12.2.16.047	Rete malleolare laterale	Lateral malleolar network
A12.2.16.048	**Arteria dorsalis pedis**	**Dorsalis pedis artery; Dorsal artery of foot**
A12.2.16.049	A. tarsalis lateralis	Lateral tarsal artery
A12.2.16.050	Aa. tarsales mediales	Medial tarsal arteries
A12.2.16.051	(A. arcuata)	(Arcuate artery)
A12.2.16.052	Aa. metatarsales dorsales	Dorsal metatarsal arteries
A12.2.16.053	Aa. digitales dorsales	Dorsal digital arteries
A12.2.16.054	A. plantaris profunda	Deep plantar artery
A12.2.16.055	**Arteria tibialis posterior**	**Posterior tibial artery**
A12.2.16.056	R. circumflexus fibularis; R. circumflexus peronealis	Circumflex fibular branch; Circumflex peroneal branch

A12.2.16.057	Rr. malleolares mediales	Medial malleolar branches
A12.2.16.058	Rete malleolare mediale	Medial malleolar network
A12.2.16.059	Rr. calcanei	Calcaneal branches
A12.2.16.060	A. nutricia tibiae; A. nutriens tibiae	Tibial nutrient artery
A12.2.16.061	**Arteria plantaris medialis**	**Medial plantar artery**
A12.2.16.062	R. profundus	Deep branch
A12.2.16.063	R. superficialis	Superficial branch
A12.2.16.064	**Arteria plantaris lateralis**	**Lateral plantar artery**
A12.2.16.065	Arcus plantaris profundus	Deep plantar arch
A12.2.16.066	Aa. metatarsales plantares	Plantar metatarsal arteries
A12.2.16.067	Rr. perforantes	Perforating branches
A12.2.16.068	Aa. digitales plantares communes	Common plantar digital arteries
A12.2.16.069	Aa. digitales plantares propriae	Plantar digital arteries proper
A12.2.16.070	(Arcus plantaris superficialis)	(Superficial plantar arch)
A12.2.16.071	**Arteria fibularis; Arteria peronea**	**Fibular artery; Peroneal artery**
A12.2.16.072	R. perforans	Perforating branch
A12.2.16.073	R. communicans	Communicating branch
A12.2.16.074	Rr. malleolares laterales	Lateral malleolar branch
A12.2.16.075	Rr. calcanei	Calcaneal branches
A12.2.16.076	Rete calcaneum	Calcaneal anastomosis
A12.2.16.077	A. nutricia fibulae; A. nutriens fibulae	Fibular nutrient artery

A12.3.00.001	**Venae**	**Veins**
A12.3.01.001	**Venae cordis**	**Veins of heart**
A12.3.01.002	**Sinus coronarius**	**Coronary sinus**
A12.3.01.003	V. cardiaca magna; V. cordis magna	Great cardiac vein
A12.3.01.004	V. interventricularis anterior	Anterior interventricular vein
A12.3.01.005	V. marginalis sinistra	Left marginal vein
A12.3.01.006	V(v). ventriculi sinistri posterior(es)	Posterior vein(s) of left ventricle
A12.3.01.007	V. obliqua atrii sinistri	Oblique vein of left atrium
A12.3.01.008	Lig. venae cavae sinistrae	Ligament of left vena cava
A12.3.01.009	V. cardiaca media; V. cordis media; V. interventricularis posterior	Middle cardiac vein; Posterior interventricular vein
A12.3.01.010	V. cardiaca parva; V. cordis parva	Small cardiac vein
A12.3.01.011	V. marginalis dextra	Right marginal vein
A12.3.01.012	V(v). ventriculi dextri anterior(es); Vv. cardiacae anteriores; Vv. cordis anteriores	Anterior vein(s) of right ventricle; Anterior cardiac veins
A12.3.01.013	Vv. cardiacae minimae; Vv. cordis minimae	Small cardiac veins
A12.3.01.014	Vv. atriales dextrae	Right atrial veins
A12.3.01.015	Vv. ventriculares dextrae	Right ventricular veins
A12.3.01.016	(Vv. atriales sinistrae)	(Left atrial veins)
A12.3.01.017	(Vv. ventriculares sinistrae)	(Left ventricular veins)

A12.3.02.001	**Venae pulmonales**	**Pulmonary veins**

A12.3.02.101	**Vena pulmonalis dextra superior**	**Right superior pulmonary vein**
A12.3.02.102	V. apicalis; R. apicalis	Apical vein; Apical branch
A12.3.02.103	Pars intrasegmentalis	Intrasegmental part
A12.3.02.104	Pars intersegmentalis	Intersegmental part
A12.3.02.105	V. anterior; R. anterior	Anterior vein; Anterior branch
A12.3.02.106	Pars intrasegmentalis	Intrasegmental part
A12.3.02.107	Pars intersegmentalis	Intersegmental part
A12.3.02.108	V. posterior; R. posterior	Posterior vein; Posterior branch
A12.3.02.109	Pars infralobaris	Infralobar part
A12.3.02.110	Pars intralobaris (intersegmentalis)	Intralobar part
A12.3.02.111	V. lobi medii; R. lobi medii	Middle lobe vein; Middle lobe branch
A12.3.02.112	Pars lateralis	Lateral part
A12.3.02.113	Pars medialis	Medial part

A12.3.02.201	**Vena pulmonalis dextra inferior**	**Right inferior pulmonary vein**
A12.3.02.202	V. superior; R. superior	Superior vein; Superior branch
A12.3.02.203	Pars intrasegmentalis	Intrasegmental part
A12.3.02.204	Pars intersegmentalis	Intersegmental part
A12.3.02.205	V. basalis communis	Common basal vein
A12.3.02.206	V. basalis superior	Superior basal vein
A12.3.02.207	V. basalis anterior; R. basalis anterior	Anterior basal vein; Anterior basal branch
A12.3.02.208	Pars intrasegmentalis	Intrasegmental part
A12.3.02.209	Pars intersegmentalis	Intersegmental part
A12.3.02.210	V. basalis inferior	Inferior basal vein

A12.3.02.301	**Vena pulmonalis sinistra superior**	**Left superior pulmonary vein**
A12.3.02.302	V. apicoposterior; R. apicoposterior	Apicoposterior vein; Apicoposterior branch
A12.3.02.303	Pars intrasegmentalis	Intrasegmental part
A12.3.02.304	Pars intersegmentalis	Intersegmental part
A12.3.02.305	V. anterior; R. anterior	Anterior vein; Anterior branch
A12.3.02.306	Pars intrasegmentalis	Intrasegmental part
A12.3.02.307	Pars intersegmentalis	Intersegmental part
A12.3.02.308	V. lingularis; R. lingularis	Lingular vein; Lingular branch
A12.3.02.309	Pars superior	Superior part
A12.3.02.310	Pars inferior	Inferior part

A12.3.02.401	**Vena pulmonalis sinistra inferior**	**Left inferior pulmonary vein**
A12.3.02.402	V. superior; R. superior	Superior vein; Superior branch
A12.3.02.403	Pars intrasegmentalis	Intrasegmental part
A12.3.02.404	Pars intersegmentalis	Intersegmental part
A12.3.02.405	V. basalis communis	Common basal vein
A12.3.02.406	V. basalis superior	Superior basal vein
A12.3.02.407	V. basalis anterior; R. basalis anterior	Anterior basal vein; Anterior basal branch
A12.3.02.408	Pars intrasegmentalis	Intrasegmental part
A12.3.02.409	Pars intersegmentalis	Intersegmental part
A12.3.02.410	V. basalis inferior	Inferior basal vein

A12.3.03.001	**VENA CAVA SUPERIOR**	**SUPERIOR VENA CAVA**
A12.3.04.001	**Vena brachiocephalica**	**Brachiocephalic vein**
A12.3.04.002	V. thyroidea inferior	Inferior thyroid vein
A12.3.04.003	Plexus thyroideus impar	Unpaired thyroid plexus
A12.3.04.004	V. laryngea inferior	Inferior laryngeal vein
A12.3.04.005	Vv. thymicae	Thymic veins
A12.3.04.006	Vv. pericardiacae	Pericardial veins
A12.3.04.007	Vv. pericardiacophrenicae	Pericardiacophrenic veins
A12.3.04.008	Vv. mediastinales	Mediastinal veins
A12.3.04.009	Vv. bronchiales	Bronchial veins
A12.3.04.010	Vv. tracheales	Tracheal veins
A12.3.04.011	Vv. oesophageales	Oesophageal veins▲
A12.3.04.012	V. vertebralis	Vertebral vein
A12.3.04.013	V. occipitalis	Occipital vein
A12.3.04.014	V. vertebralis anterior	Anterior vertebral vein
A12.3.04.015	(V. vertebralis accessoria)	(Accessory vertebral vein)
A12.3.04.016	Plexus venosus suboccipitalis	Suboccipital venous plexus
A12.3.04.017	V. cervicalis profunda; V. colli profunda	Deep cervical vein
A12.3.04.018	Vv. thoracicae internae	Internal thoracic veins
A12.3.04.019	Vv. epigastricae superiores	Superior epigastric veins
A12.3.04.020	Vv. subcutaneae abdominis	Subcutaneous abdominal veins
A12.3.04.021	Vv. musculophrenicae	Musculophrenic veins
A12.3.04.022	Vv. intercostales anteriores	Anterior intercostal veins
A12.3.04.023	V. intercostalis suprema	Supreme intercostal vein
A12.3.04.024	V. intercostalis superior sinistra	Left superior intercostal vein

A12.3.05.001	**Vena jugularis interna**	**Internal jugular vein**
A12.3.05.002	Bulbus superior venae jugularis	Superior bulb of jugular vein
A12.3.05.003	Glomus jugulare	Jugular body; Tympanic body
A12.3.05.004	V. aqueductus cochleae	Vein of cochlear aqueduct
A12.3.05.005	Bulbus inferior venae jugularis	Inferior bulb of jugular vein
A12.3.05.006	Plexus pharyngeus	Pharyngeal plexus
A12.3.05.007	Vv. pharyngeae	Pharyngeal veins
A12.3.05.008	Vv. meningeae	Meningeal veins
A12.3.05.009	V. lingualis	Lingual vein
A12.3.05.010	Vv. dorsales linguae	Dorsal lingual veins
A12.3.05.011	V. comitans nervi hypoglossi	Vena comitans of hypoglossal nerve
A12.3.05.012	V. sublingualis	Sublingual vein
A12.3.05.013	V. profunda linguae	Deep lingual vein
A12.3.05.014	V. thyroidea superior	Superior thyroid vein
A12.3.05.015	Vv. thyroideae mediae	Middle thyroid veins
A12.3.05.016	V. sternocleidomastoidea	Sternocleidomastoid vein
A12.3.05.017	V. laryngea superior	Superior laryngeal vein
A12.3.05.018	**Vena facialis**	**Facial vein**
A12.3.05.019	V. angularis	Angular vein
A12.3.05.020	Vv. supratrochleares	Supratrochlear veins
A12.3.05.021	V. supraorbitalis	Supra-orbital vein
A12.3.05.022	Vv. palpebrales superiores	Superior palpebral veins
A12.3.05.023	Vv. nasales externae	External nasal veins
A12.3.05.024	Vv. palpebrales inferiores	Inferior palpebral veins
A12.3.05.025	V. labialis superior	Superior labial vein
A12.3.05.026	Vv. labiales inferiores	Inferior labial veins
A12.3.05.027	V. profunda faciei	Deep facial vein
A12.3.05.028	Vv. parotideae; Rr. parotidei	Parotid veins; Parotid branches
A12.3.05.029	V. palatina externa	External palatine vein
A12.3.05.030	V. submentalis	Submental vein
A12.3.05.031	**Vena retromandibularis**	**Retromandibular vein**
A12.3.05.032	Vv. temporales superficiales	Superficial temporal veins
A12.3.05.033	V. temporalis media	Middle temporal vein
A12.3.05.034	V. transversa faciei	Transverse facial vein
A12.3.05.035	Vv. maxillares	Maxillary veins
A12.3.05.036	Plexus pterygoideus	Pterygoid plexus
A12.3.05.037	Vv. meningeae mediae	Middle meningeal veins
A12.3.05.038	Vv. temporales profundae	Deep temporal veins
A12.3.05.039	V. canalis pterygoidei	Vein of pterygoid canal
A12.3.05.040	Vv. auriculares anteriores	Anterior auricular veins
A12.3.05.041	Vv. parotideae	Parotid veins
A12.3.05.042	Vv. articulares	Articular veins
A12.3.05.043	Vv. tympanicae	Tympanic veins
A12.3.05.044	V. stylomastoidea	Stylomastoid vein
A12.3.05.045	**Vena jugularis externa**	**External jugular vein**
A12.3.05.046	V. auricularis posterior	Posterior auricular vein
A12.3.05.047	V. jugularis anterior	Anterior jugular vein
A12.3.05.048	Arcus venosus jugularis	Jugular venous arch
A12.3.05.049	V. suprascapularis	Suprascapular vein
A12.3.05.050	Vv. transversae cervicis; Vv. transversae colli	Transverse cervical veins
A12.3.05.101	**Sinus durae matris**	**Dural venous sinuses**
A12.3.05.102	Sinus transversus	Transverse sinus
A12.3.05.103	Confluens sinuum	Confluence of sinuses
A12.3.05.104	Sinus marginalis	Marginal sinus
A12.3.05.105	Sinus occipitalis	Occipital sinus
A12.3.05.106	Plexus basilaris	Basilar plexus
A12.3.05.107	Sinus petrosquamosus	Petrosquamous sinus
A12.3.05.108	Sinus sigmoideus	Sigmoid sinus
A12.3.05.109	Sinus sagittalis superior	Superior sagittal sinus

A12.3.05.110	Lacunae laterales	Lateral lacunae
A12.3.05.111	Sinus sagittalis inferior	Inferior sagittal sinus
A12.3.05.112	Sinus rectus	Straight sinus
A12.3.05.113	Sinus petrosus inferior	Inferior petrosal sinus
A12.3.05.114	Vv. labyrinthi	Labyrinthine veins
A12.3.05.115	Sinus petrosus superior	Superior petrosal sinus
A12.3.05.116	Sinus cavernosus	Cavernous sinus
A12.3.05.117	Sinus intercavernosus anterior	Anterior intercavernous sinus
A12.3.05.118	Sinus intercavernosus posterior	Posterior intercavernous sinus
A12.3.05.119	Sinus sphenoparietalis	Sphenoparietal sinus
A12.3.05.201	**Venae diploicae**	**Diploic veins**
A12.3.05.202	V. diploica frontalis	Frontal diploic vein
A12.3.05.203	V. diploica temporalis anterior	Anterior temporal diploic vein
A12.3.05.204	V. diploica temporalis posterior	Posterior temporal diploic vein
A12.3.05.205	V. diploica occipitalis	Occipital diploic vein
A12.3.05.301	**Venae emissariae**	**Emissary veins**
A12.3.05.302	V. emissaria parietalis	Parietal emissary vein
A12.3.05.303	V. emissaria mastoidea	Mastoid emissary vein
A12.3.05.304	V. emissaria condylaris	Condylar emissary vein
A12.3.05.305	V. emissaria occipitalis	Occipital emissary vein
A12.3.05.306	Plexus venosus canalis nervi hypoglossi	Venous plexus of hypoglossal canal
A12.3.05.307	Plexus venosus foraminis ovalis	Venous plexus of foramen ovale
A12.3.05.308	Plexus venosus caroticus internus	Internal carotid venous plexus
A12.3.05.309	Vv. portales hypophysiales	Portal veins of hypophysis

A12.3.06.001	Venae encephali	Cerebral veins
A12.3.06.002	**Venae superficiales cerebri**	**Superficial cerebral veins**
A12.3.06.003	Vv. superiores cerebri	Superior cerebral veins
A12.3.06.004	Vv. prefrontales	Prefrontal veins
A12.3.06.005	Vv. frontales	Frontal veins
A12.3.06.006	Vv. parietales	Parietal veins
A12.3.06.007	Vv. temporales	Temporal veins
A12.3.06.008	Vv. occipitales	Occipital veins
A12.3.06.009	V. media superficialis cerebri	Superficial middle cerebral vein
A12.3.06.010	V. anastomotica inferior	Inferior anastomotic vein
A12.3.06.012	V. anastomotica superior	Superior anastomotic vein
A12.3.06.013	Vv. inferiores cerebri	Inferior cerebral veins
A12.3.06.014	V. uncalis	Vein of uncus
A12.3.06.015	Vv. orbitae	Orbital veins
A12.3.06.016	Vv. temporales	Temporal veins
A12.3.06.017	**Venae profundae cerebri**	**Deep cerebral veins**
A12.3.06.018	V. basalis	Basal vein
A12.3.06.019	Vv. anteriores cerebri	Anterior cerebral veins
A12.3.06.020	V. media profunda cerebri	Deep middle cerebral vein
A12.3.06.021	Vv. insulares	Insular veins
A12.3.06.022	Vv. thalamostriatae inferiores	Inferior thalamostriate veins
A12.3.06.023	V. gyri olfactorii	Vein of olfactory gyrus
A12.3.06.024	V. ventricularis inferior	Inferior ventricular vein
A12.3.06.025	V. choroidea inferior	Inferior choroid vein
A12.3.06.026	Vv. pedunculares	Peduncular veins
A12.3.06.027	V. magna cerebri	Great cerebral vein
A12.3.06.028	Vv. internae cerebri	Internal cerebral veins
A12.3.06.029	V. choroidea superior	Superior choroid vein
A12.3.06.030	V. thalamostriata superior; V. terminalis	Superior thalamostriate vein
A12.3.06.031	V. anterior septi pellucidi	Anterior vein of septum pellucidum
A12.3.06.032	V. posterior septi pellucidi	Posterior vein of septum pellucidum
A12.3.06.033	V. medialis ventriculi lateralis	Medial vein of lateral ventricle
A12.3.06.034	V. lateralis ventriculi lateralis	Lateral vein of lateral ventricle

A12.3.06.035	Vv. nuclei caudati	Veins of caudate nucleus
A12.3.06.036	Vv. directae laterales	Lateral direct veins
A12.3.06.037	V. posterior corporis callosi; V. dorsalis corporis callosi	Posterior vein of corpus callosum; Dorsal vein of corpus callosum
A12.3.06.038	**Venae trunci encephali**	**Veins of brainstem**
A12.3.06.039	V. pontomesencephalica	Pontomesencephalic vein
A12.3.06.040	Vv. interpedunculares	Interpeduncular veins
A12.3.06.041	V. intercollicularis	Intercollicular vein
A12.3.06.042	V. mesencephalica lateralis	Lateral mesencephalic vein
A12.3.06.043	Vv. pontis	Pontine veins
A12.3.06.044	V. pontis anteromediana	Anteromedian pontine vein
A12.3.06.045	V. pontis anterolateralis	Anterolateral pontine vein
A12.3.06.046	Vv. pontis transversae	Transverse pontine veins
A12.3.06.047	V. pontis lateralis	Lateral pontine vein
A12.3.06.048	Vv. medullae oblongatae	Veins of medulla oblongata
A12.3.06.049	V. medullaris anteromediana	Anteromedian medullary vein
A12.3.06.050	V. medullaris anterolateralis	Anterolateral medullary vein
A12.3.06.051	Vv. medullares transversae	Transverse medullary veins
A12.3.06.052	Vv. medullares dorsales	Dorsal medullary veins
A12.3.06.053	V. medullaris posteromediana	Posteromedian medullary vein
A12.3.06.054	V. recessus lateralis ventriculi quarti	Vein of lateral recess of fourth ventricle
A12.3.06.055	V. cisternae cerebellomedullaris	Vein of cerebellomedullary cistern
A12.3.06.056	**Venae cerebelli**	**Cerebellar veins**
A12.3.06.057	V. superior vermis	Superior vein of vermis
A12.3.06.058	V. inferior vermis	Inferior vein of vermis
A12.3.06.059	Vv. superiores cerebelli	Superior veins of cerebellar hemisphere
A12.3.06.060	Vv. inferiores cerebelli	Inferior veins of cerebellar hemisphere
A12.3.06.061	V. precentralis cerebelli	Precentral cerebellar vein
A12.3.06.062	V. petrosa	Petrosal vein

A12.3.06.101	**Venae orbitae**	**Orbital veins**
A12.3.06.102	**Vena ophthalmica superior**	**Superior ophthalmic vein**
A12.3.06.103	V. nasofrontalis	Nasofrontal vein
A12.3.06.104	Vv. ethmoidales	Ethmoidal veins
A12.3.06.105	V. lacrimalis	Lacrimal vein
A12.3.06.106	Vv. vorticosae	Vorticose veins
A12.3.06.107	Vv. ciliares	Ciliary veins
A12.3.06.108	Vv. ciliares anteriores	Anterior ciliary veins
A12.3.06.109	Sinus venosus sclerae	Scleral venous sinus
A12.3.06.110	Vv. sclerales	Scleral veins
A12.3.06.111	V. centralis retinae	Central retinal vein
A12.3.06.112	Pars extraocularis	Extraocular part
A12.3.06.113	Pars intraocularis	Intraocular part
A12.3.06.114	Vv. episclerales	Episcleral veins
A12.3.06.115	Vv. palpebrales	Palpebral veins
A12.3.06.116	Vv. conjunctivales	Conjunctival veins
A12.3.06.117	**Vena ophthalmica inferior**	**Inferior ophthalmic vein**

A12.3.07.001	**Vena azygos**	**Azygos vein**
A12.3.07.002	Arcus venae azygos	Arch of azygos vein
A12.3.07.003	V. intercostalis superior dextra	Right superior intercostal vein
A12.3.07.004	V. hemiazygos	Hemi-azygos vein; Inferior hemi-azygos vein
A12.3.07.005	V. hemiazygos accessoria	Accessory hemi-azygos vein; Superior hemi-azygos vein
A12.3.07.006	Vv. oesophageales	Oesophageal veins▲
A12.3.07.007	Vv. bronchiales	Bronchial veins
A12.3.07.008	Vv. pericardiacae	Pericardial veins
A12.3.07.009	Vv. mediastinales	Mediastinal veins

A12.3.07.010	Vv. phrenicae superiores	Superior phrenic veins
A12.3.07.011	V. lumbalis ascendens	Ascending lumbar vein
A12.3.07.012	Vv. lumbales	Lumbar veins
A12.3.07.013	V. subcostalis	Subcostal vein
A12.3.07.014	Vv. intercostales posteriores	Posterior intercostal veins
A12.3.07.015	V. dorsalis; R. dorsalis	Dorsal vein; Dorsal branch
A12.3.07.016	V. intervertebralis	Intervertebral vein
A12.3.07.017	V. spinalis; R. spinalis	Spinal vein; Spinal branch
A12.3.07.018	**Venae columnae vertebralis**	**Veins of vertebral column**
A12.3.07.019	Plexus venosus vertebralis externus anterior	Anterior external vertebral venous plexus
A12.3.07.020	Plexus venosus vertebralis externus posterior	Posterior external vertebral venous plexus
A12.3.07.021	Plexus venosus vertebralis internus anterior	Anterior internal vertebral venous plexus
A12.3.07.022	Vv. basivertebrales	Basivertebral veins
A12.3.07.023	Vv. medullae spinalis	Veins of spinal cord
A12.3.07.024	Vv. spinales anteriores	Anterior spinal veins
A12.3.07.025	Vv. spinales posteriores	Posterior spinal veins
A12.3.07.026	Plexus venosus vertebralis internus posterior	Posterior internal vertebral venous plexus

A12.3.08.001	**VENAE MEMBRI SUPERIORIS**	**VEINS OF UPPER LIMB**
A12.3.08.002	**Vena subclavia**	**Subclavian vein**
A12.3.08.003	Vv. pectorales	Pectoral veins
A12.3.08.004	V. scapularis dorsalis	Dorsal scapular vein
A12.3.08.005	**Vena axillaris**	**Axillary vein**
A12.3.08.006	V. subscapularis	Subscapular vein
A12.3.08.007	V. circumflexa scapulae	Circumflex scapular vein
A12.3.08.008	V. thoracodorsalis	Thoracodorsal vein
A12.3.08.009	V. circumflexa humeri posterior	Posterior circumflex humeral vein
A12.3.08.010	V. circumflexa humeri anterior	Anterior circumflex humeral vein
A12.3.08.011	V. thoracica lateralis	Lateral thoracic vein
A12.3.08.012	Vv. thoracoepigastricae	Thoraco-epigastric veins
A12.3.08.013	Plexus venosus areolaris	Areolar venous plexus
A12.3.08.014	**Venae superficiales membri superioris**	**Superficial veins of upper limb**
A12.3.08.015	V. cephalica	Cephalic vein
A12.3.08.016	V. thoracoacromialis	Thoraco-acromial vein
A12.3.08.017	(V. cephalica accessoria)	(Accessory cephalic vein)
A12.3.08.018	V. basilica	Basilic vein
A12.3.08.019	V. mediana cubiti	Median cubital vein
A12.3.08.020	V. mediana antebrachii	Median antebrachial vein; Median vein of forearm
A12.3.08.021	V. cephalica antebrachii	Cephalic vein of forearm
A12.3.08.022	V. basilica antebrachii	Basilic vein of forearm
A12.3.08.023	Rete venosum dorsale manus	Dorsal venous network of hand
A12.3.08.024	Vv. intercapitulares	Intercapitular veins
A12.3.08.025	Vv. metacarpales dorsales	Dorsal metacarpal veins
A12.3.08.026	Arcus venosus palmaris superficialis	Superficial venous palmar arch
A12.3.08.027	Vv. digitales palmares	Palmar digital veins
A12.3.08.028	**Venae profundae membri superioris**	**Deep veins of upper limb**
A12.3.08.029	Vv. brachiales	Brachial veins
A12.3.08.030	Vv. ulnares	Ulnar veins
A12.3.08.031	Vv. radiales	Radial veins
A12.3.08.032	Vv. interosseae anteriores	Anterior interosseous veins
A12.3.08.033	Vv. interosseae posteriores	Posterior interosseous veins
A12.3.08.034	Arcus venosus palmaris profundus	Deep venous palmar arch
A12.3.08.035	Vv. metacarpales palmares	Palmar metacarpal veins

A12.3.09.001	**VENA CAVA INFERIOR**	**INFERIOR VENA CAVA**
A12.3.09.002	Vv. phrenicae inferiores	Inferior phrenic veins
A12.3.09.003	Vv. lumbales	Lumbar veins

A12.3.09.004	V. lumbalis ascendens	Ascending lumbar vein
A12.3.09.005	Vv. hepaticae	Hepatic veins
A12.3.09.006	V. hepatica dextra	Right hepatic vein
A12.3.09.007	V. hepatica intermedia	Intermediate hepatic vein
A12.3.09.008	V. hepatica sinistra	Left hepatic vein
A12.3.09.009	Vv. renales	Renal veins
A12.3.09.010	Vv. capsulares	Capsular veins
A12.3.09.011	V. suprarenalis sinistra	Left suprarenal vein
A12.3.09.012	V. ovarica sinistra ♀	Left ovarian vein ♀
A12.3.09.012	V. testicularis sinistra ♂	Left testicular vein ♂
* **A08.1.04.001**	Vv. intrarenales	Intrarenal veins
A12.3.09.013	V. suprarenalis dextra	Right suprarenal vein
A12.3.09.014	V. ovarica dextra ♀	Right ovarian vein ♀
A12.3.09.014	V. testicularis dextra ♂	Right testicular vein ♂
A12.3.09.015	Plexus pampiniformis	Pampiniform plexus

A12.3.10.001	**Vena iliaca communis**	**Common iliac vein**
A12.3.10.002	V. sacralis mediana	Median sacral vein
A12.3.10.003	V. iliolumbalis	Iliolumbar vein

A12.3.10.004	**Vena iliaca interna**	**Internal iliac vein**
A12.3.10.005	Vv. gluteae superiores	Superior gluteal veins
A12.3.10.006	Vv. gluteae inferiores	Inferior gluteal veins
A12.3.10.007	Vv. obturatoriae	Obturator veins
A12.3.10.008	Vv. sacrales laterales	Lateral sacral veins
A12.3.10.009	Plexus venosus sacralis	Sacral venous plexus
A12.3.10.010	Plexus venosus rectalis	Rectal venous plexus
A12.3.10.011	Vv. vesicales	Vesical veins
A12.3.10.012	Plexus venosus vesicalis	Vesical venous plexus
A12.3.10.013	Plexus venosus prostaticus ♂	Prostatic venous plexus ♂
A12.3.10.014	V. dorsalis profunda clitoridis ♀	Deep dorsal vein of clitoris ♀
A12.3.10.014	V. dorsalis profunda penis ♂	Deep dorsal vein of penis ♂
A12.3.10.015	Vv. uterinae ♀	Uterine veins ♀
A12.3.10.016	Plexus venosus uterinus ♀	Uterine venous plexus ♀
A12.3.10.017	Plexus venosus vaginalis ♀	Vaginal venous plexus ♀
A12.3.10.018	Vv. rectales mediae	Middle rectal veins
A12.3.10.019	V. pudenda interna	Internal pudendal vein
A12.3.10.020	Vv. profundae clitoridis ♀	Deep veins of clitoris ♀
A12.3.10.020	Vv. profundae penis ♂	Deep veins of penis ♂
A12.3.10.021	Vv. rectales inferiores	Inferior rectal veins
A12.3.10.022	Vv. labiales posteriores ♀	Posterior labial veins ♀
A12.3.10.022	Vv. scrotales posteriores ♂	Posterior scrotal veins ♂
A12.3.10.023	V. bulbi vestibuli ♀	Vein of bulb of vestibule ♀
A12.3.10.023	V. bulbi penis ♂	Vein of bulb of penis ♂

A12.3.10.024	**Vena iliaca externa**	**External iliac vein**
A12.3.10.025	V. epigastrica inferior	Inferior epigastric vein
A12.3.10.026	V. pubica; R. pubicus (V. obturatoria accessoria)	Pubic vein; Pubic branch (Accessory obturator vein)
A12.3.10.027	V. circumflexa ilium profunda	Deep circumflex iliac vein

* **A08.1.04.001** *Arteriae/venae intrarenales* For further details regarding the nomenclature of renal blood vessels, see the publications mentioned above in A08.1.01.015.

A12.3.11.001	**VENAE MEMBRI INFERIORIS**	**VEINS OF LOWER LIMB**
A12.3.11.002	**Venae superficiales membri inferioris**	**Superficial veins of lower limb**
A12.3.11.003	**V. saphena magna**	**Great saphenous vein; Long saphenous vein**
A12.3.11.004	Vv. pudendae externae	External pudendal veins
A12.3.11.005	V. circumflexa ilium superficialis	Superficial circumflex iliac vein
A12.3.11.006	V. epigastrica superficialis	Superficial epigastric vein
A12.3.11.007	V. saphena accessoria	Accessory saphenous vein
A12.3.11.008	Vv. dorsales superficiales clitoridis ♀	Superficial dorsal veins of clitoris ♀
A12.3.11.008	Vv. dorsales superficiales penis ♂	Superficial dorsal veins of penis ♂
A12.3.11.009	Vv. labiales anteriores ♀	Anterior labial veins ♀
A12.3.11.009	Vv. scrotales anteriores ♂	Anterior scrotal veins ♂
A12.3.11.010	**V. saphena parva**	**Small saphenous vein; Short saphenous vein**
A12.3.11.011	Rete venosum dorsale pedis	Dorsal venous network of foot
A12.3.11.012	Arcus venosus dorsalis pedis	Dorsal venous arch of foot
A12.3.11.013	Vv. metatarsales dorsales	Dorsal metatarsal veins
A12.3.11.014	Vv. digitales dorsales pedis	Dorsal digital veins
A12.3.11.015	Rete venosum plantare	Plantar venous network
A12.3.11.016	Arcus venosus plantaris	Plantar venous arch
A12.3.11.017	Vv. metatarsales plantares	Plantar metatarsal veins
A12.3.11.018	Vv. digitales plantares	Plantar digital veins
A12.3.11.019	Vv. intercapitulares	Intercapitular veins
A12.3.11.020	V. marginalis lateralis	Lateral marginal vein
A12.3.11.021	V. marginalis medialis	Medial marginal vein

A12.3.11.022	**Venae profundae membri inferioris**	**Deep veins of lower limb**
A12.3.11.023	**V. femoralis**	**Femoral vein**
A12.3.11.024	**V. profunda femoris**	**Profunda femoris vein; Deep vein of thigh**
A12.3.11.025	Vv. circumflexae femoris mediales	Medial circumflex femoral veins
A12.3.11.026	Vv. circumflexae femoris laterales	Lateral circumflex femoral veins
A12.3.11.027	Vv. perforantes	Perforating veins
A12.3.11.028	**V. poplitea**	**Popliteal vein**
A12.3.11.029	Vv. surales	Sural veins
A12.3.11.030	Vv. geniculares	Genicular veins
A12.3.11.031	Vv. tibiales anteriores	Anterior tibial veins
A12.3.11.032	Vv. tibiales posteriores	Posterior tibial veins
A12.3.11.033	Vv. fibulares; Vv. peroneae	Fibular veins; Peroneal veins

A12.3.12.001	**VENA PORTAE HEPATIS**	**HEPATIC PORTAL VEIN**
A12.3.12.002	R. dexter	Right branch
A12.3.12.003	R. anterior	Anterior branch
A12.3.12.004	R. posterior	Posterior branch
A12.3.12.005	R. sinister	Left branch
A12.3.12.006	Pars transversa	Transverse part
A12.3.12.007	Rr. lobi caudati	Caudate branches
A12.3.12.008	Pars umbilicalis	Umbilical part
A05.8.01.011	Lig. venosum	Ligamentum venosum
A12.3.12.009	Rr. laterales	Lateral branches
A12.3.12.010	V. umbilicalis	Umbilical vein
A05.8.01.015	Lig. teres hepatis	Round ligament of liver
A12.3.12.011	Rr. mediales	Medial branches
A12.3.12.012	V. cystica	Cystic vein
A12.3.12.013	Vv. paraumbilicales	Para-umbilical veins
A12.3.12.014	V. pancreaticoduodenalis superior posterior	Superior posterior pancreaticoduodenal vein
A12.3.12.015	V. gastrica sinistra	Left gastric vein
A12.3.12.016	V. gastrica dextra	Right gastric vein
A12.3.12.017	V. prepylorica	Prepyloric vein
A12.3.12.018	**Vena mesenterica superior**	**Superior mesenteric vein**
A12.3.12.019	Vv. jejunales	Jejunal veins

A12.3.12.020	Vv. ileales	Ileal veins
A12.3.12.021	V. gastroomentalis dextra; V. gastroepiploica dextra	Right gastro-omental vein; Right gastro-epiploic vein
A12.3.12.022	Vv. pancreaticae	Pancreatic veins
A12.3.12.023	Vv. pancreaticoduodenales	Pancreaticoduodenal veins
A12.3.12.024	V. ileocolica	Ileocolic vein
A12.3.12.025	V. appendicularis	Appendicular vein
A12.3.12.026	V. colica dextra	Right colic vein
A12.3.12.027	V. colica media	Middle colic vein
A12.3.12.028	**Vena splenica; V. lienalis**	**Splenic vein**
A12.3.12.029	Vv. pancreaticae	Pancreatic veins
A12.3.12.030	Vv. gastricae breves	Short gastric veins
A12.3.12.031	V. gastroomentalis sinistra; V. gastroepiploica sinistra	Left gastro-omental vein; Left gastro-epiploic vein
A12.3.12.032	V. mesenterica inferior	Inferior mesenteric vein
A12.3.12.033	V. colica sinistra	Left colic vein
A12.3.12.034	Vv. sigmoideae	Sigmoid veins
A12.3.12.035	V. rectalis superior	Superior rectal vein

A12.4.01.001	**Trunci et ductus lymphatici**	**Lymphatic trunks and ducts**
A12.4.01.002	Truncus jugularis	Jugular trunk
A12.4.01.003	Truncus subclavius	Subclavian trunk
A12.4.01.004	Plexus lymphaticus axillaris	Axillary lymphatic plexus
A12.4.01.005	Truncus bronchomediastinalis	Bronchomediastinal trunk
A12.4.01.006	Ductus lymphaticus dexter; Ductus thoracicus dexter	Right lymphatic duct; Right thoracic duct
A12.4.01.007	Ductus thoracicus	Thoracic duct
A12.4.01.008	Arcus ductus thoracici	Arch of thoracic duct
A12.4.01.009	Pars cervicalis; Pars colli	Cervical part
A12.4.01.010	Pars thoracica	Thoracic part
A12.4.01.011	Pars abdominalis	Abdominal part
A12.4.01.012	Cisterna chyli	Cisterna chyli; Chyle cistern
A12.4.01.013	Truncus lumbalis	Lumbar trunk
A12.4.01.014	Trunci intestinales	Intestinal trunks
A12.4.02.001	Nodi lymphoidei regionales {vide paginam 101}	Regional lymph nodes {see page 101}

A13.0.00.000 Systema lymphoideum — Lymphoid system

A13.1.00.001	**ORGANA LYMPHOIDEA PRIMARIA**	**PRIMARY LYMPHOID ORGANS**
A13.1.01.001	**Medulla ossium**	**Bone marrow**
A13.1.02.001	**Thymus**	**Thymus**
A13.1.02.002	Lobus	Lobe
A13.1.02.003	Lobuli thymi	Lobules of thymus
A13.1.02.004	Cortex thymi	Cortex of thymus
A13.1.02.005	Medulla thymi	Medulla of thymus
A13.1.02.006	(Lobuli thymici accessorii)	(Accessory thymic lobules)

A13.2.00.001	**ORGANA LYMPHOIDEA SECUNDARIA**	**SECONDARY LYMPHOID ORGANS**
A13.2.01.001	**Splen; Lien**	**Spleen**
A13.2.01.002	Capsula; Tunica fibrosa	Fibrous capsule
A13.2.01.003	Trabeculae splenicae	Splenic trabeculae
A13.2.01.004	Pulpa splenica; Pulpa lienalis	Splenic pulp
A13.2.01.005	Pulpa rubra	Red pulp
A13.2.01.006	Pulpa alba	White pulp
A13.2.01.007	Facies diaphragmatica	Diaphragmatic surface
A13.2.01.008	Facies visceralis	Visceral surface
A13.2.01.009	Facies renalis	Renal impression
A13.2.01.010	Facies gastrica	Gastric impression
A13.2.01.011	Facies colica	Colic impression
A13.2.01.012	(Facies pancreatica)	(Pancreatic impression)
A13.2.01.013	Extremitas anterior	Anterior extremity
A13.2.01.014	Extremitas posterior	Posterior extremity
A13.2.01.015	Margo inferior	Inferior border
A13.2.01.016	Margo superior	Superior border
A13.2.01.017	Hilum splenicum; Hilum lienale	Splenic hilum
A13.2.01.018	Tunica serosa	Serosa; Serous coat
A13.2.01.019	Sinus splenicus; Sinus lienalis	Splenic sinus
A13.2.01.020	Penicilli	Penicilli
A13.2.01.021	Noduli lymphoidei splenici; Noduli lymphoidei lienales	Splenic lymphoid nodules
A13.2.01.022	(Splen accessorius)	(Accessory spleen)

A13.2.02.001	**Anulus lymphoideus pharyngis**	**Pharyngeal lymphoid ring**
A05.1.04.022	Tonsilla lingualis	Lingual tonsil
A13.2.02.002	Cryptae tonsillares	Tonsillar crypts
A05.1.04.023	Noduli lymphoidei	Lymphoid nodules
A05.2.01.011	Tonsilla palatina	Palatine tonsil
A05.2.01.014	Fossulae tonsillares	Tonsillar pits
A05.2.01.015	Cryptae tonsillares	Tonsillar crypts
A05.2.01.012	Capsula tonsillaris	Tonsillar capsule
A05.3.01.006	Tonsilla pharyngea	Pharyngeal tonsil
A05.3.01.007	Fossulae tonsillares	Tonsillar pits
A05.3.01.008	Cryptae tonsillares	Tonsillar crypts
A05.3.01.009	Noduli lymphoidei	Lymphoid nodules
A05.3.01.016	Tonsilla tubaria	Tubal tonsil
A13.2.02.003	Cryptae tonsillares	Tonsillar crypts

A13.2.03.001	**Nodus lymphoideus; Nodus lymphaticus; Lymphonodus**	**Lymph node**
A13.2.03.002	Capsula	Capsule
A13.2.03.003	Trabeculae	Trabeculae
A13.2.03.004	Hilum	Hilum
A13.2.03.005	Cortex	Cortex

A13.2.03.006	Medulla	Medulla
A05.6.01.013	Noduli lymphoidei solitarii	Solitary lymphoid nodules
A05.6.01.014	Noduli lymphoidei aggregati	Aggregated lymphoid nodules
A05.7.02.009	Noduli lymphoidei aggregati appendicis vermiformis	Lymph nodules of vermiform appendix

A12.4.02.001	Nodi lymphoidei regionales	Regional lymph nodes
A13.3.00.001	**Nodi lymphoidei capitis et colli**	**Lymph nodes of head and neck**
A13.3.00.002	Nodi occipitales	Occipital nodes
A13.3.00.003	Nodi mastoidei	Mastoid nodes
A13.3.00.004	Nodi parotidei superficiales	Superficial parotid nodes
A13.3.00.005	Nodi parotidei profundi	Deep parotid nodes
A13.3.00.006	Nodi preauriculares	Pre-auricular nodes
A13.3.00.007	Nodi infraauriculares	Infra-auricular nodes
A13.3.00.008	Nodi intraglandulares	Intraglandular nodes
A13.3.00.009	Nodi faciales	Facial nodes
A13.3.00.010	Nodus buccinatorius	Buccinator node
A13.3.00.011	Nodus nasolabialis	Nasolabial node
A13.3.00.012	Nodus malaris	Malar node
A13.3.00.013	Nodus mandibularis	Mandibular node
A13.3.00.014	Nodi linguales	Lingual nodes
A13.3.00.015	Nodi submentales	Submental nodes
A13.3.00.016	Nodi submandibulares	Submandibular nodes
A13.3.00.017	Nodi cervicales anteriores; Nodi colli anteriores	Anterior cervical nodes
A13.3.00.018	Nodi superficiales; Nodi jugulares anteriores	Superficial nodes; Anterior jugular nodes
A13.3.00.019	Nodi profundi	Deep nodes
A13.3.00.020	Nodi infrahyoidei	Infrahyoid nodes
A13.3.00.021	Nodi prelaryngei	Prelaryngeal nodes
A13.3.00.022	Nodi thyroidei	Thyroid nodes
A13.3.00.023	Nodi pretracheales	Pretracheal nodes
A13.3.00.024	Nodi paratracheales	Paratracheal nodes
A13.3.00.025	Nodi retropharyngeales	Retropharyngeal nodes
A13.3.00.026	Nodi cervicales laterales; Nodi colli laterales	Lateral cervical nodes
A13.3.00.027	Nodi superficiales	Superficial nodes
A13.3.00.028	Nodi profundi superiores	Superior deep nodes
A13.3.00.029	Nodus jugulodigastricus	Jugulodigastric node
A13.3.00.030	Nodus lateralis	Lateral node
A13.3.00.031	Nodus anterior	Anterior node
A13.3.00.032	Nodi profundi inferiores	Inferior deep nodes
A13.3.00.033	Nodus juguloomohyoideus	Jugulo-omohyoid node
A13.3.00.034	Nodus lateralis	Lateral node
A13.3.00.035	Nodi anteriores	Anterior nodes
A13.3.00.036	Nodi supraclaviculares	Supraclavicular nodes
A13.3.00.037	Nodi accessorii	Accessory nodes
A13.3.00.038	Nodi retropharyngeales	Retropharyngeal nodes
A13.3.01.001	**Nodi lymphoidei membri superioris**	**Lymph nodes of upper limb**
A13.3.01.002	Nodi lymphoidei axillares	Axillary lymph nodes
A13.3.01.003	Nodi apicales	Apical nodes
A13.3.01.004	Nodi humerales; Nodi laterales	Humeral nodes; Lateral nodes
A13.3.01.005	Nodi subscapulares; Nodi posteriores	Subscapular nodes; Posterior nodes
A13.3.01.006	Nodi pectorales; Nodi anteriores	Pectoral nodes; Anterior nodes
A13.3.01.007	Nodi centrales	Central nodes
A13.3.01.008	Nodi interpectorales	Interpectoral nodes
A13.3.01.009	Nodi deltopectorales; Nodi infraclaviculares	Deltopectoral nodes; Infraclavicular nodes
A13.3.01.010	Nodi brachiales	Brachial nodes
A13.3.01.011	Nodi cubitales	Cubital nodes
A13.3.01.012	Nodi supratrochleares	Supratrochlear nodes

A13.3.01.013	Nodi superficiales	Superficial nodes
A13.3.01.014	Nodi profundi	Deep nodes
A13.3.02.001	**Nodi lymphoidei thoracis**	**Thoracic lymph nodes**
A13.3.02.002	Nodi paramammarii	Paramammary nodes
A13.3.02.003	Nodi parasternales	Parasternal nodes
A13.3.02.004	Nodi intercostales	Intercostal nodes
A13.3.02.005	Nodi phrenici superiores	Superior diaphragmatic nodes
A13.3.02.006	Nodi prepericardiaci	Prepericardial nodes
A13.3.02.007	Nodi brachiocephalici	Brachiocephalic nodes
A13.3.02.008	(Nodus ligamenti arteriosi)	(Node of ligamentum arteriosum)
A13.3.02.009	(Nodus arcus venae azygos)	(Node of arch of azygos vein)
A13.3.02.010	Nodi pericardiaci laterales	Lateral pericardial nodes
A13.3.02.011	Nodi paratracheales	Paratracheal nodes
A13.3.02.012	Nodi tracheobronchiales	Tracheobronchial nodes
A13.3.02.013	Nodi tracheobronchiales superiores	Superior tracheobronchial nodes
A13.3.02.014	Nodi tracheobronchiales inferiores	Inferior tracheobronchial nodes
A13.3.02.015	Nodi bronchopulmonales	Bronchopulmonary nodes
A13.3.02.016	Nodi intrapulmonales	Intrapulmonary nodes
A13.3.02.017	Nodi juxtaoesophageales	Juxta-oesophageal nodes▲
A13.3.02.018	Nodi prevertebrales	Prevertebral nodes
A13.3.03.001	**Nodi lymphoidei abdominis**	**Abdominal lymph nodes**
A13.3.03.002	Nodi lymphoidei parietales	Parietal lymph nodes
A13.3.03.003	Nodi lumbales sinistri	Left lumbar nodes
A13.3.03.004	Nodi aortici laterales	Lateral aortic nodes
A13.3.03.005	Nodi preaortici	Pre-aortic nodes
A13.3.03.006	Nodi retroaortici; Nodi postaortici	Postaortic nodes
A13.3.03.007	Nodi lumbales intermedii	Intermediate lumbar nodes
A13.3.03.008	Nodi lumbales dextri	Right lumbar nodes
A13.3.03.009	Nodi cavales laterales	Lateral caval nodes
A13.3.03.010	Nodi precavales	Precaval nodes
A13.3.03.011	Nodi retrocavales; Nodi postcavales	Postcaval nodes
A13.3.03.012	Nodi phrenici inferiores	Inferior diaphragmatic nodes
A13.3.03.013	Nodi epigastrici inferiores	Inferior epigastric nodes
A13.3.03.014	Nodi lymphoidei viscerales	Visceral lymph nodes
A13.3.03.015	Nodi coeliaci	Coeliac nodes▲
A13.3.03.016	Nodi gastrici dextri/sinistri	Right/left gastric nodes
A13.3.03.017	(Anulus lymphaticus cardiae)	(Nodes around cardia)
A13.3.03.018	Nodi gastroomentales dextri/sinistri	Right/left gastro-omental nodes
A13.3.03.019	Nodi pylorici	Pyloric nodes
A13.3.03.020	(Nodus suprapyloricus)	(Suprapyloric node)
A13.3.03.021	(Nodi subpylorici)	(Subpyloric nodes)
A13.3.03.022	(Nodi retropylorici)	(Retropyloric nodes)
A13.3.03.023	Nodi pancreatici	Pancreatic nodes
A13.3.03.024	Nodi superiores	Superior nodes
A13.3.03.025	Nodi inferiores	Inferior nodes
A13.3.03.026	Nodi splenici; Nodi lienales	Splenic nodes
A13.3.03.027	Nodi pancreaticoduodenales	Pancreaticoduodenal nodes
A13.3.03.028	Nodi superiores	Superior nodes
A13.3.03.029	Nodi inferiores	Inferior nodes
A13.3.03.030	Nodi hepatici	Hepatic nodes
A13.3.03.031	Nodus cysticus	Cystic node
A13.3.03.032	Nodus foraminalis	Node of anterior border of omental foramen
A13.3.03.033	Nodi mesenterici superiores	Superior mesenteric nodes
A13.3.03.034	Nodi juxtaintestinales	Juxta-intestinal mesenteric nodes
A13.3.03.035	Nodi superiores centrales	Central superior mesenteric nodes
A13.3.03.036	Nodi ileocolici	Ileocolic nodes
A13.3.03.037	Nodi precaecales	Precaecal nodes▲
A13.3.03.038	Nodi retrocaecales	Retrocaecal nodes▲
A13.3.03.039	Nodi appendiculares	Appendicular nodes

A13.3.03.040	Nodi mesocolici	Mesocolic nodes
A13.3.03.041	Nodi paracolici	Paracolic nodes
A13.3.03.042	Nodi colici dextri/medii/sinistri	Right/middle/left colic nodes
A13.3.03.043	Nodi mesenterici inferiores	Inferior mesenteric nodes
A13.3.03.044	Nodi sigmoidei	Sigmoid nodes
A13.3.03.045	Nodi rectales superiores	Superior rectal nodes
A13.3.04.001	**Nodi lymphoidei pelvis**	**Pelvic lymph nodes**
A13.3.04.002	Nodi lymphoidei parietales	Parietal nodes
A13.3.04.003	Nodi iliaci communes	Common iliac nodes
A13.3.04.004	Nodi mediales	Medial nodes
A13.3.04.005	Nodi intermedii	Intermediate nodes
A13.3.04.006	Nodi laterales	Lateral nodes
A13.3.04.007	Nodi subaortici	Subaortic nodes
A13.3.04.008	Nodi promontorii	Promontorial nodes
A13.3.04.009	Nodi iliaci externi	External iliac nodes
A13.3.04.010	Nodi mediales	Medial nodes
A13.3.04.011	Nodi intermedii	Intermediate nodes
A13.3.04.012	Nodi laterales	Lateral nodes
A13.3.04.013	(Nodus lacunaris medialis)	(Medial lacunar node)
A13.3.04.014	(Nodus lacunaris intermedius)	(Intermediate lacunar node)
A13.3.04.015	(Nodus lacunaris lateralis)	(Lateral lacunar node)
A13.3.04.016	Nodi interiliaci	Interiliac nodes
A13.3.04.017	Nodi obturatorii	Obturator nodes
A13.3.04.018	Nodi iliaci interni	Internal iliac nodes
A13.3.04.019	Nodi gluteales	Gluteal nodes
A13.3.04.020	Nodi superiores	Superior nodes
A13.3.04.021	Nodi inferiores	Inferior nodes
A13.3.04.022	Nodi sacrales	Sacral nodes
A13.3.04.023	Nodi lymphoidei viscerales	Visceral lymph nodes
A13.3.04.024	Nodi paravesicales	Paravesical nodes
A13.3.04.025	Nodi prevesicales	Prevesical nodes
A13.3.04.026	Nodi retrovesicales; Nodi postvesicales	Postvesical nodes
A13.3.04.027	Nodi vesicales laterales	Lateral vesical nodes
A13.3.04.028	Nodi parauterini ♀	Para-uterine nodes ♀
A13.3.04.029	Nodi paravaginales ♀	Paravaginal nodes ♀
A13.3.04.030	Nodi pararectales; Nodi anorectales	Pararectal nodes
A13.3.05.001	**Nodi lymphoidei membri inferioris**	**Lymph nodes of lower limb**
A13.3.05.002	Nodi lymphoidei inguinales	Inguinal lymph nodes
A13.3.05.003	Nodi inguinales superficiales	Superficial inguinal nodes
A13.3.05.004	Nodi superomediales	Superomedial nodes
A13.3.05.005	Nodi superolaterales	Superolateral nodes
A13.3.05.006	Nodi inferiores	Inferior nodes
A13.3.05.007	Nodi inguinales profundi	Deep inguinal nodes
A13.3.05.008	(Nodus proximalis)	(Proximal node)
A13.3.05.009	(Nodus intermedius)	(Intermediate node)
A13.3.05.010	Nodus distalis	Distal node
A13.3.05.011	Nodi poplitei	Popliteal nodes
A13.3.05.012	Nodi superficiales	Superficial nodes
A13.3.05.013	Nodi profundi	Deep nodes
A13.3.05.014	(Nodus tibialis anterior)	(Anterior tibial node)
A13.3.05.015	(Nodus tibialis posterior)	(Posterior tibial node)
A13.3.05.016	(Nodus fibularis)	(Fibular node; Peroneal node)

A14.0.00.000 Systema nervosum — Nervous system

	Nomina generalia	*General terms*
A14.0.00.001	Neurofibra	Nerve fibre▲
A14.0.00.002	Neuron	Neuron
A14.0.00.003	Perikaryon	Perikaryon
A14.0.00.004	Synapsis	Synapse
A14.0.00.005	Neuroglia	Neuroglia

A14.1.00.001 Pars centralis; Systema nervosum centrale — Central nervous system

	Nomina generalia	*General terms*
A14.1.00.002	Substantia grisea	Grey matter; Grey substance▲
A14.1.00.003	Nucleus	Nucleus
A14.1.00.004	Nucleus nervi cranialis	Nucleus of cranial nerve
A14.1.00.005	Nucleus originis	Nucleus of origin
A14.1.00.006	Nucleus terminationis	Terminal nucleus
A14.1.00.007	Columna	Column
A14.1.00.008	Lamina	Lamina
A14.1.00.009	Substantia alba	White matter; White substance
A14.1.00.010	Funiculus	Funiculus
A14.1.00.011	Tractus	Tract
A14.1.00.012	Fasciculus	Fasciculus; Fascicle
A14.1.00.013	Commissura	Commissure
A14.1.00.014	Lemniscus	Lemniscus
A14.1.00.015	Fibra	Fibre▲
A14.1.00.016	Fibra associationis	Association fibre▲
A14.1.00.017	Fibra commissuralis	Commissural fibre▲
A14.1.00.018	Fibra projectionis	Projection fibre▲
A14.1.00.019	Decussatio	Decussation
A14.1.00.020	Stria	Stria
A14.1.00.021	Formatio reticularis	Reticular formation
A14.1.00.022	Ependyma	Ependyma

A14.1.01.001	**MENINGES**	**MENINGES**
A14.1.01.002	Pachymeninx; Dura mater	Pachymeninx; Dura mater
A14.1.01.003	Leptomeninx; Arachnoidea mater et pia mater	Leptomeninx; Arachnoid mater and pia mater
A14.1.01.101	**Dura mater**	**Dura mater**
A14.1.01.102	Dura mater cranialis; Dura mater encephali	Cranial dura mater
A14.1.01.103	Falx cerebri	Falx cerebri; Cerebral falx
A14.1.01.104	Tentorium cerebelli	Tentorium cerebelli; Cerebellar tentorium
A14.1.01.105	Incisura tentorii	Tentorial notch; Incisura of tentorium
A14.1.01.106	Falx cerebelli	Falx cerebelli; Cerebellar falx
A14.1.01.107	Diaphragma sellae	Diaphragma sellae; Sellar diaphragm
A14.1.01.108	Cavum trigeminale	Trigeminal cave; Trigeminal cavity
* **A14.1.01.109**	(Spatium subdurale)	(Subdural space)
* **A14.1.01.110**	(Spatium epidurale; Spatium extradurale)	(Extradural space; Epidural space)
A14.1.01.111	Dura mater spinalis	Spinal dura mater
A14.1.01.112	Spatium epidurale; Spatium peridurale	Epidural space
A14.1.01.201	**Arachnoidea mater**	**Arachnoid mater**
* **A14.1.01.202**	Spatium subarachnoideum; Spatium leptomeningeum	Subarachnoid space; Leptomeningeal space

* **A14.1.01.109 / A14.1.01.110** *Spatium subdurale* and *spatium epidurale/extradurale* Although these terms are in common usage, under normal conditions the arachnoid is attached to the dura and the dura is attached to the skull; there are no naturally occurring spaces at these interfaces at all. The occurrence of these spaces is the result of trauma or of pathological process that artifactually separates the arachnoid from the dura or the dura from the skull. Haines D. E. 1991. "On the Question of a Subdural Space." *Anat Rec* 230: 3–21. Van Denabeele F., Creemans J., and Lambrichts I. 1996. "Ultrastructure of the Human Spinal Arachnoid Mater and Dura Mater." *J Anat* 189: 417–430.

* **A14.1.01.202** *Spatium subarachnoideum* This is the space deep to the outer layer of the leptomeninx and containing the arachnoid trabeculae. The spatium is bounded internally by the outer layer of the *pia mater*, however, and the most appropriate designation is therefore *spatium leptomeningeum*, leptomeningeal space.

A14.1.01.203	Liquor cerebrospinalis	Cerebrospinal fluid
A14.1.01.204	Arachnoidea mater cranialis; Arachnoidea mater encephali	Cranial arachnoid mater
A14.1.01.205	Granulationes arachnoideae	Arachnoid granulations
A14.1.01.206	Trabeculae arachnoideae	Arachnoid trabeculae
A14.1.01.207	Cisternae subarachnoideae	Subarachnoid cisterns
A14.1.01.208	Cisterna cerebellomedullaris posterior; Cisterna magna	Posterior cerebellomedullary cistern; Cisterna magna
A14.1.01.209	Cisterna cerebellomedullaris lateralis	Lateral cerebellomedullary cistern
A14.1.01.210	Cisterna fossae lateralis cerebri	Cistern of lateral cerebral fossa
A14.1.01.211	Cisterna chiasmatica	Chiasmatic cistern
A14.1.01.212	Cisterna interpeduncularis	Interpeduncular cistern
A14.1.01.213	Cisterna ambiens	Cisterna ambiens; Ambient cistern
A14.1.01.214	Cisterna pericallosa	Pericallosal cistern
A14.1.01.215	Cisterna pontocerebellaris	Pontocerebellar cistern
A14.1.01.216	Cisterna laminae terminalis	Cistern of lamina terminalis
A14.1.01.217	Cisterna quadrigeminalis; Cisterna venae magnae cerebri	Quadrigeminal cistern; Cistern of great cerebral vein
A14.1.01.218	Arachnoidea mater spinalis	Spinal arachnoid mater
A14.1.01.219	Cisterna lumbalis	Lumbar cistern
A14.1.01.301	**Pia mater**	**Pia mater**
A14.1.01.302	Pia mater cranialis; Pia mater encephali	Cranial pia mater
A14.1.01.303	Tela choroidea ventriculi quarti	Tela choroidea of fourth ventricle
A14.1.01.304	Plexus choroideus ventriculi quarti	Choroid plexus of fourth ventricle
A14.1.01.305	Tela choroidea ventriculi tertii	Tela choroidea of third ventricle
A14.1.01.306	Plexus choroideus ventriculi tertii	Choroid plexus of third ventricle
A14.1.01.307	Plexus choroideus ventriculi lateralis	Choroid plexus of lateral ventricle
A14.1.01.308	Glomus choroideum	Choroidal enlargement
A14.1.01.309	Pia mater spinalis	Spinal pia mater
A14.1.01.310	Lig. denticulatum	Denticulate ligament
A14.1.01.311	Septum cervicale intermedium	Intermediate cervical septum
A14.1.01.401	**Filum terminale**	**Filum terminale; Terminal filum**
A14.1.01.402	Pars duralis	Dural part; Coccygeal ligament; Filum terminale externum
A14.1.01.403	Pars pialis	Pial part; Pial filament; Filum terminale internum

A14.1.02.001	**Medulla spinalis**	**Spinal cord**
	Morphologia externa	*External features*
A14.1.02.002	Intumescentia cervicalis	Cervical enlargement
A14.1.02.003	Intumescentia lumbosacralis	Lumbosacral enlargement
A14.1.02.004	Conus medullaris	Conus medullaris; Medullary cone
A14.1.02.005	Pars spinalis fili terminalis	Spinal part of filum terminale
A14.1.02.006	Ventriculus terminalis	Terminal ventricle
A14.1.02.007	Fissura mediana anterior	Anterior median fissure; Ventral median fissure
A14.1.02.008	Sulcus medianus posterior	Posterior median sulcus; Dorsal median sulcus
A14.1.02.009	Septum medianum posterius	Posterior median septum; Dorsal median septum
A14.1.02.010	Sulcus anterolateralis	Anterolateral sulcus; Ventrolateral sulcus
A14.1.02.011	Sulcus posterolateralis	Posterolateral sulcus; Dorsolateral sulcus
A14.1.02.012	Sulcus intermedius posterior	Posterior intermediate sulcus; Dorsal intermediate sulcus
A14.1.02.013	Funiculi medullae spinalis	Funiculi of spinal cord
A14.1.02.014	Pars cervicalis; Segmenta cervicalia [1–8]	Cervical part; Cervical segments [1–8]
A14.1.02.015	Pars thoracica; Segmenta thoracica [1–12]	Thoracic part; Thoracic segments [1–12]
A14.1.02.016	Pars lumbalis; Segmenta lumbalia [1–5]	Lumbar part; Lumbar segments [1–5]
A14.1.02.017	Pars sacralis; Segmenta sacralia [1–5]	Sacral part; Sacral segments [1–5]
A14.1.02.018	Pars coccygea; Segmenta coccygea [1–3]	Coccygeal part; Coccygeal segments [1–3]

	Morphologia interna	*Internal features*
A14.1.02.019	Canalis centralis	Central canal
A14.1.02.020	Substantia grisea	Grey substance▲
A14.1.02.021	Cornu anterius	Anterior horn; Ventral horn
A14.1.02.022	Cornu laterale	Lateral horn
A14.1.02.023	Cornu posterius	Posterior horn; Dorsal horn
A14.1.02.024	Substantia alba	White substance
A14.1.02.025	Substantia gelatinosa centralis	Central gelatinous substance

A14.1.02.101	**Columnae griseae**	**Grey columns▲**
A14.1.02.102	**Columna anterior**	**Anterior column; Ventral column**
A14.1.02.103	Cornu anterius	Anterior horn; Ventral horn
* **A14.1.02.104**	Laminae spinales VII–IX	Spinal laminae VII–IX
A14.1.02.105	Nucleus anterolateralis	Anterolateral nucleus; Ventrolateral nucleus
A14.1.02.106	Nucleus anterior	Anterior nucleus
A14.1.02.107	Nucleus anteromedialis	Anteromedial nucleus; Ventromedial nucleus
A14.1.02.108	Nucleus posterolateralis	Posterolateral nucleus; Dorsolateral nucleus
A14.1.02.109	Nucleus retroposterolateralis	Retroposterior lateral nucleus; Retrodorsal lateral nucleus
A14.1.02.110	Nucleus posteromedialis	Posteromedial nucleus; Dorsomedial nucleus
A14.1.02.111	Nucleus centralis	Central nucleus
A14.1.02.112	Nucleus nervi accessorii	Nucleus of accessory nerve
A14.1.02.113	Nucleus nervi phrenici	Nucleus of phrenic nerve; Phrenic nucleus
A14.1.02.114	**Columna posterior**	**Posterior column; Dorsal column**
A14.1.02.115	Cornu posterius	Posterior horn; Dorsal horn
A14.1.02.116	Apex	Apex
A14.1.02.117	Nucleus marginalis; Lamina spinalis I	Marginal nucleus; Spinal lamina I
A14.1.02.118	Caput	Head
A14.1.02.119	Substantia gelatinosa; Lamina spinalis II	Gelatinous substance; Spinal lamina II
A14.1.02.120	Cervix	Neck
A14.1.02.121	Nucleus proprius; Laminae spinales III et IV	Nucleus proprius; Spinal laminae III and IV
A14.1.02.122	Lamina spinalis V	Spinal lamina V
A14.1.02.123	Basis	Base
A14.1.02.124	Lamina spinalis VI	Spinal lamina VI
A14.1.02.125	Substantia visceralis secundaria	Secondary visceral grey substance▲
A14.1.02.126	Nucleus basilaris internus	Internal basilar nucleus
A14.1.02.127	Nucleus cervicalis lateralis	Lateral cervical nucleus
A14.1.02.128	Nucleus cervicalis medialis	Medial cervical nucleus
A14.1.02.129	Nucleus posterior funiculi lateralis	Posterior nucleus of lateral funiculus
A14.1.02.130	**Columna intermedia**	**Intermediate column; Intermediate zone**
A14.1.02.131	Lamina spinalis VII	Spinal lamina VII
A14.1.02.132	Cornu laterale	Lateral horn
A14.1.02.133	Nucleus intermediolateralis	Intermediolateral nucleus
A14.1.02.134	Substantia intermedia centralis	Central intermediate substance
A14.1.02.135	Nucleus thoracicus posterior; Nucleus dorsalis	Posterior thoracic nucleus; Dorsal thoracic nucleus
A14.1.02.136	Substantia intermedia lateralis	Lateral intermediate substance
A14.1.02.137	Nucleus intermediomedialis	Intermediomedial nucleus
A14.1.02.138	Nuclei parasympathici sacrales	Sacral parasympathetic nuclei
A14.1.02.139	Nucleus nervi pudendi	Nucleus of pudendal nerve
A14.1.02.140	Formatio reticularis spinalis	Spinal reticular formation
A14.1.02.141	Nucleus medialis anterior	Anterior medial nucleus; Ventral medial nucleus

* **A14.1.02.104** *Laminae spinales VII–IX* At most cervical and lumbosacral levels the cells comprising spinal lamina VII extend into the anterior horn. At other levels spinal lamina VII is restricted to the intermediate zone.

* **A14.1.02.201**	**Substantia alba**	**White substance**
A14.1.02.202	**Funiculus anterior**	**Anterior funiculus; Ventral funiculus**
A14.1.02.203	Fasciculus proprius anterior	Anterior fasciculus proprius; Ventral fasciculus proprius
A14.1.02.204	Fasciculus sulcomarginalis	Sulcomarginal fasciculus
A14.1.02.205	Tractus corticospinalis anterior	Anterior corticospinal tract; Ventral corticospinal tract
A14.1.02.206	Tractus vestibulospinalis lateralis	Lateral vestibulospinal tract
A14.1.02.207	Tractus vestibulospinalis medialis	Medial vestibulospinal tract
A14.1.02.208	Fibrae reticulospinales	Reticulospinal fibres▲
A14.1.02.209	Tractus pontoreticulospinalis	Pontoreticulospinal tract; Medial reticulospinal tract
A14.1.02.210	Tractus interstitiospinalis	Interstitiospinal tract
A14.1.02.211	Tractus tectospinalis	Tectospinal tract
A14.1.02.212	Tractus raphespinalis anterior	Anterior raphespinal tract; Ventral raphespinal tract
A14.1.02.213	Fibrae olivospinales	Olivospinal fibres▲
* **A14.1.02.214**	Tractus spinothalamicus anterior	Anterior spinothalamic tract; Ventral spinothalamic tract
A14.1.02.215	**Funiculus lateralis**	**Lateral funiculus**
A14.1.02.216	Fasciculus proprius lateralis	Lateral fasciculus proprius
A14.1.02.217	Tractus fastigiospinalis	Fastigiospinal tract
A14.1.02.218	Tractus interpositospinalis	Interpositospinal tract
A14.1.02.219	Tractus corticospinalis lateralis	Lateral corticospinal tract
A14.1.02.220	Tractus rubrospinalis	Rubrospinal tract
A14.1.02.221	Tractus bulboreticulospinalis	Bulboreticulospinal tract; Medullary reticulospinal tract; Lateral reticulospinal tract
A14.1.02.223	Fibrae olivospinales	Olivospinal fibres▲
A14.1.02.224	Tractus spinotectalis	Spinotectal tract
* **A14.1.02.225**	Tractus spinothalamicus lateralis	Lateral spinothalamic tract
A14.1.02.226	Tractus spinocerebellaris anterior	Anterior spinocerebellar tract; Ventral spinocerebellar tract
A14.1.02.227	Tractus spinocerebellaris posterior	Posterior spinocerebellar tract; Dorsal spinocerebellar tract
A14.1.02.228	Tractus posterolateralis	Posterolateral tract; Dorsolateral tract
A14.1.02.229	Pars posterior funiculi lateralis	Posterior part of lateral funiculus
A14.1.02.230	Tractus spinoolivaris	Spino-olivary tract
A14.1.02.231	Tractus spinoreticularis	Spinoreticular tract
A14.1.02.232	Tractus caeruleospinalis	Caeruleospinal tract
A14.1.02.233	Fibrae hypothalamospinales	Hypothalamospinal fibres▲
A14.1.02.234	Tractus raphespinalis lateralis	Lateral raphespinal tract
A14.1.02.235	Tractus solitariospinalis	Solitariospinal tract
A14.1.02.236	Tractus spinocervicalis	Spinocervical tract
A14.1.02.237	Tractus spinovestibularis	Spinovestibular tract
A14.1.02.238	Tractus trigeminospinalis	Trigeminospinal tract
A14.1.02.239	**Funiculus posterior**	**Posterior funiculus; Dorsal funiculus**
A14.1.02.240	Fasciculus proprius posterior	Posterior fasciculus proprius; Dorsal fasciculus proprius
A14.1.02.241	Fasciculus septomarginalis	Septomarginal fasciculus
A14.1.02.242	Fasciculus interfascicularis; Fasciculus semilunaris	Interfascicular fasciculus
* **A14.1.02.243**	Fasciculus gracilis	Gracile fasciculus
* **A14.1.02.244**	Fasciculus cuneatus	Cuneate fasciculus

* **A14.1.02.201** *Substantia alba* Within the white matter of the spinal cord, *tractus corticospinales, raphespinalis, spinocerebellares*, and *vestibulospinales* are referred to as "anterior," "lateral," "medial," or "posterior" according to their relative positions in the spinal-cord white matter.

* **A14.1.02.214 / A14.1.02.225** *Tractus spinothalamicus anterior* and *tractus spinothalamicus lateralis* These terms are retained in this edition. However, it is acknowledged that the combined area of the spinal-cord white matter occupied by these two tracts, as classically described, represent what is now known as the anterolateral system (see A14.1.04.137).

* **A14.1.02.243 / A14.1.02.244** *Fasciculus gracilis, fasciculus cuneatus, nucleus gracilis* and *nucleus cuneatus* are commonly, and collectively, referred to as the dorsal column nuclei and fasciculi.

	A14.1.02.245	Fibrae cuneospinales	Cuneospinal fibres▲
	A14.1.02.246	Fibrae gracilispinales	Gracilespinal fibres▲
*	A14.1.02.247	Fibrae spinocuneatae	Spinocuneate fibres▲
*	A14.1.02.248	Fibrae spinograciles	Spinogracile fibres▲

	A14.1.02.301	**Structurae centrales medullae spinalis**	**Central cord structures**
*	A14.1.02.302	Area spinalis X; Lamina spinalis X	Spinal area X; Spinal lamina X
*	A14.1.02.303	Commissura grisea anterior	Anterior grey commissure; Ventral grey commissure▲
*	A14.1.02.304	Commissura grisea posterior	Posterior grey commissure; Dorsal grey commissure▲
	A14.1.02.305	Commissura alba anterior	Anterior white commissure; Ventral white commissure
	A14.1.02.306	Commissura alba posterior	Posterior white commissure; Dorsal white commissure
	A14.1.02.019	Canalis centralis	Central canal

	A14.1.03.001	**Encephalon**	**Brain**
	A14.1.03.002	Rhombencephalon	Rhombencephalon; Hindbrain
*	A14.1.03.003	Myelencephalon; Medulla oblongata; Bulbus	Myelencephalon; Medulla oblongata; Bulb
	A14.1.03.004	Metencephalon; Pons et cerebellum	Metencephalon; Pons and cerebellum
	A14.1.03.005	Mesencephalon	Mesencephalon; Midbrain
	A14.1.03.006	Prosencephalon	Prosencephalon; Forebrain
	A14.1.03.007	Diencephalon	Diencephalon
	A14.1.03.008	Telencephalon	Telencephalon
	A14.1.03.009	**Truncus encephali**	**Brainstem**
*	A14.1.03.003	Myelencephalon; Medulla oblongata; Bulbus	Myelencephalon; Medulla oblongata; Bulb
	A14.1.03.010	Pons	Pons
	A14.1.03.005	Mesencephalon	Midbrain

	A14.1.03.003	**MYELENCEPHALON; MEDULLA OBLONGATA; BULBUS**	**MYELENCEPHALON; MEDULLA OBLONGATA; BULB**
		Morphologia externa	*External features*
	A14.1.04.001	Fissura mediana anterior	Anterior median fissure; Ventral median fissure
	A14.1.04.002	Foramen caecum medullae oblongatae	Foramen caecum of medulla oblongata▲
	A14.1.04.003	Pyramis medullae oblongatae; Pyramis bulbi	Pyramid
	A14.1.04.004	Decussatio pyramidum	Decussation of pyramids; Motor decussation
	A14.1.04.005	Sulcus anterolateralis	Anterolateral sulcus; Ventrolateral sulcus
	A14.1.04.006	Sulcus preolivaris	Pre-olivary groove
	A14.1.04.007	Funiculus lateralis	Lateral funiculus
	A14.1.04.008	Oliva	Inferior olive
	A14.1.04.009	Fibrae arcuatae externae anteriores	Anterior external arcuate fibres; Ventral external arcuate fibres▲
	A14.1.04.010	Sulcus retroolivaris	Retro-olivary groove
	A14.1.04.011	Area retroolivaris	Retro-olivary area
	A14.1.04.012	Sulcus posterolateralis	Posterolateral sulcus; Dorsolateral sulcus

* **A14.1.02.247 / A14.1.02.248** *Fibrae spinocuneatae* and *fibrae spinograciles* These terms designate those fibres that arise from cells in the dorsal horn of the spinal cord and ascend in the cuneate and gracile fasciculi to terminate in their respective nuclei in the medulla. These are commonly, and collectively, referred to as postsynaptic dorsal column fibres.

* **A14.1.02.302** *Area spinalis X* This region of the spinal cord was called an "area" in the original description. Consequently, "area" is preferred over "lamina." Rexed B. 1954. "A Cytoarchitectonic Atlas of the Spinal Cord in the Cat." *J Comp Neurol* 100: 297–379.

* **A14.1.02.303 / A14.1.02.304** *Commissura grisea anterior* and *commissura grisea posterior* These are thin sheets of grey matter that extend across the midline adjacent to the central canal.

* **A14.1.03.003** *Bulbus* The portion between the spinal cord and the caudal border of the pons, this being the *medulla oblongata.* Strong O. S., and Elwyn A. 1943. *Human Neuroanatomy.* Baltimore, Maryland: Williams & Wilkins; Kuhlenbeck H. 1975. *The Central Nervous System of Vertebrates.* Vol. 4. "Spinal Cord and deuterencephalon." Basel: S. Karger.

A14.1.04.013	Pedunculus cerebellaris inferior	Inferior cerebellar peduncle
A14.1.04.014	Corpus restiforme	Restiform body
A14.1.04.015	Tuberculum trigeminale	Trigeminal tubercle
A14.1.04.016	Fasciculus cuneatus	Cuneate fasciculus
A14.1.04.017	Tuberculum cuneatum	Cuneate tubercle
A14.1.04.018	Fasciculus gracilis	Gracile fasciculus
A14.1.04.019	Tuberculum gracile	Gracile tubercle
A14.1.04.020	Sulcus medianus posterior	Posterior median sulcus; Dorsal median sulcus
A14.1.04.021	Obex	Obex

	Morphologia interna	*Internal features*
A14.1.04.101	**Substantia alba**	**White substance**
A14.1.04.102	Tractus pyramidalis	Pyramidal tract
A14.1.04.103	Fibrae corticospinales	Corticospinal fibres▲
A14.1.04.104	Fibrae corticonucleares bulbi	Bulbar corticonuclear fibres▲
A14.1.04.105	Fibrae corticoreticulares	Corticoreticular fibres▲
A14.1.04.106	Decussatio pyramidum	Decussation of pyramids; Motor decussation
A14.1.04.107	Fasciculus gracilis	Gracile fasciculus
A14.1.04.108	Fasciculus cuneatus	Cuneate fasciculus
A14.1.04.109	Fibrae arcuatae internae	Internal arcuate fibres▲
A14.1.04.110	Decussatio lemnisci medialis	Decussation of medial lemniscus; Sensory decussation
A14.1.04.111	Lemniscus medialis	Medial lemniscus
A14.1.04.112	Tractus tectospinalis	Tectospinal tract
A14.1.04.113	Fasciculus longitudinalis medialis	Medial longitudinal fasciculus
A14.1.04.114	Fasciculus longitudinalis posterior; Fasciculus longitudinalis dorsalis	Posterior longitudinal fasciculus; Dorsal longitudinal fasciculus
A14.1.04.115	Tractus spinalis nervi trigemini	Spinal tract of trigeminal nerve
A14.1.04.116	Amiculum olivare	Amiculum of olive
A14.1.04.117	Tractus spinoolivaris	Spino-olivary tract
A14.1.04.118	Tractus olivocerebellaris	Olivocerebellar tract
A14.1.04.013	Pedunculus cerebellaris inferior	Inferior cerebellar peduncle
A14.1.04.119	Corpus juxtarestiforme	Juxtarestiform body
A14.1.04.014	Corpus restiforme	Restiform body
A14.1.04.120	Tractus solitarius	Solitary tract
A14.1.04.009	Fibrae arcuatae externae anteriores	Anterior external arcuate fibres; Ventral external arcuate fibres▲
A14.1.04.121	Fibrae arcuatae externae posteriores	Posterior external arcuate fibres; Dorsal external arcuate fibres▲
A14.1.04.122	Raphe medullae oblongatae	Raphe of medulla oblongata
A14.1.04.123	Tractus raphespinalis anterior	Anterior raphespinal tract
A14.1.04.124	Tractus reticulospinalis anterior	Anterior reticulospinal tract; Ventral reticulospinal tract
A14.1.04.125	Tractus spinocerebellaris anterior	Anterior spinocerebellar tract; Ventral spinocerebellar tract
A14.1.04.126	Fibrae hypothalamospinales	Hypothalamospinal fibres▲
A14.1.04.127	Tractus interstitiospinalis	Interstitiospinal tract
A14.1.04.128	Tractus raphespinalis lateralis	Lateral raphespinal tract
A14.1.04.129	Tractus bulboreticulospinalis lateralis	Lateral bulboreticulospinal tract

A14.1.04.013 *Pedunculus cerebellaris inferior* and *corpus restiforme* In previous terminology lists these two structures were considered synonyms. However the *pedunculus cerebellaris inferior* is composed of two functionally/structurally distinct parts. *corpus restiforme* is located on the dorsolateral aspect of the *medulla oblongata* and contains a variety of cerebellar afferent fibres. *Corpus juxtarestiforme* joins the *corpus restiforme* as they enter the cerebellum and contains only interconnections between vestibular structures and the *cortex cerebellae* and *nucleus fastigii*. Haines D. E. 1975. "Cerebellar Corticovestibular Fibers of the Posterior Lobe in a Prosimian Primate, the Lesser Bushbaby (Galgo Senegalensis)." *J Comp Neurol* 160: 363–398.

A14.1.04.104 *Fibrae corticonucleares bulbi* The term corticobulbar, as commonly used in the past, refers to axons originating in the cerebral cortex and innervating motor nuclei of cranial nerves of the *medulla oblongata*, pons, and by extension, the midbrain. Since bulbus specifically refers to the *medulla oblongata*, application of the term corticobulbar to these fibres in the midbrain is incorrect. The term *corticonuclearis* followed by *bulbi, pontinis* (see A14.1.05.105), or *mesencephali* (see A14.1.06.202) replaces corticobulbar and specifies cortical axons that innervate motor and/ or sensory nuclei of cranial nerves.

A14.1.04.130	Fibrae medulloreticulospinales	Medullary reticulospinal fibres▲
A14.1.04.131	Tractus vestibulospinalis lateralis	Lateral vestibulospinal tract
A14.1.04.132	Tractus spinocerebellaris posterior	Posterior spinocerebellar tract; Dorsal spinocerebellar tract
A14.1.04.133	Fibrae cuneocerebellares	Cuneocerebellar fibres▲
A14.1.04.134	Tractus rubrobulbaris	Rubrobulbar tract
A14.1.04.135	Tractus rubroolivaris	Rubro-olivary tract
A14.1.04.136	Tractus rubrospinalis	Rubrospinal tract
* A14.1.04.137	Lemniscus spinalis; Tractus anterolaterales	Spinal lemniscus; Anterolateral tracts; Anterolateral system
A14.1.04.138	Fibrae spinothalamicae	Spinothalamic fibres▲
A14.1.04.139	Fibrae spinoreticulares	Spinoreticular fibres▲
A14.1.04.140	Fibrae spinomesencephalicae	Spinomesencephalic fibres▲
A14.1.04.141	Fibrae spinotectales	Spinotectal fibres▲
A14.1.04.142	Fibrae spinoperiaqueductales	Spinoperiaqueductal fibres▲
A14.1.04.143	Fibrae spinohypothalamicae	Spinohypothalamic fibres▲
A14.1.04.144	Fibrae spinobulbares	Spinobulbar fibres▲
A14.1.04.145	Fibrae spinoolivares	Spino-olivary fibres▲
A14.1.04.146	Tractus spinovestibularis	Spinovestibular tract
A14.1.04.147	Tractus tectobulbaris	Tectobulbar tract

A14.1.04.201	**Substantia grisea**	**Grey substance▲**
* A14.1.04.202	Nucleus gracilis	Gracile nucleus
A14.1.04.203	Pars centralis	Central part; Cell nest region
A14.1.04.204	Pars rostralis	Rostral part; Shell region
A14.1.04.205	Subnucleus rostrodorsalis	Rostrodorsal subnucleus; Cell group Z
* A14.1.04.206	Nucleus cuneatus	Cuneate nucleus
A14.1.04.207	Pars centralis	Central part; Cell nest region
A14.1.04.208	Pars rostralis	Rostral part; Shell region
A14.1.04.209	Nucleus cuneatus accessorius	Accessory cuneate nucleus
A14.1.04.210	Nucleus precuneatus accessorius	Preaccessory cuneate nucleus; Cell group X
A14.1.04.211	Nucleus spinalis nervi trigemini {vide etiam paginam 113}	Spinal nucleus of trigeminal nerve {see also page 113}
A14.1.04.212	Pars caudalis	Caudal part
A14.1.04.213	Subnucleus zonalis	Zonal subnucleus
A14.1.04.214	Subnucleus gelatinosus	Gelatinous subnucleus
A14.1.04.215	Subnucleus magnocellularis	Magnocellular subnucleus
A14.1.04.216	Pars interpolaris	Interpolar part
A14.1.04.217	Nucleus retrotrigeminalis	Retrotrigeminal nucleus
A14.1.04.218	Nucleus retrofacialis	Retrofacial nucleus
A14.1.04.219	Complexus olivaris inferior; Nuclei olivares inferiores	Inferior olivary complex
A14.1.04.220	Nucleus olivaris principalis	Principal olivary nucleus
A14.1.04.221	Lamella posterior	Dorsal lamella
A14.1.04.222	Lamella anterior	Ventral lamella
A14.1.04.223	Lamella lateralis	Lateral lamella
A14.1.04.224	Hilum nuclei olivaris inferioris	Hilum of inferior olivary nucleus
A14.1.04.225	Nucleus olivaris accessorius posterior	Posterior accessory olivary nucleus; Dorsal accessory olivary nucleus
A14.1.04.226	Nucleus olivaris accessorius medialis	Medial accessory olivary nucleus
A14.1.04.227	Nucleus nervi hypoglossi	Nucleus of hypoglossal nerve
A14.1.04.228	Nucleus paramedianus posterior	Posterior paramedian nucleus; Dorsal paramedian nucleus
A14.1.04.229	Nucleus posterior nervi vagi; Nucleus dorsalis nervi vagi	Posterior nucleus of vagus nerve; Dorsal nucleus of vagus nerve

* **A14.1.04.137** *Lemniscus spinalis* Contains a variety of ascending axons and, in this respect, contains essentially the same population of axons that comprise the *tractus anterolaterales*. These are synonymous terms.
* **A14.1.04.202 / A14.1.04.206** *Fasciculus gracilis, fasciculus cuneatus, nucleus gracilis* and *nucleus cuneatus* are commonly, and collectively, referred to as the dorsal column nuclei and fasciculi.

A14.1.04.230	Nuclei tractus solitarii	Nuclei of solitary tract; Solitary nuclei
A14.1.04.231	Nucleus parasolitarius	Parasolitary nucleus
A14.1.04.232	Nucleus commissuralis	Commissural nucleus
A14.1.04.233	Nucleus gelatinosus solitarius	Gelatinous solitary nucleus
A14.1.04.234	Nucleus intermedius solitarius	Intermediate solitary nucleus
A14.1.04.235	Nucleus interstitialis solitarius	Interstitial solitary nucleus
A14.1.04.236	Nucleus medialis solitarius	Medial solitary nucleus
A14.1.04.237	Nucleus paracommissuralis solitarius	Paracommissural solitary nucleus
A14.1.04.238	Nucleus solitarius posterior	Posterior solitary nucleus; Dorsal solitary nucleus
A14.1.04.239	Nucleus solitarius posterolateralis	Posterolateral solitary nucleus; Dorsolateral solitary nucleus
A14.1.04.240	Nucleus solitarius anterior	Anterior solitary nucleus; Ventral solitary nucleus
A14.1.04.241	Nucleus solitarius anterolateralis	Anterolateral solitary nucleus; Ventrolateral solitary nucleus
A14.1.04.242	Nuclei vestibulares {vide etiam paginam 114}	Vestibular nuclei {see also page 114}
A14.1.04.243	Nucleus vestibularis inferior	Inferior vestibular nucleus
A14.1.04.244	Pars magnocellularis nuclei vestibularis inferioris	Magnocellular part of inferior vestibular nucleus; Cell group F
A14.1.04.245	Nucleus vestibularis medialis	Medial vestibular nucleus
A14.1.04.246	Nucleus marginalis corporis restiformis	Marginal nucleus of restiform body; Cell group Y
A14.1.04.247	Nuclei cochleares {vide etiam paginam 114}	Cochlear nuclei {see also page 114}
A14.1.04.248	Nucleus cochlearis posterior	Posterior cochlear nucleus; Dorsal cochlear nucleus
A14.1.04.249	Nucleus cochlearis anterior	Anterior cochlear nucleus; Ventral cochlear nucleus
A14.1.04.250	Pars anterior	Anterior part
A14.1.04.251	Pars posterior	Posterior part
A14.1.04.252	Nucleus commissuralis nervi vagi	Commissural nucleus of vagus nerve
A14.1.04.253	Nucleus ambiguus	Nucleus ambiguus
A14.1.04.254	Nucleus retroambiguus	Retro-ambiguus nucleus
A14.1.04.255	Nucleus salivatorius inferior	Inferior salivatory nucleus
A14.1.04.256	Nucleus arcuatus	Arcuate nucleus
A14.1.04.257	Nuclei raphes	Raphe nuclei
A14.1.04.258	Area postrema	Area postrema
A14.1.04.259	Nucleus endolemniscalis	Endolemniscal nucleus
A14.1.04.260	Nucleus pericuneatus medialis	Medial pericuneate nucleus
A14.1.04.261	Nucleus pericuneatus lateralis	Lateral pericuneate nucleus
A14.1.04.262	Nuclei perihypoglossales	Perihypoglossal nuclei
A14.1.04.263	Nucleus subhypoglossalis	Subhypoglossal nucleus
A14.1.04.264	Nucleus intercalatus	Intercalated nucleus
A14.1.04.265	Nucleus prepositus	Prepositus nucleus
A14.1.04.266	Nucleus peritrigeminalis	Peritrigeminal nucleus
A14.1.04.267	Nucleus pontobulbaris	Pontobulbar nucleus
A14.1.04.268	Nucleus supraspinalis	Supraspinal nucleus
A14.1.04.301	**Nuclei reticulares**	**Reticular nuclei**
* A14.1.04.302	Nucleus gigantocellularis	Gigantocellular reticular nucleus
* A14.1.04.303	Pars alpha	Pars alpha
A14.1.04.304	Nucleus gigantocellularis anterior	Anterior gigantocellular reticular nucleus; Ventral gigantocellular reticular nucleus
A14.1.04.305	Nucleus paragigantocellularis lateralis	Lateral paragigantocellular reticular nucleus
A14.1.04.306	Nucleus interfascicularis nervi hypoglossi	Interfascicular nucleus of hypoglossal nerve
* A14.1.04.307	Nucleus reticularis intermedius	Intermediate reticular nucleus
A14.1.04.308	Nucleus reticularis lateralis	Lateral reticular nucleus

* **A14.1.04.302 / A14.1.04.303** *Nucleus gigantocellularis, pars alpha*, and *nucleus reticularis pontis caudalis* These have been modified from previous nomenclature lists to conform with the more widely accepted and used terminology of Olszewski J. and D. Baxter. 1982. *Cytoarchitecture of the Human Brain Stem*. Basel: Karger.

* **A14.1.04.307** *Nucleus reticularis intermedius* This has been described in the human brain. Paxinos G. and Huang X.-F. 1995. *Atlas of the Human Brain Stem*. New York: Academic Press.

A14.1.04.309	Pars magnocellularis	Magnocellular part
A14.1.04.310	Pars parvocellularis	Parvocellular part
A14.1.04.311	Pars subtrigeminalis	Subtrigeminal part
A14.1.04.312	Nucleus reticularis parvocellularis	Parvocellular reticular nucleus
A14.1.04.313	Nucleus paragigantocellularis posterior	Posterior paragigantocellular reticular nucleus; Dorsal paragigantocellular reticular nucleus
A14.1.04.314	Nucleus reticularis centralis	Central reticular nucleus
A14.1.04.315	Pars dorsalis	Dorsal part
A14.1.04.316	Pars ventralis	Ventral part
A14.1.04.317	Nucleus reticularis medialis	Medial reticular nucleus
A14.1.04.318	**Nuclei raphes**	**Raphe nuclei**
A14.1.04.319	Nucleus raphes obscurus	Obscurus raphe nucleus
A14.1.04.320	Nucleus raphes pallidus	Pallidal raphe nucleus
A14.1.04.321	Nucleus raphes magnus	Magnus raphe nucleus

A14.1.03.010	**PONS**	**PONS**
	Morphologia externa	*External features*
A14.1.05.001	Sulcus bulbopontinus	Medullopontine sulcus
A14.1.05.002	Sulcus basilaris	Basilar sulcus
A14.1.05.003	Pedunculus cerebellaris medius	Middle cerebellar peduncle
A14.1.05.004	Angulus pontocerebellaris	Cerebellopontine angle
A14.1.05.005	Frenulum veli	Frenulum veli
A14.1.05.006	Pedunculus cerebellaris superior	Superior cerebellar peduncle
A14.1.05.007	Velum medullare superius	Superior medullary velum

	Morphologia interna	*Internal features*
A14.1.05.101	**Pars basilaris pontis**	**Basilar part of pons**
A14.1.05.102	**Substantia alba**	**White substance**
A14.1.05.103	Fibrae pontis longitudinales	Longitudinal pontine fibres▲
A14.1.05.104	Fibrae corticospinales	Corticospinal fibres▲
A14.1.05.105	Fibrae corticonucleares pontis	Pontine corticonuclear fibres▲
A14.1.05.106	Fibrae corticoreticulares	Corticoreticular fibres▲
A14.1.05.107	Fibrae corticopontinae	Corticopontine fibres▲
A14.1.05.108	Fibrae tectopontinae	Tectopontine fibres▲
A14.1.05.109	Fibrae pontis transversae	Transverse pontine fibres▲
A14.1.05.110	Fibrae pontocerebellares	Pontocerebellar fibres▲

A14.1.05.201	**Substantia grisea**	**Grey substance▲**
A14.1.05.202	Nuclei pontis	Pontine nuclei
A14.1.05.203	Nucleus anterior	Anterior nucleus; Ventral nucleus
A14.1.05.204	Nucleus lateralis	Lateral nucleus
A14.1.05.205	Nucleus medianus	Median nucleus
A14.1.05.206	Nucleus paramedianus	Paramedian nucleus
A14.1.05.207	Nucleus peduncularis	Peduncular nucleus; Peripeduncular nucleus
A14.1.05.208	Nucleus posterior	Posterior nucleus; Dorsal nucleus
A14.1.05.209	Nucleus posterior lateralis	Posterolateral nucleus; Dorsolateral nucleus
A14.1.05.210	Nucleus posterior medialis	Posteromedial nucleus; Dorsomedial nucleus
A14.1.05.211	Nucleus reticularis tegmenti pontis	Reticulotegmental nucleus

A14.1.05.301	**Tegmentum pontis**	**Tegmentum of pons**
A14.1.05.302	**Substantia alba**	**White substance**
A14.1.05.303	Raphe pontis	Raphe of pons
A14.1.05.304	Fasciculus longitudinalis medialis	Medial longitudinal fasciculus
A14.1.05.305	Fasciculus longitudinalis posterior; Fasciculus longitudinalis dorsalis	Posterior longitudinal fasciculus; Dorsal longitudinal fasciculus
A14.1.04.111	Lemniscus medialis	Medial lemniscus

A14.1.04.112	Tractus tectospinalis	Tectospinal tract
A14.1.05.306	Fibrae pretectoolivares	Pretecto-olivary fibres▲
A14.1.05.307	Fibrae tectoolivares	Tecto-olivary fibres▲
A14.1.05.308	Fibrae tectoreticulares	Tectoreticular fibres▲
* **A14.1.04.137**	Lemniscus spinalis; Tractus anterolaterales	Spinal lemniscus; Anterolateral tracts; Anterolateral system
A14.1.04.138	Fibrae spinothalamicae	Spinothalamic fibres▲
A14.1.04.139	Fibrae spinoreticulares	Spinoreticular fibres▲
A14.1.04.140	Fibrae spinomesencephalicae	Spinomesencephalic fibres▲
A14.1.04.141	Fibrae spinotectales	Spinotectal fibres▲
A14.1.04.142	Fibrae spinoperiaqueductales	Spinoperiaqueductal fibres▲
A14.1.04.143	Fibrae spinohypothalamicae	Spinohypothalamic fibres▲
A14.1.04.144	Fibrae spinobulbares	Spinobulbar fibres▲
A14.1.04.145	Fibrae spinoolivares	Spino-olivary fibres▲
A14.1.05.309	Tractus spinalis nervi trigemini	Spinal tract of trigeminal nerve
* **A14.1.05.310**	Lemniscus trigeminalis; Tractus trigeminothalamicus	Trigeminal lemniscus; Trigeminothalamic tract
A14.1.05.311	Tractus trigeminothalamicus anterior	Anterior trigeminothalamic tract; Ventral trigeminothalamic tract
A14.1.05.312	Tractus trigeminothalamicus posterior	Posterior trigeminothalamic tract; Dorsal trigeminothalamic tract
A14.1.05.313	Tractus mesencephalicus nervi trigemini	Mesencephalic tract of trigeminal nerve
A14.1.05.314	Genu nervi facialis	Genu of facial nerve
A14.1.05.315	Corpus trapezoideum	Trapezoid body
A14.1.05.316	Tractus olivocochlearis	Olivocochlear tract
A14.1.05.317	Lemniscus lateralis	Lateral lemniscus
A14.1.05.318	Striae medullares ventriculi quarti	Medullary striae of fourth ventricle
A14.1.05.319	Stria cochlearis anterior	Anterior acoustic stria; Ventral acoustic stria
A14.1.05.320	Stria cochlearis intermedia	Intermediate acoustic stria
A14.1.05.321	Stria cochlearis posterior	Posterior acoustic stria; Dorsal acoustic stria
A14.1.05.322	Tractus pontoreticulospinalis anterior	Anterior pontoreticulospinal tract; Ventral pontoreticulospinal tract
A14.1.05.323	Tractus spinocerebellaris anterior	Anterior spinocerebellar tract; Ventral spinocerebellar tract
A14.1.05.324	Commissura cochlearis pontis	Auditory commissure of pons
A14.1.05.325	Tractus tegmentalis centralis	Central tegmental tract
A14.1.05.326	Fibrae rubroolivares	Rubro-olivary fibres▲
A14.1.05.327	Fibrae anuloolivares	Anulo-olivary fibres▲
A14.1.05.328	Fibrae cerebelloolivares	Cerebello-olivary fibres▲
A14.1.05.329	Tractus hypothalamospinalis	Hypothalamospinal tract
A14.1.05.330	Tractus interstitiospinalis	Interstitiospinal tract
A14.1.05.331	Tractus rubropontinus	Rubropontine tract
A14.1.05.332	Tractus rubrospinalis	Rubrospinal tract
A14.1.05.333	Tractus tectobulbaris	Tectobulbar tract
A14.1.05.334	Tractus tectopontinus	Tectopontine tract

A14.1.05.401	**Substantia grisea**	**Grey substance▲**
A14.1.05.402	Nuclei raphes	Raphe nuclei
A14.1.05.403	Formatio reticularis	Reticular formation
A14.1.05.404	Nucleus spinalis nervi trigemini {vide etiam paginam 110}	Spinal nucleus of trigeminal nerve {see also page 110}
A14.1.05.405	Subnucleus oralis	Oral subnucleus
* **A14.1.05.406**	Nucleus principalis nervi trigemini	Principal sensory nucleus of trigeminal nerve

* **A14.1.04.137** *Lemniscus spinalis* Contains a variety of ascending axons and, in this respect, contains essentially the same population of axons that comprise the *tractus anterolateralis*. These are synonymous terms.

* **A14.1.05.310** *Lemniscus trigeminalis* As used here, this contains axons which originate within all sensory nuclei of the trigeminal nerve. These axons form posterior (dorsal, crossed) and anterior (ventral, uncrossed) trigeminothalamic tracts.

* **A14.1.05.406** *Nucleus principalis nervi trigemini* This term is recommended, rather than *nucleus pontinus nervi trigeminalis*, to distinguish it more clearly from the oral part of the spinal trigeminal nucleus which is also found in the *tegmentum pontis*.

A14.1.05.407	Nucleus posteromedialis	Posteromedial nucleus; Dorsomedial nucleus
A14.1.05.408	Nucleus anterolateralis	Anterolateral nucleus; Ventrolateral nucleus
A14.1.05.409	Nucleus mesencephalicus nervi trigemini	Mesencephalic nucleus of trigeminal nerve
A14.1.05.410	Nucleus motorius nervi trigemini	Motor nucleus of trigeminal nerve
A14.1.05.411	Nucleus nervi abducentis	Nucleus of abducens nerve
A14.1.05.412	Nucleus nervi facialis	Motor nucleus of facial nerve
A14.1.05.413	Nucleus salivatorius superior	Superior salivatory nucleus
A14.1.05.414	Nucleus lacrimalis	Lacrimal nucleus
A14.1.05.415	Nucleus olivaris superior	Superior olivary nucleus; Superior olivary complex
A14.1.05.416	Nucleus olivaris superior lateralis	Lateral superior olivary nucleus
A14.1.05.417	Nucleus olivaris superior medialis	Medial superior olivary nucleus
A14.1.05.418	Nuclei periolivares	Peri-olivary nuclei
A14.1.05.419	Nuclei mediales	Medial nuclei
A14.1.05.420	Nuclei laterales	Lateral nuclei
A14.1.05.421	Nuclei corporis trapezoidei	Nuclei of trapezoid body
A14.1.05.422	Nucleus anterior corporis trapezoidei	Anterior nucleus of trapezoid body; Ventral nucleus of trapezoid body
A14.1.05.423	Nucleus lateralis corporis trapezoidei	Lateral nucleus of trapezoid body
A14.1.05.424	Nucleus medialis corporis trapezoidei	Medial nucleus of trapezoid body
A14.1.05.425	Nuclei vestibulares {vide etiam paginam 111}	Vestibular nuclei {see also page 111}
A14.1.05.426	Nucleus vestibularis medialis	Medial vestibular nucleus
A14.1.05.427	Nucleus vestibularis lateralis	Lateral vestibular nucleus
A14.1.05.428	Pars parvocellularis	Parvocellular part; Cell group L
A14.1.05.429	Nucleus vestibularis superior	Superior vestibular nucleus
A14.1.05.430	Nuclei cochleares {vide etiam paginam 111}	Cochlear nuclei {see also page 111}
A14.1.05.431	Nuclei lemnisci lateralis	Nuclei of lateral lemniscus
A14.1.05.432	Nucleus posterior lemnisci lateralis	Posterior nucleus of lateral lemniscus; Dorsal nucleus of lateral lemniscus
A14.1.05.433	Nucleus intermedius lemnisci lateralis	Intermediate nucleus of lateral lemniscus
A14.1.05.434	Nucleus anterior lemnisci lateralis	Anterior nucleus of lateral lemniscus; Ventral nucleus of lateral lemniscus
A14.1.05.435	Nucleus tegmentalis anterior	Anterior tegmental nucleus; Ventral tegmental nucleus
A14.1.05.436	Nucleus caeruleus	Caerulean nucleus
A14.1.05.437	Nucleus subcaeruleus	Subcaerulean nucleus
A14.1.05.438	Nuclei interstitiales fasciculi longitudinalis medialis	Interstitial nuclei of medial longitudinal fasciculus
A14.1.05.439	Nuclei parabrachiales	Parabrachial nuclei
A14.1.05.440	Nucleus subparabrachialis	Subparabrachial nucleus
A14.1.05.441	Nucleus parabrachialis lateralis	Lateral parabrachial nucleus
A14.1.05.442	Pars lateralis	Lateral part; Lateral subnucleus
A14.1.05.443	Pars medialis	Medial part; Medial subnucleus
A14.1.05.444	Pars posterior	Posterior part; Dorsal part; Posterior subnucleus; Dorsal subnucleus
A14.1.05.445	Pars anterior	Anterior part; Ventral part; Anterior subnucleus; Ventral subnucleus
A14.1.05.446	Nucleus parabrachialis medialis	Medial parabrachial nucleus
A14.1.05.447	Pars medialis	Medial part; Medial subnucleus
A14.1.05.448	Pars lateralis	Lateral part; Lateral subnucleus
A14.1.05.449	Nucleus tegmentalis posterior	Posterior tegmental nucleus; Dorsal tegmental nucleus
A14.1.05.450	Nucleus supralemniscalis	Supralemniscal nucleus
A14.1.05.501	**Nuclei reticulares**	**Reticular nuclei**
* **A14.1.05.502**	Nucleus reticularis pontis caudalis	Caudal pontine reticular nucleus
A14.1.05.503	Nucleus reticularis pontis rostralis	Oral pontine reticular nucleus
A14.1.05.504	Nucleus paralemniscalis	Paralemniscal nucleus

* **A14.1.05.502** *Nucleus gigantocellularis, pars alpha*, and *nucleus reticularis pontis caudalis* These have been modified from previous nomenclature lists to conform with the more widely accepted and used terminology of Olszewski J. and D. Baxter. 1982. *Cytoarchitecture of the Human Brain Stem*. Basel: Karger.

A14.1.05.505	Nucleus reticularis paramedianus	Paramedian reticular nucleus
A14.1.05.506	Nucleus reticularis tegmenti pontis	Reticulotegmental nucleus
A14.1.05.601	**Nuclei raphes**	**Raphe nuclei**
A14.1.04.321	Nucleus raphes magnus	Magnus raphe nucleus
A14.1.05.602	Nucleus raphes pontis	Pontine raphe nucleus
A14.1.05.603	Nucleus raphes medianus	Median raphe nucleus; Superior central nucleus
A14.1.05.604	Nucleus raphes posterior	Posterior raphe nucleus; Dorsal raphe nucleus
A14.1.05.701	**Ventriculus quartus**	**Fourth ventricle**
A14.1.05.702	Fossa rhomboidea	Rhomboid fossa; Floor of fourth ventricle
A14.1.05.703	Sulcus medianus	Median sulcus
A14.1.05.704	Eminentia medialis	Medial eminence
A14.1.05.705	Colliculus facialis	Facial colliculus
A14.1.05.706	Locus caeruleus	Locus caeruleus
A14.1.05.707	Striae medullares ventriculi quarti	Medullary stria of fourth ventricle
A14.1.05.708	Trigonum nervi hypoglossi	Hypoglossal trigone; Trigone of hypoglossal nerve
A14.1.05.709	Trigonum nervi vagi; Trigonum vagale	Vagal trigone; Trigone of vagus nerve
A14.1.05.710	Area vestibularis	Vestibular area
A14.1.05.711	Funiculus separans	Funiculus separans
A14.1.05.712	Taenia cinerea	Grey line; Taenia cinerea▲
A14.1.05.713	Tegmen ventriculi quarti	Roof of fourth ventricle
A14.1.05.714	Fastigium	Fastigium
A14.1.05.715	Plexus choroideus	Choroid plexus
A14.1.05.716	Tela choroidea	Choroid membrane
A14.1.05.717	Recessus lateralis	Lateral recess
A14.1.05.718	Apertura lateralis	Lateral aperture
A14.1.05.719	Velum medullare superius	Superior medullary velum
A14.1.05.720	Frenulum veli medullaris superioris	Frenulum of superior medullary vellum
A14.1.05.721	Velum medullare inferius	Inferior medullary velum
A14.1.05.722	Apertura mediana	Median aperture
A14.1.04.258	Area postrema	Area postrema
A14.1.05.723	Obex	Obex
A14.1.05.724	Sulcus limitans	Sulcus limitans
A14.1.05.725	Fovea superior	Superior fovea
A14.1.05.726	Fovea inferior	Inferior fovea

A14.1.03.005	**MESENCEPHALON**	**MESENCEPHALON; MIDBRAIN**
	Morphologia externa	*External features*
A14.1.06.001	Fossa interpeduncularis	Interpeduncular fossa
A14.1.06.002	Substantia perforata posterior	Posterior perforated substance
A14.1.06.003	Sulcus nervi oculomotorii	Oculomotor sulcus
A14.1.06.004	Pedunculus cerebri	Cerebral peduncle
* **A14.1.06.005**	Crus cerebri	Cerebral crus
A14.1.06.006	Sulcus lateralis mesencephali	Lateral groove
A14.1.06.007	Tegmentum mesencephali	Tegmentum of midbrain
A14.1.06.008	Trigonum lemnisci lateralis	Trigone of lateral lemniscus
A14.1.06.009	Pedunculus cerebellaris superior	Superior cerebellar peduncle
A14.1.06.010	Frenulum veli medullaris superioris	Frenulum
A14.1.06.011	Lamina tecti; Lamina quadrigemina	Tectal plate; Quadrigeminal plate
A14.1.06.012	Brachium colliculi inferioris	Brachium of inferior colliculus
A14.1.06.013	Brachium colliculi superioris	Brachium of superior colliculus
A14.1.06.014	Colliculus inferior	Inferior colliculus
* **A14.1.06.015**	Colliculus superior	Superior colliculus

* **A14.1.06.005** *Crus cerebri* This term is preferred to the former *pedunculus cerebri pars anterior* for clarity.
* **A14.1.06.015** *Colliculus superior* Includes two cellular layers and one layer of axons within the intermediate grey layer.

	Morphologia interna	Internal features
A14.1.06.004	**Pedunculus cerebri**	**Cerebral peduncle**
A14.1.06.101	Basis pedunculi	Base of peduncle
* **A14.1.06.005**	**Crus cerebri**	**Cerebral crus**
A14.1.06.102	Tractus pyramidalis	Pyramidal tract
A14.1.06.103	Fibrae corticospinales	Corticospinal fibres▲
A14.1.06.104	Fibrae corticonucleares	Corticonuclear fibres▲
A14.1.06.105	Tractus corticopontinus	Corticopontine fibres▲
A14.1.06.106	Fibrae frontopontinae	Frontopontine fibres▲
A14.1.06.107	Fibrae occipitopontinae	Occipitopontine fibres▲
A14.1.06.108	Fibrae parietopontinae	Parietopontine fibres▲
A14.1.06.109	Fibrae temporopontinae	Temporopontine fibres▲
A14.1.06.110	Fibrae corticoreticulares	Corticoreticular fibres▲
* **A14.1.06.111**	**Substantia nigra**	**Substantia nigra**
A14.1.06.112	Pars compacta	Compact part
A14.1.06.113	Pars lateralis	Lateral part
A14.1.06.114	Pars reticularis	Reticular part
A14.1.06.115	Pars retrorubralis	Retrorubral part

A14.1.06.007	**Tegmentum mesencephali**	**Tegmentum of midbrain**
A14.1.06.201	**Substantia alba**	**White substance**
A14.1.05.325	Tractus tegmentalis centralis	Central tegmental tract
A14.1.05.326	Fibrae rubroolivares	Rubro-olivary fibres▲
A14.1.05.328	Fibrae cerebelloolivares	Cerebello-olivary fibres▲
A14.1.06.202	Fibrae corticonucleares mesencephali	Mesencephalic corticonuclear fibres▲
A14.1.06.203	Fibrae hypothalamospinales	Hypothalamospinal fibres▲
A14.1.06.204	Lemniscus lateralis	Lateral lemniscus
A14.1.06.205	Tractus tectopontinus	Tectopontine tract
A14.1.06.206	Tractus tectobulbaris lateralis	Lateral tectobulbar tract
A14.1.06.207	Lemniscus medialis	Medial lemniscus
A14.1.06.208	Lemniscus trigeminalis	Trigeminal lemniscus
A14.1.06.209	Fasciculus longitudinalis medialis	Medial longitudinal fasciculus
A14.1.06.210	Tractus mesencephalicus nervi trigemini	Mesencephalic tract of trigeminal nerve
A14.1.06.211	Fasciculus longitudinalis posterior; Fasciculus longitudinalis dorsalis	Posterior longitudinal fasciculus; Dorsal longitudinal fasciculus
A14.1.06.212	Tractus rubronuclearis	Rubronuclear tract
A14.1.06.213	Tractus rubrospinalis	Rubrospinal tract
A14.1.06.214	Tractus rubroolivaris	Rubro-olivary tract
* **A14.1.06.215**	Lemniscus spinalis; Tractus anterolaterales	Spinal lemniscus; Anterolateral tracts; Anterolateral system
A14.1.04.138	Fibrae spinothalamicae	Spinothalamic fibres▲
A14.1.04.139	Fibrae spinoreticulares	Spinoreticular fibres▲
A14.1.04.140	Fibrae spinomesencephalicae	Spinomesencephalic fibres▲
A14.1.04.141	Fibrae spinotectales	Spinotectal fibres▲
A14.1.04.142	Fibrae spinoperiaqueductales	Spinoperiaqueductal fibres▲
A14.1.04.143	Fibrae spinohypothalamicae	Spinohypothalamic fibres▲
A14.1.06.216	Pedunculus cerebellaris superior	Superior cerebellar peduncle
A14.1.06.217	Decussatio pedunculorum cerebellarium superiorum	Decussation of superior cerebellar peduncles
A14.1.06.218	Tractus tectobulbaris	Tectobulbar tract
A14.1.06.219	Tractus tectopontinus	Tectopontine tract
A14.1.04.112	Tractus tectospinalis	Tectospinal tract
A14.1.05.306	Fibrae pretectoolivares	Pretecto-olivary fibres▲

* **A14.1.06.005** *Crus cerebri* This term is preferred to the former *pedunculus cerebri pars anterior* for clarity.

* **A14.1.06.111** *Substantia nigra* This is not a component of the *tegmentum mesencephali*. It is ventrolateral to the *tegmentum* and separates this area from the fibre bundles of the *crus cerebri*. Some authors include the *substantia nigra* as part of the *basis pedunculi*, a convention followed here.

* **A14.1.06.215** *Lemniscus spinalis* Contains a variety of ascending axons and, in this respect, contains essentially the same population of axons that comprise the *tractus anterolateralis*. These are synonymous terms.

A14.1.05.307	Fibrae tectoolivares	Tecto-olivary fibres▲
A14.1.06.220	Decussationes tegmentales	Tegmental decussations
A14.1.06.221	Decussatio tegmentalis posterior	Posterior tegmental decussation; Dorsal tegmental decussation
A14.1.06.222	Decussatio tegmentalis anterior	Anterior tegmental decussation; Ventral tegmental decussation
* A14.1.06.223	Fibrae corticomesencephalicae	Corticomesencephalic fibres▲

A14.1.06.301	**Substantia grisea**	**Grey substance▲**
A14.1.06.302	Nucleus nervi oculomotorii	Nucleus of oculomotor nerve
A14.1.06.303	Nuclei accessorii nervi oculomotorii	Accessory nuclei of oculomotor nerve
A14.1.06.304	Nuclei viscerales; Nuclei autonomici	Visceral nuclei; Autonomic nuclei
A14.1.06.305	Nucleus anteromedialis	Anterior medial nucleus; Ventral medial nucleus
A14.1.06.306	Nucleus dorsalis	Posterior nucleus; Dorsal nucleus
A14.1.06.307	Nucleus interstitialis	Interstitial nucleus
A14.1.06.308	Nucleus precommissuralis centralis	Central precommissural nucleus
A14.1.06.309	Nucleus commissurae posterioris	Nucleus of posterior commissure
A14.1.06.310	Pars ventralis	Ventral subdivision
A14.1.06.311	Pars interstitialis	Interstitial subdivision
A14.1.06.312	Pars dorsalis	Dorsal subdivision
A14.1.06.313	Nucleus interpeduncularis	Interpeduncular nucleus
A14.1.06.314	Nuclei accessorii tractus optici	Accessory nuclei of optic tract
A14.1.06.315	Nucleus posterior	Posterior nucleus; Dorsal nucleus
A14.1.06.316	Nucleus lateralis	Lateral nucleus
A14.1.06.317	Nucleus medialis	Medial nucleus
A14.1.06.318	Nucleus tegmentalis posterolateralis	Lateroposterior tegmental nucleus; Laterodorsal tegmental nucleus
A14.1.05.409	Nucleus mesencephalicus nervi trigemini	Mesencephalic nucleus of trigeminal nerve
A14.1.06.319	Nucleus nervi trochlearis	Nucleus of trochlear nerve
* A14.1.06.320	Nucleus parabigeminalis	Parabigeminal nucleus
A14.1.06.321	Substantia grisea centralis	Periaqueductal grey substance; Central grey substance▲
A14.1.06.322	Nucleus peripeduncularis	Peripeduncular nucleus
A14.1.06.323	Nucleus ruber	Red nucleus
A14.1.06.324	Pars magnocellularis	Magnocellular part
A14.1.06.325	Pars parvocellularis	Parvocellular part
A14.1.06.326	Pars posteromedialis; Pars dorsomedialis	Posteromedial part; Dorsomedial part
A14.1.06.327	Formatio reticularis {vide nuclei reticulares paginam 118}	Reticular formation {see Reticular nuclei page 118}
A14.1.06.328	Nucleus saguli; Sagulum	Sagulum nucleus
A14.1.06.329	Nucleus subbrachialis	Subbrachial nucleus
A14.1.06.330	Nuclei tegmentales anteriores	Anterior tegmental nuclei; Ventral tegmental nuclei
A14.1.06.331	Nucleus interfascicularis	Interfascicular nucleus
A14.1.06.332	Nucleus pigmentosus parabrachialis	Parabrachial pigmented nucleus
A14.1.06.333	Nucleus paranigralis	Paranigral nucleus
A14.1.06.334	Nucleus cuneiformis	Cuneiform nucleus
A14.1.06.335	Nucleus subcuneiformis	Subcuneiform nucleus
A14.1.06.336	Nucleus tegmentalis pedunculopontinus	Pedunculopontine tegmental nucleus
A14.1.06.337	Pars compacta	Compact part; Compact subnucleus
A14.1.06.338	Pars dissipata	Dissipated part; Dissipated subnucleus
A14.1.06.401	**Nuclei raphes**	**Raphe nuclei**
A14.1.05.604	Nucleus raphes posterior	Posterior raphe nucleus; Dorsal raphe nucleus
A14.1.06.402	Nucleus linearis inferioris	Inferior linear nucleus

* **A14.1.06.223** *Fibrae corticomesencephalicae* Axons arising in the cerebral cortex that innervate mesencephalic structures such as the *substantia nigra, tegmentum mesencephali,* and the *tectum.*
* **A14.1.06.320** *Nucleus parabigeminalis* Located on the lateral aspect of the midbrain, adjacent to the inferior colliculus. It receives inputs from, and projects to, the superior colliculus.

A14.1.06.403	Nucleus linearis intermedius	Intermediate linear nucleus
A14.1.06.404	Nucleus linearis superior	Superior linear nucleus
A14.1.06.501	**Aqueductus mesencephali; Aqueductus cerebri**	**Aqueduct of midbrain; Cerebral aqueduct**
A14.1.06.502	Apertura aqueductus mesencephali; Apertura aqueductus cerebri	Opening of aqueduct of midbrain; Opening of cerebral aqueduct
A14.1.06.601	**Tectum mesencephali**	**Tectum of midbrain**
A14.1.06.011	Lamina tecti; Lamina quadrigemina	Tectal plate; Quadrigeminal plate
A14.1.06.014	Colliculus inferior	Inferior colliculus
A14.1.06.602	Nuclei colliculi inferioris	Nuclei of inferior colliculus
A14.1.06.603	Nucleus centralis	Central nucleus
A14.1.06.604	Nucleus externus; Nucleus lateralis	External nucleus
A14.1.06.605	Nucleus pericentralis	Pericentral nucleus
* A14.1.06.015	Colliculus superior	Superior colliculus
A14.1.06.606	Stratum zonale; Lamina I	Zonal layer; Layer I
A14.1.06.607	Stratum griseum superficiale; Lamina II	Superficial grey layer; Layer II▲
A14.1.06.608	Stratum opticum; Lamina III	Optic layer; Layer III
A14.1.06.609	Stratum griseum intermedium; Lamina IV	Intermediate grey layer; Layer IV▲
A14.1.06.610	Stratum medullare intermedium; Lamina V	Intermediate white layer; Layer V
A14.1.06.611	Stratum griseum profundum; Lamina VI	Deep grey layer; Layer VI▲
A14.1.06.612	Stratum medullare profundum; Lamina VII	Deep white layer; Layer VII
A14.1.06.012	Brachium colliculi inferioris	Brachium of inferior colliculus
A14.1.06.013	Brachium colliculi superioris	Brachium of superior colliculus
A14.1.06.613	Commissura colliculi inferioris	Commissure of inferior colliculus
A14.1.06.614	Commissura colliculi superioris	Commissure of superior colliculus
A14.1.06.615	Decussatio fibrarum nervorum trochlearium	Decussation of trochlear nerve fibres▲
A14.1.06.701	**Nuclei reticulares**	**Reticular nuclei**
A14.1.06.334	Nucleus cuneiformis	Cuneiform nucleus
A14.1.06.335	Nucleus subcuneiformis	Subcuneiform nucleus
A14.1.06.336	Nucleus tegmentalis pedunculopontinus	Pedunculopontine tegmental nucleus
A14.1.06.337	Pars compacta	Compact part; Compact subnucleus
A14.1.06.338	Pars dissipata	Dissipated part; Dissipated subnucleus
A14.1.06.702	Nucleus parapeduncularis	Parapeduncular nucleus

A14.1.07.001	CEREBELLUM	CEREBELLUM
	Nomina generalia	*General terms*
A14.1.07.002	Fissurae cerebelli	Cerebellar fissures
A14.1.07.003	Folia cerebelli	Folia of cerebellum
A14.1.07.004	Hemispherium cerebelli [H II – H X]	Hemisphere of cerebellum [H II – H X]
A14.1.07.005	Vallecula cerebelli	Vallecula of cerebellum
A14.1.07.006	Vermis cerebelli [I–X]	Vermis of cerebellum [I–X]
* A14.1.07.007	Vestibulocerebellum	Vestibulocerebellum
* A14.1.07.008	Spinocerebellum	Spinocerebellum
* A14.1.07.009	Pontocerebellum	Pontocerebellum
* A14.1.07.010	Archicerebellum	Archicerebellum
* A14.1.07.011	Paleocerebellum	Paleocerebellum
* A14.1.07.012	Neocerebellum	Neocerebellum

	Morphologia externa	*External features*
A14.1.07.101	**Corpus cerebelli**	**Body of cerebellum**
A14.1.07.102	**Lobus cerebelli anterior**	**Anterior lobe of cerebellum**
A14.1.07.103	Lingula cerebelli [I]	Lingula [I]

* **A14.1.06.015** *Colliculus superior* Includes two cellular layers and one layer of axons within the intermediate grey layer.

* **A14.1.07.007 – A14.1.07.012** *Vestibulocerebellum-neocerebellum* The terms *vestibulocerebellum* and *spinocerebellum* reflect the fact that neurons in the vestibular nuclei and ganglia, and the nuclei of the spinal cord project directly to cerebellar structures. Since nuclei of the *pars basilaris pontis* project directly to the cerebellum, the term *pontocerebellum* is preferred over *cerebrocerebellum*, and is, consequently, consistent with *vestibulocerebellum* and *spinocerebellum*. As originally conceived, the terms *archicerebellum, paleocerebellum* and *neocerebellum* referred to the flocculonodular, vermis, and hemisphere respectively. Experimental studies reveal that these terms do not correlate with the terms *vestibulocerebellum, spinocerebellum* and *pontocerebellum* and do not identify cerebellar regions that have their own unique connections. Their continued use is not encouraged.

A14.1.07.104	Fissura precentralis; Fissura postlingualis	Precentral fissure; Post-lingual fissure
A14.1.07.105	Lobulus centralis [II et III]	Central lobule [II and III]
A14.1.07.106	Pars anterior; Pars ventralis [II]	Anterior part; Ventral part [II]
A14.1.07.107	Pars posterior; Pars dorsalis [III]	Posterior part; Dorsal part [III]
A14.1.07.108	Ala lobuli centralis	Wing of central lobule
A14.1.07.109	Pars inferior; Pars ventralis [H II]	Inferior part; Ventral part [H II]
A14.1.07.110	Pars superior; Pars dorsalis [H III]	Superior part; Dorsal part [H III]
A14.1.07.111	Fissura preculminalis; Fissura postcentralis	Preculminate fissure; Post-central fissure
A14.1.07.112	Culmen [IV et V]	Culmen [IV and V]
A14.1.07.113	Pars anterior; Pars ventralis [IV]	Anterior part; Ventral part [IV]
A14.1.07.114	Fissura intraculminalis	Intraculminate fissure
A14.1.07.115	Pars posterior; Pars dorsalis [V]	Posterior part; Dorsal part [V]
A14.1.07.116	Lobulus quadrangularis anterior [H IV et H V]	Anterior quadrangular lobule [H IV and H V]
A14.1.07.117	Pars anterior; Pars ventralis [H IV]	Anterior part; Ventral part [H IV]
A14.1.07.118	Pars posterior; Pars dorsalis [H V]	Posterior part; Dorsal part [H V]
A14.1.07.119	Fissura prima; Fissura preclivalis	Primary fissure; Preclival fissure
A14.1.07.201	**Lobus cerebelli posterior**	**Posterior lobe of cerebellum**
A14.1.07.202	Lobulus simplex [H VI et VI]	Simple lobule [H VI and VI]
A14.1.07.203	Declive [VI]	Declive [VI]
A14.1.07.204	Lobulus quadrangularis posterior [H VI]	Posterior quadrangular lobule [H VI]
A14.1.07.205	Fissura posterior superior; Fissura post clivalis	Posterior superior fissure; Post-clival fissure
A14.1.07.206	Folium vermis [VII A]	Folium of vermis [VII A]
A14.1.07.207	Lobuli semilunares; Lobulus ansiformis [H VII A]	Semilunar lobules; Ansiform lobule [H VII A]
A14.1.07.208	Lobulus semilunaris superior; Crus primum lobuli ansiformis [H VII A]	Superior semilunar lobule; First crus of ansiform lobule [H VII A]
A14.1.07.209	Fissurae horizontalis; Fissura intercruralis	Horizontal fissure; Intercrural fissure
A14.1.07.210	Lobulus semilunaris inferior; Crus secundum lobuli ansiformis [H VII A]	Inferior semilunar lobule; Second crus of ansiform lobule [H VII A]
A14.1.07.211	Fissura lunogracilis; Fissura ansoparamedianis	Lunogracile fissure; Ansoparamedian fissure
A14.1.07.212	Tuber [VII B]	Tuber [VII B]
A14.1.07.213	Lobulus gracilis; Lobulus paramedianus [H VII B]	Gracile lobule; Paramedian lobule [H VII B]
A14.1.07.214	Fissura prebiventralis; Fissura prepyramidalis	Prebiventral fissure; Prepyramidal fissure
A14.1.07.215	Pyramis [VIII]	Pyramis [VIII]
A14.1.07.216	Lobulus biventer [H VIII]	Biventral lobule [H VIII]
A14.1.07.217	Pars lateralis lobuli biventralis; Pars copularis lobuli paramediani [H VIII A]	Lateral part; Pars copularis [H VIII A]
A14.1.07.218	Fissura intrabiventralis; Fissura anterior inferior	Intrabiventral fissure; Anterior inferior fissure
A14.1.07.219	Pars medialis lobuli biventralis; Lobulus parafloccularis dorsalis [H VIII B]	Medial Part; Dorsal paraflocculars [H VIII B]
A14.1.07.220	Fissura secunda; Fissura postpyramidalis	Secondary fissure; Post-pyramidal fissure
A14.1.07.221	Uvula [IX]	Uvula [IX]
A14.1.07.222	Tonsilla cerebelli; Paraflocculus ventralis [H IX]	Tonsil of cerebellum; Ventral paraflocculus [H IX]
A14.1.07.223	Fissura posterolateralis	Posterolateral fissure
A14.1.07.301	**Lobus flocculonodularis**	**Flocculonodular lobe**
A14.1.07.302	Nodulus [X]	Nodule [X]
A14.1.07.303	Pedunculus flocculi	Peduncle of flocculus
A14.1.07.304	Flocculus [H X]	Flocculus [H X]

	Morphologia interna	*Internal features*
A14.1.07.401	Arbor vitae	Arbor vitae
A14.1.07.402	**Cortex cerebelli**	**Cerebellar cortex**
A14.1.07.403	Stratum granulosum	Granular layer
A14.1.07.404	Stratum purkinjense	Purkinje cell layer
A14.1.07.405	Stratum moleculare	Molecular layer

A14.1.07.404 *Stratum purkinjense* This term is recommended rather than *stratum neurium piriformium*. This layer of morphologically specialized cells is universally recognised by this particular term. The previous term (i.e., *stratum neurium piriformium* = layer of pear-shaped neurons) is rarely used in many countries (or texts for that matter) and it has never gained significant or wide usage. Use of the small p (*purkinjense*) changes *Purkinje* from the nominative form to the adjectival form, the latter modifying *stratum*.

* A14.1.07.406	**Nuclei cerebelli**	**Cerebellar nuclei**
A14.1.07.407	Nucleus dentatus; Nucleus lateralis cerebelli	Dentate nucleus; Nucleus lateralis cerebelli
A14.1.07.408	Hilum nuclei dentati	Hilum of dentate nucleus
A14.1.07.409	Nucleus interpositus anterior; Nucleus emboliformis	Anterior interpositus nucleus; Emboliform nucleus
A14.1.07.410	Nucleus interpositus posterior; Nucleus globosus	Posterior interpositus nucleus; Globose nucleus
A14.1.07.411	Nucleus fastigii; Nucleus medialis cerebelli	Fastigial nucleus; Nucleus medialis cerebelli
A14.1.07.412	**Pedunculi cerebellares**	**Cerebellar peduncles**
A14.1.07.413	Pedunculus cerebellaris inferior	Inferior cerebellar peduncle
A14.1.07.414	Corpus restiforme	Restiform body
A14.1.07.415	Corpus juxtarestiforme	Juxtarestiform body
A14.1.07.416	Pedunculus cerebellaris medius	Middle cerebellar peduncle
A14.1.07.417	Pedunculus cerebellaris superior	Superior cerebellar peduncle
A14.1.07.418	Corpus medullare cerebelli	White substance of cerebellum
A14.1.07.419	Commissura cerebelli	Cerebellar commissure
A14.1.07.420	Fasciculus uncinatus cerebelli	Uncinate fasciculus of cerebellum

A14.1.08.001	**DIENCEPHALON**	**DIENCEPHALON**
	Morphologia externa	*External features*
A14.1.08.002	**Epithalamus**	**Epithalamus**
A14.1.08.003	Habenula	Habenula
A14.1.08.004	Sulcus habenularis	Habenular sulcus
A14.1.08.005	Trigonum habenulare	Habenular trigone
A11.2.00.001	Glandula pinealis	Pineal gland

A14.1.08.101	**Thalamus**	**Thalamus; Dorsal thalamus**
A14.1.08.102	Tuberculum anterius thalami	Anterior thalamic tubercle
A14.1.08.103	Adhesio interthalamica	Interthalamic adhesion; Massa intermedia
A14.1.08.104	Pulvinar thalami	Pulvinar
A14.1.08.105	Taenia thalami	Taenia thalami▴
A14.1.08.106	Stria medullaris thalami	Stria medullaris of thalamus

A14.1.08.201	**Subthalamus**	**Subthalamus; Ventral thalamus**

A14.1.08.301	**Metathalamus**	**Metathalamus**
A14.1.08.302	Corpus geniculatum laterale	Lateral geniculate body
A14.1.08.303	Corpus geniculatum mediale	Medial geniculate body

A14.1.08.401	**Hypothalamus**	**Hypothalamus**
A14.1.08.402	Corpus mammillare	Mammillary body
A11.1.00.006	Neurohypophysis	Neurohypophysis
A11.1.00.007	Infundibulum	Infundibulum
A11.1.00.008	Pars nervosa	Pars nervosa
A14.1.08.403	Chiasma opticum	Optic chiasm; Optic chiasma
A14.1.08.404	Tractus opticus	Optic tract
A14.1.08.405	Radix lateralis	Lateral root
A14.1.08.406	Radix medialis	Medial root
A14.1.08.407	Area preoptica	Preoptic area
A14.1.08.408	Tuber cinereum	Tuber cinereum
A14.1.08.409	Eminentia mediana	Median eminence
A14.1.08.410	**Ventriculus tertius**	**Third ventricle**
A14.1.08.411	Foramen interventriculare	Interventricular foramen

* **A14.1.07.406** *Nuclei cerebelli* The terms "dentate," "emboliform," "globose," and "fastigial" are used for the nuclei of the human cerebellum and, frequently, for these nuclei in nonhuman primates. The terms "lateral," "anterior interpositus," "posterior interpositus," and "medial cerebellar nuclei" are, respectively, synonymous with the above terms and are commonly used to describe the cerebellar nuclei in nonprimate mammals and, occasionally, in primates. Rudeberg S.-I. 1961. *Morphogenetic Studies on the Cerebellar Nuclei and their Homologization in Different Vertebrates Including Man.* Diss., Tornblad Institute of Comparative Embryology and Institute of Zoology, University of Lund, Lund, Sweden: pp. 1–148.

A14.1.08.412	Organum subfornicale	Subfornical organ
A14.1.08.105	Taenia thalami	Taenia thalami▲
A14.1.01.305	Tela choroidea	Choroid membrane
A14.1.01.306	Plexus choroideus	Choroid plexus
A14.1.08.106	Stria medullaris thalami	Stria medullaris thalami
A14.1.08.413	Recessus suprapinealis	Suprapineal recess
A14.1.08.414	Commissura habenularum	Habenular commissure
A14.1.08.415	Recessus pinealis	Pineal recess
A14.1.08.416	Commissura posterior; Commissura epithalamica	Posterior commissure
A14.1.06.502	Apertura aqueductus mesencephali; Apertura aqueductus cerebri	Opening of aqueduct of midbrain; Opening of cerebral aqueduct
A14.1.08.417	Recessus infundibuli; Recessus infundibularis	Infundibular recess
A14.1.08.418	Recessus supraopticus	Supra-optic recess
A14.1.08.419	Lamina terminalis	Lamina terminalis
A14.1.08.420	Columna fornicis	Column of fornix
A14.1.08.421	Commissura anterior	Anterior commissure
A14.1.08.422	Sulcus hypothalamicus	Hypothalamic sulcus
A14.1.08.103	Adhesio interthalamica	Interthalamic adhesion; Massa intermedia

	Morphologia interna	*Internal features*
A14.1.08.501	**Epithalamus**	**Epithalamus**
A14.1.08.414	Commissura habenularum	Habenular commissure
A14.1.08.502	Tractus habenulointerpeduncularis;fasciculus retroflexus	Habenulo-interpeduncular tract; Fasciculus retroflexus
A14.1.08.503	Nucleus habenularis lateralis	Lateral habenular nucleus
A14.1.08.504	Nucleus habenularis medialis	Medial habenular nucleus
A14.1.08.416	Commissura posterior; Commissura epithalamica	Posterior commissure
A14.1.08.505	Area pretectalis	Pretectal area
A14.1.08.506	Nuclei pretectales	Pretectal nuclei
A14.1.08.507	Nucleus pretectalis anterior	Anterior pretectal nucleus
A14.1.08.508	Nucleus tractus optici	Nucleus of optic tract
A14.1.08.509	Nucleus pretectalis olivaris	Olivary pretectal nucleus
A14.1.08.510	Nucleus pretectalis posterior	Posterior pretectal nucleus
A14.1.08.511	Organum subcommissurale	Subcommissural organ

A14.1.08.601	**Thalamus**	**Thalamus**
A14.1.08.602	**Substantia grisea thalami**	**Grey substance of thalamus▲**
A14.1.08.603	Nuclei anteriores thalami	Anterior nuclei of thalamus
A14.1.08.604	Nucleus anterodorsalis	Anterodorsal nucleus
A14.1.08.605	Nucleus anteromedialis	Anteromedial nucleus
A14.1.08.606	Nucleus anteroventralis	Anteroventral nucleus
A14.1.08.607	Nuclei dorsales thalami	Dorsal nuclei of thalamus
A14.1.08.608	Nucleus dorsalis lateralis	Lateral dorsal nucleus
A14.1.08.609	Nucleus lateralis posterior	Lateral posterior nucleus
A14.1.08.610	Nuclei pulvinares	Pulvinar nuclei
A14.1.08.611	Nucleus pulvinaris anterior	Anterior pulvinar nucleus
A14.1.08.612	Nucleus pulvinaris inferior	Inferior pulvinar nucleus
A14.1.08.613	Nucleus pulvinaris lateralis	Lateral pulvinar nucleus
A14.1.08.614	Nucleus pulvinaris medialis	Medial pulvinar nucleus
A14.1.08.615	Nuclei intralaminares thalami	Intralaminar nuclei of thalamus
A14.1.08.616	Nucleus centralis lateralis	Central lateral nucleus
A14.1.08.617	Nucleus centralis medialis	Central medial nucleus
A14.1.08.618	Nucleus centromedianus	Centromedian nucleus
A14.1.08.619	Nucleus paracentralis	Paracentral nucleus
A14.1.08.620	Nucleus parafascicularis	Parafascicular nucleus
A14.1.08.621	Nuclei mediales thalami	Medial nuclei of thalamus

A14.1.08.622	Nucleus mediodorsalis	Medial dorsal nucleus; Dorsomedial nucleus
A14.1.08.623	Pars parvocellularis lateralis	Lateral nucleus; Parvocellular nucleus
A14.1.08.624	Pars magnocellularis medialis	Medial nucleus; Magnocellular nucleus
A14.1.08.625	Pars paralaminaris	Paralaminar part; Pars laminaris
A14.1.08.626	Nucleus medioventralis	Medial ventral nucleus
A14.1.08.627	Nuclei mediani thalami	Median nuclei of thalamus
A14.1.08.628	Nucleus parataenialis	Parataenial nucleus▲
A14.1.08.629	Nuclei paraventriculares thalami	Paraventricular nuclei of thalamus
A14.1.08.630	Nucleus paraventricularis anterior	Anterior paraventricular nucleus
A14.1.08.631	Nucleus paraventricularis posterior	Posterior paraventricular nucleus
A14.1.08.632	Nucleus reuniens	Nucleus reuniens
A14.1.08.633	Nucleus commissuralis rhomboidalis	Rhomboid nucleus
A14.1.08.634	Nuclei posteriores thalami	Posterior nuclear complex of thalamus
A14.1.08.635	Nucleus limitans	Nucleus limitans
A14.1.08.636	Nucleus posterior	Posterior nucleus
A14.1.08.637	Nucleus suprageniculatus	Suprageniculate nucleus
A14.1.08.638	Nucleus reticularis thalami	Reticular nucleus of thalamus
A14.1.08.639	Nuclei ventrales thalami	Ventral nuclei of thalamus
A14.1.08.640	Nuclei ventrobasales	Ventrobasal complex
A14.1.08.641	Nucleus ventralis posterolateralis	Ventral posterolateral nucleus
A14.1.08.642	Nucleus ventralis posteromedialis	Ventral posteromedial nucleus
A14.1.08.643	Pars parvocellularis	Parvocellular part
A14.1.08.644	Nuclei ventrales mediales	Ventral medial complex
A14.1.08.645	Nucleus basalis ventralis medialis	Basal ventral medial nucleus
A14.1.08.646	Nucleus principalis ventralis medialis	Principal ventral medial nucleus
A14.1.08.647	Nucleus submedialis	Submedial nucleus
A14.1.08.648	Nucleus ventralis posterior inferior	Ventral posterior inferior nucleus
A14.1.08.649	Nuclei ventrales laterales	Ventral lateral complex
A14.1.08.650	Nucleus anterior ventrolateralis	Anterior ventrolateral nucleus
A14.1.08.651	Nucleus posterior ventrolateralis	Posterior ventrolateral nucleus
A14.1.08.652	Nucleus ventralis anterior	Ventral anterior nucleus
A14.1.08.653	Pars magnocellularis	Magnocellular division
A14.1.08.654	Pars principalis	Principal division
A14.1.08.655	Nucleus ventralis intermedius	Ventral intermediate nucleus
A14.1.08.656	Nucleus ventralis posterolateralis	Ventral posterolateral nucleus
A14.1.08.657	Nucleus ventralis posterior internus	Ventral posterior internal nucleus
A14.1.08.658	Nucleus ventroposterior parvocellularis	Ventral posterior parvocellular nucleus
A14.1.08.659	**Substantia alba thalami**	**White substance of thalamus**
A14.1.08.660	Lamina medullaris lateralis	External medullary lamina
A14.1.08.661	Lamina medullaris medialis	Internal medullary lamina
A14.1.08.662	Radiatio acustica	Acoustic radiation
A14.1.08.663	Ansa lenticularis	Ansa lenticularis
A14.1.08.664	Fasciculus lenticularis	Lenticular fasciculus
A14.1.08.665	Ansa peduncularis	Ansa peduncularis
A14.1.08.666	Radiatio anterior thalami	Anterior radiation of thalamus
A14.1.06.012	Brachium colliculi inferioris	Brachium of inferior colliculus
A14.1.06.013	Brachium colliculi superioris	Brachium of superior colliculus
A14.1.08.667	Radiatio centralis thalami	Central thalamic radiation
A14.1.08.668	Radiatio inferior thalami	Inferior thalamic radiation
A14.1.08.669	Fibrae intrathalamicae	Intrathalamic fibres▲
A14.1.08.670	Lemniscus lateralis	Lateral lemniscus
A14.1.08.671	Fasciculus mammillothalamicus	Mammillothalamic fasciculus
A14.1.08.672	Lemniscus medialis	Medial lemniscus
A14.1.08.673	Radiatio optica	Optic radiation
A14.1.08.674	Fibrae periventriculares	Periventricular fibres▲
A14.1.08.675	Radiatio posterior thalami	Posterior thalamic radiation
A14.1.08.676	Lemniscus spinalis	Spinal lemniscus
A14.1.08.677	Fasciculus subthalamicus	Subthalamic fasciculus
A14.1.08.678	Pedunculus cerebellaris superior	Superior cerebellar peduncle

A14.1.08.679	Fasciculus thalamicus	Thalamic fasciculus
A14.1.08.680	Lemniscus trigeminalis	Trigeminal lemniscus

A14.1.08.701	**Subthalamus**	**Subthalamus**
A14.1.08.702	Nucleus subthalamicus	Subthalamic nucleus
* A14.1.08.703	Nuclei campi perizonalis [H, H1, H2]	Nuclei of perizonal fields [H, H1, H2]
A14.1.08.704	Nucleus campi medialis [H]	Nucleus of medial field [H]
A14.1.08.705	Nucleus campi dorsalis [H1]	Nucleus of dorsal field [H1]
A14.1.08.706	Nucleus campi ventralis [H2]	Nucleus of ventral field [H2]
A14.1.08.707	Zona incerta	Zona incerta

A14.1.08.801	**Metathalamus**	**Metathalamus**
A14.1.08.802	Nucleus dorsalis corporis geniculati lateralis	Dorsal lateral geniculate nucleus
A14.1.08.803	Stratum koniocellulare	Koniocellular layer
A14.1.08.804	Strata magnocellularia	Magnocellular layers
A14.1.08.805	Strata parvocellularia	Parvocellular layers
A14.1.08.806	Nucleus ventralis corporis geniculati lateralis; Nucleus pregeniculatus	Ventral lateral geniculate nucleus; Pregeniculate nucleus
A14.1.08.807	Folium intergeniculatum	Intergeniculate leaf
A14.1.08.808	Nuclei corporis geniculati medialis	Medial geniculate nuclei
A14.1.08.809	Nucleus ventralis	Ventral principal nucleus
A14.1.08.810	Nucleus dorsalis	Dorsal nucleus
A14.1.08.811	Nucleus medialis magnocellularis	Medial magnocellular nucleus

A14.1.08.901	**Hypothalamus**	**Hypothalamus**
A14.1.08.902	Area hypothalamica rostralis	Anterior hypothalamic area; Anterior hypothalamic region
A14.1.08.903	Nucleus anterior hypothalami	Anterior hypothalamic nucleus
A14.1.08.904	Nucleus periventricularis ventralis	Anterior periventricular nucleus
A14.1.08.905	Nuclei interstitiales hypothalami anteriores	Interstitial nuclei of anterior hypothalamus
A14.1.08.906	Nucleus preopticus lateralis	Lateral preoptic nucleus
A14.1.08.907	Nucleus preopticus medialis	Medial preoptic nucleus
A14.1.08.908	Nucleus preopticus medianus	Median preoptic nucleus
A14.1.08.909	Nucleus paraventricularis hypothalami	Paraventricular nucleus
A14.1.08.910	Nucleus preopticus periventricularis	Periventricular preoptic nucleus
A14.1.08.911	Nucleus suprachiasmaticus	Suprachiasmatic nucleus
A14.1.08.912	Nucleus supraopticus	Supra-optic nucleus
A14.1.08.913	Pars dorsolateralis	Dorsolateral part
A14.1.08.914	Pars dorsomedialis	Dorsomedial part
A14.1.08.915	Pars ventromedialis	Ventromedial part
A14.1.08.916	Area hypothalamica dorsalis	Dorsal hypothalamic area; Dorsal hypothalamic region
A14.1.08.917	Nucleus dorsomedialis	Dorsomedial nucleus
A14.1.08.918	Nucleus endopeduncularis	Endopeduncular nucleus
A14.1.08.919	Nucleus ansae lenticularis	Nucleus of ansa lenticularis
A14.1.08.920	Area hypothalamica intermedia	Intermediate hypothalamic area; Intermediate hypothalamic region
A14.1.08.921	Nucleus dorsalis hypothalami	Dorsal nucleus
A14.1.08.922	Nucleus dorsomedialis	Dorsomedial nucleus
A14.1.08.923	Nucleus arcuatus; Nucleus semilunaris; Nucleus infundibularis	Arcuate nucleus; Infundibular nucleus
A14.1.08.924	Nucleus periventricularis	Periventricular nucleus
A14.1.08.925	Nucleus periventricularis posterior	Posterior periventricular nucleus
A14.1.08.926	Area retrochiasmatica	Retrochiasmatic area; Retrochiasmatic region
A14.1.08.927	Nuclei tuberales laterales	Lateral tuberal nuclei

A14.1.08.703 *Nuclei campi perizonalis* Fibres in the medial field (also called the prerubral field or area) and in the dorsal field (*fasciculus thalamicus*) and ventral field (*fasciculus lenticularis*) comprise, respectively, the fields of Forel H, H1, and H2. Cell bodies insinuated among these fasciculi constitute the nuclei listed here.

A14.1.08.928	Nucleus ventromedialis hypothalami	Ventromedial nucleus of hypothalamus
A14.1.08.929	Area hypothalamica lateralis	Lateral hypothalamic area
A14.1.08.407	Area preoptica	Preoptic area
A14.1.08.930	Nuclei tuberales laterales	Lateral tuberal nuclei
A14.1.08.931	Nucleus perifornicalis	Perifornical nucleus
A14.1.08.932	Nucleus tuberomammillaris	Tuberomammillary nucleus
A14.1.08.933	Area hypothalamica posterior	Posterior hypothalamic area; Posterior hypothalamic region
A14.1.08.934	Nucleus premammillaris dorsalis	Dorsal premammillary nucleus
A14.1.08.935	Nucleus mammillaris lateralis	Lateral nucleus of mammillary body
A14.1.08.936	Nucleus mammillaris medialis	Medial nucleus of mammillary body
A14.1.08.937	Nucleus supramammillaris	Supramammillary nucleus
A14.1.08.938	Nucleus premammillaris ventralis	Ventral premammillary nucleus
A14.1.08.939	Nucleus posterior hypothalami	Posterior nucleus of hypothalamus
A14.1.08.940	Organum vasculosum laminae terminalis	Vascular organ of lamina terminalis
A14.1.08.941	Zonae hypothalamicae	Zones of hypothalamus
A14.1.08.942	Zona periventricularis	Periventricular zone
A14.1.08.943	Zona medialis	Medial zone
A14.1.08.944	Zona lateralis	Lateral zone
A11.1.00.006	**Neurohypophysis {vide paginam 74}**	**Neurohypophysis {see page 74}**
A14.1.08.945	**Substantia alba hypothalami**	**White substance of hypothalamus**
A14.1.08.946	Fasciculus longitudinalis posterior; Fasciculus longitudinalis dorsalis	Posterior longitudinal fasciculus; Dorsal longitudinal fasciculus
A14.1.08.947	Commissura supraoptica dorsalis	Dorsal supra-optic commissure
A14.1.08.948	Fibrae striae terminalis	Fibres of stria terminalis▲
A14.1.08.949	Fornix	Fornix
A14.1.08.950	Tractus hypothalamohypophysialis	Hypothalamohypophysial tract
A14.1.08.951	Fibrae paraventriculohypophysiales	Paraventricular fibres▲
A14.1.08.952	Fibrae supraopticohypophysiales	Supra-optic fibres▲
A14.1.08.953	Fasciculus mammillotegmentalis	Mammillotegmental fasciculus
A14.1.08.954	Fasciculus mammillothalamicus	Mammillothalamic fasciculus
A14.1.08.955	Fasciculus medialis telencephali	Medial forebrain bundle
A14.1.08.956	Tractus paraventriculohypophysialis	Paraventriculohypophysial tract
A14.1.08.957	Fibrae periventriculares	Periventricular fibres▲
A14.1.08.958	Tractus supraopticohypophysialis	Supra-opticohypophysial tract
A14.1.08.959	Commissura supraoptica ventralis	Ventral supra-optic commissure
A14.1.08.960	Tractus retinohypothalamicus	Retinohypothalamic tract

A14.1.09.001	**TELENCEPHALON; CEREBRUM**	**TELENCEPHALON; CEREBRUM**
	Nomina generalia	*General terminology*
A14.1.09.002	**Hemispherium cerebri**	**Cerebral hemisphere**
A14.1.09.003	Pallium	Cerebral cortex
A14.1.09.004	Gyri cerebri	Cerebral gyri
A14.1.09.005	Lobi cerebri	Cerebral lobes
A14.1.09.006	Sulci cerebri	Cerebral sulci
A14.1.09.007	Fissura longitudinalis cerebri	Longitudinal cerebral fissure
A14.1.09.008	Fissura transversa cerebri	Transverse cerebral fissure
A14.1.09.009	Fossa lateralis cerebri	Lateral cerebral fossa
A14.1.09.010	Margo superior	Superior margin
A14.1.09.011	Margo inferomedialis	Inferomedial margin
A14.1.09.012	Margo inferolateralis	Inferolateral margin

A14.1.09.101	**Facies superolateralis hemispherii cerebri**	**Superolateral face of cerebral hemisphere**
A14.1.09.102	Sulci interlobares	Interlobar sulci
A14.1.09.103	Sulcus centralis	Central sulcus
A14.1.09.104	Sulcus lateralis	Lateral sulcus
A14.1.09.105	Ramus posterior	Posterior ramus
A14.1.09.106	Ramus ascendens	Ascending ramus

A14.1.09.107	Ramus anterior	Anterior ramus
A14.1.09.108	Sulcus parietooccipitalis	Parieto-occipital sulcus
A14.1.09.109	Incisura preoccipitalis	Preoccipital notch
A14.1.09.110	**Lobus frontalis**	**Frontal lobe**
A14.1.09.111	Polus frontalis	Frontal pole
A14.1.09.112	Operculum frontale	Frontal operculum
A14.1.09.113	Gyrus frontalis inferior	Inferior frontal gyrus
A14.1.09.114	Pars orbitalis	Orbital part
A14.1.09.115	Pars triangularis	Triangular part
A14.1.09.116	Pars opercularis	Opercular part
A14.1.09.117	Sulcus frontalis inferior	Inferior frontal sulcus
A14.1.09.118	Gyrus frontalis medius	Middle frontal gyrus
A14.1.09.119	Gyrus precentralis	Precentral gyrus
A14.1.09.120	Sulcus precentralis	Precentral sulcus
A14.1.09.121	Gyrus frontalis superior	Superior frontal gyrus
A14.1.09.122	Sulcus frontalis superior	Superior frontal sulcus
A14.1.09.123	**Lobus parietalis**	**Parietal lobe**
A14.1.09.124	Gyrus angularis	Angular gyrus
A14.1.09.125	Lobulus parietalis inferior	Inferior parietal lobule
A14.1.09.126	Operculum parietale	Parietal operculum
A14.1.09.127	Sulcus intraparietalis	Intraparietal sulcus
A14.1.09.128	Gyrus postcentralis	Postcentral gyrus
A14.1.09.129	Sulcus postcentralis	Postcentral sulcus
A14.1.09.130	Lobulus parietalis superior	Superior parietal lobule
A14.1.09.131	Gyrus supramarginalis	Supramarginal gyrus
A14.1.09.132	**Lobus occipitalis**	**Occipital lobe**
A14.1.09.133	Polus occipitalis	Occipital pole
A14.1.09.134	Sulcus lunatus	Lunate sulcus
A14.1.09.109	Incisura preoccipitalis	Preoccipital notch
A14.1.09.135	Sulcus occipitalis transversus	Transverse occipital sulcus
A14.1.09.136	**Lobus temporalis**	**Temporal lobe**
A14.1.09.137	Polus temporalis	Temporal pole
A14.1.09.138	Gyrus temporalis superior	Superior temporal gyrus
A14.1.09.139	Operculum temporale	Temporal operculum
A14.1.09.140	Gyri temporales transversi	Transverse temporal gyri
A14.1.09.141	Gyrus temporalis transversus anterior	Anterior transverse temporal gyrus
A14.1.09.142	Gyrus temporalis transversus posterior	Posterior transverse temporal gyrus
A14.1.09.143	Planum temporale	Temporal plane
A14.1.09.144	Sulcus temporalis transversus	Transverse temporal sulcus
A14.1.09.145	Sulcus temporalis superior	Superior temporal sulcus
A14.1.09.146	Gyrus temporalis medius	Middle temporal gyrus
A14.1.09.147	Sulcus temporalis inferior	Inferior temporal sulcus
A14.1.09.148	Gyrus temporalis inferior	Inferior temporal gyrus
A14.1.09.149	**Insula; Lobus insularis**	**Insula; Insular lobe**
A14.1.09.150	Gyri insulae	Insular gyri
A14.1.09.151	Gyrus longus insulae	Long gyrus of insula
A14.1.09.152	Gyri breves insulae	Short gyri of insula
A14.1.09.153	Sulcus centralis insulae	Central sulcus of insula
A14.1.09.154	Sulcus circularis insulae	Circular sulcus of insula
A14.1.09.155	Limen insulae	Limen insulae; Insular threshold

* **A14.1.09.201**	**Facies medialis et inferior hemispherii cerebri**	**Medial and inferior surfaces of cerebral hemisphere**
A14.1.09.102	Sulci interlobares	Interlobar sulci

* **A14.1.09.201** *Facies medialis et inferior hemispherii cerebri* The term rhinencephalon has been omitted because it is no longer in common use and the areas/structures listed under this designation in previous terminologies subserve considerably more than just olfactory functions. These structures now appear under headings which specify their proper anatomical location (A14.1.09.110 – *Lobus frontalis*, A14.1.09.401 – *Pars basalis telencephali*).

A14.1.09.202	Sulcus corporis callosi	Sulcus of corpus callosum
A14.1.09.203	Sulcus cinguli	Cingulate sulcus
A14.1.09.204	Ramus marginalis; Sulcus marginalis	Marginal branch; Marginal sulcus
A14.1.09.205	Sulcus subparietalis	Subparietal sulcus
A14.1.09.108	Sulcus parietooccipitalis	Parieto-occipital sulcus
A14.1.09.206	Sulcus collateralis	Collateral sulcus
A14.1.09.103	Sulcus centralis	Central sulcus
A14.1.09.110	**Lobus frontalis**	**Frontal lobe**
A14.1.09.207	Gyrus frontalis medialis	Medial frontal gyrus
A14.1.09.208	Sulcus paracentralis	Paracentral sulcus
A14.1.09.209	Lobulus paracentralis	Paracentral lobule
A14.1.09.210	Gyrus paracentralis anterior	Anterior paracentral gyrus
A14.1.09.103	Sulcus centralis	Central sulcus
A14.1.09.211	Area subcallosa	Subcallosal area; Subcallosal gyrus
A14.1.09.212	Gyrus paraterminalis	Paraterminal gyrus
A14.1.09.213	Area paraolfactoria	Paraolfactory area
A14.1.09.214	Gyri paraolfactorii	Paraolfactory gyri
A14.1.09.215	Sulci paraolfactorii	Paraolfactory sulci
A14.1.09.216	Gyri orbitales	Orbital gyri
A14.1.09.217	Sulci orbitales	Orbital sulci
A14.1.09.218	Gyrus rectus	Straight gyrus
A14.1.09.219	Sulcus olfactorius	Olfactory sulcus
A14.1.09.220	Gyrus olfactorius lateralis	Lateral olfactory gyrus
A14.1.09.221	Gyrus olfactorius medialis	Medial olfactory gyrus
A14.1.09.123	**Lobus parietalis**	**Parietal lobe**
A14.1.09.209	Lobulus paracentralis	Paracentral lobule
A14.1.09.222	Gyrus paracentralis posterior	Posterior paracentral gyrus
A14.1.09.223	Precuneus	Precuneus
A14.1.09.205	Sulcus subparietalis	Subparietal sulcus
A14.1.09.108	Sulcus parietooccipitalis	Parieto-occipital sulcus
A14.1.09.204	Ramus marginalis; Sulcus marginalis	Marginal branch; Marginal sulcus
A14.1.09.132	**Lobus occipitalis**	**Occipital lobe**
A14.1.09.224	Cuneus	Cuneus
A14.1.09.225	Sulcus calcarinus	Calcarine sulcus
A14.1.09.226	Gyrus lingualis	Lingual gyrus
A14.1.09.227	Gyrus occipitotemporalis lateralis	Lateral occipitotemporal gyrus
A14.1.09.228	Gyrus occipitotemporalis medialis	Medial occipitotemporal gyrus
A14.1.09.229	Sulcus occipitotemporalis	Occipitotemporal sulcus
A14.1.09.108	Sulcus parietooccipitalis	Parieto-occipital sulcus
A14.1.09.136	**Lobus temporalis**	**Temporal lobe**
A14.1.09.206	Sulcus collateralis	Collateral sulcus
A14.1.09.228	Gyrus occipitotemporalis medialis	Medial occipitotemporal gyrus
A14.1.09.229	Sulcus occipitotemporalis	Occipitotemporal sulcus
A14.1.09.227	Gyrus occipitotemporalis lateralis	Lateral occipitotemporal gyrus
A14.1.09.147	Sulcus temporalis inferior	Inferior temporal sulcus
A14.1.09.148	Gyrus temporalis inferior	Inferior temporal gyrus
* A14.1.09.230	**Lobus limbicus**	**Limbic lobe**
A14.1.09.203	Sulcus cinguli	Cingulate sulcus
A14.1.09.231	Gyrus cinguli	Cingulate gyrus
A14.1.09.232	Isthmus gyri cinguli	Isthmus of cingulate gyrus
A14.1.09.233	Gyrus fasciolaris	Fasciolar gyrus
A14.1.09.234	Gyrus parahippocampalis	Parahippocampal gyrus
A14.1.09.235	Uncus	Uncus
A14.1.09.236	Sulcus hippocampalis	Hippocampal sulcus

* **A14.1.09.230** *Lobus limbicus* Consists of structures which form a continuum on the most medial aspect of the cerebral hemisphere. These structures are not located internal to a bone of the same name and, therefore, do not share this feature with most other lobes of the hemisphere. However, structures forming the limbic lobe, as is the case for other lobes of the cerebral hemisphere, have functions that are characteristic of, and unique to, that lobe and are separated from adjacent structures by named fissures. When the term *lobus limbicus* is not used, its constituent parts are considered as the medial portions of the frontal, parietal, and temporal lobes.

A14.1.09.237	Gyrus dentatus	Dentate gyrus
A14.1.09.238	Sulcus fimbriodentatus	Fimbriodentate sulcus
A14.1.09.239	Fimbria hippocampi	Fimbria of hippocampus
A14.1.09.206	Sulcus collateralis	Collateral sulcus
A14.1.09.240	Sulcus rhinalis	Rhinal sulcus
A14.1.09.241	**Corpus callosum**	**Corpus callosum**
A14.1.09.242	Rostrum	Rostrum
A14.1.09.243	Genu	Genu
A14.1.09.244	Truncus	Trunk; Body
A14.1.09.245	Splenium	Splenium
A14.1.09.246	Indusium griseum	Indusium griseum
A14.1.09.247	Stria longitudinalis lateralis	Lateral longitudinal stria
A14.1.09.248	Stria longitudinalis medialis	Medial longitudinal stria
A14.1.09.249	Radiatio corporis callosi	Radiation of corpus callosum
A14.1.09.250	Forceps minor; Forceps frontalis	Minor forceps; Frontal forceps
A14.1.09.251	Forceps major; Forceps occipitalis	Major forceps; Occipital forceps
A14.1.09.252	Tapetum	Tapetum
A14.1.08.419	**Lamina terminalis**	**Lamina terminalis**
A14.1.08.940	Organum vasculosum laminae terminalis	Vascular organ of lamina terminalis
A14.1.08.421	**Commissura anterior**	**Anterior commissure**
A14.1.09.253	Pars anterior	Anterior part
A14.1.09.254	Pars posterior	Posterior part
A14.1.09.255	**Fornix**	**Fornix**
A14.1.08.420	Columna	Column
A14.1.09.256	Fibrae precommissurales	Precommissural fibres▲
A14.1.09.257	Fibrae postcommissurales	Postcommissural fibres▲
A14.1.09.258	Corpus	Body
A14.1.09.259	Crus	Crus
A14.1.09.260	Commissura	Commissure
A14.1.09.261	Taenia fornicis	Taenia▲
A14.1.09.262	**Septum pellucidum**	**Septum pellucidum**
A14.1.09.263	Cavum	Cave
A14.1.09.264	Lamina	Lamina
A14.1.09.265	Nucleus septalis precommissuralis	Precommissural septal nucleus
* A14.1.09.266	**Nuclei septales et structurae pertinentes**	**Septal nuclei and related structures**
A14.1.09.267	Nucleus septalis dorsalis	Dorsal septal nucleus
A14.1.09.268	Nucleus septalis lateralis	Lateral septal nucleus
A14.1.09.269	Nucleus septalis medialis	Medial septal nucleus
A14.1.09.270	Nucleus septofimbrialis	Septofimbrial nucleus
A14.1.08.412	Organum subfornicale	Subfornical organ
A14.1.09.271	Nucleus triangularis	Triangular nucleus
A14.1.09.272	**Ventriculus lateralis**	**Lateral ventricle**
A14.1.09.273	Cornu frontale; Cornu anterius	Frontal horn; Anterior horn
A14.1.08.411	Foramen interventriculare	Interventricular foramen
A14.1.09.274	Pars centralis	Central part; Body
A14.1.09.275	Stria terminalis	Stria terminalis
A14.1.09.276	Lamina affixa	Lamina affixa
A14.1.09.277	Taenia choroidea	Choroid line
A14.1.09.278	Fissura choroidea	Choroidal fissure
A14.1.09.279	Plexus choroideus	Choroid plexus
A14.1.09.280	Trigonum collaterale	Collateral trigone
* A14.1.09.281	Atrium	Atrium
A14.1.09.282	Eminentia collateralis	Collateral eminence
A14.1.09.283	Glomus choroideum	Choroid enlargement
A14.1.09.284	Bulbus cornus posterioris	Bulb of occipital horn

* **A14.1.09.266** *Nuclei septales et structurae pertinentes* This newly created section has been added to make it easier to locate nuclei normally grouped under this general designation.

* **A14.1.09.281** *Atrium* The expansion of the *ventriculus lateralis* where the *pars centralis* meets the *cornu occipitale* and the *cornu temporale*.

A14.1.09.285	Calcar avis	Calcarine spur
A14.1.09.286	Cornu occipitale; Cornu posterius	Occipital horn; Posterior horn
A14.1.09.287	Cornu temporale; Cornu inferius	Temporal horn; Inferior horn
A14.1.09.301	**Cortex cerebri**	**Cerebral cortex**
A14.1.09.302	Archicortex	Archicortex
A14.1.09.303	Paleocortex	Paleocortex
A14.1.09.304	Neocortex	Neocortex
A14.1.09.305	Allocortex	Allocortex
A14.1.09.306	Mesocortex	Mesocortex
A14.1.09.307	Isocortex	Isocortex
A14.1.09.308	Strata isocorticis	Layers of isocortex
A14.1.09.309	Lamina molecularis [Lamina I]	Molecular layer [layer I]
A14.1.09.310	Lamina granularis externa [Lamina II]	External granular layer [layer II]
A14.1.09.311	Lamina pyramidalis externa [Lamina III]	External pyramidal layer [layer III]
A14.1.09.312	Lamina granularis interna [Lamina IV]	Internal granular layer [layer IV]
A14.1.09.313	Lamina pyramidalis interna [Lamina V]	Internal pyramidal layer [layer V]
A14.1.09.314	Lamina multiformis [Lamina VI]	Multiform layer [layer VI]
A14.1.09.315	Stria laminae molecularis	Stria of molecular layer
A14.1.09.316	Stria laminae granularis externae	Stria of external granular layer
A14.1.09.317	Stria laminae granularis internae	Stria of internal granular layer
A14.1.09.318	Stria occipitalis	Occipital stripe; Occipital line
A14.1.09.319	Stria laminae pyramidalis internae	Stria of internal pyramidal layer
A14.1.09.320	Neurofibrae tangentiales	Tangential fibres▲
A14.1.09.321	**Hippocampus**	**Hippocampus**
A14.1.09.322	Parasubiculum	Parasubiculum
A14.1.09.323	Pes hippocampi	Pes
A14.1.09.324	Digitationes hippocampi	Hippocampal digitations
A14.1.09.325	Presubiculum	Presubiculum
A14.1.09.326	Subiculum	Subiculum
A14.1.09.327	Hippocampus proprius; Cornu ammonis	Hippocampus proper; Ammon's horn
A14.1.09.328	Regio I hippocampi proprii; Regio I cornus ammonis; CA1	Region I; CA1
A14.1.09.329	Regio II hippocampi proprii; Regio II cornus ammonis; CA2	Region II; CA2
A14.1.09.330	Regio III hippocampi proprii; Regio III cornus ammonis; CA3	Region III; CA3
A14.1.09.331	Regio IV hippocampi proprii; Regio IV cornus ammonis; CA4	Region IV; CA4
A14.1.09.332	Fimbria hippocampi	Fimbria
A14.1.09.333	Alveus hippocampi	Alveus
A14.1.09.334	Strata hippocampi; Strata cornus ammonis	Layers of hippocampus; Layers of ammon's horn
A14.1.09.335	Stratum moleculare et substratum lacunosum	Lacunar-molecular layer
A14.1.09.336	Stratum oriens	Oriens layer
A14.1.09.337	Stratum pyramidale	Pyramidal layer
A14.1.09.338	Stratum radiatum	Radiate layer
A14.1.09.339	Gyrus dentatus	Dentate gyrus
A14.1.09.340	Strata gyri dentati	Layers of dentate gyrus
A14.1.09.341	Stratum moleculare	Molecular layer
A14.1.09.342	Stratum granulare	Granular layer
A14.1.09.343	Stratum multiforme	Multiform layer

* **A14.1.09.401**	**Pars basalis telencephali**	**Basal forebrain**
* **A14.1.09.402**	**Corpus amygdaloideum**	**Amygdaloid body; Amygdaloid complex**
A14.1.09.403	Area amygdaloclaustralis	Amygdaloclaustral area
A14.1.09.404	Area parahippocampalis	Amygdalohippocampal area
A14.1.09.405	Area transitionis amygdalopiriformis	Amygdalopiriform transition area
A14.1.09.406	Area amygdaloidea anterior	Anterior amygdaloid area
A14.1.09.407	Nucleus amygdalae basalis lateralis	Basolateral amygdaloid nucleus
A14.1.09.408	Nucleus amygdalae basalis medialis	Basomedial amygdaloid nucleus
A14.1.09.409	Nucleus amygdalae centralis	Central amygdaloid nucleus
A14.1.09.410	Nucleus amygdalae corticalis	Cortical amygdaloid nucleus
A14.1.09.411	Nucleus amygdalae interstitialis	Interstitial amygdaloid nucleus
A14.1.09.412	Nucleus amygdalae lateralis	Lateral amygdaloid nucleus
A14.1.09.413	Nucleus amygdalae medialis	Medial amygdaloid nucleus
A14.1.09.414	Nucleus tractus olfactorii lateralis	Nucleus of lateral olfactory tract
A14.1.09.415	Cortex periamygdaloideus	Periamygdaloid cortex
A14.1.09.416	Nucleus olfactorius anterior	Anterior olfactory nucleus
A14.1.09.417	Substantia basalis	Basal substance
A14.1.09.418	Nucleus basalis	Basal nucleus
* **A14.1.09.419**	Nucleus striae terminalis	Bed nucleus of stria terminalis
* **A14.1.09.420**	Pars sublenticularis amygdalae	Sublenticular extended amygdala
A14.1.09.421	Claustrum	Claustrum
A14.1.09.422	Stria diagonalis	Diagonal band
A14.1.09.423	Crus horizontale	Horizontal limb
A14.1.09.424	Crus verticale	Vertical limb
A14.1.09.425	Nucleus striae diagonalis	Nucleus of diagonal band
* **A14.1.09.426**	Substantia innominata	Innominate substance
A14.1.09.427	Fasciculus peduncularis	Fasciculus peduncularis
A14.1.09.428	Insulae olfactoriae	Olfactory islets
A14.1.09.429	Bulbus olfactorius	Olfactory bulb
A14.1.09.430	Pedunculus olfactorius	Olfactory peduncle
A14.1.09.431	Tractus olfactorius	Olfactory tract
A14.1.09.432	Trigonum olfactorium	Olfactory trigone
A14.1.09.433	Tuberculum olfactorium	Olfactory tubercle
A14.1.09.434	Striae olfactoriae	Olfactory striae
A14.1.09.435	Stria olfactoria medialis	Medial stria
A14.1.09.436	Stria olfactoria lateralis	Lateral stria
A14.1.09.437	Substantia perforata anterior; Substantia perforata rostralis	Anterior perforated substance
A14.1.09.438	Pallidum ventrale	Ventral pallidum
A14.1.09.439	Striatum ventrale; Corpus striatum ventrale	Ventral striatum
A14.1.09.440	Nucleus accumbens	Nucleus accumbens
A14.1.09.441	Pars lateralis	Lateral part; Core region
A14.1.09.442	Pars medialis	Medial part; Shell region
A14.1.08.665	Ansa peduncularis	Peduncular loop
A14.1.09.443	Area septalis	Septal area
A14.1.09.444	Nucleus septalis dorsalis	Dorsal septal nucleus
A14.1.09.445	Nucleus septalis lateralis	Lateral septal nucleus
A14.1.09.446	Nucleus septalis medialis	Medial septal nucleus
A14.1.09.447	Nucleus septofimbrialis	Septofimbrial nucleus
A14.1.09.448	Nucleus triangularis septi	Triangular nucleus of septum
A14.1.09.449	Organum subfornicale	Subfornical organ

* **A14.1.09.401** *Pars basalis telencephali* This new section includes structures that in previous terminology lists have been scattered throughout other sections. It is noted, however, that the *pars basalis telencephali* includes some structures that may also be referred to as parts of the *nuclei basalis* (e.g., *pallidum ventrale, striatum ventrale*).

* **A14.1.09.402** *Corpus amygdaloideum* This was listed as a component part of the *nuclei basalis* in previous terminologies, and functions largely outside activities governed by the *nuclei basalis*. Consequently, it is listed here in the correct location within the *pars basalis telencephali* (see A14.1.09.401).

* **A14.1.09.419 / A14.1.09.420 / A14.1.09.426** *Nucleus striae terminalis/pars sublenticularis amygdalae/substantia innominata* In the *pars basalis telencephali*, the *pars sublenticularis amygdalae* (which includes the *nuclei amygdalarum centralis et medialis*), the *nuclei striae terminalis*, the *substantia innominata, the striatum ventrale* and the *pallidum ventrale* form a continuous grey complex.

* A14.1.09.501	**Nuclei basales et structurae pertinentes**	**Basal nuclei and related structures**
A14.1.09.502	**Nucleus caudatus**	**Caudate nucleus**
A14.1.09.503	Caput	Head
A14.1.09.504	Corpus	Body
A14.1.09.505	Cauda	Tail
A14.1.09.506	**Nucleus lentiformis**	**Lentiform nucleus; Lenticular nucleus**
A14.1.09.507	Putamen	Putamen
A14.1.09.508	Lamina medullaris lateralis; Lamina medullaris externa	Lateral medullary lamina; External medullary lamina
A14.1.09.509	Globus pallidus lateralis	Globus pallidus lateral segment; Globus pallidus external segment
A14.1.09.510	Lamina medullaris medialis; Lamina medullaris interna	Medial medullary lamina; Internal medullary lamina
A14.1.09.511	Globus pallidus medialis	Globus pallidus medial segment; Globus pallidus internal segment
A14.1.09.512	Pars lateralis	Lateral part
A14.1.09.513	Lamina medullaris accessoria	Accessory medullary lamina
A14.1.09.514	Pars medialis	Medial part
A14.1.09.515	**Corpus striatum**	**Corpus striatum**
A14.1.09.516	Striatum	Striatum; Neostriatum
A14.1.09.517	Striatum dorsale	Dorsal striatum
A14.1.09.439	Striatum ventrale; Corpus striatum ventrale	Ventral striatum
A14.1.09.518	Pallidum	Pallidum; Paleostriatum
A14.1.09.519	Pallidum dorsale	Dorsal pallidum
A14.1.09.438	Pallidum ventrale	Ventral pallidum
A14.1.09.520	Ansa lenticularis	Ansa lenticularis
A14.1.09.521	Fasciculus lenticularis	Lenticular fasciculus
A14.1.09.522	Fasciculus subthalamicus	Subthalamic fasciculus
A14.1.09.523	Fasciculus thalamicus	Thalamic fasciculus
A14.1.09.524	**Capsula interna**	**Internal capsule**
A14.1.09.525	Pontes grisei caudatolenticulares	Caudolenticular grey bridges; Transcapsular grey bridges▲
A14.1.09.526	Crus anterius	Anterior limb
A14.1.09.527	Radiatio thalami anterior	Anterior thalamic radiation
A14.1.09.528	Tractus frontopontinus	Frontopontine fibres▲
A14.1.09.529	Genu capsulae internae	Genu of internal capsule
* A14.1.09.530	Fibrae corticonucleares	Corticonuclear fibres▲
* A14.1.09.531	Crus posterius	Posterior limb
A14.1.09.532	Radiatio thalami centralis	Central thalamic radiation
A14.1.09.533	Fibrae corticoreticulares	Corticoreticular fibres▲
A14.1.09.534	Fibrae corticorubrales	Corticorubral fibres▲
A14.1.09.535	Fibrae corticospinales	Corticospinal fibres▲
A14.1.09.536	Fibrae corticothalamici	Corticothalamic fibres▲
A14.1.09.537	Fibrae parietopontinae	Parietopontine fibres▲
A14.1.09.538	Fibrae thalamoparietales	Thalamoparietal fibres▲
A14.1.09.539	Pars retrolentiformis	Retrolentiform limb; Retrolenticular limb
A14.1.09.540	Fibrae occipitopontinae	Occipitopontine fibres▲
A14.1.09.541	Fibrae occipitotectales	Occipitotectal fibres▲
A14.1.09.542	Radiatio optica; Fibrae geniculocalcarinae	Optic radiation; Geniculocalcarine fibres▲

* **A14.1.09.501** *Nuclei basales et structurae pertinentes* Some textbooks state, without qualification, that the *substantia nigra* and *nucleus subthalamicus* are parts of the basal nuclei of the telencephalon. Since this affiliation is based on functional, not structural or developmental, grounds it is inappropriate to include these structures under this heading. The *substantia nigra* and the *nucleus subthalamicus* are parts of the mesencephalon and diencephalon, respectively.
* **A14.1.09.530** *Fibrae corticonucleares bulbi* The term corticobulbar, as commonly used in the past, refers to axons originating in the cerebral cortex and innervating motor nuclei of cranial nerves of the *medulla oblongata*, pons, and by extension, the midbrain. Since bulbus specifically refers to the *medulla oblongata*, application of the term corticobulbar to these fibres in the midbrain is incorrect. The term *corticonuclearis* followed by *bulbi*, *pontinis* (see A14.1.05.105), or *mesencephali* (see A14.1.06.202) replaces corticobulbar and specifies cortical axons that innervate motor and/or sensory nuclei of cranial nerves.
* **A14.1.09.531** *Crus posterius* of *Capsula interna* Consists of what were historically called thalamolentiform, sublentiform, and retrolentiform parts. However, as each contains different and functionally unique fibre populations, these parts are frequently called, respectively, the posterior limb, the sublentiform (or sublenticular) limb, and the retrolentiform (or retrolenticular) limb of the internal capsule.

A14.1.09.543	Radiatio thalamica posterior	Posterior thalamic radiation
A14.1.09.544	Pars sublentiformis	Sublentiform limb; Sublenticular limb
A14.1.09.545	Radiatio acustica; Fibrae geniculotemporales	Acoustic radiation; Geniculotemporal fibres▲
A14.1.09.546	Fibrae corticotectales	Corticotectal fibres▲
A14.1.09.547	Radiatio optica	Optic radiation
A14.1.09.548	Fibrae temporopontinae	Temporopontine fibres▲
A14.1.09.549	Fibrae corticothalamicae	Corticothalamic fibres▲
A14.1.09.550	**Corona radiata**	**Corona radiata**
A14.1.09.551	Capsula externa	External capsule
A14.1.09.552	Capsula extrema	Extreme capsule
A14.1.08.421	Commissura anterior	Anterior commissure
A14.1.09.253	Pars anterior	Anterior part
A14.1.09.254	Pars posterior	Posterior part
A14.1.09.553	**Fibrae associationis telencephali**	**Association fibres of telencephalon▲**
A14.1.09.554	Fibrae arcuatae cerebri	Arcuate fibres▲
A14.1.09.555	Cingulum	Cingulum
A14.1.09.556	Fasciculus longitudinalis inferior	Inferior longitudinal fasciculus
A14.1.09.557	Fasciculus longitudinalis superior; Fasciculus arcuatus	Superior longitudinal fasciculus; Arcuate fasciculus
A14.1.09.558	Fibrae associationis longae	Long association fibres▲
A14.1.09.559	Fibrae associationis breves	Short association fibres▲
A14.1.09.560	Fasciculus uncinatus	Uncinate fasciculus
A14.1.09.561	Fasciculus occipitofrontalis inferior	Inferior occipitofrontal fasciculus
A14.1.09.562	Fasciculus occipitofrontalis superior; Fasciculus subcallosus	Superior occipitofrontal fasciculus; Subcallosal fasciculus
A14.1.09.563	Fasciculi occipitales verticales	Vertical occipital fasciculi
A14.1.09.564	Fibrae laterales	Lateral fibres▲
A14.1.09.565	Fibrae caudales	Caudal fibres▲
A14.1.09.566	Fasciculi occipitales horizontales	Transverse occipital fasciculi
A14.1.09.567	Fibrae cuneatae	Cuneus fibres▲
A14.1.09.568	Fibrae linguales	Lingual fibres▲
A14.1.09.569	**Fibrae commissurales telencephali**	**Commissural fibres of telencephalon▲**
A14.1.09.570	Fibrae corporis callosi	Corpus callosum fibres▲
A14.1.09.571	Commissura hippocampi	Hippocampal commissure
A14.1.08.421	Commissura anterior	Anterior commissure

A14.1.09.601	Aggregationes cellularum chemergicarum	Chemically-defined cell groups
A14.1.09.602	**Cellulae aminergicae**	**Aminergic cells**
A14.1.09.603	Cellulae noradrenergicae medullae oblongatae [A1, A2]	Noradrenergic cells in medulla; Norepinephric cells in medulla [A1, A2]
A14.1.09.604	Cellulae noradrenergicae nuclei lemnisci lateralis [A7]	Noradrenergic cells in nucleus of lateral lemniscus; Norepinephric cells in nucleus of lateral lemniscus [A7]
A14.1.09.605	Cellulae noradrenergicae loci caerulei [A6]	Noradrenergic cells in locus caeruleus; Norepinephric cells in locus caeruleus [A6]
A14.1.09.606	Cellulae noradrenergicae caudalis lateralis [A5]	Noradrenergic cells in caudolateral pons; Norepinephric cells in caudolateral pons [A5]
A14.1.09.607	Cellulae aminergicae formationis reticularis; Nucleus retrobulbaris [A8]	Aminergic cells in reticular formation; Retrobulbar nucleus [A8]
A14.1.09.608	Cellulae dopaminergicae	Dopaminergic cells
A14.1.09.609	Cellulae noradrenergicae	Noradrenergic cells; Norepinephric cells
A14.1.09.610	Cellulae aminergicae partis compactae substantiae nigrae [A9]	Aminergic cells in compact part of substantia nigra [A9]
A14.1.09.611	Cellulae dopaminergicae	Dopaminergic cells
A14.1.09.612	Cellulae noradrenergicae	Noradrenergic cells; Norepinephric cells
A14.1.09.613	Cellulae aminergicae areae tegmentalis ventralis [A10]	Aminergic cells in ventral tegmental area [A10]
A14.1.09.614	Cellulae dopaminergicae	Dopaminergic cells
A14.1.09.615	Cellulae noradrenergicae	Noradrenergic cells; Norepinephric cells

A14.1.09.616	Cellulae dopaminergicae areae hypothalamicae posterioris [A11]	Dopaminergic cells in posterior hypothalamus [A11]
A14.1.09.617	Cellulae dopaminergicae nuclei arcuati [A12]	Dopaminergic cells in arcuate nucleus [A12]
A14.1.09.618	Cellulae dopaminergicae zonae incertae [A13]	Dopaminergic cells in zona incerta [A13]
A14.1.09.619	Cellulae dopaminergicae zonae medialis et areae anterioris hypothalamicae [A14]	Dopaminergic cells in medial zone and anterior area of hypothalamus [A14]
A14.1.09.620	Cellulae dopaminergicae bulbi olfactorii [A15]	Dopaminergic cells in olfactory bulb [A15]
A14.1.09.621	Cellulae serotoninergicae nuclei raphes pallidi [B1]	Serotoninergic cells in pallidal raphe nucleus [B1]
A14.1.09.622	Cellulae serotoninergicae nuclei raphes obscuri [B2]	Serotoninergic cells in obscurus raphe nucleus [B2]
A14.1.09.623	Cellulae serotoninergicae nuclei raphes magni [B3]	Serotoninergic cells in magnus raphe nucleus [B3]
A14.1.09.624	Cellulae serotoninergicae vicinae nuclei vestibularis medialis et nuclei prepositi [B4]	Serotoninergic cells adjacent to medial vestibular nucleus and prepositus nucleus [B4]
A14.1.09.625	Cellulae serotoninergicae nuclei raphes pontis [B5]	Serotoninergic cells in pontine raphe nucleus [B5]
A14.1.09.626	Cellulae serotoninergicae nuclei raphes mediani [B6]	Serotoninergic cells in median raphe nucleus [B6]
A14.1.09.627	Cellulae serotoninergicae nuclei raphes dorsalis [B7]	Serotoninergic cells in dorsal raphe nucleus [B7]
A14.1.09.628	Cellulae adrenergicae areae postremae et nuclei reticularis anterioris [C1, C2]	Adrenergic cells in area postrema and anterior reticular nucleus; Epinephric cells in area postrema and anterior reticular nucleus [C1, C2]
A14.1.09.629	**Cellulae cholinergicae**	**Cholinergic cells**
A14.1.09.630	Cellulae cholinergicae nuclei septi medialis [Ch1]	Cholinergic cells of medial septal nuclei [Ch1]
A14.1.09.631	Cellulae cholinergicae globi pallidi, nuclei accumbentis et gyri diagonalis [Ch2]	Cholinergic cells of globus pallidus, accumbens nucleus and diagonal gyrus [Ch2]
A14.1.09.632	Cellulae cholinergicae globi pallidi, nuclei accumbentis et striae diagonalis [Ch3]	Cholinergic cells of globus pallidus, accumbens nucleus and diagonal band [Ch3]
A14.1.09.633	Cellulae cholinergicae substantiae innominatae, nuclei basalis, corporis amygdaloidei et tuberculi olfactorii [Ch4]	Cholinergic cells of substantia innominata, basal nucleus, amygdaloid body and olfactory tubercle [Ch4]
A14.1.09.634	Cellulae cholinergicae areae tegmentalis dorsalis [Ch5, Ch6, Ch8]	Cholinergic cells of dorsal tegmental area [Ch5, Ch6, Ch8]
A14.1.09.635	Cellulae cholinergicae epithalamicae [Ch7]	Cholinergic cells of epithalamus [Ch7]

A14.2.00.001 Pars peripherica; Systema nervosum periphericum — Peripheral nervous system

	Nomina generalia	*General terms*
A14.2.00.002	Ganglion	Ganglion
A14.2.00.003	Capsula ganglii	Capsule of ganglion
A14.2.00.004	Stroma ganglii	Stroma of ganglion
A14.2.00.005	Ganglion craniospinale sensorium	Craniospinal sensory ganglion
A14.2.00.006	Ganglion sensorium nervi spinalis	Spinal ganglion; Dorsal root ganglion
A14.2.00.007	Ganglion sensorium nervi cranialis	Cranial sensory ganglion
A14.2.00.008	Ganglion autonomicum	Autonomic ganglion
A14.2.00.009	Neurofibrae preganglionicae	Preganglionic nerve fibres▲
A14.2.00.010	Neurofibrae postganglionicae	Postganglionic nerve fibres▲
A14.2.00.011	Ganglion sympathicum	Sympathetic ganglion
A14.2.00.012	Ganglion parasympathicum	Parasympathetic ganglion
A14.2.00.013	Nervus	Nerve
A14.2.00.014	Endoneurium	Endoneurium
A14.2.00.015	Perineurium	Perineurium
A14.2.00.016	Epineurium	Epineurium
A14.2.00.017	Neurofibrae afferentes	Afferent nerve fibres▲
A14.2.00.018	Neurofibrae efferentes	Efferent nerve fibres▲
A14.2.00.019	Neurofibrae somaticae	Somatic nerve fibres▲
A14.2.00.020	Neurofibrae autonomicae	Autonomic nerve fibres▲

A14.2.00.021	N. motorius	Motor nerve
A14.2.00.022	N. sensorius	Sensory nerve
A14.2.00.023	N. mixtus	Mixed nerve
A14.2.00.024	R. cutaneus	Cutaneous branch
A14.2.00.025	R. articularis	Articular branch
A14.2.00.026	R. muscularis	Muscular branch
A14.2.00.027	N. spinalis	Spinal nerve
A14.2.00.028	Fila radicularia	Rootlets
A14.2.00.029	Radix anterior; Radix motoria	Anterior root; Motor root; Ventral root
A14.2.00.030	Radix posterior; Radix sensoria	Posterior root; Sensory root; Dorsal root
A14.2.00.031	Truncus nervi spinalis	Trunk of spinal nerve
A14.2.00.032	R. meningeus; R. recurrens	Meningeal branch; Recurrent branch
A14.2.00.033	R. communicans	Ramus communicans
A14.2.00.034	R. anterior	Anterior ramus
A14.2.00.035	R. posterior	Posterior ramus
A14.2.00.036	Cauda equina	Cauda equina
A14.2.00.037	Plexus nervorum spinalium	Spinal nerve plexus
A14.2.00.038	N. cranialis	Cranial nerve
A14.2.00.039	N. autonomicus	Autonomic nerve
A14.2.00.040	R. autonomicus	Autonomic branch
A14.2.00.041	Plexus autonomicus	Autonomic plexus
A14.2.00.042	Plexus visceralis	Visceral plexus
A14.2.00.043	Plexus vascularis	Vascular plexus
A14.2.00.044	Plexus periarterialis	Periarterial plexus
A14.2.00.045	Nn. vasorum	Vascular nerves

A14.2.01.001	**Nervi craniales**	**Cranial nerves**
A14.2.01.002	**Nervus terminalis [0]**	**Terminal nerve [0]**
A14.2.01.003	Ganglion terminale	Terminal ganglion

A14.2.01.004	**Nervus olfactorius [I]**	**Olfactory nerve [I]**
A14.2.01.005	Fila olfactoria	Olfactory nerves

A14.2.01.006	**Nervus opticus [II]**	**Optic nerve [II]**

A14.2.01.007	**Nervus oculomotorius [III]**	**Oculomotor nerve [III]**
A14.2.01.008	R. superior	Superior branch
A14.2.01.009	R. inferior	Inferior branch
A14.2.01.010	Ramus ad ganglion ciliare;radix parasympathica ganglii ciliaris; Radix oculomotoria ganglii ciliaris	Branch to ciliary ganglion; Parasympathetic root of ciliary ganglion; Oculomotor root of ciliary ganglion

A14.2.01.011	**Nervus trochlearis [IV]**	**Trochlear nerve [IV]**

A14.2.01.012	**Nervus trigeminus [V]**	**Trigeminal nerve [V]**
A14.2.01.013	Radix sensoria	Sensory root
A14.2.01.014	Ganglion trigeminale	Trigeminal ganglion
A14.2.01.015	Radix motoria	Motor root
A14.2.01.016	**Nervus ophthalmicus [Va; V_1]**	**Ophthalmic nerve; Ophthalmic division[Va; V_1]**
A14.2.01.017	R. meningeus recurrens; R. tentorius	Tentorial nerve
A14.2.01.018	N. lacrimalis	Lacrimal nerve
A14.2.01.019	R. communicans cum nervo zygomatico	Communicating branch with zygomatic nerve
A14.2.01.020	N. frontalis	Frontal nerve
A14.2.01.021	N. supraorbitalis	Supra-orbital nerve
A14.2.01.022	R. lateralis	Lateral branch
A14.2.01.023	R. medialis	Medial branch
A14.2.01.024	N. supratrochlearis	Supratrochlear nerve
A14.2.01.025	N. nasociliaris	Nasociliary nerve

A14.2.01.026	R. communicans cum ganglio ciliari; Radix sensoria ganglii ciliaris; Radix nasociliaris ganglii ciliaris	Communicating branch with ciliary ganglion; Sensory root of ciliary ganglion; Nasociliary root of ciliary ganglion
A14.2.01.027	Nn. Ciliares longi	Long ciliary nerves
A14.2.01.028	N. ethmoidalis posterior	Posterior ethmoidal nerve
A14.2.01.029	R. meningeus anterior	Anterior meningeal branch
A14.2.01.030	N. ethmoidalis anterior	Anterior ethmoidal nerve
A14.2.01.031	Rr. nasales interni	Internal nasal branches
A14.2.01.032	Rr. nasales laterales	Lateral nasal branches
A14.2.01.033	Rr. nasales mediales	Medial nasal branches
A14.2.01.034	R. nasalis externus	External nasal nerve
A14.2.01.035	N. infratrochlearis	Infratrochlear nerve
A14.2.01.036	Rr. palpebrales	Palpebral branches
A14.2.01.037	**Nervus maxillaris [Vb; V_2]**	**Maxillary nerve; Maxillary division [Vb; V_2]**
A14.2.01.038	R. meningeus	Meningeal branch
A14.2.01.039	Rr. ganglionares ad ganglion pterygopalatinum; Radix sensoria ganglii pterygopalatini	Ganglionic branches to pterygopalatine ganglion; Sensory root of pterygopalatine ganglion
A14.2.01.040	Rr. orbitales	Orbital branches
A14.2.01.041	Rr. nasales posteriores superiores laterales	Posterior superior lateral nasal branches
A14.2.01.042	Rr. nasales posteriores superiores mediales	Posterior superior medial nasal branches
A14.2.01.043	N. nasopalatinus	Nasopalatine nerve
A14.2.01.044	N. pharyngeus	Pharyngeal nerve
A14.2.01.045	N. palatinus major	Greater palatine nerve
A14.2.01.046	Rr. nasales posteriores inferiores	Posterior inferior nasal nerves
A14.2.01.047	Nn. palatini minores	Lesser palatine nerves
A14.2.01.048	Rr. tonsillares	Tonsillar branches
A14.2.01.049	Nn. alveolares superiores	Superior alveolar nerves
A14.2.01.050	Rr. alveolares superiores posteriores	Posterior superior alveolar branches
A14.2.01.051	R. alveolaris superior medius	Middle superior alveolar branch
A14.2.01.052	Rr. alveolares superiores anteriores	Anterior superior alveolar branches
A14.2.01.053	Plexus dentalis superior	Superior dental plexus
A14.2.01.054	Rr. dentales superiores	Superior dental branches
A14.2.01.055	Rr. gingivales superiores	Superior gingival branches
A14.2.01.056	N. zygomaticus	Zygomatic nerve
A14.2.01.057	R. zygomaticotemporalis	Zygomaticotemporal branch
A14.2.01.058	R. zygomaticofacialis	Zygomaticofacial branch
A14.2.01.059	N.infraorbitalis	Infra-orbital nerve
A14.2.01.060	Rr. palpebrales inferiores	Inferior palpebral branches
A14.2.01.061	Rr. nasales externi	External nasal branches
A14.2.01.062	Rr. nasales interni	Internal nasal branches
A14.2.01.063	Rr. labiales superiores	Superior labial branches
A14.2.01.064	**Nervus mandibularis [Vc; V_3]**	**Mandibular nerve; Mandibular division [Vc; V_3]**
A14.2.01.065	R. meningeus; N. spinosus	Meningeal branch; Nervus spinosus
A14.2.01.066	N. pterygoideus medialis	Nerve to medial pterygoid
A14.2.01.067	Rr. ganglionares ad ganglion oticum; Radix sensoria ganglii otici	Branches to otic ganglion; Sensory root of otic ganglion
A14.2.01.068	N. musculi tensoris veli palatini	Nerve to tensor veli palatini
A14.2.01.069	N. musculi tensoris tympani	Nerve to tensor tympani
A14.2.01.070	N. massetericus	Masseteric nerve
A14.2.01.071	Nn. temporales profundi	Deep temporal nerves
A14.2.01.072	N. pterygoideus lateralis	Nerve to lateral pterygoid
A14.2.01.073	N. buccalis	Buccal nerve
A14.2.01.074	N. auriculotemporalis	Auriculotemporal nerve
A14.2.01.075	N. meatus acustici externi	Nerve to external acoustic meatus
A14.2.01.076	Rr. membranae tympani	Branches to tympanic membrane
A14.2.01.077	Rr. parotidei	Parotid branches
A14.2.01.078	Rr. communicantes cum nervo faciale	Communicating branches with facial nerve
A14.2.01.079	Nn. auriculares anteriores	Anterior auricular nerves

A14.2.01.080	Rr. temporales superficiales	Superficial temporal branches
A14.2.01.081	N. lingualis	Lingual nerve
A14.2.01.082	Rr. isthmi faucium	Branches to isthmus of fauces
A14.2.01.083	Rr. communicantes cum nervo hypoglosso	Communicating branches with hypoglossal nerve
A14.2.01.084	Chorda tympani	Chorda tympani
A14.2.01.085	N. sublingualis	Sublingual nerve
A14.2.01.086	Rr. linguales	Lingual branches
A14.2.01.087	Rr. ganglionares ad ganglion submandibulare; Radix sensoria ganglii submandibularis	Ganglionic branches to submandibular ganglion; Sensory root of submandibular ganglion
A14.2.01.088	Rr. ganglionares ad ganglion sublinguale; Radix sensoria ganglii sublingualis	Ganglionic branches to sublingual ganglion; Sensory root of sublingual ganglion
A14.2.01.089	N. alveolaris inferior	Inferior alveolar nerve
A14.2.01.090	N. mylohyoideus	Nerve to mylohyoid
A14.2.01.091	Plexus dentalis inferior	Inferior dental plexus
A14.2.01.092	Rr. dentales inferiores	Inferior dental branches
A14.2.01.093	Rr. gingivales inferiores	Inferior gingival branches
A14.2.01.094	N. mentalis	Mental nerve
A14.2.01.095	Rr. mentales	Mental branches
A14.2.01.096	Rr. labiales	Labial branches
A14.2.01.097	Rr. gingivales	Gingival branches

A14.2.01.098	**Nervus abducens [VI]**	**Abducent nerve; Abducens nerve [VI]**

A14.2.01.099	**Nervus facialis [VII]**	**Facial nerve [VII]**
A14.2.01.100	Geniculum	Geniculum
A14.2.01.101	N. stapedius	Nerve to stapedius
A14.2.01.102	N. auricularis posterior	Posterior auricular nerve
A14.2.01.103	R. occipitalis	Occipital branch
A14.2.01.104	R. auricularis	Auricular branch
A14.2.01.105	R. digastricus	Digastric branch
A14.2.01.106	R. stylohyoideus	Stylohyoid branch
A14.2.01.107	R. communicans cum nervo glossopharyngeo	Communicating branch with glossopharyngeal nerve
A14.2.01.108	Plexus intraparotideus	Parotid plexus
A14.2.01.109	Rr. temporales	Temporal branches
A14.2.01.110	Rr. zygomatici	Zygomatic branches
A14.2.01.111	Rr. buccales	Buccal branches
A14.2.01.112	(R. lingualis)	(Lingual branch)
A14.2.01.113	R. marginalis mandibularis	Marginal mandibular branch
A14.2.01.114	R. colli; R. cervicalis	Cervical branch
A14.2.01.115	**Nervus intermedius**	**Intermediate nerve**
A14.2.01.116	Ganglion geniculi; Ganglion geniculatum	Geniculate ganglion
A14.2.01.117	N. petrosus major; Radix parasympathica ganglii pterygopalatini; Radix intermedia ganglii pterygopalatini	Greater petrosal nerve; Parasympathetic root of pterygopalatine ganglion
A14.2.01.118	Chorda tympani; Radix parasympathica ganglii submandibularis	Chorda tympani; Parasympathetic root of submandibular ganglion
A14.2.01.119	R. communicans cum plexu tympanico	Communicating branch with tympanic plexus
A14.2.01.120	R. communicans cum nervo vago	Communicating branch with vagus nerve

A14.2.01.121	**Nervus vestibulocochlearis [VIII]**	**Vestibulocochlear nerve [VIII]**
A14.2.01.122	**Nervus vestibularis**	**Vestibular nerve**
A14.2.01.123	Ganglion vestibulare	Vestibular ganglion
A14.2.01.124	R. communicans cochlearis	Cochlear communicating branch
A14.2.01.125	Pars superior	Superior part
A14.2.01.126	N. utriculoampullaris	Utriculo-ampullary nerve
A14.2.01.127	N. utricularis	Utricular nerve
A14.2.01.128	N. ampullaris anterior	Anterior ampullary nerve

A14.2.01.129	N. ampullaris lateralis	Lateral ampullary nerve
A14.2.01.130	Pars inferior	Inferior part
A14.2.01.131	N. ampullaris posterior	Posterior ampullary nerve
A14.2.01.132	N. saccularis	Saccular nerve
A14.2.01.133	**Nervus cochlearis**	**Cochlear nerve**
A14.2.01.134	Ganglion cochleare; Ganglion spirale cochleae	Cochlear ganglion; Spiral ganglion

A14.2.01.135	**Nervus glossopharyngeus [IX]**	**Glossopharyngeal nerve [IX]**
A14.2.01.136	Ganglion superius	Superior ganglion
A14.2.01.137	Ganglion inferius	Inferior ganglion
A14.2.01.138	N. tympanicus	Tympanic nerve
A14.2.01.139	Intumescentia tympanica; Ganglion tympanicum	Tympanic enlargement; Tympanic ganglion
A14.2.01.140	Plexus tympanicus	Tympanic plexus
A14.2.01.141	R. tubarius	Tubal branch
A14.2.01.142	Nn. caroticotympanici	Caroticotympanic nerves
A14.2.01.143	R. communicans cum ramo auriculare nervi vagi	Communicating branch with auricular branch of vagus nerve
A14.2.01.144	Rr. pharyngei	Pharyngeal branches
A14.2.01.145	R. musculi stylopharyngei	Stylopharyngeal branch
A14.2.01.146	R. sinus carotici	Carotid branch
A14.2.01.147	Rr. tonsillares	Tonsillar branches
A14.2.01.148	Rr. linguales	Lingual branches
A14.2.01.149	N. petrosus minor; Radix parasympathica ganglii otici	Lesser petrosal nerve; Parasympathetic root of otic ganglion
A14.2.01.150	R. communicans cum ramo meningeo	Communicating branch with meningeal branch
A14.2.01.151	R. communicans cum nervo auriculotemporali	Communicating branch with auriculotemporal nerve
A14.2.01.152	R. communicans cum chorda tympani	Communicating branch with chorda tympani

A14.2.01.153	**Nervus vagus [X]**	**Vagus nerve [X]**
A14.2.01.154	Ganglion superius	Superior ganglion
A14.2.01.155	R. meningeus	Meningeal branch
A14.2.01.156	R. auricularis	Auricular branch
A14.2.01.157	Ganglion inferius	Inferior ganglion
A14.2.01.143	R. communicans cum nervo glossopharyngeo	Communicating branch with glossopharyngeal nerve
A14.2.01.158	R. pharyngeus	Pharyngeal branch
A14.2.01.159	Plexus pharyngeus	Pharyngeal plexus
A14.2.01.160	N. laryngeus superior	Superior laryngeal nerve
A14.2.01.161	R. externus	External branch
A14.2.01.162	R. internus	Internal branch
A14.2.01.163	R. communicans cum nervo laryngeo recurrente	Communicating branch with recurrent laryngeal nerve
A14.2.01.164	Rr. cardiaci cervicales superiores	Superior cervical cardiac branches
A14.2.01.165	Rr. cardiaci cervicales inferiores	Inferior cervical cardiac branches
A14.2.01.166	N. laryngeus recurrens	Recurrent laryngeal nerve
A14.2.01.167	Rr. tracheales	Tracheal branches
A14.2.01.168	Rr. oesophagei	Oesophageal branches▲
A14.2.01.169	Rr. pharyngei	Pharyngeal branches
A14.2.01.170	Rr. cardiaci thoracici	Thoracic cardiac branches
A14.2.01.171	Rr. bronchiales	Bronchial branches
A14.2.01.172	Plexus pulmonalis	Pulmonary plexus
A14.2.01.173	Plexus oesophageus	Oesophageal plexus▲
A14.2.01.174	Truncus vagalis anterior	Anterior vagal trunk
A14.2.01.175	Rr. gastrici anteriores	Anterior gastric branches
A14.2.01.176	N. curvaturae minoris anterior	Anterior nerve of lesser curvature
A14.2.01.177	Rr. hepatici	Hepatic branches
A14.2.01.178	R. pyloricus	Pyloric branch

A14.2.01.179	Truncus vagalis posterior	Posterior vagal trunk
A14.2.01.180	Rr. gastrici posteriores	Posterior gastric branches
A14.2.01.181	N. curvaturae minoris posterior	Posterior nerve of lesser curvature
A14.2.01.182	Rr. coeliaci	Coeliac branches▲
A14.2.01.183	Rr. renales	Renal branches

A14.2.01.184	**Nervus accessorius [XI]**	**Accessory nerve [XI]**
A14.2.01.185	Radix cranialis; Pars vagalis	Cranial root; Vagal part
A14.2.01.186	Radix spinalis; Pars spinalis	Spinal root; Spinal part
A14.2.01.187	Truncus nervi accessorii	Trunk of accessory nerve
A14.2.01.188	R. internus	Internal branch
A14.2.01.189	R. externus	External branch
A14.2.01.190	Rr. musculares	Muscular branches

A14.2.01.191	**Nervus hypoglossus [XII]**	**Hypoglossal nerve [XII]**
A14.2.01.192	Rr. linguales	Lingual branches

A14.2.02.001	**Nervi spinales**	**Spinal nerves**
A14.2.02.002	**NERVI CERVICALES [C1–C8]**	**CERVICAL NERVES [C1–C8]**
A14.2.02.003	**Rami posteriores; Rami dorsales**	**Posterior rami; Dorsal rami**
A14.2.02.004	R. medialis	Medial branch
A14.2.02.005	R. lateralis	Lateral branch
A14.2.02.006	R. cutaneus posterior	Posterior cutaneous branch
A14.2.02.007	N. suboccipitalis	Suboccipital nerve
A14.2.02.008	N. occipitalis major	Greater occipital nerve
A14.2.02.009	N. occipitalis tertius	Third occipital nerve
A14.2.02.010	Plexus cervicalis posterior	Posterior cervical plexus

A14.2.02.011	**Rami anteriores; Rami ventrales**	**Anterior rami; Ventral rami**
A14.2.02.012	**Plexus cervicalis**	**Cervical plexus**
A14.2.02.013	Ansa cervicalis	Ansa cervicalis
A14.2.02.014	Radix superior	Superior root; Superior limb
A14.2.02.015	Radix inferior	Inferior root; Inferior limb
A14.2.02.016	R. thyrohyoideus	Thyrohyoid branch
A14.2.02.017	N. occipitalis minor	Lesser occipital nerve
A14.2.02.018	N. auricularis magnus	Great auricular nerve
A14.2.02.019	R. posterior	Posterior branch
A14.2.02.020	R. anterior	Anterior branch
A14.2.02.021	N. transversus colli; N. transversus cervicalis	Transverse cervical nerve
A14.2.02.022	Rr. superiores	Superior branches
A14.2.02.023	Rr. inferiores	Inferior branches
A14.2.02.024	Nn. supraclaviculares	Supraclavicular nerves
A14.2.02.025	Nn. supraclaviculares mediales	Medial supraclavicular nerves
A14.2.02.026	Nn. supraclaviculares intermedii	Intermediate supraclavicular nerves
A14.2.02.027	Nn. supraclaviculares laterales	Lateral supraclavicular nerves
A14.2.02.028	**Nervus phrenicus**	**Phrenic nerve**
A14.2.02.029	R. pericardiacus	Pericardial branch
A14.2.02.030	Rr. phrenicoabdominales	Phrenico-abdominal branches
A14.2.02.031	(Nn. phrenici accessorii)	(Accessory phrenic nerves)

A14.2.03.001	**Plexus brachialis**	**Brachial plexus**
	Nomina generalia	*General terms*
A14.2.03.002	Radices	Roots
A14.2.03.003	Trunci	Trunks
A14.2.03.004	Truncus superior	Superior trunk; Upper trunk
A14.2.03.005	Truncus medius	Middle trunk

A14.2.03.006	Truncus inferior	Inferior trunk; Lower trunk
A14.2.03.007	Divisiones anteriores	Anterior divisions
A14.2.03.008	Divisiones posteriores	Posterior divisions
A14.2.03.009	Fasciculi	Cords

A14.2.03.010	**Pars supraclavicularis**	**Supraclavicular part**
A14.2.03.011	N. dorsalis scapulae	Dorsal scapular nerve
A14.2.03.012	N. thoracicus longus	Long thoracic nerve
A14.2.03.013	N. subclavius	Subclavian nerve
A14.2.03.014	N. suprascapularis	Suprascapular nerve
A14.2.03.015	Nn. subscapulares	Subscapular nerves
A14.2.03.016	N. thoracodorsalis	Thoracodorsal nerve
A14.2.03.017	N. pectoralis medialis	Medial pectoral nerve
A14.2.03.018	N. pectoralis lateralis	Lateral pectoral nerve
A14.2.03.019	Rr. musculares	Muscular branches

A14.2.03.020	**Pars infraclavicularis**	**Infraclavicular part**
A14.2.03.021	Fasciculus lateralis	Lateral cord
A14.2.03.022	Fasciculus medialis	Medial cord
A14.2.03.023	Fasciculus posterior	Posterior cord
A14.2.03.024	**N. musculocutaneus**	**Musculocutaneous nerve**
A14.2.03.025	Rr. musculares	Muscular branches
A14.2.03.026	N. cutaneus antebrachii lateralis	Lateral cutaneous nerve of forearm; Lateral antebrachial cutaneous nerve
A14.2.03.027	**N. cutaneus brachii medialis**	**Medial cutaneous nerve of arm; Medial brachial cutaneous nerve**
A14.2.03.028	**N. cutaneus antebrachii medialis**	**Medial cutaneous nerve of forearm; Medial antebrachial cutaneous nerve**
A14.2.03.029	R. anterior	Anterior branch
A14.2.03.030	R. posterior	Posterior branch
A14.2.03.031	**N. medianus**	**Median nerve**
A14.2.03.032	Radix medialis nervi mediani	Medial root of median nerve
A14.2.03.033	Radix lateralis nervi mediani	Lateral root of median nerve
A14.2.03.034	N. interosseus antebrachii anterior	Anterior interosseous nerve
A14.2.03.035	Rr. musculares	Muscular branches
A14.2.03.036	R. palmaris	Palmar branch
A14.2.03.037	R. communicans cum nervo ulnari	Communicating branch with ulnar nerve
A14.2.03.038	Nn. digitales palmares communes	Common palmar digital nerves
A14.2.03.039	Nn. digitales palmares proprii	Proper palmar digital nerves
A14.2.03.040	**N. ulnaris**	**Ulnar nerve**
A14.2.03.041	Rr. musculares	Muscular branches
A14.2.03.042	R. dorsalis	Dorsal branch
A14.2.03.043	Nn. digitales dorsales	Dorsal digital nerves
A14.2.03.044	R. palmaris	Palmar branch
A14.2.03.045	R. superficialis	Superficial branch
A14.2.03.046	Nn. digitales palmares communes	Common palmar digital nerves
A14.2.03.047	Nn. digitales palmares proprii	Proper palmar digital nerves
A14.2.03.048	R. profundus	Deep branch
A14.2.03.049	**N. radialis**	**Radial nerve**
A14.2.03.050	N. cutaneus brachii posterior	Posterior cutaneous nerve of arm; Posterior brachial cutaneous nerve
A14.2.03.051	N. cutaneus brachii lateralis inferior	Inferior lateral cutaneous nerve of arm; Inferior lateral brachial cutaneous nerve
A14.2.03.052	N. cutaneus antebrachii posterior	Posterior cutaneous nerve of forearm; Posterior antebrachial cutaneous nerve
A14.2.03.053	Rr. musculares	Muscular branches
A14.2.03.054	R. profundus	Deep branch
A14.2.03.055	N. interosseus antebrachii posterior	Posterior interosseous nerve
A14.2.03.056	R. superficialis	Superficial branch

A14.2.03.057	R. communicans ulnaris	Communicating branch with ulnar nerve
A14.2.03.058	Nn. digitales dorsales	Dorsal digital branches
A14.2.03.059	**N. axillaris**	**Axillary nerve**
A14.2.03.060	Rr. musculares	Muscular branches
A14.2.03.061	N. cutaneus brachii lateralis superior	Superior lateral cutaneous nerve of arm; Superior lateral brachial cutaneous nerve
A14.2.04.001	**NERVI THORACICI [T1–T12]**	**THORACIC NERVES [T1–T12]**
A14.2.04.002	**Rami posteriores; Rami dorsales**	**Posterior rami; Dorsal rami**
A14.2.04.003	R. medialis	Medial branch
A14.2.04.004	R. lateralis	Lateral branch
A14.2.04.005	R. cutaneus posterior	Posterior cutaneous branch; Posterior cutaneous nerve
A14.2.04.006	**Nn. intercostales; Rami anteriores; Rami ventrales**	**Intercostal nerves; Anterior rami; Ventral rami**
A14.2.04.007	Rr. musculares	Muscular branches
A14.2.04.008	R. collateralis	Collateral branch
A14.2.04.009	R. cutaneus lateralis pectoralis	Lateral pectoral cutaneous branch
A14.2.04.010	Rr. mammarii laterales	Lateral mammary branches
A14.2.04.011	R. cutaneus lateralis abdominalis	Lateral abdominal cutaneous branch
A14.2.04.012	Nn. intercostobrachiales	Intercostobrachial nerves
A14.2.04.013	R. cutaneus anterior pectoralis	Anterior pectoral cutaneous branch
A14.2.04.014	Rr. mammarii mediales	Medial mammary branches
A14.2.04.015	R. cutaneus anterior abdominalis	Anterior abdominal cutaneous branch
A14.2.04.016	N. subcostalis	Subcostal nerve
A14.2.05.001	**NERVI LUMBALES [L1–L5]**	**LUMBAR NERVES [L1–L5]**
A14.2.05.002	**Rami posteriores; Rami dorsales**	**Posterior rami; Dorsal rami**
A14.2.05.003	R. medialis	Medial branch
A14.2.05.004	R. lateralis	Lateral branch
A14.2.05.005	R. cutaneus posterior	Posterior cutaneous branch; Posterior cutaneous nerve
A14.2.05.006	Nn. clunium superiores	Superior clunial nerves
A14.2.05.007	Plexus posterior	Posterior plexus
A14.2.05.008	**Rami anteriores; Rami ventrales**	**Anterior rami; Ventral rami**
A14.2.06.001	**NERVI SACRALES ET NERVUS COCCYGEUS [S1–S5, Co]**	**SACRAL NERVES AND COCCYGEAL NERVE [S1–S5, Co]**
A14.2.06.002	**Rami posteriores; Rami dorsales**	**Posterior rami; Dorsal rami**
A14.2.06.003	R. medialis	Medial branch
A14.2.06.004	R. lateralis	Lateral branch
A14.2.06.005	R. cutaneus posterior	Posterior cutaneous branch; Posterior cutaneous nerve
A14.2.06.006	Nn. clunium medii	Medial clunial nerves
A14.2.06.007	**Rami anteriores; Rami ventrales**	**Anterior rami; Ventral rami**
A14.2.07.001	**Plexus lumbosacralis**	**Lumbosacral plexus**
A14.2.07.002	**Plexus lumbalis**	**Lumbar plexus**
A14.2.07.003	**N. iliohypogastricus; N. iliopubicus**	**Iliohypogastric nerve; Iliopubic nerve**
A14.2.07.004	R. cutaneus lateralis	Lateral cutaneous branch
A14.2.07.005	R. cutaneus anterior	Anterior cutaneous branch
A14.2.07.006	**N. ilioinguinalis**	**Ilio-inguinal nerve**
A14.2.07.007	Nn. labiales anteriores ♀	Anterior labial nerves ♀
A14.2.07.007	Nn. scrotales anteriores ♂	Anterior scrotal nerves ♂
A14.2.07.008	**N. genitofemoralis**	**Genitofemoral nerve**

A14.2.07.009	R. genitalis	Genital branch
A14.2.07.010	R. femoralis	Femoral branch
A14.2.07.011	**N. cutaneus femoris lateralis**	**Lateral cutaneous nerve of thigh; Lateral femoral cutaneous nerve**
A14.2.07.012	**N. obturatorius**	**Obturator nerve**
A14.2.07.013	R. anterior	Anterior branch
A14.2.07.014	R. cutaneus	Cutaneous branch
A14.2.07.015	Rr. musculares	Muscular branches
A14.2.07.016	R. posterior	Posterior branch
A14.2.07.017	Rr. musculares	Muscular branches
A14.2.07.018	R. articularis	Articular branch
A14.2.07.019	**N. obturatorius accessorius**	**Accessory obturator nerve**
A14.2.07.020	**N. femoralis**	**Femoral nerve**
A14.2.07.021	Rr. musculares	Muscular branches
A14.2.07.022	Rr. cutanei anteriores	Anterior cutaneous branches
A14.2.07.023	N. saphenus	Saphenous nerve
A14.2.07.024	R. infrapatellaris	Infrapatellar branch
A14.2.07.025	Rr. cutanei cruris mediales	Medial cutaneous nerve of leg; Medial crural cutaneous nerve
A14.2.07.026	**Truncus lumbosacralis**	**Lumbosacral trunk**

A14.2.07.027	**Plexus sacralis**	**Sacral plexus**
A14.2.07.028	N. musculi obturatorii interni	Nerve to obturator internus
A14.2.07.029	N. musculi piriformis	Nerve to piriformis
A14.2.07.030	N. musculi quadrati femoris	Nerve to quadratus femoris
A14.2.07.031	N. gluteus superior	Superior gluteal nerve
A14.2.07.032	N. gluteus inferior	Inferior gluteal nerve
A14.2.07.033	N. cutaneus femoris posterior	Posterior cutaneous nerve of thigh; Posterior femoral cutaneous nerve
A14.2.07.034	Nn. clunium inferiores	Inferior clunial nerves
A14.2.07.035	Rr. perineales	Perineal branches
A14.2.07.036	N. cutaneus perforans	Perforating cutaneous nerve
A14.2.07.037	**N. pudendus**	**Pudendal nerve**
A14.2.07.038	Nn. anales inferiores; Nn. rectales inferiores	Inferior anal nerves; Inferior rectal nerves
A14.2.07.039	Nn. perineales	Perineal nerves
A14.2.07.040	Nn. labiales posteriores ♀	Posterior labial nerves ♀
A14.2.07.040	Nn. scrotales posteriores ♂	Posterior scrotal nerves ♂
A14.2.07.041	Rr. musculares	Muscular branches
A14.2.07.042	N. dorsalis clitoridis ♀	Dorsal nerve of clitoris ♀
A14.2.07.042	N. dorsalis penis ♂	Dorsal nerve of penis ♂
A14.2.07.043	**N. coccygeus**	**Coccygeal nerve**
A14.2.07.044	Plexus coccygeus	Coccygeal plexus
A14.2.07.045	N. anococcygeus	Anococcygeal nerve

A14.2.07.046	**N. ischiadicus**	**Sciatic nerve**
A14.2.07.047	**N. fibularis communis; N. peroneus communis**	**Common fibular nerve; Common peroneal nerve**
A14.2.07.048	N. cutaneus surae lateralis	Lateral sural cutaneous nerve
A14.2.07.049	R. communicans fibularis; R. communicans peroneus	Sural communicating branch
A14.2.07.050	N. fibularis superficialis; N. peroneus superficialis	Superficial fibular nerve; Superficial peroneal nerve
A14.2.07.051	Rr. musculares	Muscular branches
A14.2.07.052	N. cutaneus dorsalis medialis	Medial dorsal cutaneous nerve
A14.2.07.053	N. cutaneus dorsalis intermedius	Intermediate dorsal cutaneous nerve
A14.2.07.054	Nn. digitales dorsales pedis	Dorsal digital nerves of foot
A14.2.07.055	N. fibularis profundus; N. peroneus profundus	Deep fibular nerve; Deep peroneal nerve
A14.2.07.056	Rr. musculares	Muscular branches
A14.2.07.057	Nn. digitales dorsales pedis	Dorsal digital nerves of foot

A14.2.07.058	**N. tibialis**	**Tibial nerve**
A14.2.07.059	Rr. musculares	Muscular branches
A14.2.07.060	N. interosseus cruris	Interosseous nerve of leg; Crural interosseous nerve
A14.2.07.061	N. cutaneus surae medialis	Medial sural cutaneous nerve
A14.2.07.062	N. suralis	Sural nerve
A14.2.07.063	N. cutaneus dorsalis lateralis	Lateral dorsal cutaneous nerve
A14.2.07.064	Rr. calcanei laterales	Lateral calcaneal branches
A14.2.07.065	Rr. calcanei mediales	Medial calcaneal branches
A14.2.07.066	N. plantaris medialis	Medial plantar nerve
A14.2.07.067	Nn. digitales plantares communes	Common plantar digital nerves
A14.2.07.068	Nn. digitales plantares proprii	Proper plantar digital nerves
A14.2.07.069	N. plantaris lateralis	Lateral plantar nerve
A14.2.07.070	R. superficialis	Superficial branch
A14.2.07.071	Nn. digitales plantares communes	Common plantar digital nerves
A14.2.07.072	Nn. digitales plantares proprii	Proper plantar digital nerves
A14.2.07.073	R. profundus	Deep branch

A14.3.00.001	**Divisio autonomica; Pars autonomica systematis nervosi peripherici**	**Autonomic division; Autonomic part of peripheral nervous system**
A14.3.01.001	PARS SYMPATHICA	SYMPATHETIC PART
A14.3.01.002	**Truncus sympathicus**	**Sympathetic trunk**
A14.3.01.003	Ganglion trunci sympathici	Ganglion of sympathetic trunk
A14.3.01.004	Rr. interganglionares	Interganglionic branches
A14.3.01.005	Rr. communicantes	Rami communicantes
A14.3.01.006	R. communicans griseus	Grey ramus communicans▲
A14.3.01.007	R. communicans albus	White ramus communicans
A14.3.01.008	Ganglia intermedia	Intermediate ganglia
A14.3.01.009	**Ganglion cervicale superius**	**Superior cervical ganglion**
A14.3.01.010	N. jugularis	Jugular nerve
A14.3.01.011	N. caroticus internus	Internal carotid nerve
A14.3.01.012	N. pinealis	Pineal nerve
A14.3.01.013	Nn. carotici externi	External carotid nerves
A14.3.01.014	Rr. laryngopharyngei	Laryngopharyngeal branches
A14.3.01.015	N. cardiacus cervicalis superior	Superior cervical cardiac nerve
A14.3.01.016	**Ganglion cervicale medium**	**Middle cervical ganglion**
A14.3.01.017	Ganglion vertebrale	Vertebral ganglion
A14.3.01.018	N. cardiacus cervicalis medius	Middle cervical cardiac nerve
A14.3.01.019	**(Ganglion cervicale inferioris)**	**(Inferior cervical ganglion)**
A14.3.01.020	**Ganglion cervicothoracicum; Ganglion stellatum**	**Cervicothoracic ganglion; Stellate ganglion**
A14.3.01.021	Ansa subclavia	Ansa subclavia
A14.3.01.022	N. cardiacus cervicalis inferior	Inferior cervical cardiac nerve
A14.3.01.023	N. vertebralis	Vertebral nerve
A14.3.01.024	**Ganglia thoracica**	**Thoracic ganglia**
A14.3.01.025	Rr. cardiaci thoracici	Thoracic cardiac branches
A14.3.01.026	Rr. pulmonales thoracici	Thoracic pulmonary branches
A14.3.01.027	Rr. oesophageales	Oesophageal branches▲
A14.3.01.028	N. splanchnicus major	Greater splanchnic nerve
A14.3.01.029	Ganglion thoracicum splanchnicum	Thoracic splanchnic ganglion
A14.3.01.030	N. splanchnicus minor	Lesser splanchnic nerve
A14.3.01.031	R. renalis	Renal branch

A14.3.00.001 *Divisio autonomica* The term *systema nervosum autonomicum* is not used in this list to avoid ambiguity. For some it parallels the somatic nervous system and has central and peripheral components; for others it is a part of the peripheral nervous system. In addition some consider it to have efferent elements only, while others recognise afferent elements as well. There are very many connections between somatic nerves and autonomic ganglia and between autonomic structures in the head. Examples are the connections between the superior cervical ganglion and the sensory trigeminal ganglion, between the nerve plexus around the internal carotid artery and cavernous plexus and the abducens nerve and between the pterygopalatine and the ciliary ganglion. Of these connections, only *n. pinealis* has been named.

A14.3.01.012 *Nervus pinealis* Previously known under the name of *n. conarii*, referring to the old name of the pineal gland, *conarium*.

A14.3.01.032	N. splanchnicus imus	Least splanchnic nerve; Lowest splanchnic nerve
A14.3.01.033	**Ganglia lumbalia**	**Lumbar ganglia**
A14.3.01.034	Nn. splanchnici lumbales	Lumbar splanchnic nerves
A14.3.01.035	**Ganglia sacralia**	**Sacral ganglia**
A14.3.01.036	Nn. splanchnici sacrales	Sacral splanchnic nerves
A14.3.01.037	Ganglion impar	Ganglion impar
A14.3.01.078	Paraganglia sympathica	Sympathetic paraganglia

A14.3.02.001	PARS PARASYMPATHICA	PARASYMPATHETIC PART
A14.3.02.002	**Pars cranialis**	**Cranial part**
A14.3.02.003	Ganglion ciliare	Ciliary ganglion
A14.2.01.010	Radix parasympathica; Radix oculomotoria; R. n. oculomotorii ad ganglion ciliare	Parasympathetic root; Oculomotor root; Branch of oculomotor nerve to ciliary ganglion
A14.3.02.004	Radix sympathica	Sympathetic root
A14.2.01.026	Radix sensoria; Radix nasociliaris; R. communicans n. nasociliaris cum ganglio ciliare	Sensory root; Nasociliary root; Communicating branch of nasociliary nerve with cilary ganglion
A14.3.02.005	Nn. ciliares breves	Short ciliary nerves
A14.3.02.006	Ganglion pterygopalatinum	Pterygopalatine ganglion
A14.3.02.007	N. canalis pterygoidei	Nerve of pterygoid canal
A14.2.01.117	Radix parasympathica; Radix intermedia; N. petrosus major	Parasympathetic root; Greater petrosal nerve
A14.3.02.008	Radix sympathica; N. petrosus profundus	Sympathetic root; Deep petrosal nerve
A14.2.01.039	Radix sensoria ganglii pterygopalatini; Rr. ganglionares n. maxillaris	Sensory root; Ganglionic branches of maxillary nerve
A14.3.02.009	Ganglion submandibulare	Submandibular ganglion
A14.2.01.118	Radix parasympathica; Chorda tympani	Parasympathetic root; Chorda tympani
A14.3.02.010	Radix sympathica	Sympathetic root
A14.2.01.087	Radix sensoria; Rr. ganglionares n. mandibularis	Sensory root; Ganglionic branches of mandibular nerve
A14.3.02.011	Ganglion sublinguale	Sublingual ganglion
A14.3.02.012	Radix parasympathica; Chorda tympani	Parasympathetic root; Chorda tympani
A14.3.02.013	Radix sympathica	Sympathetic root
A14.2.01.088	Radix sensoria; Rr. ganglionares n. mandibularis	Sensory root; Ganglionic branches of mandibular nerve
A14.3.02.014	Ganglion oticum	Otic ganglion
A14.2.01.149	Radix parasympathica; N. petrosus minor	Parasympathetic root; Lesser petrosal nerve
A14.3.02.015	Radix sympathica	Sympathetic root
A14.2.01.067	Radix sensoria; Rr. ganglionares n. mandibularis	Sensory root; Ganglionic branches of mandibular nerve
A14.3.02.016	**Pars pelvica**	**Pelvic part**
A14.3.02.017	Ganglia pelvica	Pelvic ganglia
A14.3.02.018	Radix parasympathica; Nn. splanchnici pelvici	Parasympathetic root; Pelvic splanchnic nerves
A14.3.02.019	Radix sympathica	Sympathetic root
A14.3.02.020	Radix sensoria	Sensory root

A14.3.03.001	PLEXUS VISCERALES ET GANGLIA VISCERALIA	PERIPHERAL AUTONOMIC PLEXUSES AND GANGLIA
A14.3.03.002	**Pars craniocervicalis**	**Craniocervical part**
A14.3.03.003	Plexus caroticus communis	Common carotid plexus
A14.3.03.004	Plexus caroticus internus	Internal carotid plexus
A14.3.02.004	Radix sympathica ganglii ciliaris	Sympathetic root of ciliary ganglion
A14.3.02.008	Radix sympathica ganglii pterygopalatini; N. petrosus profundus	Sympathetic root of pterygopalatine ganglion; Deep petrosal nerve
A14.3.02.010	Radix sympathica ganglii submandibularis	Sympathetic root of submandibular ganglion
A14.3.03.005	Radix sympathica ganglii sublingualis	Sympathetic root of sublingual ganglion
A14.3.02.015	Radix sympathica ganglii otici	Sympathetic root of otic ganglion
A14.2.01.142	Nn. caroticotympanici	Caroticotympanic nerves

A14.3.03.006	Plexus cavernosus	Cavernous plexus
A14.3.03.007	Plexus caroticus externus	External carotid plexus
A14.3.03.008	Plexus subclavius	Subclavian plexus
A14.3.03.009	Plexus autonomicus brachialis	Brachial autonomic plexus
A14.3.03.010	Plexus vertebralis	Vertebral plexus
A14.3.03.011	**Pars thoracica**	**Thoracic part**
A14.3.03.012	Plexus aorticus thoracicus	Thoracic aortic plexus
A14.3.03.013	Plexus cardiacus	Cardiac plexus
A14.3.03.014	Ganglia cardiaca	Cardiac ganglia
A14.3.03.015	Plexus oesophageus	Oesophageal plexus▲
A14.3.03.016	Plexus pulmonalis	Pulmonary plexus
A14.3.03.017	Rr. pulmonales	Pulmonary branches
A14.3.03.018	**Pars abdominalis**	**Abdominal part**
A14.3.03.019	Plexus aorticus abdominalis	Abdominal aortic plexus
A14.3.03.020	Ganglia phrenica	Phrenic ganglia
A14.3.03.021	Plexus coeliacus	Coeliac plexus▲
A14.3.03.022	Plexus hepaticus	Hepatic plexus
A14.3.03.023	Plexus splenicus; Plexus lienalis	Splenic plexus
A14.3.03.024	Plexus gastrici	Gastric plexuses
A14.3.03.025	Plexus pancreaticus	Pancreatic plexus
A14.3.03.026	Plexus suprarenalis	Suprarenal plexus
A14.3.03.027	Ganglia coeliaca	Coeliac ganglia▲
A14.3.03.028	Ganglia aorticorenalia	Aorticorenal ganglia
A14.3.03.029	Plexus mesentericus superior	Superior mesenteric plexus
A14.3.03.030	Ganglion mesentericum superius	Superior mesenteric ganglion
A14.3.03.031	Plexus intermesentericus	Intermesenteric plexus
A14.3.03.032	Plexus renalis	Renal plexus
A14.3.03.033	Ganglia renalia	Renal ganglia
A14.3.03.034	Plexus uretericus	Ureteric plexus
A14.3.03.035	Plexus ovaricus ♀	Ovarian plexus ♀
A14.3.03.035	Plexus testicularis ♂	Testicular plexus ♂
A14.3.03.036	Plexus mesentericus inferior	Inferior mesenteric plexus
A14.3.03.037	Ganglion mesentericum inferius	Inferior mesenteric ganglion
A14.3.03.038	Plexus rectalis superior	Superior rectal plexus
A14.3.03.039	Plexus entericus	Enteric plexus
A14.3.03.040	Plexus subserosus	Subserous plexus
A14.3.03.041	Plexus myentericus	Myenteric plexus
A14.3.03.042	Plexus submucosus	Submucous plexus
A14.3.03.043	Plexus iliacus	Iliac plexus
A14.3.03.044	Plexus femoralis	Femoral plexus
A14.3.03.045	**Pars pelvica**	**Pelvic part**
A14.3.03.046	Plexus hypogastricus superior; N. presacralis	Superior hypogastric plexus; Presacral nerve
A14.3.03.047	N. hypogastricus	Hypogastric nerve
A14.3.03.048	Plexus hypogastricus inferior; Plexus pelvicus	Inferior hypogastric plexus; Pelvic plexus
A14.3.03.049	Plexus rectalis medius	Middle rectal plexus
A14.3.03.050	Plexus rectalis inferior	Inferior rectal plexus
A14.3.03.051	Nn. anales superiores	Superior anal nerves
A14.3.03.052	Plexus uterovaginalis ♀	Uterovaginal plexus ♀
A14.3.03.053	Nn. vaginales ♀	Vaginal nerves ♀
A14.3.03.052	Plexus prostaticus ♂	Prostatic plexus ♂
A14.3.03.054	Plexus deferentialis ♂	Deferential plexus; Plexus of ductus deferens ♂
A14.3.03.055	Plexus vesicalis	Vesical plexus
A14.3.03.056	Nn. cavernosi clitoridis ♀	Cavernous nerves of clitoris ♀
A14.3.03.056	Nn. cavernosi penis ♂	Cavernous nerves of penis ♂

A15.0.00.000	**Organa sensuum**	**Sense organs**
A15.1.00.001	**Organum olfactorium; Organum olfactus**	**Olfactory organ**
A15.1.00.002	Pars olfactoria tunicae mucosae nasi	Olfactory part of nasal mucosa; Olfactory area
A15.1.00.003	Glandulae olfactoriae	Olfactory glands
A15.2.00.001	**Oculus et structurae pertinentes**	**Eye and related structures**
A15.2.01.001	BULBUS OCULI	EYEBALL
A15.2.01.002	Polus anterior	Anterior pole
A15.2.01.003	Polus posterior	Posterior pole
A15.2.01.004	Equator	Equator
A15.2.01.005	Meridiani	Meridians
A15.2.01.006	Axis bulbi externus	External axis of eyeball
A15.2.01.007	Axis bulbi internus	Internal axis of eyeball
A15.2.01.008	Axis opticus	Optic axis
A15.2.01.009	Segmentum anterius	Anterior segment
A15.2.01.010	Segmentum posterius	Posterior segment
A15.2.02.001	**Tunica fibrosa bulbi**	**Fibrous layer of eyeball**
A15.2.02.002	**Sclera**	**Sclera**
A15.2.02.003	Sulcus sclerae	Sulcus sclerae
A15.2.02.004	Reticulum trabeculare	Trabecular tissue
A15.2.02.005	Pars corneoscleralis	Corneoscleral part
A15.2.02.006	Pars uvealis	Uveal part
A15.2.02.007	Calcar sclerae	Scleral spur
A12.3.06.109	Sinus venosus sclerae	Scleral venous sinus
A15.2.02.008	Lamina episcleralis	Episcleral layer
A15.2.02.009	Substantia propria sclerae	Substantia propria
A15.2.02.010	Lamina fusca sclerae	Suprachoroid lamina
A15.2.02.011	Lamina cribrosa sclerae	Lamina cribrosa of sclera
A15.2.02.012	**Cornea**	**Cornea**
A15.2.02.013	Anulus conjunctivae	Conjunctival ring
A15.2.02.014	Limbus corneae	Corneoscleral junction; Corneal limbus
A15.2.02.015	Vertex corneae	Corneal vertex
A15.2.02.016	Facies anterior	Anterior surface
A15.2.02.017	Facies posterior	Posterior surface
A15.2.02.018	Epithelium anterius	Corneal epithelium
A15.2.02.019	Lamina limitans anterior	Anterior limiting lamina
A15.2.02.020	Substantia propria	Substantia propria
A15.2.02.021	Lamina limitans posterior	Posterior limiting lamina
A15.2.02.022	Epithelium posterius	Endothelium of anterior chamber
A15.2.03.001	**Tunica vasculosa bulbi**	**Vascular layer of eyeball**
A15.2.03.002	**Choroidea**	**Choroid**
A15.2.03.003	Lamina suprachoroidea	Suprachoroid lamina
A15.2.03.004	Spatium perichoroideum	Perichoroidal space
A15.2.03.005	Lamina vasculosa	Vascular lamina
A15.2.03.006	Lamina choroidocapillaris	Capillary lamina
A15.2.03.007	Lamina basalis	Basal lamina
A15.2.03.008	Vasa sanguinea choroideae	Choroid blood vessels
A15.2.03.009	**Corpus ciliare**	**Ciliary body**
A15.2.03.010	Corona ciliaris	Corona ciliaris
A15.2.03.011	Processus ciliares	Ciliary processes
A15.2.03.012	Plicae ciliares	Ciliary plicae
A15.2.03.013	Orbiculus ciliaris	Orbiculus ciliaris
A15.2.03.014	M. ciliaris	Ciliary muscle
A15.2.03.015	Fibrae meridionales	Meridional fibres▲

A15.2.03.016	Fibrae longitudinales	Longitudinal fibres▲
A15.2.03.017	Fibrae radiales	Radial fibres▲
A15.2.03.018	Fibrae circulares	Circular fibres▲
A15.2.03.019	Lamina basalis	Basal lamina
A15.2.03.020	**Iris**	**Iris**
A15.2.03.021	Margo pupillaris	Pupillary margin
A15.2.03.022	Margo ciliaris	Ciliary margin
A15.2.03.023	Facies anterior	Anterior surface
A15.2.03.024	Facies posterior	Posterior surface
A15.2.03.025	Anulus iridis major	Outer border of iris
A15.2.03.026	Anulus iridis minor	Inner border of iris
A15.2.03.027	Plicae iridis	Folds of iris
A15.2.03.028	Pupilla	Pupil
A15.2.03.029	M. sphincter pupillae	Sphincter pupillae
A15.2.03.030	M. dilatator pupillae	Dilator pupillae
A15.2.03.031	Stroma iridis	Stroma of iris
A15.2.03.032	Epithelium pigmentosum	Pigmented epithelium
A15.2.03.033	Spatia anguli iridocornealis	Spaces of iridocorneal angle
A15.2.03.034	Circulus arteriosus iridis major	Major circulus arteriosus of iris
A15.2.03.035	Circulus arteriosus iridis minor	Minor circulus arteriosus of iris
A15.2.03.036	(Membrana pupillaris)	(Pupillary membrane)

A15.2.04.001	**Tunica interna bulbi**	**Inner layer of eyeball**
A15.2.04.002	**Retina**	**Retina**
A15.2.04.003	Pars caeca retinae	Nonvisual retina
A15.2.04.004	Pars ciliaris retinae	Ciliary part of retina
A15.2.04.005	Pars iridica retinae	Iridial part of retina
A15.2.04.006	Ora serrata	Ora serrata
A15.2.04.007	Pars optica retinae	Optic part of retina
A15.2.04.008	Stratum pigmentosum	Pigmented layer
A15.2.04.009	Stratum nervosum	Neural layer
* **A15.2.04.010**	Stratum segmentorum externorum et internorum	Layer of inner and outer segments
A15.2.04.011	Stratum limitans externum	Outer limiting layer
A15.2.04.012	Stratum nucleare externum	Outer nuclear layer
A15.2.04.013	Stratum plexiforme externum	Outer plexiform layer
A15.2.04.014	Stratum nucleare internum	Inner nuclear layer
A15.2.04.015	Stratum plexiforme internum	Inner plexiform layer
A15.2.04.016	Stratum ganglionicum	Ganglionic layer
A15.2.04.017	Stratum neurofibrarum	Layer of nerve fibres▲
A15.2.04.018	Stratum limitans internum	Inner limiting layer
A15.2.04.019	Discus nervi optici	Optic disc
A15.2.04.020	Excavatio disci	Depression of optic disc; Physiological cup
A15.2.04.021	Macula lutea	Macula
A15.2.04.022	Fovea centralis	Fovea centralis
A15.2.04.023	Foveola	Foveola
A15.2.04.024	**Nervus opticus**	**Optic nerve**
A15.2.04.025	Pars intracranialis	Intracranial part
A15.2.04.026	Pars canalis	Part in canal
A15.2.04.027	Pars orbitalis	Orbital part
A15.2.04.028	Pars intraocularis	Intra-ocular part
A15.2.04.029	Pars postlaminaris	Postlaminar part
A15.2.04.030	Pars intralaminaris	Intralaminar part
A15.2.04.031	Pars prelaminaris	Prelaminar part
A15.2.04.032	Vagina externa	Outer sheath

* **A15.2.04.010** *Stratum segmentorum externorum et internorum* Previously, this layer was termed *stratum neuroepitheliale*. This has led to terminological inconsistencies between textbooks, because neuroepithelium in its full sense includes more structures than this layer. The recommended term is based on the major structural components of this layer.

A15.2.04.033	Vagina interna	Inner sheath
A15.2.04.034	Spatium intervaginale subarachnoidale; Spatium leptomeningeum	Subarachnoid space; Leptomeningeal space
A15.2.04.035	**Vasa sanguinea retinae**	**Retinal blood vessels**
A12.2.06.026	A. centralis retinae, pars intraocularis	Central retinal artery, intraocular part
A15.2.04.036	Circulus vasculosus nervi optici	Vascular circle of optic nerve
A15.2.04.037	Arteriola temporalis retinae superior	Superior temporal retinal arteriole
A15.2.04.038	Arteriola temporalis retinae inferior	Inferior temporal retinal arteriole
A15.2.04.039	Arteriola nasalis retinae superior	Superior nasal retinal arteriole
A15.2.04.040	Arteriola nasalis retinae inferior	Inferior nasal retinal arteriole
A15.2.04.041	Arteriola macularis superior	Superior macular arteriole
A15.2.04.042	Arteriola macularis inferior	Inferior macular arteriole
A15.2.04.043	Arteriola macularis media	Middle macular arteriole
A12.3.06.113	V. centralis retinae, pars intraocularis	Central retinal vein, intraocular part
A15.2.04.044	Venula temporalis retinae superior	Superior temporal retinal venule
A15.2.04.045	Venula temporalis retinae inferior	Inferior temporal retinal venule
A15.2.04.046	Venula nasalis retinae superior	Superior nasal retinal venule
A15.2.04.047	Venula nasalis retinae inferior	Inferior nasal retinal venule
A15.2.04.048	Venula macularis superior	Superior macular venule
A15.2.04.049	Venula macularis inferior	Inferior macular venule
A15.2.04.050	Venula macularis media	Middle macular venule

A15.2.05.001	**Lens**	**Lens**
A15.2.05.002	Substantia lentis	Lens substance
A15.2.05.003	Cortex lentis	Cortex of lens
A15.2.05.004	Nucleus lentis	Nucleus of lens
A15.2.05.005	Fibrae lentis	Lens fibres▲
A15.2.05.006	Epithelium lentis	Lens epithelium
A15.2.05.007	Capsula lentis	Capsule of lens
A15.2.05.008	Polus anterior	Anterior pole
A15.2.05.009	Polus posterior	Posterior pole
A15.2.05.010	Facies anterior	Anterior surface
A15.2.05.011	Facies posterior	Posterior surface
A15.2.05.012	Axis	Axis
A15.2.05.013	Equator	Equator
A15.2.05.014	Radii	Radii
A15.2.05.015	Zonula ciliaris	Ciliary zonule
A15.2.05.016	Fibrae zonulares	Zonular fibres▲
A15.2.05.017	Spatia zonularia	Zonular spaces

A15.2.06.001	**Camerae bulbi**	**Chambers of eyeball**
A15.2.06.002	Humor aquosus	Aqueous humor
A15.2.06.003	Camera anterior	Anterior chamber
A15.2.06.004	Angulus iridocornealis	Iridocorneal angle
A15.2.06.005	Camera posterior	Posterior chamber
* A15.2.06.006	Camera postrema; Camera vitrea	Postremal chamber; Vitreous chamber
* A15.2.06.007	Spatium retrozonulare	Retrozonular space
A15.2.06.008	Corpus vitreum	Vitreous body
A15.2.06.009	(A. hyaloidea)	(Hyaloid artery)
A15.2.06.010	Canalis hyaloideus	Hyaloid canal
A15.2.06.011	Fossa hyaloidea	Hyaloid fossa
A15.2.06.012	Membrana vitrea	Vitreous membrane
A15.2.06.013	Stroma vitreum	Vitreous stroma
A15.2.06.014	Humor vitreus	Vitreous humor

* **A15.2.06.006** *Camera postrema* This new term is consistent with the terms used for the other chambers of the eye, which are based on their position.

* **A15.2.06.007** *Spatium retrozonulare* This new term describes the part of the *camera postrema* immediately behind the *zonula ciliaris* which contains *humor aquosus* and communicates with the *camera posterior* via the *spatia zonulares*.

A15.2.07.001	STRUCTURAE OCULI ACCESSORIAE	ACCESSORY VISUAL STRUCTURES
A15.2.07.002	Periorbita	Periorbita
A15.2.07.003	Septum orbitale	Orbital septum
A15.2.07.004	Vagina bulbi	Fascial sheath of eyeball
A15.2.07.005	Lig. suspensorium bulbi	Suspensory ligament of eyeball
A15.2.07.006	Spatium episclerale	Episcleral space
A15.2.07.007	Corpus adiposum orbitae	Retrobulbar fat; Orbital fat body
A15.2.07.008	Fasciae musculares	Muscular fascia
A04.1.01.001	**Musculi externi bulbi oculi**	**Extra-ocular muscles; Extrinsic muscles of eyeball**
A15.2.07.009	M. orbitalis	Orbitalis; Orbital muscle
A15.2.07.010	M. rectus superior	Superior rectus
A15.2.07.011	M. rectus inferior	Inferior rectus
A15.2.07.012	M. rectus medialis	Medial rectus
A15.2.07.013	M. rectus lateralis	Lateral rectus
A15.2.07.014	Lacertus musculi recti lateralis	Check ligament of lateral rectus muscle
A15.2.07.015	Anulus tendineus communis	Common tendinous ring; Common anular tendon
A15.2.07.016	M. obliquus superior	Superior oblique
A15.2.07.017	Trochlea	Trochlea
A15.2.07.018	Vagina tendinis musculi obliqui superioris	Tendinous sheath of superior oblique
A15.2.07.019	M. obliquus inferior	Inferior oblique
A15.2.07.020	M. levator palpebrae superioris	Levator palpebrae superioris
A15.2.07.021	Lamina superficialis	Superficial layer
A15.2.07.022	Lamina profunda	Deep layer
A15.2.07.023	**Supercilium**	**Eyebrow**
A15.2.07.024	**Palpebrae**	**Eyelids**
A15.2.07.025	Palpebra superior	Superior eyelid; Upper eyelid
A15.2.07.026	Palpebra inferior	Inferior eyelid; Lower eyelid
A15.2.07.027	Facies anterior palpebrae	Anterior surface of eyelid
A15.2.07.028	Plica palpebronasalis	Palpebronasal fold; Medial canthic fold
A15.2.07.029	Facies posterior palpebrae	Posterior surface of eyelid
A15.2.07.030	Rima palpebrarum	Palpebral fissure
A15.2.07.031	Commissura lateralis palpebrarum	Lateral palpebral commissure
A15.2.07.032	Commissura medialis palpebrarum	Medial palpebral commissure
A15.2.07.033	Angulus oculi lateralis	Lateral angle of eye
A15.2.07.034	Angulus oculi medialis	Medial angle of eye
A15.2.07.035	Limbus anterior palpebrae	Anterior palpebral margin
A15.2.07.036	Limbus posterior palpebrae	Posterior palpebral margin
A15.2.07.037	Cilia	Eyelash
A15.2.07.038	Tarsus superior	Superior tarsus
A15.2.07.039	Tarsus inferior	Inferior tarsus
A15.2.07.040	Lig. palpebrale laterale	Lateral palpebral ligament
A15.2.07.041	Lig. palpebrale mediale	Medial palpebral ligament
A15.2.07.042	Glandulae tarsales	Tarsal glands
A15.2.07.043	Glandulae ciliares	Ciliary glands
A15.2.07.044	Glandulae sebaceae	Sebaceous glands
A15.2.07.045	M. tarsalis superior	Superior tarsal muscle
A15.2.07.046	M. tarsalis inferior	Inferior tarsal muscle
A15.2.07.047	**Tunica conjunctiva**	**Conjunctiva**
A15.2.07.048	Plica semilunaris	Plica semilunaris
A15.2.07.049	Caruncula lacrimalis	Lacrimal caruncle
A15.2.07.050	Tunica conjunctiva bulbi	Bulbar conjunctiva
A15.2.07.051	Tunica conjunctiva palpebrarum	Palpebral conjunctiva
A15.2.07.052	Fornix conjunctivae superior	Superior conjunctival fornix
A15.2.07.053	Fornix conjunctivae inferior	Inferior conjunctival fornix
A15.2.07.054	Saccus conjunctivalis	Conjunctival sac
A15.2.07.055	Glandulae conjunctivales	Conjunctival glands
A15.2.07.056	**Apparatus lacrimalis**	**Lacrimal apparatus**

A15.2.07.057	Glandula lacrimalis	Lacrimal gland
A15.2.07.058	Pars orbitalis	Orbital part
A15.2.07.059	Pars palpebralis	Palpebral part
A15.2.07.060	Ductuli excretorii	Excretory ducts
A15.2.07.061	(Glandulae lacrimales accessoriae)	(Accessory lacrimal glands)
A15.2.07.062	Rivus lacrimalis	Lacrimal pathway
A15.2.07.063	Lacus lacrimalis	Lacus lacrimalis; Lacrimal lake
A15.2.07.064	Papilla lacrimalis	Lacrimal papilla
A15.2.07.065	Punctum lacrimale	Lacrimal punctum
A15.2.07.066	Canaliculus lacrimalis	Lacrimal canaliculus
A15.2.07.067	Ampulla canaliculi lacrimalis	Ampulla of lacrimal canaliculus
A15.2.07.068	Saccus lacrimalis	Lacrimal sac
A15.2.07.069	Fornix sacci lacrimalis	Fornix of lacrimal sac
A15.2.07.070	Ductus nasolacrimalis	Nasolacrimal duct
A15.2.07.071	Plica lacrimalis	Lacrimal fold

A15.3.00.001	Auris	Ear
A15.3.01.001	AURIS EXTERNA	EXTERNAL EAR
A15.3.01.002	**Auricula**	**Auricle; Pinna**
A15.3.01.003	Lobulus auriculae	Lobule of auricle; Lobe of ear
A15.3.01.004	Cartilago auriculae	Auricular cartilage
A15.3.01.005	Helix	Helix
A15.3.01.006	Crus helicis	Crus of helix
A15.3.01.007	Spina helicis	Spine of helix
A15.3.01.008	Cauda helicis	Tail of helix
A15.3.01.009	Antihelix	Antihelix
A15.3.01.010	Fossa triangularis	Triangular fossa
A15.3.01.011	Crura antihelicis	Crura of antihelix
A15.3.01.012	Scapha	Scapha
A15.3.01.013	Concha auriculae	Concha of auricle
A15.3.01.014	Cymba conchae	Cymba conchae
A15.3.01.015	Cavitas conchae; Cavum conchae	Cavity of concha
A15.3.01.016	Antitragus	Antitragus
A15.3.01.017	Tragus	Tragus
A15.3.01.018	Incisura anterior	Anterior notch
A15.3.01.019	Incisura intertragica	Intertragic incisure; Intertragic notch
A15.3.01.020	(Tuberculum auriculare)	(Auricular tubercle)
A15.3.01.021	(Apex auriculae)	(Apex of auricle; Tip of ear)
A15.3.01.022	Sulcus posterior auriculae	Posterior auricular groove
A15.3.01.023	(Tuberculum supratragicum)	(Supratragic tubercle)
A15.3.01.024	Isthmus cartilaginis auricularis	Isthmus of cartilaginous auricle
A15.3.01.025	Incisura terminalis auricularis	Terminal notch of auricle
A15.3.01.026	Fissura antitragohelicina	Fissura antitragohelicina
A15.3.01.027	Sulcus cruris helicis	Groove of crus of helix
A15.3.01.028	Fossa antihelica	Fossa antihelica; Antihelical fossa
A15.3.01.029	Eminentia conchae	Eminentia conchae
A15.3.01.030	Eminentia scaphae	Eminentia scaphae
A15.3.01.031	Eminentia fossae triangularis	Eminentia fossae triangularis
A15.3.01.032	**Ligg. auricularia**	**Ligaments of auricle**
A15.3.01.033	Lig. auriculare anterius	Anterior ligament of auricle
A15.3.01.034	Lig. auriculare superius	Superior ligament of auricle
A15.3.01.035	Lig. auriculare posterius	Posterior ligament of auricle
A15.3.01.036	**Mm. auriculares**	**Auricular muscles**
A15.3.01.037	M. helicis major	Helicis major
A15.3.01.038	M. helicis minor	Helicis minor
A15.3.01.039	M. tragicus	Tragicus
A15.3.01.040	(M. incisurae terminalis)	(Muscle of terminal notch)
A15.3.01.041	M. pyramidalis auriculae	Pyramidal muscle of auricle

A15.3.01.042	M. antitragicus	Antitragicus
A15.3.01.043	M. transversus auriculae	Transverse muscle of auricle
A15.3.01.044	M. obliquus auriculae	Oblique muscle of auricle
A15.3.01.045	**Meatus acusticus externus**	**External acoustic meatus**
A15.3.01.046	Porus acusticus externus	External acoustic pore; External acoustic aperture
A15.3.01.047	Incisura tympanica	Tympanic notch
A15.3.01.048	Meatus acusticus externus cartilagineus	Cartilaginous external acoustic meatus
A15.3.01.049	Cartilago meatus acustici	Cartilage of acoustic meatus
A15.3.01.050	Incisura cartilaginis meatus acustici	Notch in cartilage of acoustic meatus
A15.3.01.051	Lamina tragi	Tragal lamina
A15.3.01.052	**Membrana tympanica**	**Tympanic membrane**
A15.3.01.053	Pars flaccida	Pars flaccida
A15.3.01.054	Pars tensa	Pars tensa
A15.3.01.055	Plica mallearis anterior	Anterior malleolar fold
A15.3.01.056	Plica mallearis posterior	Posterior malleolar fold
A15.3.01.057	Prominentia mallearis	Malleolar prominence
A15.3.01.058	Stria mallearis	Malleolar stria
A15.3.01.059	Umbo membranae tympanicae	Umbo of tympanic membrane
A15.3.01.060	Anulus fibrocartilagineus	Fibrocartilaginous ring

A15.3.02.001	**AURIS MEDIA**	**MIDDLE EAR**
A15.3.02.002	**Cavitas tympani**	**Tympanic cavity**
A15.3.02.003	Paries tegmentalis	Tegmental wall; Tegmental roof
A15.3.02.004	Recessus epitympanicus	Epitympanic recess
A15.3.02.005	Pars cupularis	Cupular part
A15.3.02.006	Paries jugularis	Jugular wall; Floor
A15.3.02.007	Prominentia styloidea	Styloid prominence
A15.3.02.008	Paries labyrinthicus	Labyrinthine wall; Medial wall
A15.3.02.009	Fenestra vestibuli	Oval window
A15.3.02.010	Fossula fenestrae vestibuli	Fossa of oval window
A15.3.02.011	Promontorium	Promontory
A15.3.02.012	Sulcus promontorii	Groove of promontory
A15.3.02.013	Subiculum promontorii	Subiculum of promontory
A15.3.02.014	Sinus tympani	Sinus tympani
A15.3.02.015	Fenestra cochleae	Round window
A15.3.02.016	Fossula fenestrae cochleae	Fossa of round window
A15.3.02.017	Crista fenestrae cochleae	Crest of round window
A15.3.02.018	Processus cochleariformis	Processus cochleariformis
A15.3.02.019	Membrana tympanica secundaria	Secondary tympanic membrane
A15.3.02.020	Paries mastoideus	Mastoid wall; Posterior wall
A15.3.02.021	Aditus ad antrum mastoideum	Aditus to mastoid antrum
A15.3.02.022	Prominentia canalis semicircularis lateralis	Prominence of lateral semicircular canal
A15.3.02.023	Prominentia canalis facialis	Prominence of facial canal
A15.3.02.024	Eminentia pyramidalis	Pyramidal eminence
A15.3.02.025	Fossa incudis	Fossa of incus
A15.3.02.026	Sinus posterior	Posterior sinus
A15.3.02.027	Apertura tympanica canaliculi chordae tympani	Tympanic aperture of canaliculus for chorda tympani
A15.3.02.028	Antrum mastoideum	Mastoid antrum
A15.3.02.029	Cellulae mastoideae	Mastoid cells
A15.3.02.030	Cellulae tympanicae	Tympanic cells
A15.3.02.031	Paries caroticus	Carotid wall
A15.3.02.032	Paries membranaceus	Membranous wall; Lateral wall

A02.1.17.001	**Ossicula auditus; Ossicula auditoria**	**Auditory ossicles**
A15.3.02.033	**Stapes**	**Stapes**
A15.3.02.034	Caput stapedis	Head of stapes

A15.3.02.035	Crus anterius	Anterior limb
A15.3.02.036	Crus posterius	Posterior limb
A15.3.02.037	Basis stapedis	Base of stapes; Footplate
A15.3.02.038	**Incus**	**Incus**
A15.3.02.039	Corpus incudis	Body of incus
A15.3.02.040	Crus longum	Long limb
A15.3.02.041	Processus lenticularis	Lenticular process
A15.3.02.042	Crus breve	Short limb
A15.3.02.043	**Malleus**	**Malleus**
A15.3.02.044	Manubrium mallei	Handle of malleus
A15.3.02.045	Caput mallei	Head of malleus
A15.3.02.046	Collum mallei	Neck of malleus
A15.3.02.047	Processus lateralis	Lateral process
A15.3.02.048	Processus anterior	Anterior process

A15.3.02.049	Articulationes ossiculorum auditus; Articulationes ossiculorum auditoriorum	Articulations of auditory ossicles
A15.3.02.050	Articulatio incudomallearis	Incudomallear joint
A15.3.02.051	Articulatio incudostapedialis	Incudostapedial joint
A15.3.02.052	Syndesmosis tympanostapedialis	Tympanostapedial syndesmosis
A15.3.02.053	**Ligg. ossiculorum auditus; Ligg. ossiculorum auditoriorum**	**Ligaments of auditory ossicles**
A15.3.02.054	Lig. mallei anterius	Anterior ligament of malleus
A15.3.02.055	Lig. mallei superius	Superior ligament of malleus
A15.3.02.056	Lig. mallei laterale	Lateral ligament of malleus
A15.3.02.057	Lig. incudis superius	Superior ligament of incus
A15.3.02.058	Lig. incudis posterius	Posterior ligament of incus
A15.3.02.059	Membrana stapedialis	Stapedial membrane
A15.3.02.060	Lig. anulare stapediale	Anular ligament of stapes

A04.1.02.001	Musculi ossiculorum auditus; Musculi ossiculorum auditoriorum	Muscles of auditory ossicles
A15.3.02.061	M. tensor tympani	Tensor tympani
A15.3.02.062	M. stapedius	Stapedius
A15.3.02.063	**Tunica mucosa cavitatis tympanicae**	**Mucosa of tympanic cavity**
A15.3.02.064	Plica mallearis posterior	Posterior fold of malleus
A15.3.02.065	Plica mallearis anterior	Anterior fold of malleus
A15.3.02.066	Plica chordae tympani	Fold of chorda tympani
A15.3.02.067	Recessus membranae tympanicae	Recesses of tympanic membrane
A15.3.02.068	Recessus anterior	Anterior recess
A15.3.02.069	Recessus superior	Superior recess
A15.3.02.070	Recessus posterior	Posterior recess
A15.3.02.071	Plica incudialis	Fold of incus
A15.3.02.072	Plica stapedialis	Fold of stapedius

A15.3.02.073	Tuba auditiva; Tuba auditoria	Pharyngotympanic tube; Auditory tube
A15.3.02.074	Ostium tympanicum tubae auditivae; Ostium tympanicum tubae auditoriae	Tympanic opening
A15.3.02.075	**Pars ossea**	**Bony part**
A15.3.02.076	Isthmus tubae auditivae; Isthmus tubae auditoriae	Isthmus
A15.3.02.077	Cellulae pneumaticae	Tubal air cells
A15.3.02.078	**Pars cartilaginea**	**Cartilaginous part**
A15.3.02.079	Cartilago tubae auditivae; Cartilago tubae auditoriae	Cartilage of tube
A15.3.02.080	Lamina medialis	Medial lamina
A15.3.02.081	Lamina lateralis	Lateral lamina
A15.3.02.082	Lamina membranacea	Membranous lamina

A15.3.02.083	Tunica mucosa	Mucosa; Mucous membrane
A15.3.02.084	Glandulae tubariae	Tubal glands
A15.3.02.085	Ostium pharyngeum tubae auditivae; Ostium pharyngeum tubae auditoriae	Pharyngeal opening

A15.3.03.001	AURIS INTERNA	INTERNAL EAR
A15.3.03.002	Organum vestibulocochleare	Vestibulocochlear organ

A15.3.03.003	**Labyrinthus osseus**	**Bony labyrinth**
A15.3.03.004	Vestibulum	Vestibule
A15.3.03.005	Recessus ellipticus; Recessus utricularis	Elliptical recess; Utricular recess
A15.3.03.006	Apertura interna canaliculi vestibuli	Internal opening of vestibular canaliculus
A15.3.03.007	Crista vestibuli	Vestibular crest
A15.3.03.008	Pyramis vestibuli	Pyramid of vestibule
A15.3.03.009	Recessus sphericus; Recessus saccularis	Spherical recess; Saccular recess
A15.3.03.010	Recessus cochlearis	Cochlear recess
A15.3.03.011	Maculae cribrosae	Maculae cribrosae
A15.3.03.012	Macula cribrosa superior	Macula cribrosa superior
A15.3.03.013	Macula cribrosa media	Macula cribrosa media
A15.3.03.014	Macula cribrosa inferior	Macula cribrosa inferior
A15.3.03.015	**Canales semicirculares**	**Semicircular canals**
A15.3.03.016	Canalis semicircularis anterior	Anterior semicircular canal
A15.3.03.017	Ampulla ossea anterior	Anterior bony ampulla
A15.3.03.018	Canalis semicircularis posterior	Posterior semicircular canal
A15.3.03.019	Ampulla ossea posterior	Posterior bony ampulla
A15.3.03.020	Crus osseum commune	Common bony limb
A15.3.03.021	Crura ossea ampullaria	Ampullary bony limbs
A15.3.03.022	Canalis semicircularis lateralis	Lateral semicircular canal
A15.3.03.023	Ampulla ossea lateralis	Lateral bony ampulla
A15.3.03.024	Crus osseum simplex	Simple bony limb
A15.3.03.025	**Cochlea**	**Cochlea**
A15.3.03.026	Cupula cochleae	Cochlear cupula
A15.3.03.027	Basis cochleae	Base of cochlea
A15.3.03.028	Canalis spiralis cochleae	Spiral canal of cochlea
A15.3.03.029	Lamina spiralis ossea	Osseous spiral lamina
A15.3.03.031	Lamella vestibularis	Vestibular lamella
A15.3.03.032	Lamella tympanica	Tympanic lamella
A15.3.03.033	Foramina nervosa	Foramina nervosa
A15.3.03.034	Hamulus laminae spiralis	Hamulus of spiral lamina
A15.3.03.035	Lamina spiralis secundaria	Secondary spiral lamina
A15.3.03.036	Apertura interna canaliculi cochleae	Internal opening of cochlear canaliculus
A15.3.03.037	Septum cochleae	Cochlear septum
A15.3.03.038	Modiolus cochleae	Modiolus
A15.3.03.039	Basis modioli	Base of modiolus
A15.3.03.040	Lamina modioli	Lamina of modiolus
A15.3.03.041	Canalis spiralis modioli	Spiral canal of modiolus
A15.3.03.042	Canales longitudinales modioli	Longitudinal canals of modiolus
A15.3.03.043	Scala vestibuli	Scala vestibuli
A15.3.03.044	Helicotrema	Helicotrema
A15.3.03.045	Scala tympani	Scala tympani
A02.1.06.033	**Meatus acusticus internus**	**Internal acoustic meatus**
A02.1.06.032	Porus acusticus internus	Internal acoustic opening
A15.3.03.046	Fundus meatus acustici interni	Fundus of internal acoustic meatus
A15.3.03.047	Crista transversa	Transverse crest
A15.3.03.048	Area nervi facialis	Facial area
A15.3.03.049	Crista verticalis	Vertical crest
A15.3.03.050	Area vestibularis superior	Superior vestibular area
A15.3.03.051	Area vestibularis inferior	Inferior vestibular area

A15.3.03.052	Foramen singulare	Foramen singulare
A15.3.03.053	Area cochlearis; Area cochleae	Cochlear area
A15.3.03.054	Tractus spiralis foraminosus	Tractus spiralis foraminosus
A15.3.03.055	**Spatium perilymphaticum**	**Perilymphatic space**
A15.3.03.056	Perilympha	Perilymph
A15.3.03.057	Aqueductus vestibuli	Vestibular aqueduct
A15.3.03.058	Aqueductus cochleae	Cochlear aqueduct

A15.3.03.059	**Labyrinthus membranaceus**	**Membranous labyrinth**
A15.3.03.060	Spatium endolymphaticum	Endolymphatic space
A15.3.03.061	Endolympha	Endolymph

A15.3.03.062	**Labyrinthus vestibularis**	**Vestibular labyrinth**
A15.3.03.063	**Utriculus**	**Utricle**
A15.3.03.064	Recessus utricularis; Recessus utriculi	Utricular recess
A15.3.03.065	**Sacculus**	**Saccule**
A15.3.03.066	**Ductus semicirculares**	**Semicircular ducts**
A15.3.03.067	Ductus semicircularis anterior	Anterior semicircular duct
A15.3.03.068	Ampulla membranacea anterior	Anterior membranous ampulla
A15.3.03.069	Ductus semicircularis posterior	Posterior semicircular duct
A15.3.03.070	Ampulla membranacea posterior	Posterior membranous ampulla
A15.3.03.071	Crus membranaceum commune	Common membranous limb
A15.3.03.072	Crura membranacea ampullaria	Ampullary membranous limbs
A15.3.03.073	Ductus semicircularis lateralis	Lateral semicircular duct
A15.3.03.074	Ampulla membranacea lateralis	Lateral membranous ampulla
A15.3.03.075	Crus membranaceum simplex	Simple membranous limb
A15.3.03.076	**Ductus utriculosaccularis**	**Utriculosaccular duct**
A15.3.03.077	Ductus utricularis	Utricular duct
A15.3.03.078	Ductus saccularis	Saccular duct
A15.3.03.079	**Ductus endolymphaticus**	**Endolymphatic duct**
A15.3.03.080	Saccus endolymphaticus	Endolymphatic sac
A15.3.03.081	Ductus reuniens	Ductus reuniens
A15.3.03.082	Maculae	Maculae
A15.3.03.083	Macula utriculi	Macula of utricle
A15.3.03.084	Macula sacculi	Macula of saccule
A15.3.03.085	Membrana statoconiorum	Otolithic membrane
A15.3.03.086	Statoconium	Otolith
A15.3.03.087	Striola	Striola
A15.3.03.088	Crista ampullaris	Ampullary crest
A15.3.03.089	Sulcus ampullaris	Ampullary groove
A15.3.03.090	Cupula ampullaris	Ampullary cupula

A15.3.03.091	**Labyrinthus cochlearis**	**Cochlear labyrinth**
A15.3.03.092	Scala media	Scala media
A15.3.03.093	**Ductus cochlearis**	**Cochlear duct**
A15.3.03.094	Paries vestibularis; Membrana vestibularis	Vestibular surface; Vestibular membrane
A15.3.03.095	Paries externus	External surface
A15.3.03.096	Stria vascularis	Stria vascularis
A15.3.03.097	Prominentia spiralis	Spiral prominence
A15.3.03.098	Vas prominens	Vas prominens
A15.3.03.099	Ligamentum spirale	Spiral ligament
A15.3.03.100	Paries tympanicus; Membrana spiralis	Tympanic surface; Spiral membrane
A15.3.03.101	Crista basilaris; Crista spiralis	Basal crest; Spiral crest
A15.3.03.102	Lamina basilaris	Basal lamina
A15.3.03.103	Vas spirale	Vas spirale
A15.3.03.104	Limbus spiralis	Spiral limbus
A15.3.03.105	Labium limbi tympanicum	Tympanic lip

A15.3.03.106	Labium limbi vestibulare	Vestibular lip
A15.3.03.107	Dentes acustici	Acoustic teeth
A15.3.03.108	Membrana tectoria	Tectorial membrane
A15.3.03.109	Caecum vestibulare	Vestibular caecum▲
A15.3.03.120	Caecum cupulare	Cupular caecum▲
A15.3.03.121	Organum spirale	Spiral organ
A15.3.03.122	Membrana reticularis	Reticular membrane
A15.3.03.123	Sulcus spiralis internus	Inner spiral sulcus
A15.3.03.124	Sulcus spiralis externus	Outer spiral sulcus
A15.3.03.125	Ganglion spirale cochleae	Spiral ganglion
A15.3.03.126	**Vasa sanguinea auris internae**	**Vessels of internal ear**
A12.2.08.020	A. labyrinthi	Labyrinthine arteries
A15.3.03.127	A. vestibularis anterior; A. vestibuli	Anterior vestibular artery
A15.3.03.128	A. cochlearis communis	Common cochlear artery
A15.3.03.129	A. vestibulocochlearis	Vestibulocochlear artery
A15.3.03.130	R. vestibularis posterior	Posterior vestibular branch
A15.3.03.131	R. cochlearis	Cochlear branch
A15.3.03.132	A. cochlearis propria	Proper cochlear artery
A15.3.03.133	A. spiralis modioli	Spiral modiolar artery
A15.3.03.134	V. aqueductus vestibuli	Vein of vestibular aqueduct
A15.3.03.135	Vv. ductuum semicircularium	Veins of semicircular ducts
A15.3.03.136	V. aqueductus cochleae	Vein of cochlear aqueduct
A15.3.03.137	V. modioli communis	Common modiolar vein
A15.3.03.138	V. scalae vestibuli	Vein of scala vestibuli
A15.3.03.139	V. scalae tympani	Vein of scala tympani
A15.3.03.140	V. vestibulocochlearis	Vestibulocochlear vein
A15.3.03.141	V. vestibularis anterior	Anterior vestibular vein
A15.3.03.142	V. vestibularis posterior	Posterior vestibular vein
A15.3.03.143	V. fenestrae cochleae	Vein of cochlear window
A12.3.05.114	Vv. labyrinthi	Labyrinthine veins

A15.4.00.001	Organum gustatorium; Organum gustus	Gustatory organ
A15.4.00.002	Caliculus gustatorius; Gemma gustatoria	Taste bud
A15.4.00.003	Porus gustatorius	Taste pore

A16.0.00.001	**Integumentum commune**	**The integument**
A16.0.00.002	**Cutis**	**Skin**
A16.0.00.003	Sulci cutis	Skin sulci
A16.0.00.004	Cristae cutis	Dermal ridges; Papillary ridges
A16.0.00.005	Retinacula cutis	Skin ligaments
A16.0.00.006	Retinaculum caudale	Retinaculum caudale
A16.0.00.007	Toruli tactiles	Tactile elevations
A16.0.00.008	Lineae distractiones	Tension lines; Cleavage lines
A16.0.00.009	**Epidermis**	**Epidermis**
A16.0.00.010	**Dermis; Corium**	**Dermis; Corium**
A16.0.00.011	Stratum papillare	Papillary layer
A16.0.00.012	Papillae	Papillae
A16.0.00.013	Stratum reticulare	Reticular layer
A16.0.00.014	Pili	Hairs
A16.0.00.015	Lanugo	Downy hair; Primary hair
A16.0.00.016	Capilli	Hairs of head
A16.0.00.017	Supercilia	Eyebrows
A15.2.07.037	Cilia	Eyelashes
A16.0.00.018	Barba	Beard
A16.0.00.019	Tragi	Hairs of tragus
A16.0.00.020	Vibrissae	Hairs of vestibule of nose
A16.0.00.021	Hirci	Axillary hairs
A16.0.00.022	Pubes	Pubic hairs
A16.0.00.023	Folliculus pili	Hair follicle
A16.0.00.024	M. arrector pili	Arrector muscle of hair
A16.0.00.025	Flumina pilorum	Hair streams
A16.0.00.026	Vortices pilorum	Hair whorls
A16.0.00.027	Cruces pilorum	Hair crosses
A16.0.00.028	Glandulae cutis	Skin glands
A16.0.00.029	Glandula sudorifera	Sweat gland
A16.0.00.030	Glandula sebacea	Sebaceous gland
A16.0.00.031	Terminationes nervorum	Nerve terminals
A16.0.01.001	**Unguis**	**Nail**
A16.0.01.002	Matrix unguis	Nail matrix
A16.0.01.003	Vallum unguis	Nail wall
A16.0.01.004	Corpus unguis	Body of nail
A16.0.01.005	Lunula	Lunule
A16.0.01.006	Margo occultus	Hidden border
A16.0.01.007	Margo lateralis	Lateral border
A16.0.01.008	Margo liber	Free border
A16.0.01.009	Perionyx	Perionyx
A16.0.01.010	Eponychium	Eponychium
A16.0.01.011	Hyponychium	Hyponychium
* A16.0.02.001	**Mamma**	**Breast**
A16.0.02.002	Sulcus intermammarius	Intermammary cleft
A16.0.02.003	(Mamma accessoria)	(Accessory breast)
A16.0.02.004	Papilla mammaria	Nipple
A16.0.02.005	Corpus mammae	Body of breast
A16.0.02.006	Glandula mammaria	Mammary gland
A16.0.02.007	Processus axillaris; Processus lateralis	Axillary process; Axillary tail
A16.0.02.008	Lobi glandulae mammariae	Lobes of mammary gland
A16.0.02.009	Lobuli glandulae mammariae	Lobules of mammary gland
A16.0.02.010	Ductus lactiferi	Lactiferous duct
A16.0.02.011	Sinus lactiferi	Lactiferous sinus
A16.0.02.012	Areola mammae	Areola

* **A16.0.02.001** *Mamma* The separate term *mamma masculina* has been omitted because the breast in the male contains no unique elements but those of the female breast developed to a lesser extent.

A16.0.02.013	Glandulae areolares	Areolar glands
A16.0.02.014	Tubercula areolae	Areolar tubercles
A16.0.02.015	Ligg. suspensoria mammaria; Retinaculum cutis mammae	Suspensory ligaments of breast; Suspensory retinaculum of breast

* **A16.0.03.001**	**Tela subcutanea; Hypodermis**	**Subcutaneous tissue**
A16.0.03.002	Panniculus adiposus	Fatty layer
A16.0.03.003	Stratum musculosum	Muscle layer
A16.0.03.004	Stratum fibrosum	Fibrous layer
A16.0.03.005	Stratum membranosum	Membranous layer
A16.0.03.006	Textus connectivus laxus	Loose connective tissue

* **A16.0.03.001** *Tela subcutanea* None of the layers of subcutaneous tissue is present throughout the body. The fatty layer is most widely present. At some sites a layer of skin muscles may be found in it. Where it is thick, it has a membranous layer on its deep surface and may be lamellated by one or more fibrous layers within it. It is absent from the eyelids, the clitoris/penis and much of the pinna and is represented only by its muscular layer in the scrotum.

History of International Anatomical Terminology

After centuries of accumulating terms to name parts of the human body, in addition to those of other animals, a group of anatomists led by internationally renowned German-speaking morphologists, including specialists in macroscopical structures, embryologists and histologists, prepared a list of names to serve as a worldwide official standard vocabulary for all health sciences. The list that appeared in 1895 became known as the *Basle Nomina Anatomica* (BNA). Such a "standard Latin anatomical nomenclature was introduced and adopted in many countries and to a large extent dispelled the confusion existing up till that time" (WOERDEMAN, 1957)[1]. In actual fact, the revision of modern anatomical terminology had been initiated in Leipzig, Germany, in 1887 and continued in the United Kingdom in 1894.

Under the leadership of HIS, the *Basle Nomina Anatomica* was published in Latin in 1895 after its unanimous approval at the IX Congress of the Anatomische Gesellschaft in Basel, Switzerland, on April 19 1895. Unfortunately it failed to be adopted worldwide because it was used only by German-speaking, Italian, US and Latin American Anatomists (BEAU, 1955)[2].

This was the first international attempt to offer a basis for universal agreement on the use of terms related to the human body, both for anatomy and the other health sciences. The adoption of the same terminology would eliminate national differences that were causing extreme confusion because the same structure was known by several names. Compounding the confusion, the anatomical terms sometimes included the name of one or more scientists to honour those who had first described, drawn attention to, demonstrated the meaning of, or correctly interpreted a particular structure.

In 1903 NICOLAS, from Nancy, France, was successful in founding the International Federation of Associations of Anatomists whose members would use the same language for communication purposes. The vocabulary for such a language would contain a list of Latin terms to be translated into the vernacular of each nation. Each term would correspond to just one anatomical structure. In other words, one of the Federation's original, and primary, objectives was the selection of a uniform nomenclature for the anatomical sciences that would be universally adopted.

In 1905 in Geneva, Switzerland, during the I Federative International Congress of Anatomy, presided over by D'ETERNOD, a resolution was approved to review the BNA (1895). In so doing, the Federation was taking a major step towards achieving its first main goal of obtaining a general agreement for the adoption of a uniform and simplified anatomical terminology. In 1910 in Brussels, under the presidency of WALDEYER, the II Federative International Congress of Anatomy was held. Its principal topic of discussion was the nomenclature, and a committee to reform the terminology of embryology was created. Two decades later during the III Federative International Congress of Anatomy, held in Amsterdam, The Netherlands, and presided over by Van den BROEK, no progress occurred in terminological issues for either anatomy or embryology.

In 1933 (according to WOERDEMAN, 1957), the Anatomical Society of Great Britain and Ireland updated the BNA, presenting the *Birmingham Revision* (BR), and the Anatomische Gesellschaft did the same in 1935, presenting the *Jenaer* or *Jenenser Nomina Anatomica* (JNA) (reported by STIEVE, 1939)[3]. Though both versions were excellent neither was universally adopted. In fact, American and Japanese anatomists had drawn up their own lists causing confusion to recur.

The IV Federative International Congress of Anatomy took place in 1936 in Milan, Italy, under the presidency of LIVINI. During this meeting, the selection of a single list of terms was attempted but no general agreement was reached. A new International Anatomical Nomenclature Com-

1 WOERDEMAN, M. W. 1957. *Nomina Anatomica Parisiensia (1955) et BNA (1895)*. Utrecht: A. Oosthoek Publ. Co.

2 BEAU, A. 1955. *Nomina Anatomica*. Revisés par le Comité International de la Nomenclature Anatomique designé lors du Cinquième Congrés International d'Anatomie réuni à Oxford en 1950. London and Colchester: Spottiswoode, Ballantyne et Cie., S.A.R.L.

3 STIEVE, H. 1939. *Nomina Anatomica*. Zusammengestellt von der im Jahre 1923 gewählten Nomenklatur-Kommission, unter Berücksichtigung der Vorschläge der Mitglieder der Anatomischen Gesellschaft, der Anatomical Society of Great Britain and Ireland, sowie der American Association of Anatomists, durch Beschluss der Anatomischen Gesellschaft auf der Tagung in Jena 1935 endgültig angenommen. Zweite, verbesserte und erweiterte Auflage. Jena: Verlag G. Fischer.

mittee was appointed but it was unable to prepare a list of terms that could be accepted universally since meetings could not take place because of the War (1939 to 1945).

When the V Federative International Congress of Anatomy was held in Oxford, England, in 1950 the question of an official list of anatomical terms was again discussed. The Federative Congress directed its President, LE GROS CLARK, to appoint a new international committee, to include three representatives of each country attending the Congress, and to invite each anatomical association or society to elect their own representatives. The British representative, JOHNSTON, was asked to convene the meetings of the Committee, the first of which took place in 1952 in London, after he had persuaded the Brazilian Society of Anatomy to wait for the report to be presented in Paris before proceeding with its own version. The main task of the Committee, according to the decision of the Oxford Federative International Congress, was to prepare a list of anatomical terms to be submitted to the subsequent Congress, scheduled to be held in Paris in 1955.

Thanks to a grant awarded by the Council for International Organizations of Medical Sciences (CIOMS), a meeting of the members of the Nomenclature Committee was held in London on May 26 to 30 1952, during which CORNER was elected chairman and JOHNSTON Honorary Secretary. Since a further meeting was necessary, the United Nations Educational, Scientific, and Cultural Organization (UNESCO), at the request of its branch the CIOMS, provided the necessary funds for holding one in London in April 1954.

The first deliberation of the Nomenclature Committee was to use the BNA (1895) as a basis for discussions, because the JNA (1936) had included a few changes that were considered too drastic and had abandoned the orthostatic attitude as the standard position of the human body for anatomical description. Several principles, almost identical to those of the BNA, were adopted unanimously. The Committee, faced with different views expressed by its members, made recommendations, only supported by the majority, such as the acceptance of the erect posture as the official position for anatomic descriptive purposes, and the use of the adjectives ventralis and dorsalis (both used for spinal nerve roots), and cranialis and caudalis, used in exceptional cases and restricted to the human trunk. The Committee then prepared a final report to be submitted to the VI Federative International Congress of Anatomy, scheduled for 1955 in Paris. A subsequent meeting of the Nomenclature Committee, already split into subcommittees, was held in London from May 31 to June 5 1954. It was to review all the recommendations concerning seven sections: (1) osteology, (2) syndesmology, Myology, and Bursae, (3) splanchnology, (4) angiology, (5) central nervous system, (6) peripheral nervous system, (7) organs of the senses and the common integument. The first final report was primarily a list of terms for macroscopic anatomy, including ontogenetic terms and a number of terms on microscopic anatomy that were contained in the BNA. In the introduction of *Nomina Anatomica*, published in 1956 by The Williams and Wilkins Co., Baltimore, USA, it is stated that "The members of the Committee were anxious to submit the final results of their deliberations to the Congress of Anatomists to be held in Paris in the Summer of 1955".

The VI Federative International Congress of Anatomy was held, as planned, in Paris, under the presidency of COLLIN, and the *Parisiensia Nomina Anatomica* (later known as the *Nomina Anatomica*), a conservative revision of the BNA, was unanimously approved by the participants on July 24 1955.[4]

The *Nomina Anatomica* had been revised by the International Anatomical Nomenclature Committee (IANC), appointed by the V Federative International Congress of Anatomy (Oxford, 1950), and included special features such as: (1) the names of structures discovered since the publication of the BNA list (1354 names), (2) the anatomicosurgical segments of the lungs, their bronchi and vessels, based on publications by CHEVALIER-JACKSON, HUBER, and BOYDEN, and on the work of the International Committee of Thoracic Surgeons, (3) the group of endocrine organs, and (4) no eponyms, the grand total reaching 5640 terms (4286 being unchanged BNA terms).

At the request of the committee membership, CORNER, chairman of the IANC, submitted a resolution to set up a permanent "Anatomical Nomenclature Committee to consider proposed additions and alterations to this list of terms, with authority to insert such additions and alterations as met with its approval, subject to confirmation by the next ensuing International Congress of Anatomists". The resolution was unanimously approved by the participants of the VI Federative International Congress of Anatomy (1955). At the VII Federative International Congress of Anatomy, held in 1960 in New York, USA, under the presi-

4 Since this was the first congress attended by the author of this report, the subsequent information was personally obtained.

dency of Bennett, the Nomenclature Committee, chaired by Corner, decided to continue updating the anatomical terminology.

It was agreed that sub-committees should be constituted to prepare *Nomina Embryologica* and *Nomina Histologica* in order to cover and provide uniformity to all biomorphological sciences. During this meeting Woerdeman was elected chairman of the Nomenclature Committee to succeed Corner, who had requested to be relieved from the chairmanship. In 1961 the second edition of *Nomina Anatomica* was published, followed by a reprint (erroneously indicated as the third edition) in 1963.

On August 9 1965, during the VIII Federative International Congress of Anatomy, which took place in Wiesbaden, Germany, under the presidency of Bargmann, the meeting of the IANC was presided over by Starck. For the first time the meeting of the Nomenclature Committee welcomed as observers a number of veterinary anatomists, who were already discussing veterinary anatomical terminology. At the time, the hope was expressed that a close relationship could be established with international committees on veterinary anatomical, embryological and histological nomenclatures. Such initial exchange resulted in further rapprochement between the committees, which led to the inclusion in the human Anatomical Nomenclature Committee of members of the veterinary counterpart (Barone, Baumel, Weber, Evans and Hullinger) and vice versa (Di Dio), a link that lasted several years.

At the same meeting Woerdeman resigned from the chairmanship and was succeeded by Bargmann, who was elected by unanimous vote. Alongside several recommendations and amendments, the use of Latin for all terms was approved. In addition, approval was granted for the inclusion of the names of the anatomicosurgical segments of the liver and of the kidney because the stage had been reached where the segments of both organs needed official sanction, previously only awarded to the segments of the lung. The future of the IANC and its subcommittees was discussed and it was decided by unanimous vote that the subcommittees on Embryology and Histology should retain their close association with the parent Federative Committee as all had essential work to do.

In order to obtain financial support for the activities of the Committee, primarily with regard to communication involving membership, an annual subvention from all the anatomical societies, based on US$ 0.25 per capita or the equivalent thereof in other currencies, was unanimously approved. Such a contribution was expected to attract additional support from UNESCO, the National Institutes of Health (NIH) of the USA and other agencies or foundations. A subcommittee on Finance was proposed (Di Dio), unanimously approved and its members selected: Zwemer (USA convener), Tuchmann-Duplessis (France) and Bachmann (Germany). Arey (USA) was elected convener of the sub-committee on Embryology, and Eliseev (USSR) was elected convener of the subcommittee on Histology.

In 1966 the third edition of *Nomina Anatomica* appeared and in 1968 a reprint was published, with an index, by the Excerpta Medica Foundation. The list of terms had been prepared by the Nomenclature Committee, appointed by the V Federative International Congress of Anatomy (Oxford, 1950), and approved at the VI Congress (Paris, 1955). It included revisions approved at the VII Congress (New York, 1960) and VIII Congress (Wiesbaden, 1965).

In 1968 the subcommittee on Embryology held a meeting in London, hosted by the Ciba Foundation, to finalize a provisional list of terms. In 1969 the subcommittee on Histology met in Moscow, sponsored by the Ministry of Public Health of the USSR.

During the IX Federative International Congress of Anatomy, held in Leningrad in 1970, and presided over by Jdanov, provisional lists of both *Nomina Embryologica* and *Nomina Histologica* were distributed to the participants. The meeting of the IANC was attended by representatives of the already official International Committees on Veterinary Anatomical Nomenclature and Avian Anatomical Nomenclature; the aim was to publish a list of consistent terms. The main decision was taken to publish as one volume the *Nominae Anatomica, Embryologica et Histologica*, corresponding to a *Nomenclature of Human Biomorphological Sciences*. When Bargmann resigned from the Chairmanship of the Nomenclature Committee, Mitchell was elected as his successor.

At the X Federative International Congress of Anatomy, held in Tokyo, Japan, in 1975, under the presidency of Nakayama, the Nomenclature Committee met and approved the lists of *Nominae Anatomica, Embryologica et Histologica*. At this meeting Arey was elected to succeed Mitchell. In 1977 the fourth edition of *Nomina Anatomica* with *Nomina Embryologica and Nomina Histologica* was published by Excerpta Medica, Amsterdam, Oxford.

On August 1 to 5 1979, the IV International Symposium on the Morphological Sciences in Toledo, Ohio, USA, presided over by Di Dio, sponsored a special meeting of the IANC. For the first time the Committee and all subcommittees met simultaneously on the same site. Accepting the invitation, Arey, chairman of the IANC, convened the members of this Committee and those of the subcommittees at the International Symposium. The members of the Committee and subcommittees of *Nomina Anatomica* and those of the subcommittee on Embryology met in sufficient numbers, but the few members of the subcommittee on Histology attending the Symposium "failed to produce a working group". After a special lecture on anatomical nomenclature, delivered by Warwick, the first formal meetings of all subcommittees for *Nomina Anatomica et Embryologica* of the Nomenclature Committee were held simultaneously to discuss suggestions submitted by interested morphologists. Such reviews were made to expedite the updating of the lists of nomenclature in preparation for the forthcoming Federative International Congress of Anatomy in Mexico (1980). The success of these meetings, in which personal exchanges of views had been possible, prompted the participants to recommend that subsequent international symposia on morphological sciences include similar events on nomenclature topics and reviews.

At the X Federative International Congress of Anatomy, held in Mexico City in 1980, and presided over by Acosta-Vidrio, the IANC and the Veterinary Anatomical Nomenclature Committee met separately. The revisions of all lists of terms were discussed and many recommendations were approved. At the end of the meeting Woodburne was elected to succeed Arey.

Following submission of the revised and updated lists by the Committee and subcommittees of the Anatomical Nomenclature and approval therefore by the XI Federative International Congress of Anatomy, the fifth edition of *Nomina Anatomica* and the second edition of *Nomina Histologica* and *Nomina Embryologica* were published in 1983 as a combined volume. This combined volume of the *Nomina* did not include an index, an important feature that most morphologists felt should be restored in future editions. *Nomina Histologica* had been approved both by the XI Federative International Congress of Anatomists and the World Associations of Veterinary Anatomists in Mexico City (1980).

At the XII Federative International Congress of Anatomy, held in London in 1985 under the presidency of Harrison, a meeting of the members of the IANC took place. The session was presided over by Woodburne and the review of the lists of terms approved in the preceding meeting (Mexico, 1980) was continued. Additional suggestions for changes were considered and some were approved for inclusion in the subsequent edition of *Nomina Anatomica*. During the administrative portion of the session, a proposal was made by Warwick, Honorary Secretary, to change the IANC into an editorial board independent of the IFAA and, consequently, not subject to approval of the Federative Member Associations. After a long discussion, the subject was dropped (no action on the proposal was taken) and the meeting was adjourned.

As the Executive Committee of the IFAA had received suggestions from many anatomical societies to restructure the IANC, the officers of the IFAA met in London and attempted to implement a smooth transition by a democratic process of election of new members. This attempt was rejected by the Chairman and the Secretary of the IANC. In his letter, the Chairman stated that "based on historical facts, the International Federation of Associations of Anatomists had no jurisdiction over the International Anatomical Nomenclature Committee." Considering that there was no historical base for such interpretation, the Executive Committee of the IFAA decided to restructure the Nomenclature Committee and to submit a proposition on the subject to the General Assembly of the IFAA, scheduled for 1989, during the XIII Federative International Congress of Anatomy.

In December 1985 Harrison was succeeded by Di Dio who, in consultation with the other officers of the IFAA and the presidents of the anatomical societies, continued to make efforts to solve the Nomenclature Committee issue. From 1985 to 1989 repeated attempts were made to bring the impasse to a resolution, but all approaches proved unsuccessful.

The IANC proceeded to work on the lists and published the sixth edition, which was not submitted to the Executive Committee of the IFAA or to the XIII Federative International Congress of Anatomy, held in Rio de Janeiro in 1989 and presided over by Moscovici.

At the General Assembly of the IFAA, during his presidential report, Di Dio reviewed in detail the problems of the Nomenclature Committee and urged the General Assembly to provide directions for the future, based on a fully democratic preparation of an official list of anatomical

terms and a democratic election of a federative committee to represent anatomists from the five continents. On August 10 1989, after a long discussion, the General Assembly unanimously approved the creation of a new Federative Committee on Anatomical Terminology (FCAT), and elected its 12 initial members:

1. Ian Whitmore (Secretary of the Anatomical Society of Great Britain and Ireland)
2. Lutz Vollrath (President of the Anatomische Gesellschaft, Germany)
3. Edward Klika (President of the Anatomical Society of Czechoslovakia)
4. Georges Grignon (Secretary General of the Association des Anatomistes, France)
5. José C. Prates (President of the Brazilian Society of Anatomy, Brazil)
6. George Martin (President of the Nomenclature Committee of the American Association of Anatomists)
7. Antoine Dhem (Delegate of the Belgian Society of Anatomy, Belgium)
8. Keith L. Moore (Delegate of the Canadian Association of Anatomists)
9. Kenjiro Yasuda (President of the Japanese Association of Anatomists, Japan)
10. Pierre Sprumont (Secretary General of the Swiss Society of Anatomy, Histology and Embryology)
11. Colin Wendell-Smith (Delegate of the Anatomical Society of Australia and New Zealand)
12. Liberato J. A. Di Dio (President of the International Federation of Associations of Anatomists, USA)

The members of the FCAT were from the following 11 countries: Australia, Belgium, Canada, Brazil, Czechoslovakia, France, Germany, Japan, Switzerland, United Kingdom and USA. After the election the president of the IFAA underlined the fact that the FCAT was an IFAA committee, and that consequently it belonged to all anatomical societies, to which it should report periodically. In addition the FCAT should democratically prepare and publish lists of terms of all biomorphological sciences. He indicated that within the budget of the IFAA, the Executive Committee thereof should finance the activities of the FCAT, and that copyrights of the publications would belong to the IFAA through the FCAT. The first officers of the FCAT were elected as follows: Chairman, Ian Whitmore; Vice-Chairman, Keith L. Moore; Secretary General, L. J. A. Di Dio; Secretaries, Georges Grignon and Lutz Vollrath.

The FCAT held meetings in the following countries: (I) France, 1990; (II) Canada, 1991; (III) England, 1992; (IV) Spain, 1993; (V) The Netherlands, 1994; (VI) Portugal, 1994; (VII) England, 1994; (VIII) Greece, 1995; (IX) Costa Rica, 1996; (X) Germany, 1996; (XI) Switzerland, 1996; (XII) USA, 1997; (XIII) Brazil, 1997.

In 1991 at the meeting held in Toronto, Canada, the following members of the FCAT were added *ad referendum* of the IFAA General Assembly: Giuseppe Balboni (Italy), Jan Drukker (The Netherlands), Domingo Ruano-Gil (Spain), Galina Satjukova (Russia) and Phillip Tobias (South Africa).

Since the first meeting, the FCAT made several contacts with the IANC aiming at the natural transition from the old approach to the approach established by the General Assembly of the IFAA. Such initiatives, however, did not result in a *modus vivendi* for harmonious collaboration.

In 1994 during the XIV Federative International Congress of Anatomy held in Lisbon, Portugal, under the presidency of Esperança-Pina, Whitmore, Chairman of the FCAT, presented its first report on the activities of the Committee. In the discussion the report was highly praised by the delegates of several anatomical societies, and was unanimously approved. Since there was a need to increase the number of members of the FCAT, the following anatomists were elected by unanimous vote for the subsequent quinquennium (until 1999):

1. David Brynmor-Thomas, United Kingdom
2. Rolando Cruz-Gutiérrez, Costa Rica
3. Antoine Dhem, Belgium
4. Liberato J. A. Di Dio, USA
5. Jan Drukker, The Netherlands
6. Georges Grignon, France
7. Duane E. Haines, USA
8. Lev L. Kolesnikov, Russia
9. Keith L. Moore, Canada
10. José C. Prates, Brazil
11. Alessandro Riva, Italy
12. Domingo Ruano-Gil, Spain
13. Harumichi Seguchi, Japan
14. Pierre Sprumont, Switzerland
15. Phillip V. Tobias, South Africa
16. Lutz Vollrath, Germany
17. Colin Wendell-Smith, Australia
18. Ian Whitmore, United Kingdom

Additional members have been nominated by the FCAT *ad referendum* of the IFAA General Assembly to be held in Rome, Italy (1999). These being Raymond Gasser (USA) and Jacques Gilloteaux (USA).

The new FCAT has representatives of anatomical societies from 16 countries of the five continents (Australia, Belgium, Brazil, Canada, Costa Rica, France, Germany, Italy, Japan, Russia, Spain, South Africa, Switzerland, The Netherlands, United Kingdom, USA). The current officers of the FCAT are: Chairman, Ian Whitmore; Vice-chairman, Lutz Vollrath; Secretary General, L. J. A. Di Dio; Secretaries, Georges Grignon and Colin Wendell-Smith.

Following previous financial support by UNESCO, universities, foundations and organizing committees of congresses and symposia, the American Association of Anatomists supported the XII FCAT meeting in New Orleans, USA. In addition, the private sector has funded recent FCAT meetings. Novartis and ZLB SRK, for example, provided partial funding for the XI meeting in Fribourg, Switzerland, and the Banco Real S.A., provided full funding for the XIII meeting in São Paulo, Brazil.

In the Fribourg meeting, it was decided to submit the preliminary list of *Terminologia Anatomica* to all associations of anatomists. The results of the review and the amendments were to be received by December 1 1996. Shortly after this date, the suggestions were grouped by systems and regions to be discussed and evaluated. The vast majority was voted upon in the XII Meeting of the FCAT in New Orleans (April 5 to 9 1997).

The FCAT accepted the invitation of the Secretary General to meet on August 24 to 28 1997 in São Paulo, Brazil for the purpose of completing the preparation of the list of anatomical terms, officially launching the new *Terminologia Anatomica*, deciding on its publications and dealing with other administrative matters. At the closing of the XIII Meeting of the FCAT on August 28 1997, Whitmore made an official announcement of the completion on the *Terminologia Anatomica* indicating that the new, updated, simplified and uniform anatomical terminology was ready for publication and that it would be available shortly. Each anatomical society would then provide its members with a translation in its own language. On behalf of the IFAA, the acting President, Thomas, complimented FCAT on the completion of the *Terminologia Anatomica*, and, on behalf of the Brazilian clinicians and surgeons, Prof. Dr. A. A. Laudanna and Prof. Dr. A. Habr-Gama respectively, expressed support for the new terminology and congratulated the IFAA on the successful work of the FCAT.

Liberato J. A. Di Dio
FCAT Secretary General

Index of Eponyms

A

Abernethy's fascia A04.5.02.009 **39**
Achilles tendon A04.7.02.048 **43**
Adam's apple A06.2.02.003 **58**
Adamkiewicz, Artery of A12.2.11.015 **87**
Addison's plane A01.2.00.007 **3**
Albarran's gland A09.3.08.015 **69**
Alcock's canal A09.5.04.003 **71**
Alderman's nerve A14.2.01.156 **136**
Ammon's horn A14.1.09.327 **128**
Andersch, Ganglion of A14.2.01.137 **136**
Andersch, Nerve of A14.2.01.138 **136**
Arantius, Bodies of A12.1.04.016 **77**
Arantius, Ligament of A05.8.01.011 **54, 98**
Arnold's ganglion A14.3.02.014 **142**
Arnold's nerves A14.2.01.017 **133**, A14.2.01.156 **136**, A14.2.02.008 **137**
Arnold, Tract of A14.1.09.528 **130**
Aschoff-Tawara node A12.1.06.004 **77**
Auerbach's plexus A14.3.03.041 **143**

B

Baillarger's external band, stripe A14.1.09.317 **128**
Baillarger's internal band, stripe A14.1.09.319 **128**
Ball's valves A05.7.05.005 **54**
Bartholin's duct A05.1.02.009 **47**
Bartholin's gland A09.2.01.016 **67**
Baudelocque's diameter A02.5.02.018 **22**
Bauhin's valve A05.7.02.003 **53**
Bechterew, Nucleus of A14.1.05.429 **114**
Bell's nerve A14.2.03.012 **138**
Berry's ligament A04.2.05.005 **36**
Bertin's bone A02.1.05.019 **11**
Bertin's columns A08.1.01.019 **63**
Bertin's ligament A03.6.07.003 **30**
Betz' cells A14.1.09.313 **128**
Bichat's fat pad A05.1.01.015 **47**
Bigelow's ligament A03.6.07.003 **30**
Blandin, Gland of A05.1.02.018 **47**
Blumenbach, Clivus of A02.1.00.051 **8**
Bochdalek's triangle A04.4.02.016 **38**
Bogros, Space of A10.1.01.004 **72**
Botallo's duct, ligament A12.2.01.202 **78**
Botallo's foramen A12.1.01.007 **76**
Botallo's node A13.3.02.008 **102**
Bourgery's ligament A03.6.08.013 **31**
Bowman's glands A15.1.00.003 **144**
Bowman's membrane A15.2.02.019 **144**
Boxer's muscle A04.4.01.008 **37**
Boyden, Four-part sphincter of A05.8.02.015 **56**, A05.8.02.016 **56**, A05.8.02.018 **56**, A05.9.01.016 **56**
Boyer's bursa A06.2.02.015 **58**
Broca's diagonal band A14.1.09.422 **129**
Brodie's bursa A04.8.05.027 **45**
Bruch's membrane A15.2.03.007 **144**
Brücke's muscle A15.2.03.015 **144**
Brunner's glands A05.6.02.017 **53**
Buck's fascia (penis) A09.4.01.026 **69**
Buck's fascia (perineum) A09.5.02.002 **71**
Burdach's nucleus A14.1.04.206 **110**
Burdach's tract A14.1.02.244 **107**
Burn's ligament A04.7.03.017 **43**
Burow's veins A12.3.09.009 **97**

C

Cajal's interstitia1 nucleus A14.1.06.306 **117**
Calleja, Olfactory islets of A14.1.09.428 **129**
Calot's triangle A10.1.02.428 **73**
Camper's fascia A04.5.02.017 **39**
Carabelli formation A05.1.03.071 **49**
Casserio's ligament A15.3.02.054 **150**
Casserio's muscle A04.6.02.018 **40**
Casserio's nerve A14.2.03.024 **138**
Chassaignac's tubercle A02.2.02.005 **16**
Chievitz, Organ of A05.1.01.016 **47**
Chopart's joint A03.6.10.201 **31**
Chopart's ligament A03.6.10.511 **31**
Clarke's column, nucleus A14.1.02.135 **106**
Cloquet's canal A15.2.06.010 **146**
Cloquet's gland, node A13.3.05.009 **103**
Colles' fascia (penis) A09.4.01.027 **70**
Colles' fascia (perineum) A09.5.00.007 **71**
Colles' fascia (scrotum) A09.4.03.003 **70**
Colles' ligament A04.5.01.012 **38**
Cooper's fascia A09.3.04.004 **68**
Cooper's ligament (groin) A04.5.01.011 **38**
Cooper's ligaments (breast) A16.0.02.015 **155**
Corti, Ganglion of A15.3.03.125 **153**
Corti, Organ of A15.3.03.121 **153**
Cowper's glands A09.3.09.001 **69**
Cruveilhier's nerve A14.2.01.112 **135**, A14.3.01.023 **141**
Cruveilhier's plexuses A14.2.02.010 **137**, A14.3.03.010 **143**

D

Darkschewitsch, Nucleus of A14.1.06.309 **117**
Darwin's tubercle A15.3.01.020 **148**
Deiters' nucleus A14.1.05.427 **114**
Denonvilliers' ligament A04.5.03.012 **39**, A04.5.03.015 **39**
Denonvilliers' fascia A04.5.03.003 **39**
Descemet's membrane A15.2.02.021 **144**
Douglas, Fold of A10.1.02.511 **73**
Douglas, Pouch of A10.1.02.512 **73**
Douglas, Semicircular line of A04.5.01.006 **38**
Drummond, Marginal artery of A12.2.12.068 **88**
Duverney's gland A09.2.01.016 **67**

E

Edinger-Westphal nucleus A14.1.06.304 **117**
Ehrenritter's ganglion A14.2.01.136 **136**
Eustachian amygdala A05.3.01.016 **50, 100**
Eustachian muscle A15.3.02.061 **150**
Eustachian tube A15.3.02.073 **150**
Eustachian valve A12.1.01.015 **76**

F

Fallopian canal A02.1.06.009 **12**
Fallopian ligament A04.5.01.009 **38**
Fallopian tube A09.1.02.001 **65**

Ferrein's pyramids A08.1.01.018 **63**
Flechsig's tract A14.1.02.227 **107**
Flechsig, Oval bundle of A14.1.02.241 **107**
Flood's ligament A03.5.08.003 **29**
Folian process A15.3.02.048 **150**
Fontana, Spaces of A15.2.03.033 **145**
Forel, Decussation of A14.1.06.222 **117**
Forel, Fields of *A14.1.08.703 **123**
Forel, Nuclei of Fields of A14.1.08.703 **123**
Frankenhäuser's ganglion ♀ A14.3.03.052 **143**
Führer's artery A12.2.16.009 **90**

G

Galen, Vein of A12.3.06.027 **94**
Gallaudet's fascia (abdomen) A04.5.02.018 **39**
Gallaudet's fascia (perineum) A09.5.02.002 **71**
Ganser's commissure A14.1.08.947 **124**
Gartner's duct A09.1.05.002 **66**
Gasserian ganglion A14.2.01.014 **133**
Gennari, Stria of, Line of A14.1.09.318 **128**
Gerdy's ligament A04.6.03.003 **41**
Gerlach's tonsil A05.3.01.016 **50, 100**
Gerota's capsule, fascia A08.1.01.010 **63**
Gierke, Respiratory bundle of A14.1.04.120 **109**
Gimbernat's ligament A04.5.01.010 **38**
Giraldès, Organ of A09.3.03.001 **68**
Glaserian fissure A02.1.06.074 **13**
Glisson's capsule A05.8.01.055 **55**
Goll's nucleus A14.1.04.202 **110**
Goll's tract A14.1.02.243 **107**
Gowers' tract A14.1.02.226 **107**
Graafian follicle A09.1.01.013 **65**
Gratiolet's radiation A14.1.08.673 **122**
Grynfelt's triangle A01.2.05.010 **4**
Gudden, von Gudden's commissure A14.1.08.959 **124**
Gudden, von Gudden's ganglion A14.1.06.312 **117**
Gudden, von Gudden's nucleus A14.1.05.449 **114**
Gudden, von Gudden's tract A14.1.08.953 **124**
Guerin's valve A09.4.02.023 **70**
Guthrie's muscle A09.2.03.006 **67, 71**, A09.5.03.004 **71**, A09.4.02.016 **70**
Guyon, loge de A03.5.11.202 **29**

H

Haller's arches A04.4.02.006 **38**, A04.4.02.007 **38**
Haller's artery A12.2.12.042 **88**
Haller's ductulus aberrans A09.3.02.009 **68**
Haller's layer A15.2.03.005 **144**
Haller's rete A09.3.01.024 **68**
Haller's tripus A12.2.12.012 **87**
Hannover's canal, spaces A15.2.05.017 **146**
Hartmann's pouch A05.8.02.004 **56**
Harvey's ligament A12.2.01.202 **78**
Hasner's valve A15.2.07.071 **148**
Haversian folds A03.0.00.029 **25**
Heister's valve A05.8.02.012 **56**
Held's bundle A14.1.04.112 **109, 113, 116**
Helweg's tract A14.1.02.230 **107**
Henle's ligament A04.5.01.020 **38**
Henle's spine A02.1.06.070 **13**
Herophilus, Torcular of A12.3.05.103 **93**
Heschl's transverse convolutions A14.1.09.140 **125**
Hesselbach's fascia A04.7.03.020 **43**
Hesselbach's ligament A04.5.02.012 **39**
Hesselbach's triangle A10.1.02.433 **73**
Heubner's recurrent artery A12.2.07.034 **83**
Hey's ligament A04.7.03.017 **43**
Highmore, Antrum of A02.1.12.023 **14**
Highmore, Body of A09.3.01.018 **67**
Hilton, Waterbed of A14.1.01.215 **105**
His, Angle of A05.5.01.011 **52**
His, Bundle of A12.1.06.005 **77**
Hoche, Bundle of, Tract of A14.1.02.242 **107**
Horner's muscle A04.1.03.016 **34**
Houston's valve (middle of three) A05.7.04.007 **54**
Humphrey, Ligament of A03.6.08.003 **30**
Hunter's ligament A09.1.03.029 **66**
Hunter's canal A04.7.03.006 **43**
Huschke's cartilage A06.1.01.016 **57**
Hyrtl's muscle A04.7.02.002 **42**

I

Ingrassia's process A02.1.05.020 **11**

J

Jackson's membrane, veil A05.7.02.010 **53**
Jacobson's canaliculus A02.1.06.049 **13**
Jacobson's cartilage A06.1.01.016 **57**
Jacobson's nerve A14.2.01.138 **136**
Jacobson's organ A06.1.02.008 **57**
Jacobson's plexus A14.2.01.140 **136**

K

Keith-Flack, Node of A12.1.06.003 **77**
Kent's bundle A12.1.06.005 **77**
Kerckring's valves A05.6.01.007 **52**
Key and Retzius, Foramen of A14.1.05.718 **115**
Klaes-Bechterew, Band of, Stripe of A14.1.09.315 **128**
Kobelt's tubules A09.1.06.001 **66**
Koch's node A12.1.06.003 **77**
Koch's triangle A12.1.00.030 **76**
Kohlrausch's fold (middle of three) A05.7.04.007 **54**
Kölliker-Fuse nucleus A14.1.05.440 **114**
Koyter's muscle A04.1.03.018 **34**
Krause, Glands of A15.2.07.061 **148**

L

Lallouette's pyramid A11.3.00.004 **74**
Labbé, Vein of A12.3.06.009 **94**
Lancisi, Stria of A14.1.09.248 **127**
Langer's lines A16.0.00.008 **154**
Langerhans. Islets of A05.9.01.019 **56, 74**
Latarjet's anterior nerve A14.2.01.176 **136**
Latarjet's posterior nerve A14.2.01.181 **137**
Lecomte's pronator of ulna A04.6.02.024 **40**
Leonardo (da Vinci)'s cord A12.1.02.020 **77**
Lesshaft's space, triangle A01.2.05.010 **4**
Lieberkühn, Crypts of A05.6.01.012 **52**
Lieutaud's trigone A08.3.01.025 **64**
Lisfranc's joint A03.6.10.601 **31**
Lisfranc's ligament (medial of) A03.6.10.604 **32**
Lisfranc's tubercle A02.3.02.015 **18**
Lissauer's tract A14.1.02.228 **107**
Lister's tubercle A02.4.05.017 **20**
Littre, Glands of A09.4.02.025 **70**
Lockwood's ligament A15.2.07.005 **147**
Louis, Angle of A02.3.03.005 **18**
Lower's tubercle A12.1.01.014 **76**
Ludwig (Ludovicus), Angle of A02.3.03.005 **18**
Luschka, Foramen of A14.1.05.718 **115**

Luschka, Glands of, Tonsil of A05.3.01.006 **50, 100**, A12.2.12.011 **87**
Luschka, Recurrent nerve of A14.2.00.032 **133**
Luys, Nucleus of (Corpus Luysii) A14.1.08.702 **123**

M

Macewen's triangle A02.1.06.069 **13**
Mackenrodt's ligament A09.1.03.031 **66**
Magendie (Majendie), Foramen of A14.1.05.722 **115**
Maier, Sinus of A15.2.07.069 **148**
Maissiat, Bandelette of A04.7.03.003 **43**
Malpighian canal A09.1.05.002 **66**
Malpighian capsule A13.2.01.002 **100**
Malpighian corpuscles A13.2.01.004 **100**
Marie, Tract of A14.1.02.204 **107**
Marshall's vein A12.3.01.007 **91**
Mauchart's ligaments A03.2.04.002 **27**
Mayo's vein A12.3.12.017 **98**
Meckel's groove A02.1.06.028 **12**
Meckel's cave A14.1.01.108 **104**
Meckel's diverticulum A05.6.03.003
Meckel's ganglion A14.3.02.006 **142**
Meibomian glands A15.2.07.042 **147**
Meissner's plexus A14.3.03.042 **143**
Mercier's bar A08.3.01.026 **64**
Meynert's commissure A14.1.08.947 **124**
Meynert's decussation A14.1.06.221 **117**
Meynert's nucleus A14.1.09.418 **129**
Meynert's retroflex bundle A14.1.08.502 **121**
Michels' artery A12.2.12.021 **87**
Mohrenheim's fossa A01.2.03.003 **4**
Moll's glands A15.2.07.043 **147**
Monakow's tract A14.1.04.136 **110**
Monro, Foramen of A14.1.08.414 **121**
Montgomery's tubercles A16.0.02.014 **155**
Morand's foramen A05.1.04.020 **49**
Morgagni, Cartilage of A06.2.06.001 **58**
Morgagni, Columns of A05.7.05.004 **54**
Morgagni, Foramen of A05.1.04.020 **49**, A15.3.03.033 **151**
Morgagni, Hydatid of A09.1.05.004 **66**, A09.3.02.010 **68**
Morgagni, Lacunae of A09.4.02.024 **70**
Morgagni, Nodules of A12.1.02.014 **77**
Morgagni, Triangle of A04.4.02.015 **38**
Morgagni, Ventricle of A06.2.09.010 **59**
Morison's pouch A10.1.02.427 **73**
Müller's muscles A15.2.03.018 **145**, A15.2.07.009 **147**, A15.2.07.045 **147**

N

Nuhn, Gland of A05.1.02.018 **47**

O

Oddi, Sphincter of A05.8.02.018 **56**
Onuf's nucleus A14.1.02.139 **106**

P

Pacchionian granulations A02.1.00.039 **8**
Parona, Space of A04.6.01.006 **40**
Passavant's ridge/bar A05.3.01.018 **50**
Pavlov's (Pawlow) nerve A14.3.01.022 **141**
Pecquet, Cistern of A12.4.01.012 **99**
Petit, Canal of, Spaces of A15.2.05.017 **146**
Petit, Ligaments of A09.1.03.032 **66**
Petit, Triangle of A01.2.05.009 **4**
Peyer's patches A05.6.01.014 **52, 101**
Phillippe-Gombault, Triangle of A14.1.02.242 **107**
Pirogoff's aponeurosis A04.6.02.017 **40**
Poupart's ligament A04.5.01.009 **38**
Purkinje cell layer A14.1.07.404 **119**
Purkinje fibres A12.1.06.008 **77**

R

Rasmussen, Bundle of A14.1.05.316 **113**
Rau's process A15.3.02.048 **150**
Reichert's membrane A15.2.02.019 **144**
Reil, Island of A14.1.09.149 **125**
Reissner's canal A15.3.03.093 **152**
Reissner's membrane A15.3.03.094 **152**
Remak's plexus A14.3.03.042 **143**
Retzius' band A04.5.02.023 **39, 67, 70**
Retzius, Cave of A10.1.01.003 **72**
Riolan, Arcade of A12.2.12.068 **88**
Riolan, Muscle of A04.1.03.015 **34**, A09.3.04.003 **68**
Rivinus, Ducts of A05.1.02.010 **47**
Rivinus' gland A05.1.02.008 **47**
Rivinus' membrane A15.3.01.052 **149**
Rivinus' notch A02.1.06.059 **13**
Robert, Ligament of A03.6.08.004 **30**
Rolando, Fissure of, Sulcus of A14.1.09.103 **124, 126**
Roller's nucleus A14.1.04.262 **111**
Rosenmüller, Fossa of A05.3.01.017 **50**
Rosenmüller's gland, node A13.3.05.008 **103**
Rosenmüller, Organ of A09.1.05.001 **66**
Rosenthal's vein A12.3.06.018 **94**
Rouget's muscle A15.2.03.017 **145**
Russell, Uncinate bundle of A14.1.07.420 **120**
Ruysch' veins A12.3.06.106 **95**

S

Santorini's muscles A04.1.03.008 **34**, A04.1.03.028 **34**, A15.3.01.040 **148**
Santorini's cartilage A06.2.05.001 **58**
Santorini's caruncle A05.6.02.016 **53**
Santorini's duct A05.9.01.017 **56**
Santorini's notch A15.3.01.050 **149**
Sappey, Veins of A12.3.12.013 **98**
Sattler's layer A15.2.03.005 **144**
Scarpa's fascia A04.5.02.022 **39**
Scarpa's ganglion A14.2.01.123 **135**
Scarpa's nerve A14.2.01.043 **134**
Scarpa's orifice A15.3.03.044 **151**
Scarpa's triangle A04.7.03.013 **43**
Schlemm, Canal of A12.3.06.109 **95, 144**
Schultze's comma tract A14.1.02.242 **107**
Schütz, Fasciculus of, Bundle of A14.1.04.114 **109**
Schwalbe's nucleus A14.1.04.244 **111**
Shrapnell's membrane A15.3.01.053 **149**
Sibson's fascia A06.6.02.018
Sibson's muscle A04.2.01.007 **35**
Skene's tubules A09.2.03.015 **67**
Soemmering's substance A14.1.06.111 **116**
Spence, Tail of A16.0.02.007 **154**
Spiegel's (Spighel's) line A04.5.01.025 **38**
Spiegelian lobe A05.8.01.030 **55**
Staderini's nucleus A14.1.04.263 **111**
Stensen's (Stenon) duct A05.1.02.007 **47**
Stenson's foramen A02.1.00.062 **9**
Stenson's canal A02.1.12.032 **14**
Stilling's canal A15.2.06.010 **146**
Stilling-Clarke's column, nucleus A14.1.02.135 **106**
Stroud's pecten A05.7.05.010 **54**

Sylvian artery A12.2.07.046 **83–84**
Sylvian fissure, sulcus A14.1.09.104 **124**
Sylvius, Aqueduct of A14.1.06.501 **118**

T

Tawara, Node of A12.1.06.004 **77**
Tenon's capsule A15.2.07.004 **147**
Testut's artery A12.2.12.043 **88**
Thebesian valve A12.1.01.016 **76**
Thebesian veins A12.3.01.013 **91**
Thiele's canal A12.1.07.001 **77**
Thiele's muscle A09.5.02.003 **71**
Tiedemann's gland A09.2.01.016 **67**
Torin's hole A02.1.06.024 **12**
Treitz, Ligament of, Muscle of A05.6.02.011 **52**
Treves, Bloodless fold of A10.1.02.421 **73**
Trolard's vein A12.3.06.010 **94**
Tsai, Tegmental area of A14.1.06.329 **117**
Türck, Bundle of A14.1.09.548 **131**
Türck, Column of A14.1.02.205 **107**
Tyrrel's fascia A04.5.03.003 **39**

V

Valsalva, Nodules of A12.1.04.016 **77**
Valsalva, Sinus of A12.2.03.002 **79**
Varolius, Pons of A14.1.03.010 **108, 112**
Vater, Ampulla of A05.8.02.017 **56**
Vater, Tubercle of A05.6.02.015 **53**
Vesalius' ligament A04.5.01.009 **38**
Vesalius, Foramen of A02.1.05.037 **11**
Vicq d'Azyr's bundle A14.1.08.671 **122**
Vicq d'Azyr's foramen A14.1.04.002 **108**
Vicq d'Azyr's stria A14.1.09.318 **128**
Vidian artery A12.2.05.082 **81**
Vidian canal A02.1.05.053 **12**
Vidian nerve A14.3.02.007 **142**
Vidian veins A12.3.05.039 **93**
Vieussens, Anulus of A14.3.01.021 **141**
von Gudden's commissure A14.1.08.959 **124**
von Gudden's ganglion A14.1.06.312 **117**
von Gudden's nucleus A14.1.05.449 **114**
von Gudden's tract A14.1.08.953 **124**

W

Waldeyer's fascia A04.5.03.020 **39**
Waldeyer's organ A09.3.03.001 **68**
Waldeyer's ring A13.2.02.001 **100**
Wernekink's decussation A14.1.06.217 **116**
Wharton's duct A05.1.02.012 **47**
Whitnall's tubercle A02.1.14.008 **15**
Wilkie's artery A12.2.12.017 **87**
Willis' nerve A14.2.01.184 **137**
Willis, Circle of A12.2.07.080 **83**
Winslow's pancreas A05.9.01.003 **56**
Winslow, Foramen of A10.1.02.403 **72**
Winslow, Ligament of A03.6.08.013 **31**
Wirsung, Duct of A05.9.01.015 **56**
Wolfring, Glands of A15.2.07.061 **148**
Wood's muscle A04.7.02.064 **43**
Wormian bone A02.1.00.043 **8**
Wrisberg, Cartilage of A06.2.06.001 **58**
Wrisberg, Ganglion of A14.3.03.014 **143**
Wrisberg, Ligament of A03.6.08.004 **30**
Wrisberg, Nerve of A14.2.01.115 **135**, A14.2.03.027 **138**

Z

Zeis, Glands of A15.2.07.044 **147**
Zinn, Anulus of A15.2.07.015 **147**
Zinn's artery A12.2.06.024 **81**
Zinn, Zonule of A15.2.05.015 **146**
Zuckerkandl, Bodies of A12.2.04.003 **79**
Zuckerkandl, Fascia of A08.1.01.010 **63**

Index of Latin Terms

A

Abdomen A01.1.00.016 **2**
Abductio A03.0.00.053 **25**
Acetabulum A02.5.01.002 **21**
Acromion A02.4.01.009 **18**
Adductio A03.0.00.054 **25**
Adenohypophysis A11.1.00.002 **74**
Adhesio interthalamica A14.1.08.103 **120, 121**
Aditus
- ad antrum mastoideum A15.3.02.021 **149**
- laryngis A06.2.09.002 **59**
- orbitalis A02.1.00.069 **9**
Adminiculum lineae albae A04.5.01.024 **38**
Agger nasi A06.1.02.021 **57**
Aggregationes cellularum chemergicarum A14.1.09.601 **131**
Ala
- cristae galli A02.1.07.005 **13**
- lobuli centralis cerebelli A14.1.07.108 **119**
- major ossis sphenoidalis A02.1.05.024 **11**
- minor ossis sphenoidalis A02.1.05.020 **11**
- nasi A06.1.01.005 **57**
- ossis
- - ilii A02.5.01.104 **21**
- - sacri A02.2.05.004 **17**
- vomeris A02.1.11.002 **14**
Allocortex A14.1.09.305 **128**
Alveolus/i
- dentalis/es A03.1.03.008 **26**, A05.1.03.074 **49**
- - mandibulae A02.1.15.018 **15**
- - maxillae A02.1.12.037 **14**
Alveus hippocampi A14.1.09.333 **128**
Amiculum olivare A14.1.04.116 **109**
Amphiarthrosis A03.0.00.052 **25**
Ampulla
- biliaropancreatica A05.8.02.017 **56**
- canaliculi lacrimalis A15.2.07.067 **148**
- ductus deferentis A09.3.05.006 **68**
- duodeni A05.6.02.003 **52**
- hepatopancreatica A05.8.02.017 **56**
- membranacea
- - anterior A15.3.03.068 **152**
- - lateralis A15.3.03.074 **152**
- - posterior A15.3.03.070 **152**
- ossea
- - anterior A15.3.03.017 **151**
- - lateralis A15.3.03.023 **151**
- - posterior A15.3.03.019 **151**
- recti A05.7.04.008 **54**
- tubae uterinae A09.1.02.006 **65**
Anastomosis
- arteriolovenularis A12.0.00.002 **75**
- arteriovenosa A12.0.00.002 **75**
Angulus
- acromii A02.4.01.011 **18**
- costae A02.3.02.010 **18**
- frontalis ossis parietalis A02.1.02.015 **10**
- inferior scapulae A02.4.01.016 **19**
- infrasternalis A02.3.04.008 **18**
- iridocornealis A15.2.06.004 **146**
- lateralis scapulae A02.4.01.017 **19**
- mandibulae A02.1.15.025 **15**
- mastoideus ossis parietalis A02.1.02.018 **10**
- occipitalis ossis parietalis A02.1.02.016 **10**
- oculi
- - lateralis A15.2.07.033 **147**
- - medialis A15.2.07.034 **147**
- oris A05.1.01.013 **47**
- pontocerebellaris A14.1.05.004 **112**
- sphenoidalis ossis parietalis A02.1.02.017 **10**
- sterni A02.3.03.005 **18**
- subpubicus A02.5.02.004 **22**
- superior scapulae A02.4.01.018 **19**
Ansa
- cervicalis A14.2.02.013 **137**
- lenticularis
- - in corpore striato A14.1.09.520 **130**
- - in thalamo A14.1.08.663 **122**
- peduncularis A14.1.08.665 **122, 129**
- subclavia A14.3.01.021 **141**
Antebrachium A01.1.00.024 **2**
Anterior A01.0.00.011 **1**
Antihelix A15.3.01.009 **148**
Antitragus A15.3.01.016 **148**
Antrum
- mastoideum A15.3.02.028 **149**
- pyloricum A05.5.01.015 **52**
Anulus
- conjunctivae A15.2.02.013 **144**
- femoralis A04.7.03.014 **43**
- fibrocartilagineus membranae tympani A15.3.01.060 **149**
- fibrosus A03.2.02.004 **27**
- - dexter/sinister cordis A12.1.00.027 **76**
- inguinalis
- - profundus A04.5.01.021 **38**
- - superficialis A04.5.01.013 **38**
- iridis
- - major A15.2.03.025 **145**
- - minor A15.2.03.026 **145**
- lymphaticus cardiae A13.3.03.017 **102**
- lymphoideus pharyngis A13.2.02.001 **100**
- tendineus communis A15.2.07.015 **147**
- tympanicus A02.1.06.053 **13**
- umbilicalis A04.5.01.023 **38**
Anus A05.7.05.013 **54**
Aorta A12.2.02.001 **79**
- abdominalis A12.2.12.001 **87**
- ascendens A12.2.03.001 **79**
- descendens A12.2.10.001 **86**
- thoracica A12.2.11.001 **86**
Apertura
- aqueductus cerebri mesencephali A14.1.06.502 **118, 121**
- canaliculi
- - cochleae A02.1.06.043 **12**
- - vestibuli A02.1.06.036 **12**
- ductus nasolacrimalis A06.1.02.030 **57**
- externa canalis carotici A02.1.06.014 **12**
- interna
- - canaliculi
- - - cochleae A15.3.03.036 **151**
- - - vestibuli A15.3.03.006 **151**
- - canalis carotici A02.1.06.015 **12**
- lateralis ventriculi quarti A14.1.05.718 **115**
- mediana ventriculi quarti A14.1.05.722 **115**
- nasalis posterior A02.1.00.096 **9**
- pelvis
- - inferior A02.5.02.009 **22**
- - superior A02.5.02.008 **22**
- piriformis A02.1.00.088 **9**
- sinus
- - frontalis A02.1.03.030 **10**
- - sphenoidalis A02.1.05.018 **11**
- thoracis
- - inferior A02.3.04.004 **18**
- - superior A02.3.04.003 **18**
- tympanica canaliculi chordae tympani A15.3.02.027 **149**
Apex A14.1.02.116 **106**
- auriculae A15.3.01.021 **148**
- capitis fibulae A02.5.07.004 **23**
- cartilaginis arytenoideae A06.2.04.012 **58**
- cordis A12.1.00.007 **76**
- cornu posterioris medullae spinalis A14.1.02.116 **106**
- cuspidis dentis A05.1.03.011 **48**

– dentis A02.2.02.203 **17**
– linguae A05.1.04.010 **49**
– nasi A06.1.01.004 **57**
– ossis sacralis/sacri A02.2.05.021 **17**
– partis petrosae ossis temporalis A02.1.06.012 **12**
– patellae A02.5.05.003 **23**
– prostatae A09.3.08.006 **69**
– pulmonis A06.5.01.005 **60**
– radicis dentis A05.1.03.032 **48**
– vesicae A08.3.01.002 **64**
Apicalis A01.0.00.022 **1**
Aponeurosis A04.0.00.047 **34**
– bicipitalis A04.6.02.016 **40**
– epicranialis A04.1.03.007 **34**
– glutea A04.7.02.009 **42**
– linguae A05.1.04.025 **49**
– m. erectoris spinae A04.3.02.003 **36**
– musculi bicipitis brachii A04.6.02.016 **40**
– palatina A05.2.01.101 **50**
– palmaris A04.6.03.012 **41**
– plantaris A04.7.03.031 **44**
Apophysis A02.0.00.023 **7**
Apparatus lacrimalis A15.2.07.056 **147**
Appendix/ces
– adiposae coli A05.7.03.010 **53**
– epididymidis A09.3.02.011 **68**
– epiploicae A05.7.03.010 **53**
– fibrosa hepatis A05.8.01.028 **55**
– omentales A05.7.03.010 **53**
– testis A09.3.02.010 **68**
– vermiformis A05.7.02.007 **53**
– vesiculosae epoophori A09.1.05.004 **66**
Aqueductus
– cerebri A14.1.06.501 **118**
– cochleae A15.3.03.058 **152**
– mesencephali A14.1.06.501 **118**
– vestibuli A15.3.03.057 **152**
Arachnoidea mater A14.1.01.201 **104**
– cranialis A14.1.01.204 **105**
– encephali A14.1.01.204 **105**
– et pia mater A14.1.01.003 **104**
– spinalis A14.1.01.218 **105**
Arbor
– bronchialis A06.4.01.002 **59**
– vitae A14.1.07.401 **119**
Archicerebellum A14.1.07.010 **118**
Archicortex A14.1.09.302 **128**
Arcus
– alveolaris
– – mandibulae A02.1.15.017 **15**
– – maxillae A02.1.12.036 **14**
– anterior atlantis A02.2.02.105 **16**
– aortae A12.2.04.001 **79**
– cartilaginis cricoideae A06.2.03.002 **58**
– costalis A02.3.04.006 **18**
– dentalis
– – inferior A05.1.03.003 **48**
– – mandibularis A05.1.03.003 **48**
– – maxillaris A05.1.03.002 **48**
– – superior A05.1.03.002 **48**
– ductus thoracici A12.4.01.008 **99**
– iliopectineus A04.5.02.010 **39, 43**
– inguinalis A04.5.01.009 **38**
– marginalis coli A12.2.12.068 **88**
– palatoglossus A05.2.01.005 **50**
– palatopharyngeus A05.2.01.007 **50**
– palmaris
– – profundus A12.2.09.038 **86**
– – superficialis A12.2.09.056 **86**
– palpebralis
– – inferior A12.2.06.046 **82**
– – superior A12.2.06.047 **82**
– pedis
– – longitudinalis A01.2.08.028 **5**
– – transversus
– – – distalis A01.2.08.032 **5**
– – – proximalis A01.2.08.031 **5**
– plantaris
– – profundus A12.2.16.065 **91**
– – superficialis A12.2.16.070 **91**
– posterior atlantis A02.2.02.108 **17**
– pubicus A02.5.02.003 **22**
– superciliaris A02.1.03.005 **10**
– tendineus A04.0.00.048 **34**
– – fasciae pelvis A04.5.03.010 **39**
– – musculi
– – – levatoris ani A04.5.04.009 **40**
– – – solei A04.7.03.024 **43**
– venae azygos A12.3.07.002 **95**
– venosus
– – dorsalis pedis A12.3.11.012 **98**
– – jugularis A12.3.05.048 **93**
– – palmaris
– – – profundus A12.3.08.034 **96**
– – – superficialis A12.3.08.026 **96**
– – plantaris A12.3.11.016 **98**
– vertebrae A02.2.01.005 **16**
– zygomaticus A02.1.00.023 **8**
Area/e
– amygdaloclaustralis A14.1.09.403 **129**
– amygdaloidea anterior A14.1.09.406 **129**
– cochleae A15.3.03.053 **152**
– cochlearis A15.3.03.053 **152**
– contingens dentis A05.1.03.043 **48**
– cribrosa papillae renalis A08.1.01.030 **63**
– gastricae A05.5.01.030 **52**
– hypothalamica
– – dorsalis A14.1.08.916 **123**
– – intermedia A14.1.08.920 **123**
– – lateralis A14.1.08.929 **124**
– – posterior A14.1.08.933 **124**
– – rostralis A14.1.08.902 **123**
– intercondylaris
– – anterior A02.5.06.006 **23**
– – posterior A02.5.06.007 **23**
– nervi facialis meati acustici interni A15.3.03.048 **151**
– nuda faciei diaphragmaticae hepatis A05.8.01.008 **54**
– parahippocampalis A14.1.09.404 **129**
– paraolfactoria A14.1.09.213 **126**
– postrema A14.1.04.258 **111, 115**
– preoptica A14.1.08.407 **120, 124**
– pretectalis A14.1.08.505 **121**
– retrochiasmatica A14.1.08.926 **123**
– retroolivaris A14.1.04.011 **108**
– septalis A14.1.09.443 **129**
– spinalis X A14.1.02.302 **108**
– subcallosa A14.1.09.211 **126**
– transitionis amygdalopiriformis A14.1.09.405 **129**
– trapezoidea infraprostica A09.3.08.021 **69**
– vestibularis A14.1.05.710 **115**
– – inferior meati acustici interni A15.3.03.051 **151**
– – superior A15.3.03.050 **151**
– – – meati acustici interni A15.3.03.050 **151**
Areola mammae A16.0.02.012 **154**
Arteria/e A12.0.00.003 **75**, A12.2.00.001 **78**
– alveolares superiores anteriores A12.2.05.079 **81**
– alveolaris
– – inferior A12.2.05.056 **80**
– – superior posterior A12.2.05.075 **81**
– angularis A12.2.05.029 **80**
– appendicularis A12.2.12.062 **88**
– arcuata A12.2.16.051 **90**
– arcuatae renis A08.1.03.003 **63**
– ascendens A12.2.12.070 **88**
– auricularis
– – posterior A12.2.05.037 **80**
– – profunda A12.2.05.054 **80**
– axillaris A12.2.09.002 **85**
– azygos vaginae ♀ A12.2.15.032 **89**
– basilaris A12.2.07.081 **84**
– brachialis A12.2.09.018 **86**
– – superficialis A12.2.09.019 **86**
– buccalis A12.2.05.074 **81**
– bulbi
– – penis ♂ A12.2.15.043 **89**
– – vestibuli ♀ A12.2.15.043 **89**
– caecalis
– – anterior A12.2.12.060 **88**
– – posterior A12.2.12.061 **88**
– callosa mediana A12.2.07.032 **83**
– callosomarginalis A12.2.07.037 **83**
– canalis pterygoidei A12.2.05.082 **81**, A12.2.06.006 **81**
– caroticotympanicae A12.2.06.005 **81**
– carotis
– – communis A12.2.04.006 **79**
– – externa A12.2.05.001 **79**
– – interna A12.2.06.001 **81, 83**
– caudae pancreatis A12.2.12.046 **88**
– centrales
– – anterolaterales A12.2.07.048 **83**
– – anteromediales
– – – a. cerebri anterior A12.2.07.024 **82**

– – – a. communicans anterior A12.2.07.024 **82**
– – posterolaterales A12.2.07.089 **84**
– – posteromediales
– – – a. cerebri posterior A12.2.07.084 **84**
– – – a. communicans posterior A12.2.07.069 **83**
– – retinae A12.2.06.024 **81**
– – – pars intraocularis A12.2.06.026 **81, 146**
– cerebri
– – anterior A12.2.07.022 **82, 83**
– – media A12.2.07.046 **83, 84**
– – posterior A12.2.07.082 **84, 85**
– cervicalis
– – ascendens A12.2.08.049 **85**
– – profunda A12.2.08.060 **85**
– choroidea anterior A12.2.06.019 **81, 82**
– ciliares
– – anteriores A12.2.06.034 **82**
– – posteriores
– – – breves A12.2.06.031 **82**
– – – longae A12.2.06.032 **82**
– circumferentiales breves A12.2.07.085 **84**
– circumflexa
– – femoris
– – – lateralis A12.2.16.027 **90**
– – – medialis A12.2.16.021 **90**
– – humeri
– – – anterior A12.2.09.016 **86**
– – – posterior A12.2.09.017 **86**
– – ilium
– – – profunda A12.2.16.008 **90**
– – – superficialis A12.2.16.012 **90**
– – scapulae A12.2.09.015 **86**
– cochlearis
– – communis A15.3.03.128 **153**
– – propria A15.3.03.132 **153**
– colica
– – dextra A12.2.12.065 **88**
– – media A12.2.12.067 **88**
– – sinistra A12.2.12.071 **88**
– collateralis
– – media A12.2.09.023 **86**
– – radialis A12.2.09.024 **86**
– – ulnaris
– – – inferior A12.2.09.026 **86**
– – – superior A12.2.09.025 **86**
– collicularis A12.2.07.087 **84**
– comitans nervi
– – ischiadici A12.2.15.019 **89**
– – mediani A12.2.09.049 **86**
– commissuralis mediana A12.2.07.031 **82**
– communicans
– – anterior A12.2.07.029 **82, 84**
– – posterior A12.2.06.018 **81, 83, 84**
– conjunctivales
– – anteriores A12.2.06.035 **82**
– – posteriores A12.2.06.045 **82**
– coronaria
– – dextra A12.2.03.101 **79**
– – sinistra A12.2.03.201 **79**
– corticales radiatae A08.1.03.004 **63**
– – renis A08.1.03.004 **63**
– cremasterica ♂ A12.2.16.007 **90**
– cystica A12.2.12.031 **87**
– descendens genus A12.2.16.017 **90**
– digitales
– – dorsales A12.2.09.035 **86**, A12.2.16.053 **90**
– – palmares
– – – communes A12.2.09.057 **86**
– – – propriae A12.2.09.058 **86**
– – plantares
– – – communes A12.2.16.068 **91**
– – – propriae A12.2.16.069 **91**
– dorsalis
– – clitoridis ♀ A12.2.15.044 **89**
– – nasi A12.2.06.049 **82**
– – pedis A12.2.16.048 **90**
– – penis ♂ A12.2.15.044 **89**
– – scapulae A12.2.08.057 **85**, A12.2.08.058 **85**
– ductus deferentis ♂ A12.2.15.022 **89**
– encephali A12.2.07.001 **82**
– epigastrica
– – inferior A12.2.16.003 **90**
– – superficialis A12.2.16.011 **90**
– – superior A12.2.08.041 **85**
– episclerales A12.2.06.036 **82**
– ethmoidalis
– – anterior A12.2.06.039 **82**
– – posterior A12.2.06.043 **82**
– facialis A12.2.05.020 **80**
– femoralis A12.2.16.010 **90**
– fibularis A12.2.16.071 **91**
– flexurae dextrae A12.2.12.066 **88**
– frontobasalis
– – lateralis A12.2.07.062 **83**
– – medialis A12.2.07.035 **83**
– gastrica
– – dextra A12.2.12.028 **87**
– – posterior A12.2.12.052 **88**
– – sinistra A12.2.12.013 **87**
– gastricae breves A12.2.12.050 **88**
– gastroduodenalis A12.2.12.016 **87**
– gastroomentalis
– – dextra A12.2.12.022 **87**
– – sinistra A12.2.12.047 **88**
– glutea
– – inferior A12.2.15.018 **89**
– – superior A12.2.15.013 **89**
– helicinae A09.4.01.024 **69**
– – penis A09.4.01.024 **69**
– hepatica
– – communis A12.2.12.015 **87**
– – propria A12.2.12.029 **87**
– hyaloidea A15.2.06.009 **146**
– hypophysialis
– – inferior A12.2.06.012 **81**
– – superior A12.2.06.017 **81**
– ileales A12.2.12.058 **88**
– ileocolica A12.2.12.059 **88**
– iliaca
– – communis A12.2.14.001 **89**
– – externa A12.2.16.002 **90**
– – interna A12.2.15.001 **89**
– iliolumbalis A12.2.15.002 **89**
– inferior
– – anterior cerebelli A12.2.08.019 **84**
– – lateralis genus A12.2.16.038 **90**
– – medialis genus A12.2.16.039 **90**
– – posterior cerebelli A12.2.08.012 **84**
– infraorbitalis A12.2.05.078 **81**
– insulares A12.2.07.054 **83**
– intercostales posteriores A12.2.11.007 **86**
– intercostalis
– – posterior
– – – prima A12.2.08.062 **85**
– – – secunda A12.2.08.063 **85**
– – suprema A12.2.08.061 **85**
– interlobares A08.1.03.002 **63**
– – renis A08.1.03.002 **63**
– interlobulares A05.8.01.057 **55**, A08.1.03.004 **63**
– – hepatis A05.8.01.057 **55**
– – renis A08.1.03.004 **63**
– interossea
– – anterior A12.2.09.048 **86**
– – communis A12.2.09.047 **86**
– – posterior A12.2.09.050 **86**
– – recurrens A12.2.09.052 **86**
– intrarenales A08.1.03.001 **63, 88**
– jejunales A12.2.12.057 **88**
– juxtacolica A12.2.12.068 **88**
– labialis
– – inferior A12.2.05.025 **80**
– – superior A12.2.05.026 **80**
– labyrinthi A12.2.08.020 **84, 153**
– lacrimalis A12.2.06.027 **81**
– laryngea
– – inferior A12.2.08.044 **85**
– – superior A12.2.05.005 **80**
– lienalis A12.2.12.040 **88**
– ligamenti teretis uteri ♀ A12.2.16.007 **90**
– lingualis A12.2.05.015 **80**
– lingularis A12.2.01.211 **78**
– – inferior A12.2.01.212 **79**
– – superior A12.2.01.213 **79**
– lobares
– – inferiores pulmonis
– – – dextri A12.2.01.113 **78**
– – – sinistri A12.2.01.214 **79**
– – superiores pulmonis
– – – dextri A12.2.01.102 **78**
– – – sinistri A12.2.01.203 **78**
– lobaris media pulmonis dextri A12.2.01.110 **78**
– lobi caudati A12.2.12.032 **87**, A12.2.12.036 **87**
– lumbales A12.2.12.004 **87**
– – imae A12.2.12.009 **87**
– malleolaris anterior
– – lateralis A12.2.16.045 **90**
– – medialis A12.2.16.046 **90**
– mammillares A12.2.07.078 **83**
– marginalis coli A12.2.12.068 **88**
– masseterica A12.2.05.070 **81**
– maxillaris A12.2.05.053 **80**

– media genus A12.2.16.036 **90**
– medullaris segmentalis
– – a. vertebralis A12.2.08.007 **84**
– – aa. intercostales posteriores A12.2.11.016 **87**
– – aa. lumbales A12.2.12.007 **87**
– membri
– – inferioris A12.2.16.001 **90**
– – superioris A12.2.09.001 **85**
– meningea
– – media A12.2.05.061 **80**
– – posterior A12.2.05.011 **80**
– mesencephalicae A12.2.08.024 **84**
– mesenterica
– – inferior A12.2.12.069 **88**
– – superior A12.2.12.053 **88**
– metacarpales
– – dorsales A12.2.09.034 **86**
– – palmares A12.2.09.039 **86**
– metatarsales
– – dorsales A12.2.16.052 **90**
– – plantares A12.2.16.066 **91**
– musculares A12.2.06.033 **82**
– musculophrenica A12.2.08.040 **85**
– nasales posteriores laterales A12.2.05.089 **81**
– nutricia/nutriens A12.0.00.004 **75**
– – fibulae A12.2.16.077 **91**
– – radii A12.2.09.029 **86**
– – tibiae A12.2.16.060 **91**
– – ulnae A12.2.09.046 **86**
– nutriciae/nutrientes
– – femoris A12.2.16.032 **90**
– – humeri A12.2.09.021 **86**
– obturatoria A12.2.15.008 **89**
– – accessoria A12.2.16.006 **90**
– occipitalis A12.2.05.030 **80**
– – lateralis A12.2.07.094 **84**
– – medialis A12.2.07.098 **84**
– ophthalmica A12.2.06.016 **81**
– orbitofrontalis
– – lateralis A12.2.07.062 **83**
– – medialis A12.2.07.035 **83**
– ovarica ♀ A12.2.12.086 **88**
– palatina
– – ascendens A12.2.05.021 **80**
– – descendens A12.2.05.084 **81**
– – major A12.2.05.085 **81**
– palatinae minores A12.2.05.086 **81**
– palpebrales
– – laterales A12.2.06.029 **82**
– – mediales A12.2.06.044 **82**
– pancreatica
– – dorsalis A12.2.12.042 **88**
– – inferior A12.2.12.043 **88**
– – magna A12.2.12.045 **88**
– pancreaticoduodenalis
– – inferior A12.2.12.054 **88**
– – superior
– – – anterior A12.2.12.025 **87**
– – – posterior A12.2.12.018 **87**
– parietalis
– – anterior A12.2.07.067 **83**
– – posterior A12.2.07.068 **83**
– perforantes A12.2.16.031 **90**
– – anteriores A12.2.07.027 **82**
– – penis ♂ A12.2.15.046 **89**
– – radiatae A08.1.03.007 **63**
– – – renis A08.1.03.007 **63**
– pericallosa A12.2.07.043 **83**
– pericardiacophrenica A12.2.08.034 **85**
– perinealis A12.2.15.040 **89**
– peronea A12.2.16.071 **91**
– pharyngea ascendens A12.2.05.010 **80**
– phrenica inferior A12.2.12.002 **87**
– phrenicae superiores A12.2.11.006 **86**
– plantaris
– – lateralis A12.2.16.064 **91**
– – medialis A12.2.16.061 **91**
– – profunda A12.2.16.054 **90**
– polaris
– – frontalis A12.2.07.036 **83**
– – temporalis A12.2.07.051 **83**
– pontis A12.2.08.021 **84**
– poplitea A12.2.16.033 **90**
– prefrontalis A12.2.07.063 **83**
– preopticae A12.2.07.028 **82**
– prepancreatica A12.2.12.044 **88**
– princeps pollicis A12.2.09.036 **86**
– profunda
– – brachii A12.2.09.020 **86**
– – clitoridis ♀ A12.2.15.045 **89**
– – femoris A12.2.16.020 **90**
– – linguae A12.2.05.019 **80**
– – penis ♂ A12.2.15.045 **89**
– pterygomeningea A12.2.05.069 **81**
– pudenda
– – externa
– – – profunda A12.2.16.014 **90**
– – – superficialis A12.2.16.013 **90**
– – interna A12.2.15.038 **89**
– pulmonalis
– – dextra A12.2.01.101 **78**
– – sinistra A12.2.01.201 **78**
– quadrigeminalis A12.2.07.087 **84**
– radialis A12.2.09.027 **86**
– – indicis A12.2.09.037 **86**
– radicularis
– – anterior A12.2.11.015 **87**
– – posterior A12.2.11.014 **87**
– rectalis
– – inferior A12.2.15.039 **89**
– – media A12.2.15.036 **89**
– – superior A12.2.12.073 **88**
– recurrens
– – radialis A12.2.09.028 **86**
– – tibialis
– – – anterior A12.2.16.043 **90**
– – – posterior A12.2.16.044 **90**
– – ulnaris A12.2.09.042 **86**
– renalis A12.2.12.075 **88**
– retroduodenales A12.2.12.021 **87**
– sacrales laterales A12.2.15.006 **89**
– sacralis mediana A12.2.12.008 **87**
– segmentalis
– – anterior pulmonis
– – – dextri A12.2.01.104 **78**
– – – sinistri A12.2.01.205 **78**
– – apicalis pulmonis
– – – dextri A12.2.01.103 **78**
– – – sinistri A12.2.01.204 **78**
– – basalis
– – – anterior pulmonis
– – – – dextri A12.2.01.116 **78**
– – – – sinistri A12.2.01.217 **79**
– – – lateralis pulmonis
– – – – dextri A12.2.01.117 **78**
– – – – sinistri A12.2.01.218 **79**
– – – medialis pulmonis
– – – – dextri A12.2.01.118 **78**
– – – – sinistri A12.2.01.219 **79**
– – – posterior pulmonis
– – – – dextri A12.2.01.119 **78**
– – – – sinistri A12.2.01.220 **79**
– – lateralis A12.2.01.112 **78**
– – medialis A12.2.01.111 **78**
– – posterior pulmonis
– – – dextri A12.2.01.107 **78**
– – – sinistri A12.2.01.208 **78**
– – superior pulmonis
– – – dextri A12.2.01.114 **78**
– – – sinistri A12.2.01.215 **79**
– segmenti
– – anterioris hepatici A12.2.12.033 **87**
– – – inferioris renalis A12.2.12.081 **88**
– – – superioris renalis A12.2.12.080 **88**
– – inferioris renalis A12.2.12.082 **88**
– – lateralis hepatici A12.2.12.038 **87**
– – medialis hepatici A12.2.12.037 **87**
– – posterioris
– – – hepatici A12.2.12.034 **87**
– – – renalis A12.2.12.084 **88**
– – superioris renalis A12.2.12.079 **88**
– sigmoideae A12.2.12.072 **88**
– sphenopalatina A12.2.05.088 **81**
– spinalis
– – anterior A12.2.08.016 **84**
– – posterior A12.2.08.013 **84**
– spiralis modioli A15.3.03.133 **153**
– splenica A12.2.12.040 **88**
– striata medialis distalis A12.2.07.034 **83**
– striatae mediales proximales A12.2.07.025 **82**
– stylomastoidea A12.2.05.038 **80**
– subclavia A12.2.08.001 **84**
– subcostalis A12.2.11.020 **87**
– sublingualis A12.2.05.018 **80**
– submentalis A12.2.05.023 **80**
– subscapularis A12.2.09.013 **85**
– sulci
– – centralis A12.2.07.065 **83**
– – postcentralis A12.2.07.066 **83**
– – precentralis A12.2.07.064 **83**
– superior
– – cerebelli A12.2.08.025 **84**

– – lateralis genus
A12.2.16.034 **90**
– – medialis genus
A12.2.16.035 **90**
– suprachiasmatica
A12.2.07.030 **82**
– supraduodenalis
A12.2.12.017 **87**
– supraoptica A12.2.07.026 **82**
– supraorbitalis A12.2.06.037 **82**
– suprarenales superiores
A12.2.12.003 **87**
– suprarenalis
– – inferior A12.2.12.077 **88**
– – media A12.2.12.074 **88**
– suprascapularis A12.2.08.051 **85**
– supratrochlearis
A12.2.06.048 **82**
– surales A12.2.16.037 **90**
– tarsales mediales
A12.2.16.050 **90**
– tarsalis lateralis A12.2.16.049 **90**
– temporalis
– – anterior A12.2.07.052 **83**
– – media A12.2.05.050 **80**
– – profunda
– – – anterior A12.2.05.071 **81**
– – – posterior A12.2.05.072 **81**
– – superficialis A12.2.05.045 **80**
– testicularis ♂ A12.2.12.086 **88**
– thalami perforans
A12.2.07.086 **84**
– thalamogeniculata
A12.2.07.090 **84**
– thalamotuberalis
A12.2.07.076 **83**
– thoracica
– – interna A12.2.08.029 **85**
– – lateralis A12.2.09.011 **85**
– – superior A12.2.09.004 **85**
– thoracoacromialis
A12.2.09.005 **85**
– thoracodorsalis A12.2.09.014 **85**
– thyroidea
– – ima A12.2.04.005 **79**
– – inferior A12.2.08.043 **85**
– – superior A12.2.05.002 **79**
– tibialis
– – anterior A12.2.16.042 **90**
– – posterior A12.2.16.055 **90**
– transversa
– – cervicis A12.2.08.053 **85**
– – colli A12.2.08.053 **85**
– – faciei A12.2.05.047 **80**
– tuberis cinerei A12.2.07.073 **83**
– tympanica
– – anterior A12.2.05.055 **80**
– – inferior A12.2.05.013 **80**
– – posterior A12.2.05.039 **80**
– – superior A12.2.05.067 **81**
– ulnaris A12.2.09.041 **86**
– umbilicalis A12.2.15.020 **89**
– uncalis A12.2.06.020 **81, 83**
– urethralis A12.2.15.042 **89**
– uterina ♀ A12.2.15.029 **89**
– vaginalis ♀ A12.2.15.035 **89**
– vermis superior A12.2.08.027 **85**
– vertebralis A12.2.08.002 **84**
– vesicales superiores
A12.2.15.024 **89**
– vesicalis inferior
A12.2.15.027 **89**
– vestibularis anterior
A15.3.03.127 **153**
– vestibuli A15.3.03.127 **153**
– vestibulocochlearis
A15.3.03.129 **153**
– zygomaticoorbitalis
A12.2.05.049 **80**
Arteriola/e A12.0.00.005 **75**
– glomerularis
– – afferens renis A08.1.03.005 **63**
– – efferens renis A08.1.03.006 **63**
– macularis
– – inferior A15.2.04.042 **146**
– – media A15.2.04.043 **146**
– – superior A15.2.04.041 **146**
– nasalis retinae
– – inferior A15.2.04.040 **146**
– – superior A15.2.04.039 **146**
– rectae renis A08.1.03.008 **63**
– temporalis retinae
– – inferior A15.2.04.038 **146**
– – superior A15.2.04.037 **146**
Articulatio/nes A03.0.00.020 **25**
– acromioclavicularis
A03.5.03.001 **28**
– atlantoaxialis
– – lateralis A03.2.05.001 **27**
– – mediana A03.2.04.001 **27**
– atlantooccipitalis
A03.1.08.001 **27**
– bicondylaris A03.0.00.047 **25**
– calcaneocuboidea
A03.6.10.204 **31**
– capitis costae A03.3.04.002 **28**
– carpi A03.5.11.101 **29**
– carpometacarpales
A03.5.11.301 **29**
– carpometacarpalis pollicis
A03.5.11.304 **29**
– cinguli
– – membri superioris
A03.5.02.001 **28**
– – pectoralis A03.5.02.001 **28**
– columnae vertebralis
A03.2.03.001 **27**
– composita A03.0.00.042 **25**
– costochondrales
A03.3.06.001 **28**
– costotransversaria
A03.3.04.005 **28**
– costovertebrales
A03.3.04.001 **28**
– cotylica A03.0.00.051 **25**
– coxae A03.6.07.001 **30**
– coxofemoralis A03.6.07.001 **30**
– cranii A03.1.06.001 **27**
– cricoarytenoidea
A06.2.04.014 **58**
– cricothyroidea A06.2.03.006 **58**
– cubiti A03.5.09.001 **29**
– cuneonavicularis
A03.6.10.301 **31**
– cylindrica A03.0.00.044 **25**
– ellipsoidea A03.0.00.049 **25**
– genus A03.6.08.001 **30**
– glenohumeralis A03.5.08.001 **29**
– humeri A03.5.08.001 **29**
– humeroradialis A03.5.09.003 **29**
– humeroulnaris A03.5.09.002 **29**
– incudomallearis
A15.3.02.050 **150**
– incudostapedialis
A15.3.02.051 **150**
– intercarpales A03.5.11.101 **29**
– interchondrales A03.3.07.001 **28**
– intercuneiformes
A03.6.10.401 **31**
– intermetacarpales
A03.5.11.401 **29**
– intermetatarsales
A03.6.10.701 **32**
– interphalangeae
– – manus A03.5.11.601 **30**
– – pedis A03.6.10.901 **32**
– lumbosacralis A03.2.07.001 **27**
– manus A03.5.11.001 **29**
– mediocarpalis A03.5.11.102 **29**
– membri
– – inferioris liberi
A03.6.06.001 **30**
– – superioris liberi
A03.5.07.001 **29**
– metacarpophalangeae
A03.5.11.501 **30**
– metatarsophalangeae
A03.6.10.801 **32**
– ossiculorum auditus/
auditoriorum
A15.3.02.049 **150**
– ossis pisiformis A03.5.11.107 **29**
– pedis A03.6.10.001 **31**
– plana A03.0.00.043 **25**
– radiocarpalis A03.5.11.002 **29**
– radioulnaris
– – distalis A03.5.10.001 **29**
– – proximalis A03.5.09.004 **29**
– sacrococcygea A03.2.08.001 **27**
– sacroiliaca A03.6.03.001 **30**
– sellaris A03.0.00.048 **25**
– simplex A03.0.00.041 **25**
– spheroidea A03.0.00.050 **25**
– sternoclavicularis
A03.5.04.001 **29**
– sternocostales A03.3.05.001 **28**
– subtalaris A03.6.10.101 **31**
– talocalcanea A03.6.10.101 **31**
– talocalcaneonavicularis
A03.6.10.202 **31**
– talocruralis A03.6.10.002 **31**
– tarsi transversa A03.6.10.201 **31**
– tarsometatarsales
A03.6.10.601 **31**
– temporomandibularis
A03.1.07.001 **27**
– thoracis A03.3.03.001 **28**
– tibiofibularis A03.6.09.001 **31**
– trochoidea A03.0.00.045 **25**
– zygapophysiales
A03.2.06.001 **27**
Asterion A02.1.00.020 **8**
Atlas [C I] A02.2.02.101 **16**
Atrium
– cordis
– – dextrum A12.1.00.017 **76**

– – sinistrum A12.1.03.001 **77**
– meatus medii A06.1.02.025 **57**
– ventriculi lateralis A14.1.09.281 **127**
Auricula A15.3.01.002 **148**
– atrii
– – dextra A12.1.01.002 **76**
– – sinistra A12.1.03.002 **77**
Auris A01.1.00.005 **2**
– externa A15.3.01.001 **148**
– interna A15.3.03.001 **151**
– media A15.3.02.001 **149**
Axialis A01.0.00.029 **1**
Axilla A01.1.00.021 **2**
Axis
– externus bulbi oculi A15.2.01.006 **144**
– internus bulbi oculi A15.2.01.007 **144**
– lentis A15.2.05.012 **146**
– opticus A15.2.01.008 **144**
– pelvis A02.5.02.010 **22**
– [C II] A02.2.02.201 **17**

B

Barba A16.0.00.018 **154**
Basalis A01.0.00.023 **1**
Basilaris A01.0.00.024 **1**
Basion A02.1.04.003 **10**
Basis
– cartilaginis arytenoideae A06.2.04.003 **58**
– cochleae A15.3.03.027 **151**
– cordis A12.1.00.002 **75**
– cornu posterioris medullae spinalis A14.1.02.123 **106**
– cranii A02.1.00.044 **8**
– – externa A02.1.00.053 **8**
– – interna A02.1.00.045 **8**
– mandibulae A02.1.15.003 **15**
– modioli A15.3.03.039 **151**
– – cochleae A15.3.03.039 **151**
– ossis
– – metacarpi A02.4.09.002 **20**
– – metatarsi A02.5.17.002 **24**
– – sacri A02.2.05.002 **17**
– patellae A02.5.05.002 **23**
– pedunculi A14.1.06.101 **116**
– phalangis
– – manus A02.4.10.006 **21**
– – pedis A02.5.18.006 **24**
– prostatae A09.3.08.002 **68**
– pulmonis A06.5.01.004 **60**
– stapedis A15.3.02.037 **150**
Bifurcatio
– aortae A12.2.13.001 **89**
– carotidis A12.2.04.009 **79**
– tracheae A06.3.01.008 **59**
– trunci pulmonalis A12.2.01.004 **78**
Brachium A01.1.00.022 **2**
– colliculi
– – inferioris A14.1.06.012 **115, 118, 122**
– – superioris A14.1.06.013 **115, 118, 122**
Bregma A02.1.00.016 **8**
Bronchioli A06.5.02.026 **61**
Bronchus/i A06.4.01.001 **59**
– cardiacus
– – dexter [B VII] A06.4.02.011 **60**
– – sinister [B VII] A06.4.02.022 **60**
– intrasegmentales A06.4.02.026 **60**
– lingularis
– – inferior [B V] A06.4.02.019 **60**
– – superior [B IV] A06.4.02.018 **60**
– lobares et segmentales A06.4.02.001 **60**
– lobaris
– – inferior
– – – dexter A06.4.02.009 **60**
– – – sinister A06.4.02.020 **60**
– – medius A06.4.02.006 **60**
– – superior
– – – dexter A06.4.02.002 **60**
– – – sinister A06.4.02.015 **60**
– principalis
– – dexter A06.4.01.003 **59**
– – sinister A06.4.01.004 **59**
– segmentalis
– – anterior
– – – dexter [B III] A06.4.02.005 **60**
– – – sinister [B III] A06.4.02.017 **60**
– – apicalis [B I] A06.4.02.003 **60**
– – apicoposterior [B I+II] A06.4.02.016 **60**
– – basalis
– – – anterior
– – – – dexter [B VIII] A06.4.02.012 **60**
– – – – sinister [B VIII] A06.4.02.023 **60**
– – – lateralis
– – – – dexter [B IX] A06.4.02.013 **60**
– – – – sinister [B IX] A06.4.02.024 **60**
– – – medialis
– – – – dexter A06.4.02.011 **60**
– – – – sinister A06.4.02.022 **60**
– – – posterior
– – – – dexter [B X] A06.4.02.014 **60**
– – – – sinister [B X] A06.4.02.025 **60**
– – lateralis [B IV] A06.4.02.007 **60**
– – medialis [B V] A06.4.02.008 **60**
– – posterior [B II] A06.4.02.004 **60**
– – superior [B VI] A06.4.02.010 **60**
Bucca A01.1.00.008 **2**, A05.1.01.014 **47**
Bulbus
– aortae A12.2.03.004 **79**
– cornus posterioris ventriculi lateralis A14.1.09.284 **127**
– duodeni A05.6.02.003 **52**
– inferior venae jugularis A12.3.05.005 **93**
– oculi A15.2.01.001 **144**
– olfactorius A14.1.09.429 **129**
– penis A09.4.01.016 **69**
– rhombencephali A14.1.03.003 **108**
– superior venae jugularis A12.3.05.002 **93**
– vestibuli A09.2.01.013 **67**
Bulla ethmoidalis A02.1.07.015 **13**, A06.1.02.026 **57**
Bursa/e
– anserina A04.8.05.022 **45**
– bicipitoradialis A04.8.03.014 **44**
– colli A04.8.02.001 **44**
– cubitalis interossea A04.8.03.015 **44**
– iliopectinea A04.8.05.011 **45**
– infrahyoidea A04.8.02.004 **44**, A06.2.02.016 **58**
– infrapatellaris profunda A04.8.05.019 **45**
– intermusculares musculorum gluteorum A04.8.05.009 **45**
– intratendinea olecrani A04.8.03.012 **44**
– ischiadica musculi
– – glutei maximi A04.8.05.010 **45**
– – obturatorii interni A04.8.05.007 **45**
– membri
– – inferioris A04.8.05.001 **45**
– – superioris A04.8.03.001 **44**
– musculi
– – bicipitis femoris superior A04.8.05.013 **45**
– – coracobrachialis A04.8.03.006 **44**
– – piriformis A04.8.05.006 **45**
– – semimembranosi A04.8.05.027 **45**
– – tensoris veli palatini A04.8.02.002 **44**
– omentalis A10.1.02.402 **72**
– pharyngealis A05.3.01.010 **50**
– retrohyoidea A04.8.02.005 **44**, A06.2.02.015 **58**
– subacromialis A04.8.03.004 **44**
– subcutanea A04.8.01.001 **44**
– – acromialis A04.8.03.003 **44**
– – calcanea A04.8.05.031 **45**
– – infrapatellaris A04.8.05.018 **45**
– – malleoli
– – – lateralis A04.8.05.028 **45**
– – – medialis A04.8.05.029 **45**
– – olecrani A04.8.03.011 **44**
– – prepatellaris A04.8.05.014 **45**
– – prominentiae laryngeae A04.8.02.003 **44**
– – trochanterica A04.8.05.002 **45**
– – tuberositatis tibiae A04.8.05.020 **45**
– subdeltoidea A04.8.03.005 **44**
– subfascialis A04.8.01.003 **44**
– – prepatellaris A04.8.05.015 **45**
– submuscularis A04.8.01.002 **44**
– subtendinea A04.8.01.004 **44**
– – iliaca A04.8.05.012 **45**
– – musculi
– – – bicipitis femoris inferior A04.8.05.023 **45**

– – – gastrocnemii
– – – – lateralis A04.8.05.025 **45**
– – – – medialis A04.8.05.026 **45**
– – – infraspinati A04.8.03.007 **44**
– – – latissimi dorsi
A04.8.03.010 **44**
– – – obturatorii interni
A04.8.05.008 **45**
– – – subscapularis
A04.8.03.008 **44**
– – – teretis majoris
A04.8.03.009 **44**
– – – tibialis anterioris
A04.8.05.030 **45**
– – – trapezii A04.8.03.002 **44**
– – – tricipitis brachii
A04.8.03.013 **44**
– – prepatellaris A04.8.05.016 **45**
– subtendineae musculi sartorii
A04.8.05.021 **45**
– suprapatellaris A04.8.05.017 **45**
– synovialis A03.0.00.039 **25, 34**
– tendinis calcanei
A04.8.05.032 **45**
– trochanterica/e musculi glutei
– – maximi A04.8.05.003 **45**
– – medii A04.8.05.004 **45**
– – minimi A04.8.05.005 **45**

C

CA1 A14.1.09.328 **128**
CA2 A14.1.09.329 **128**
CA3 A14.1.09.330 **128**
CA4 A14.1.09.331 **128**
Caecum A05.7.02.001 **53**
– cupulare A15.3.03.120 **153**
– vestibulare A15.3.03.109 **153**
Calcaneus A02.5.11.001 **24**
Calcar
– avis A14.1.09.285 **128**
– sclerae A15.2.02.007 **144**
Calices renales
– majores A08.1.05.003 **64**
– minores A08.1.05.007 **64**
Caliculus gustatorius
A15.4.00.002 **153**
Calvaria A02.1.00.032 **8**
Calx A01.1.00.042 **2**
Calyx/ces
– inferior renis A08.1.05.006 **64**
– medius renis A08.1.05.005 **64**
– superior renis A08.1.05.004 **64**
Camera/e
– anterior bulbi oculi
A15.2.06.003 **146**
– bulbi oculi A15.2.06.001 **146**
– posterior bulbi oculi
A15.2.06.005 **146**
– postrema bulbi oculi
A15.2.06.006 **146**
– vitrea bulbi oculi
A15.2.06.006 **146**
Canaliculus/i
– caroticotympanici
A02.1.06.016 **12**
– chordae tympani
A02.1.06.011 **12**
– cochleae A02.1.06.042 **12**
– lacrimalis A15.2.07.066 **148**
– mastoideus A02.1.06.044 **13**
– tympanicus A02.1.06.049 **13**
– vestibuli A02.1.06.035 **12**
Canalis/es
– adductorius A04.7.03.006 **43**
– alveolares corporis maxillae
A02.1.12.015 **14**
– analis A05.7.05.001 **54**
– arteriae vertebralis
A02.2.02.110 **17**
– caroticus A02.1.06.013 **12**
– carpi A03.5.11.201 **29**
– centralis medullae spinalis
A14.1.02.019 **106, 108**
– cervicis uteri A09.1.03.018 **66**
– condylaris A02.1.04.015 **10**
– diploici A02.1.00.036 **8**
– femoralis A04.7.03.012 **43**
– gastricus A05.5.01.013 **52**
– hyaloideus A15.2.06.010 **146**
– incisivi A02.1.00.061 **9, 14**
– infraorbitalis A02.1.12.004 **14**
– inguinalis A04.5.01.026 **38**
– longitudinales modioli cochleae
A15.3.03.042 **151**
– mandibulae A02.1.15.030 **15**
– musculotubarius
A02.1.06.017 **12**
– nasolacrimalis A02.1.00.085 **9**
– nervi
– – facialis A02.1.06.009 **12**
– – hypoglossi A02.1.04.016 **10**
– nutricius/nutriens
A02.0.00.042 **7**
– obturatorius A03.6.01.003 **30**
– opticus A02.1.05.021 **11**
– palatini minores A02.1.13.008 **15**
– palatinus major A02.1.00.057 **9**
– palatovaginalis A02.1.00.064 **9**
– pterygoideus A02.1.05.053 **12**
– pudendalis A09.5.04.003 **71**
– pyloricus A05.5.01.016 **52**
– radicis dentis A05.1.03.049 **48**
– sacralis A02.2.05.019 **17**
– semicirculares A15.3.03.015 **151**
– semicircularis
– – anterior A15.3.03.016 **151**
– – lateralis A15.3.03.022 **151**
– – posterior A15.3.03.018 **151**
– spiralis
– – cochleae A15.3.03.028 **151**
– – modioli A15.3.03.041 **151**
– ulnaris A03.5.11.202 **29**
– vertebralis A02.2.00.009 **16**
– vomerorostralis A02.1.00.066 **9**
– vomerovaginalis A02.1.00.065 **9**
Capilli A16.0.00.016 **154**
Capitulum humeri
A02.4.04.022 **19**
Capsula
– adiposa perirenalis
A08.1.01.012 **63**
– articularis A03.0.00.026 **25**
– – cricoarytenoidea
A06.2.04.015 **58**
– – cricothyroidea
A06.2.03.007 **58**
– externa A14.1.09.551 **131**
– extrema A14.1.09.552 **131**
– fibrosa
– – glandulae thyroideae
A11.3.00.006 **74**
– – perivascularis hepatis
A05.8.01.055 **55**
– – renis A08.1.01.013 **63**
– ganglii A14.2.00.003 **132**
– interna A14.1.09.524 **130**
– lentis A15.2.05.007 **146**
– nodi lymphoidei
A13.2.03.002 **100, 137**
– prostatica A09.3.08.017 **69**
– splenica A13.2.01.002 **100**
– tonsillae/tonsillaris
A05.2.01.012 **50, 100**
Caput A01.1.00.001 **2**,
A04.0.00.001 **33**
– articulare A03.0.00.024 **25**
– breve m. bicipitis
– – brachii A04.6.02.015 **40**
– – femoris A04.7.02.034 **42**
– cornu posterioris medullae
spinalis A14.1.02.118 **106**
– costae A02.3.02.002 **18**
– epididymidis A09.3.02.002 **68**
– femoris A02.5.04.002 **22**
– fibulae A02.5.07.002 **23**
– humerale
– – m. extensoris carpi ulnaris
A04.6.02.046 **41**
– – m. flexoris carpi ulnaris
A04.6.02.031 **41**
– – m. pronatoris teretis
A04.6.02.026 **40**
– humeri A02.4.04.002 **19**
– humeroulnare m. flexoris digitorum superficialis
A04.6.02.034 **41**
– inferius m. pterygoidei lateralis
A04.1.04.008 **35**
– laterale
– – m. flexoris hallucis brevis
A04.7.02.059 **43**
– – m. gastrocnemii
A04.7.02.045 **43**
– – m. tricipitis brachii
A04.6.02.021 **40**
– longum
– – m. bicipitis
– – – brachii A04.6.02.014 **40**
– – – femoris A04.7.02.033 **42**
– – m. tricipitis brachii
A04.6.02.020 **40**
– mallei A15.3.02.045 **150**
– mandibulae A02.1.15.036 **16**
– mediale
– – m. flexoris hallucis brevis
A04.7.02.058 **43**
– – m. gastrocnemii
A04.7.02.046 **43**
– – m. tricipitis brachii
A04.6.02.022 **40**
– nuclei caudati A14.1.09.503 **130**
– obliquum m. adductoris
– – hallucis A04.7.02.061 **43**
– – pollicis A04.6.02.060 **41**
– ossis
– – metacarpi A02.4.09.004 **20**

– – metatarsi A02.5.17.004 **24**
– pancreatis A05.9.01.002 **56**
– phalangis
– – manus A02.4.10.008 **21**
– – pedis A02.5.18.008 **24**
– profundum A04.6.02.022 **40**, A04.6.02.057 **41**
– – m. flexoris pollicis brevis A04.6.02.057 **41**
– – m. tricipitis brachii A04.6.02.022 **40**
– radiale m. flexoris digitorum superficialis A04.6.02.035 **41**
– radii A02.4.05.002 **19**
– rectum m. rectus femoris A04.7.02.019 **42**
– reflexum m. rectus femoris A04.7.02.020 **42**
– stapedis A15.3.02.034 **149**
– superficiale m. flexoris pollicis brevis A04.6.02.056 **41**
– superius m. pterygoidea lateralis A04.1.04.007 **35**
– tali A02.5.10.002 **23**
– transversum m. adductoris
– – hallucis A04.7.02.062 **43**
– – pollicis A04.6.02.061 **41**
– ulnae A02.4.06.015 **20**
– ulnare
– – m. extensoris carpi ulnaris A04.6.02.047 **41**
– – m. flexoris carpi ulnaris A04.6.02.032 **41**
– – m. pronatoris teretis A04.6.02.027 **41**
Cardia A05.5.01.007 **51**
Carina
– tracheae A06.3.01.009 **59**
– urethralis vaginae A09.1.04.016 **66**
Carpus A01.1.00.026 **2**
Cartilago/ines
– alares minores nasi A06.1.01.011 **57**
– alaris major nasi A06.1.01.007 **57**
– arytenoidea A06.2.04.001 **58**
– auriculae A15.3.01.004 **148**
– corniculata A06.2.05.001 **58**
– costalis A02.3.01.005 **17**
– cricoidea A06.2.03.001 **58**
– cuneiformis A06.2.06.001 **58**
– epiglottica A06.2.07.002 **58**
– epiphysialis A02.0.00.019 **7**, A03.0.00.018 **25**
– et articulationes laryngis A06.2.02.001 **58**
– meatus acustici A15.3.01.049 **149**
– nasi A06.1.01.006 **57**
– – accessoriae A06.1.01.012 **57**
– septi nasi A06.1.01.013 **57**
– sesamoidea lig. cricopharyngei A06.2.04.018 **58**
– thyroidea A06.2.02.002 **58**
– tracheales A06.3.01.004 **59**
– triticea A06.2.02.018 **58**
– tubae auditivae/auditoriae A15.3.02.079 **150**
– vomeronasalis A06.1.01.016 **57**
Caruncula/e
– hymenales A09.1.04.009 **66**
– lacrimalis A15.2.07.049 **147**
– sublingualis A05.1.01.112 **47**
Cauda
– epididymidis A09.3.02.005 **68**
– equina A14.2.00.036 **133**
– helicis A15.3.01.008 **148**
– nuclei caudati A14.1.09.505 **130**
– pancreatis A05.9.01.014 **56**
Caudalis A01.0.00.020 **1**
Cavea thoracis A02.3.04.001 **18**
Cavernae
– corporis spongiosi A09.4.01.023 **69**
– corporum cavernosorum A09.4.01.022 **69**
Cavitas/tes A01.1.00.047 **2**
– abdominis/abdominalis A01.1.00.051 **2**, A10.1.00.001 **72**
– – et pelvis A01.1.00.050 **2**, A10.1.00.000 **72**
– articularis A03.0.00.022 **25**
– conchae A15.3.01.015 **148**
– coronae A05.1.03.048 **48**
– cranii A01.1.00.048 **2**, A02.1.00.012 **8**
– dentis A05.1.03.047 **48**
– glenoidalis scapulae A02.4.01.019 **19**
– infraglottica A06.2.09.018 **59**
– laryngis A06.2.09.001 **59**
– medullaris A02.0.00.037 **7**
– nasalis ossea A02.1.00.086 **9**
– nasi A06.1.02.001 **57**
– orbitalis A02.1.00.068 **9**
– oris A05.1.01.001 **47**
– – propria A05.1.01.101 **47**
– pelvina A10.1.00.002 **72**
– pelvis A01.1.00.052 **2**, A02.5.02.002 **22**, A10.1.00.002 **72**
– pericardiaca/pericardialis A07.1.03.001 **62**, A06.6.03.001 **77**
– peritonealis A10.1.02.001 **72**
– pharyngis A05.3.01.002 **50**
– pleuralis A07.1.01.001 **62**
– pulparis A05.1.03.047 **48**
– thoracica/thoracis A01.1.00.049 **2**, A02.3.04.002 **18, 62**
– tympani A02.1.06.051 **13**, A15.3.02.002 **149**
– uteri A09.1.03.007 **65**
Cavum A14.1.09.263 **127**
– conchae A15.3.01.015 **148**
– septi pellucidi A14.1.09.263 **127**
– trigeminale A14.1.01.108 **104**
Cellulae
– adrenergicae areae postremae et nuclei reticularis anterioris [C1, C2] A14.1.09.628 **132**
– aminergicae A14.1.09.602 **131**
– – areae tegmentalis ventralis [A10] A14.1.09.613 **131**
– – formationis reticularis A14.1.09.607 **131**
– – partis compactae substantiae nigrae [A9] A14.1.09.610 **131**
– cholinergicae A14.1.09.629 **132**
– – areae tegmentalis dorsalis [Ch5, Ch6, Ch8] A14.1.09.634 **132**
– – epithalamicae [Ch7] A14.1.09.635 **132**
– – globi pallidi, nuclei accumbentis et
– – – gyri diagonalis [Ch2] A14.1.09.631 **132**
– – – striae diagonalis [Ch3] A14.1.09.632 **132**
– – nuclei septi medialis [Ch1] A14.1.09.630 **132**
– – substantiae innominatae, nuclei basalis, corporis amygdaloidei et tuberculi olfactorii [Ch4] A14.1.09.633 **132**
– dopaminergicae
– – areae
– – – hypothalamicae posterioris [A11] A14.1.09.616 **132**
– – – tegmentalis ventralis A14.1.09.614 **131**
– – bulbi olfactorii [A15] A14.1.09.620 **132**
– – formationis reticularis A14.1.09.608 **131**
– – nuclei arcuati [A12] A14.1.09.617 **132**
– – partis compactae substantiae nigrae A14.1.09.611 **131**
– – zonae
– – – incertae [A13] A14.1.09.618 **132**
– – – medialis et areae anterioris hypothalamicae [A14] A14.1.09.619 **132**
– ethmoidales A06.1.03.005 **57**
– – anteriores A02.1.07.008 **13**, A06.1.03.006 **57**
– – mediae A02.1.07.009 **13**, A06.1.03.007 **58**
– – posteriores A02.1.07.010 **13**, A06.1.03.008 **58**
– mastoideae A15.3.02.029 **149**
– noradrenergicae
– – areae tegmentalis ventralis A14.1.09.615 **131**
– – caudalis lateralis [A5] A14.1.09.606 **131**
– – formationis reticularis A14.1.09.609 **131**
– – loci caerulei [A6] A14.1.09.605 **131**
– – medullae oblongatae [A1, A2] A14.1.09.603 **131**
– – nuclei lemnisci lateralis [A7] A14.1.09.604 **131**
– – partis compactae substantiae nigrae A14.1.09.612 **131**
– pneumaticae A15.3.02.077 **150**
– serotoninergicae
– – nuclei raphes
– – – dorsalis [B7] A14.1.09.627 **132**
– – – magni [B3] A14.1.09.623 **132**

– – – mediani [B6] A14.1.09.626 **132**
– – – obscuri [B2] A14.1.09.622 **132**
– – – pallidi [B1] A14.1.09.621 **132**
– – – pontis [B5] A14.1.09.625 **132**
– – vicinae nuclei vestibularis medialis et nuclei prepositi [B4] A14.1.09.624 **132**
– tympanicae A15.3.02.030 **149**
Cementum A03.1.03.007 **26**, A05.1.03.057 **48**
Centralis A01.0.00.037 **1**
Centrum
– ossificationis A02.0.00.043 **7**
– perinei A09.5.00.005 **71**
– tendineum diaphragmatis A04.4.02.013 **38**
Cerebellum A14.1.07.001 **118**
Cerebrum A14.1.09.001 **124**
Cervix A01.1.00.012 **2**
– cornu posterioris medullae spinalis A14.1.02.120 **106**
– dentis A05.1.03.030 **48**
– uteri A09.1.03.010 **65**
– vesicae A08.3.01.005 **64**
Chiasma
– opticum A14.1.08.403 **120**
– tendinum digitorum manus A04.6.03.014 **41**
Choana/e A02.1.00.096 **9**, A06.1.02.003 **57**
Chondrocranium A02.1.00.009 **8**
Chorda/e
– a. umbilicalis A12.2.15.026 **89**
– obliqua membranae interossei antebrachii A03.5.06.003 **29**
– tendineae cordis A12.1.00.023 **76**
– – falsae A12.1.00.024 **76**
– – spuriae A12.1.00.024 **76**
– tympani A14.2.01.084 **135**, A14.2.01.118 **135, 142**, A14.3.02.012 **142**
Choroidea A15.2.03.002 **144**
Cilia A15.2.07.037 **147**, A15.2.07.038 **147, 154**
Cingulum
– dentis A05.1.03.044 **48**
– membri
– – inferioris A01.1.00.032 **2**, A02.5.00.002 **21**
– – superioris A01.1.00.020 **2**, A02.4.00.002 **18**
– pectorale A01.1.00.020 **2**, A02.4.00.002 **18**
– pelvicum A01.1.00.032 **2**, A02.5.00.002 **21**
– prosencephali A14.1.09.555 **131**
Circulus
– arteriosus A12.0.00.006 **75**
– – cerebri A12.2.07.080 **83**
– – iridis
– – – major A15.2.03.034 **145**
– – – minor A15.2.03.035 **145**
– vasculosus A12.0.00.007 **75**
– – nervi optici A15.2.04.036 **146**
Circumductio A03.0.00.057 **26**
Circumferentia articularis capitis
– radii A02.4.05.004 **20**
– ulnae A02.4.06.016 **20**
Cisterna/e A12.0.00.008 **75**
– ambiens A14.1.01.213 **105**
– cerebellomedullaris
– – lateralis A14.1.01.209 **105**
– – posterior A14.1.01.208 **105**
– chiasmatica A14.1.01.211 **105**
– chyli A12.4.01.012 **99**
– fossae lateralis cerebri A14.1.01.210 **105**
– interpeduncularis A14.1.01.212 **105**
– laminae terminalis A14.1.01.216 **105**
– lumbalis A14.1.01.219 **105**
– magna A14.1.01.208 **105**
– pericallosa A14.1.01.214 **105**
– pontocerebellaris A14.1.01.215 **105**
– quadrigeminalis A14.1.01.217 **105**
– subarachnoideae A14.1.01.207 **105**
– venae magnae cerebri A14.1.01.217 **105**
Claustrum A14.1.09.421 **129**
Clavicula A02.4.02.001 **19**
Clitoris A09.2.02.001 **67**
Clivus A02.1.00.051 **8**, A02.1.04.006 **10**
Clunes A01.1.00.033 **2**
Coccyx [vertebrae coccygeae I–IV] A02.2.06.001 **17**
Cochlea A15.3.03.025 **151**
Colliculus A06.2.04.007 **58**
– cartilaginis arytenoideae A06.2.04.007 **58**
– facialis A14.1.05.705 **115**
– inferior A14.1.06.014 **115, 118**
– seminalis A09.4.02.008 **70**
– superior A14.1.06.015 **115, 118**
Collum A01.1.00.012 **2**
– anatomicum humeri A02.4.04.003 **19**
– chirurgicum humeri A02.4.04.004 **19**
– costae A02.3.02.005 **18**
– femoris A02.5.04.004 **22**
– fibulae A02.5.07.005 **23**
– glandis penis A09.4.01.010 **69**
– mallei A15.3.02.046 **150**
– mandibulae A02.1.15.037 **16**
– pancreatis A05.9.01.005 **56**
– radii A02.4.05.005 **20**
– scapulae A02.4.01.022 **19**
– tali A02.5.10.007 **24**
– vesicae A08.3.01.005 **64**
– – biliaris/felleae A05.8.02.005 **56**
Colon A05.7.03.001 **53**
– ascendens A05.7.03.002 **53**
– descendens A05.7.03.006 **53**
– sigmoideum A05.7.03.007 **53**
– transversum A05.7.03.004 **53**
Columna/e A14.1.00.007 **104**
– anales A05.7.05.004 **54**
– anterior A14.1.02.102 **106**
– fornicis A14.1.08.420 **121, 127**
– grisea/e
– – anterior medullae spinalis A14.1.02.102 **106**
– – intermedia medullae spinalis A14.1.02.130 **106**
– – medullae spinalis A14.1.02.101 **106**
– – posterior medullae spinalis A14.1.02.114 **106**
– renales A08.1.01.019 **63**
– rugarum A09.1.04.013 **66**
– – anterior A09.1.04.014 **66**
– – posterior A09.1.04.015 **66**
– vertebralis A02.2.00.001 **16**
Commissura/e A14.1.00.013 **104**
– alba
– – anterior medullae spinalis A14.1.02.305 **108**
– – posterior medullae spinalis A14.1.02.306 **108**
– anterior A14.1.08.421 **121, 127, 131**
– bulborum vestibuli A09.2.01.014 **67**
– cerebelli A14.1.07.419 **120**
– cochlearis pontis A14.1.05.324 **113**
– colliculi
– – inferioris A14.1.06.613 **118**
– – superioris A14.1.06.614 **118**
– epithalamica A14.1.08.416 **121**
– fornicis A14.1.09.260 **127**
– grisea
– – anterior medullae spinalis A14.1.02.303 **108**
– – posterior medullae spinalis A14.1.02.304 **108**
– habenularum A14.1.08.414 **121**
– hippocampi A14.1.09.571 **131**
– labiorum
– – anterior A09.2.01.004 **66**
– – oris A05.1.01.012 **47**
– – posterior A09.2.01.005 **66**
– lateralis palpebrarum A15.2.07.031 **147**
– medialis palpebrarum A15.2.07.032 **147**
– posterior A14.1.08.416 **121**
– prostatae A09.3.08.016 **69**
– supraoptica
– – dorsalis A14.1.08.947 **124**
– – ventralis A14.1.08.959 **124**
– valvularum semilunarium valvae
– – aortae A12.1.04.018 **77**
– – trunci pulmonalis A12.1.02.016 **77**
Compartimentum/a A04.0.00.030 **33**, A04.6.01.001 **40**, A04.7.01.001 **42**
– antebrachii
– – anterius A04.6.01.004 **40**
– – extensorum A04.6.01.007 **40**
– – flexorum A04.6.01.004 **40**
– – posterius A04.6.01.007 **40**
– brachii
– – anterius A04.6.01.002 **40**
– – extensorum A04.6.01.003 **40**
– – flexorum A04.6.01.002 **40**
– – posterius A04.6.01.003 **40**

– cruris
– – anterius A04.7.01.005 **42**
– – extensorum A04.7.01.005 **42**
– – fibularium A04.7.01.009 **42**
– – flexorum A04.7.01.006 **42**
– – laterale A04.7.01.009 **42**
– – peroneorum A04.7.01.009 **42**
– – posterius A04.7.01.006 **42**
– femoris
– – adductorum A04.7.01.004 **42**
– – anterius A04.7.01.002 **42**
– – extensorum A04.7.01.002 **42**
– – flexorum A04.7.01.003 **42**
– – mediale A04.7.01.004 **42**
– – posterius A04.7.01.003 **42**
– superficiale perinei A09.5.02.001 **71**
Complexus
– olivaris inferior A14.1.04.219 **110**
– stimulans cordis A12.1.06.002 **77**
Concha
– auriculae A15.3.01.013 **148**
– nasalis/nasi
– – inferior A02.1.08.001 **13**, A06.1.02.015 **57**
– – media A02.1.07.014 **13**, A06.1.02.014 **57**
– – superior A02.1.07.013 **13**, A06.1.02.013 **57**
– – suprema A02.1.07.012 **13**, A06.1.02.012 **57**
– sphenoidalis A02.1.05.019 **11**
Condylus A02.0.00.029 **7**
– humeri A02.4.04.021 **19**
– lateralis
– – femoris A02.5.04.024 **22**
– – tibiae A02.5.06.004 **23**
– mandibulae A02.1.15.036 **16**
– medialis
– – femoris A02.5.04.021 **22**
– – tibiae A02.5.06.003 **23**
– occipitalis A02.1.04.014 **10**
Confluens sinuum A12.3.05.103 **93**
Conjugata
– anatomica A02.5.02.013 **22**
– diagonalis A02.5.02.015 **22**
– externa A02.5.02.018 **22**
– mediana A02.5.02.017 **22**
– recta A02.5.02.016 **22**
– vera A02.5.02.014 **22**
Connexus intertendinei m. extensoris digitorum A04.6.02.043 **41**
Constrictio
– bronchoaortica oesophageae A05.4.01.004 **51**
– diaphragmatica oesophageae A05.4.01.005 **51**
– partis thoracicae oesophageae A05.4.01.004 **51**
– pharyngooesophagealis A05.3.01.026 **50**
– phrenica oesophageae A05.4.01.005 **51**
Conus/i
– arteriosus A12.1.02.008 **76**
– elasticus A06.2.09.024 **59**
– epididymidis A09.3.02.003 **68**
– medullaris A14.1.02.004 **105**
Cor A12.1.00.001 **75**
Corium A16.0.00.010 **154**
Cornea A15.2.02.012 **144**
Cornu
– ammonis A14.1.09.327 **128**
– anterius
– – medullae spinalis A14.1.02.021 **106**, A14.1.02.103 **106**
– – ventriculi lateralis A14.1.09.273 **127**
– coccygeum A02.2.06.002 **17**
– frontale ventriculi lateralis A14.1.09.273 **127**
– inferius
– – cartilaginis thyroidea A06.2.02.011 **58**
– – marginis falciformis hiatus saphenus A04.7.03.019 **43**
– – ventriculi lateralis A14.1.09.287 **128**
– laterale medullae spinalis A14.1.02.022 **106**, A14.1.02.132 **106**
– majus ossis hyoidei A02.1.16.004 **16**
– minus ossis hyoidei A02.1.16.003 **16**
– occipitale ventriculi lateralis A14.1.09.286 **128**
– posterius
– – medullae spinalis A14.1.02.023 **106**, A14.1.02.115 **106**
– – ventriculi lateralis A14.1.09.286 **128**
– sacrale A02.2.05.018 **17**
– superius
– – cartilaginis thyroideae A06.2.02.010 **58**
– – marginis falciformis hiatus saphenus A04.7.03.018 **43**
– temporale ventriculi lateralis A14.1.09.287 **128**
– uteri A09.1.03.004 **65**
Corona
– ciliaris A15.2.03.010 **144**
– clinica dentis A05.1.03.029 **48**
– dentis A05.1.03.009 **48**
– glandis penis A09.4.01.008 **69**
– radiata A14.1.09.550 **131**
Coronalis A01.0.00.004 **1**
Corpus/ora
– adiposum
– – buccae A05.1.01.015 **47**
– – fossae ischioanalis A09.5.04.002 **71**
– – infrapatellare A03.6.08.018 **31**
– – orbitae A15.2.07.007 **147**
– – pararenale A08.1.01.011 **63**
– – preepiglotticum A06.2.07.007 **59**
– albicans A09.1.01.016 **65**
– amygdaloideum A14.1.09.402 **129**
– anococcygeum A04.5.04.016 **40**, **71**
– callosum A14.1.09.241 **127**
– cavernosum
– – clitoridis A09.2.02.005 **67**
– – penis A09.4.01.014 **69**
– cerebelli A14.1.07.101 **118**
– ciliare A15.2.03.009 **144**
– claviculae A02.4.02.005 **19**
– clitoridis A09.2.02.003 **67**
– costae A02.3.02.007 **18**
– epididymidis A09.3.02.004 **68**
– femoris A02.5.04.012 **22**
– fibulae A02.5.07.006 **23**
– fornicis A14.1.09.258 **127**
– gastricum A05.5.01.012 **52**
– geniculatum
– – laterale A14.1.08.302 **120**
– – mediale A14.1.08.303 **120**
– humeri A02.4.04.010 **19**
– incudis A15.3.02.039 **150**
– juxtarestiforme A14.1.04.119 **109**, A14.1.07.415 **120**
– linguae A05.1.04.002 **49**
– luteum A09.1.01.015 **65**
– mammae A16.0.02.005 **154**
– mammillare A14.1.08.402 **120**
– mandibulae A02.1.15.002 **15**
– maxillae A02.1.12.002 **14**
– medullare cerebelli A14.1.07.418 **120**
– nuclei caudati A14.1.09.504 **130**
– ossis
– – hyoidei A02.1.16.002 **16**
– – ilii A02.5.01.102 **21**
– – ischii A02.5.01.202 **21**
– – metacarpi A02.4.09.003 **20**
– – metatarsi A02.5.17.003 **24**
– – pubis A02.5.01.302 **21**
– – sphenoidalis A02.1.05.002 **11**
– pancreatis A05.9.01.006 **56**
– paraaortica A12.2.04.003 **79**
– penis A09.4.01.003 **69**
– perineale A09.5.00.005 **71**
– phalangis
– – manus A02.4.10.007 **21**
– – pedis A02.5.18.007 **24**
– pineale A11.2.00.001 **74, 120**
– radii A02.4.05.006 **20**
– restiforme A14.1.04.014 **109**, A14.1.07.414 **120**
– rubrum A09.1.01.014 **65**
– spongiosum penis A09.4.01.015 **69**
– sterni A02.3.03.006 **18**
– striatum A14.1.09.515 **130**
– – ventrale A14.1.09.439 **129, 130**
– tali A02.5.10.010 **24**
– tibiae A02.5.06.011 **23**
– trapezoideum A14.1.05.315 **113**
– ulnae A02.4.06.007 **20**
– unguis A16.0.01.004 **154**
– uteri A09.1.03.003 **65**
– vertebrae A02.2.01.002 **16**
– vesicae A08.3.01.003 **64**
– – biliaris/felleae A05.8.02.004 **56**
– vitreum A15.2.06.008 **146**
Cortex
– cerebelli A14.1.07.402 **119**
– cerebri A14.1.09.301 **128**

– corticis renalis A08.1.01.017 **63**
– glandulae suprarenalis A11.5.00.007 **74**
– lentis A15.2.05.003 **146**
– nodi lymphoidei A13.2.03.005 **100**
– ovarii A09.1.01.011 **65**
– periamygdaloideus A14.1.09.415 **129**
– renalis A08.1.01.015 **63**
– thymi A13.1.02.004 **100**
Costa/e [I–XII] A02.3.02.001 **17**
– cervicalis A02.3.02.013 **18**
– colli A02.3.02.013 **18**
– fluctuantes [XI–XII] A02.3.01.004 **17**
– lumbalis A02.3.02.020 **18**
– prima [I] A02.3.02.014 **18**
– secunda [II] A02.3.02.018 **18**
– spuriae [VIII–XII] A02.3.01.003 **17**
– verae [I–VII] A02.3.01.002 **17**
Coxa A01.1.00.034 **2**
Cranialis A01.0.00.019 **1**
Cranium A02.1.00.001 **8**
Crena
– analis/ani A01.2.08.003 **5**
– interglutealis A01.2.08.003 **5**
Crista/e A02.0.00.031 **7**
– ampullaris A15.3.03.088 **152**
– arcuata cartilaginis arytenoideae A06.2.04.006 **58**
– basilaris ductus cochlearis A15.3.03.101 **152**
– capitis costae A02.3.02.004 **18**
– choanalis vomeris A02.1.11.004 **14**
– colli costae A02.3.02.006 **18**
– conchalis
– – corporis maxillae A02.1.12.019 **14**
– – ossis palatini A02.1.13.009 **15**
– corporis costae A02.3.02.012 **18**
– costae A02.3.02.012 **18**
– cutis A16.0.00.004 **154**
– ethmoidalis
– – maxillae A02.1.12.027 **14**
– – ossis palatini A02.1.13.010 **15**
– fenestrae cochleae A15.3.02.017 **149**
– frontalis A02.1.03.016 **10**
– galli A02.1.07.004 **13**
– iliaca A02.5.01.106 **21**
– infratemporalis alaris majoris ossis sphenoidalis A02.1.05.028 **11**
– intertrochanterica A02.5.04.010 **22**
– lacrimalis
– – anterior A02.1.12.025 **14**
– – posterior A02.1.09.002 **14**
– marginalis dentis A05.1.03.045 **48**
– medialis fibulae A02.5.07.010 **23**
– musculi supinatoris A02.4.06.014 **20**
– nasalis
– – laminae horizontalis ossis palatini A02.1.13.018 **15**
– – maxillae A02.1.12.030 **14**
– obliqua dentis A05.1.03.016 **48**
– obturatoria A02.5.01.309 **21**
– occipitalis
– – externa A02.1.04.023 **11**
– – interna A02.1.04.030 **11**
– palatina laminae horizontalis ossis palatini A02.1.13.019 **15**
– palatopharyngea A05.3.01.018 **50**
– pubica A02.5.01.305 **21**
– renalis A08.1.01.028 **63**
– sacralis
– – lateralis A02.2.05.017 **17**
– – medialis A02.2.05.016 **17**
– – mediana A02.2.05.014 **17**
– sphenoidalis A02.1.05.014 **11**
– spiralis ductus cochlearis A15.3.03.101 **152**
– supracondylaris
– – lateralis A02.4.04.019 **19**
– – medialis A02.4.04.016 **19**
– supraepicondylaris
– – lateralis A02.4.04.019 **19**
– – medialis A02.4.04.016 **19**
– supramastoidea A02.1.06.068 **13**
– suprastyloidea A02.4.05.016 **20**
– supravalvularis A12.2.01.003 **78**, A12.2.03.003 **79**
– supraventricularis A12.1.02.007 **76**
– temporalis mandibulae A02.1.15.033 **15**
– terminalis atrii dextri A12.1.01.003 **76**
– transversa meati acustici interni A15.3.03.047 **151**
– transversalis dentis A05.1.03.014 **48**
– triangularis dentis A05.1.03.015 **48**
– tuberculi
– – majoris A02.4.04.008 **19**
– – minoris A02.4.04.009 **19**
– urethralis A09.2.03.004 **67**, A09.4.02.007 **70**
– verticalis meati acustici interni A15.3.03.049 **151**
– vestibuli A15.3.03.007 **151**
Cruces pilorum A16.0.00.027 **154**
Crus/ra A01.1.00.038 **2**
– anterius
– – capsulae internae A14.1.09.526 **130**
– – stapedis A15.3.02.035 **150**
– antihelicis A15.3.01.011 **148**
– breve incudis A15.3.02.042 **150**
– cerebri A14.1.06.005 **115, 116**
– clitoridis A09.2.02.002 **67**
– dextrum
– – diaphragmatis A04.4.02.003 **38**
– – fasciculi atrioventricularis A12.1.06.006 **77**
– fornicis A14.1.09.259 **127**
– helicis A15.3.01.006 **148**
– horizontale striae diagonalis A14.1.09.423 **129**
– inferius marginis falciformis hiatus saphenus A04.7.03.019 **43**
– laterale
– – anuli inguinalis superficialis A04.5.01.015 **38**
– – cartilaginis alaris majoris nasi A06.1.01.010 **57**
– longum incudis A15.3.02.040 **150**
– mediale
– – anuli inguinalis superficialis A04.5.01.014 **38**
– – cartilaginis alaris majoris nasi A06.1.01.008 **57**
– membranacea ampullaria ductus semicircularis A15.3.03.072 **152**
– membranaceum
– – commune ductus semicircularis A15.3.03.071 **152**
– – simplex ductus semicircularis A15.3.03.075 **152**
– ossea ampullaria canalis semicircularis A15.3.03.021 **151**
– osseum
– – commune canalis semicircularis A15.3.03.020 **151**
– – simplex canalis semicircularis A15.3.03.024 **151**
– penis A09.4.01.004 **69**
– posterius
– – capsulae internae A14.1.09.531 **130**
– – stapedis A15.3.02.036 **150**
– primum lobuli ansiformis cerebelli [H VII A] A14.1.07.208 **119**
– secundum lobuli ansiformis cerebelli [H VII A] A14.1.07.210 **119**
– sinistrum
– – diaphragmatis A04.4.02.004 **38**
– – fasciculi atrioventricularis A12.1.06.007 **77**
– superius marginis falciformis hiatus saphenus A04.7.03.018 **43**
– verticale striae diagonalis A14.1.09.424 **129**
Cryptae tonsillae/res
– lingualis A13.2.02.002 **100**
– palatini A05.2.01.015 **50, 100**
– pharyngealis A05.2.01.008 **50, 100**
– tubariae A13.2.02.003 **100**
Cubitus A01.1.00.023 **2**
Culmen [IV et V] A14.1.07.112 **119**
Cuneus A14.1.09.224 **126**
Cupula
– ampullaris A15.3.03.090 **152**
– cochleae A15.3.03.026 **151**
– pleurae A07.1.02.006 **62**
Curvatura/e
– major gastricae A05.5.01.004 **51**
– minor gastricae A05.5.01.005 **51**
– primaria A02.2.00.002 **16**
– secundariae A02.2.00.005 **16**
Curvea occlusalis A05.1.03.075 **49**
Cuspis/des A12.0.00.022 **75**
– acessoria dentis A05.1.03.012 **48**

– anterior valvae atrioventricularis
– – dextrae A12.1.02.004 **76**
– – sinistri A12.1.04.004 **77**
– buccalis A05.1.03.019 **48**
– commissurales valvae atrioventricularis sinistri A12.1.04.006 **77**
– dentis A05.1.03.010 **48**
– – distalis A05.1.03.028 **48**
– – distobuccalis A05.1.03.025 **48**
– – distolingualis A05.1.03.027 **48**
– – distopalatinalis A05.1.03.026 **48**
– – lingualis A05.1.03.021 **48**
– – mesiobuccalis A05.1.03.022 **48**
– – mesiolingualis A05.1.03.024 **48**
– – mesiopalatalis A05.1.03.023 **48**
– – palatinalis A05.1.03.020 **48**
– – paramolaris A05.1.03.072 **49**
– posteriorvalvae atrioventricularis
– – dextrae A12.1.02.005 **76**
– – sinistri A12.1.04.005 **77**
– septalis valvae atrioventricularis dextrae A12.1.02.006 **76**
Cutis A16.0.00.002 **154**
Cymba conchae A15.3.01.014 **148**

D

Declive [VI] A14.1.07.203 **119**
Decussatio/nes A14.1.00.019 **104**
– fibrarum nervorum trochlearium A14.1.06.615 **118**
– lemnisci medialis A14.1.04.110 **109**
– pedunculorum cerebellarium superiorum A14.1.06.217 **116**
– pyramidum A14.1.04.004 **108**, A14.1.04.106 **109**
– tegmentales A14.1.06.220 **117**
– – anterior A14.1.06.222 **117**
– – posterior A14.1.06.221 **117**
Dens/tes A05.1.03.001 **48**
– acustici A15.3.03.107 **153**
– axis A02.2.02.202 **17**
– caninus A05.1.03.005 **48**
– decidui A05.1.03.076 **49**
– incisivus A05.1.03.004 **48**
– molaris A05.1.03.007 **48**
– – tertius A05.1.03.008 **48**
– permanentes A05.1.03.077 **49**
– premolaris A05.1.03.006 **48**
– serotinus A05.1.03.008 **48**
Dentinum A05.1.03.055 **48**
Dermis A16.0.00.010 **154**
Desmocranium A02.1.00.010 **8**
Desmodontium A03.1.03.006 **26**
Dexter A01.0.00.006 **1**
Diameter
– obliqua pelvis A02.5.02.012 **22**
– transversa pelvis A02.5.02.011 **22**
Diaphragma A04.4.02.001 **38**
– pelvis A04.5.04.001 **39**
– sellae A14.1.01.107 **104**
Diaphysis A02.0.00.017 **7**
Diarthrosis A03.0.00.020 **25**
Diastema A05.1.03.078 **49**
Diencephalon A14.1.03.007 **108**, A14.1.08.001 **120**
Digitationes hippocampi A14.1.09.324 **128**
Digitus/i
– anularis A01.2.07.030 **5**
– manus [I–V] A01.1.00.030 **2**, A01.2.07.026 **5**
– medius A01.2.07.029 **5**
– minimus
– – manus A01.2.07.031 **5**
– – pedis A01.2.08.040 **6**
– pedis [I–V] A01.1.00.046 **2**, A01.2.08.035 **6**
– primus [I] manus A01.2.07.027 **5**
– primus [I] pedis A01.2.08.036 **6**
– quartus [IV] manus A01.2.07.030 **5**
– quartus [IV] pedis A01.2.08.039 **6**
– quintus [V] manus A01.2.07.031 **5**
– quintus [V] pedis A01.2.08.040 **6**
– secundus [II] manus A01.2.07.028 **5**
– secundus [II] pedis A01.2.08.037 **6**
– tertius [III] manus A01.2.07.029 **5**
– tertius [III] pedis A01.2.08.038 **6**
Diploe A02.1.00.035 **8**
Discus
– articularis/articulationis A03.0.00.032 **25**
– – acromioclavicularis A03.5.03.003 **28**
– – radioulnaris distalis A03.5.10.002 **29**
– – sternoclavicularis A03.5.04.002 **29**
– – temporomandibularis A03.1.07.002 **27**
– interpubicus A03.6.02.002 **30**
– intervertebralis A03.2.02.003 **27**
– nervi optici A15.2.04.019 **145**
Distalis A01.0.00.036 **1**
Distantia
– intercristalis A02.5.02.020 **22**
– interspinosa A02.5.02.019 **22**
– intertrochanterica A02.5.02.021 **22**
Diverticula ampullae ductus deferentis A09.3.05.007 **68**
Diverticulum ilei A05.6.04.003 **53**
Divisio/nes
– anteriores plexus brachialis A14.2.03.007 **138**
– autonomica A14.3.00.001 **141**
– lateralis
– – dextra hepatis A05.8.01.049 **55**
– – m. erectoris spinae lumborum A04.3.02.007 **36**
– – sinistrahepatis A05.8.01.038 **55**
– medialis
– – dextrahepatis A05.8.01.046 **55**
– – m. erectoris spinae lumborum A04.3.02.012 **36**
– – sinistra hepatis A05.8.01.041 **55**
– posteriores plexus brachialis A14.2.03.008 **138**
Dorsalis A01.0.00.014 **1**
Dorsum A01.1.00.018 **2**
– linguae A05.1.04.004 **49**
– manus A01.1.00.029 **2**
– nasi A06.1.01.003 **57**
– pedis A01.1.00.045 **2**, A01.2.08.024 **5**
– penis A09.4.01.005 **69**
– sellae A02.1.05.010 **11**
Ductulus/i
– aberrans/tes
– – epididymi A09.3.02.007 **68**
– – inferior epididymi A09.3.02.009 **68**
– – superior epididymi A09.3.02.008 **68**
– efferentes testis A09.3.01.025 **68**
– excretoriic glandulae lacrimalis A15.2.07.060 **148**
– prostatici A09.3.08.019 **69**
– transversi epoophori A09.1.05.003 **66**
Ductus
– biliaris A05.8.02.013 **56**
– biliferi interlobulares A05.8.01.060 **56**
– choledochus A05.8.02.013 **56**
– cochlearis A15.3.03.093 **152**
– cysticus A05.8.02.011 **56**
– deferens A09.3.05.001 **68**
– – vestigialis A09.1.06.002 **66**
– ejaculatorius A09.3.07.001 **68**
– endolymphaticus A15.3.03.079 **152**
– epididymidis A09.3.02.006 **68**
– excretorius glandulae vesiculosae A09.3.06.005 **68**
– glandulae bulbourethralis A09.3.09.002 **69**
– hepaticus
– – communis A05.8.01.061 **56**
– – dexter A05.8.01.062 **56**
– – sinister A05.8.01.065 **56**
– incisivus A06.1.02.033 **57**
– lactiferi A16.0.02.010 **154**
– lobi caudati
– – dexter hepatis A05.8.01.068 **56**
– – sinister hepatis A05.8.01.069 **56**
– longitudinalis epoophori A09.1.05.002 **66**
– lymphaticus dexter A12.4.01.006 **99**
– nasolacrimalis A15.2.07.070 **148**
– pancreaticus A05.9.01.015 **56**
– – accessorius A05.9.01.017 **56**
– paraurethrales A09.2.03.015 **67**, A09.4.02.026 **70**
– parotideus A05.1.02.007 **47**
– reuniens A15.3.03.081 **152**
– saccularis A15.3.03.078 **152**
– semicirculares A15.3.03.066 **152**
– – anterior A15.3.03.067 **152**
– – lateralis A15.3.03.073 **152**
– – posterior A15.3.03.069 **152**

– sublinguales minores A05.1.02.010 **47**
– sublingualis major A05.1.02.009 **47**
– submandibularis A05.1.02.012 **47**
– thoracicus A12.4.01.007 **99**
– – dexter A12.4.01.006 **99**
– thyroglossalis A05.1.04.021 **49**
– utricularis A15.3.03.077 **152**
– utriculosaccularis A15.3.03.076 **152**
Duodenum A05.6.02.001 **52**
Dura mater A14.1.01.002 **104**, A14.1.01.101 **104**
– cranialis A14.1.01.102 **104**
– encephali A14.1.01.102 **104**
– spinalis A14.1.01.111 **104**

E

Eminentia A02.0.00.027 **7**
– arcuata A02.1.06.023 **12**
– collateralis ventriculi lateralis A14.1.09.282 **127**
– conchae A15.3.01.029 **148**
– cruciformis A02.1.04.028 **11**
– fossae triangularis A15.3.01.031 **148**
– frontalis A02.1.03.004 **10**
– hypothenaris A01.2.07.024 **5**
– iliopubica A02.5.01.307 **21**
– intercondylaris A02.5.06.008 **23**
– maxillae A02.1.12.016 **14**
– medialis fossae rhomboideae A14.1.05.704 **115**
– mediana hypothalami A14.1.08.409 **120**
– parietalis A02.1.02.010 **9**
– pyramidalis A15.3.02.024 **149**
– scaphae A15.3.01.030 **148**
– thenaris A01.2.07.023 **5**
Enamelum A05.1.03.056 **48**
Enarthrosis A03.0.00.050 **25**
Encephalon A14.1.03.001 **108**
Endocardium A12.1.05.001 **77**
Endolympha A15.3.03.061 **152**
Endometrium A09.1.03.027 **66**
Endomysium A04.0.00.043 **34**
Endoneurium A14.2.00.014 **132**
Endorotatio A03.0.00.056 **26**
Endosteum A02.0.00.038 **7**
Ependyma A14.1.00.022 **104**
Epicardium A12.1.08.007 **78**
Epicondylus A02.0.00.030 **7**
– lateralis
– – femoris A02.5.04.025 **22**
– – humeri A02.4.04.029 **19**
– medialis
– – femoris A02.5.04.022 **22**
– – humeri A02.4.04.027 **19**
Epidermis A16.0.00.009 **154**
Epididymis A09.3.02.001 **68**
Epigastrium A01.2.04.003 **4**
Epiglottis A06.2.07.001 **58**
Epimysium A04.0.00.041 **34**
Epineurium A14.2.00.016 **132**
Epiphysis A02.0.00.018 **7**
– anularis A02.2.01.004 **16**
Epithalamus A14.1.08.002 **120**, A14.1.08.501 **121**
Epithelium
– anterius corneae A15.2.02.018 **144**
– lentis A15.2.05.006 **146**
– pigmentosum iridis A15.2.03.032 **145**
– posterius corneae A15.2.02.022 **144**
Eponychium A16.0.01.010 **154**
Epoophoron A09.1.05.001 **66**
Equator
– bulbi oculi A15.2.01.004 **144**
– lentis A15.2.05.013 **146**
Excavatio
– disci A15.2.04.020 **145**
– rectouterina ♀ A10.1.02.512 **73**
– rectovesicalis ♂ A10.1.02.513 **73**
– vesicouterina ♀ A10.1.02.504 **73**
Exorotatio A03.0.00.055 **25**
Extensio A03.0.00.059 **26**
Extensor A01.0.00.046 **1**
Externus A01.0.00.030 **1**
Extremitas
– acromialis claviculae A02.4.02.007 **19**
– anterior splenica A13.2.01.013 **100**
– inferior
– – renis A08.1.01.009 **63**
– – testis A09.3.01.003 **67**
– posterior splenica A13.2.01.014 **100**
– sternalis claviculae A02.4.02.002 **19**
– superior
– – renis A08.1.01.008 **63**
– – testis A09.3.01.002 **67**
– tubaria ovarii A09.1.01.007 **65**
– uterina ovarii A09.1.01.008 **65**

F

Facies A01.1.00.006 **2**
– anterior
– – cordis A12.1.00.003 **75**
– – corneae A15.2.02.016 **144**
– – corporis maxillae A02.1.12.007 **14**
– – glandulae suprarenalis A11.5.00.002 **74**
– – iridis A15.2.03.023 **145**
– – lentis A15.2.05.010 **146**
– – palpebrae A15.2.07.027 **147**
– – partis petrosae ossis temporalis A02.1.06.021 **12**
– – patellae A02.5.05.005 **23**
– – prostatae A09.3.08.007 **69**
– – radii A02.4.05.008 **20**
– – renis A08.1.01.006 **63**
– – scapulae A02.4.01.002 **18**
– – ulnae A02.4.06.008 **20**
– – uteri A09.1.03.008 **65**
– anteroinferior corporis pancreatis A05.9.01.009 **56**
– anterolateralis
– – cartilaginis arytenoideae A06.2.04.004 **58**
– – humeri A02.4.04.012 **19**
– anteromedialis humeri A02.4.04.011 **19**
– anterosuperior corporis pancreatis A05.9.01.007 **56**
– approximalis dentis A05.1.03.042 **48**
– articularis
– – acromialis claviculae A02.4.02.008 **19**
– – anterior dentis A02.2.02.204 **17**
– – arytenoidea cricoideae A06.2.03.004 **58**
– – calcanea
– – – anterior tali A02.5.10.006 **23**
– – – media tali A02.5.10.008 **24**
– – – posterior tali A02.5.10.020 **24**
– – capitis
– – – costae A02.3.02.003 **18**
– – – fibulae A02.5.07.003 **23**
– – carpalis radii A02.4.05.020 **20**
– – cartilaginis arytenoideae A06.2.04.002 **58**
– – clavicularis scapulae A02.4.01.010 **18**
– – cuboidea calcanei A02.5.11.015 **24**
– – fibularis tibiae A02.5.06.005 **23**
– – fossae mandibularis ossis temporalis A02.1.06.072 **13**
– – inferior
– – – atlantis A02.2.02.104 **16**
– – – tibiae A02.5.06.024 **23**
– – – vertebrae A02.2.01.017 **16**
– – ligamenti calcaneonavicularis plantaris tali A02.5.10.004 **23**
– – malleoli
– – – lateralis A02.5.07.015 **23**
– – – medialis tibiae A02.5.06.022 **23**
– – navicularis tali A02.5.10.003 **23**
– – partis calcaneonavicularis ligamenti bifurcati tali A02.5.10.005 **23**
– – patellae A02.5.05.004 **23**
– – posterior dentis A02.2.02.205 **17**
– – sternalis claviculae A02.4.02.003 **19**
– – superior
– – – atlantis A02.2.02.103 **16**
– – – tibiae A02.5.06.002 **23**
– – – vertebrae A02.2.01.015 **16**
– – talaris
– – – anterior calcanei A02.5.11.010 **24**
– – – media calcanei A02.5.11.011 **24**
– – – posterior calcanei A02.5.11.012 **24**
– – thyroidea cricoideae A06.2.03.005 **58**
– – tuberculi costae A02.3.02.009 **18**

– auricularis ossis
– – ilii A02.5.01.121 **21**
– – sacri A02.2.05.007 **17**
– buccalis dentis A05.1.03.036 **48**
– cerebralis
– – alaris majoris ossis sphenoidalis A02.1.05.025 **11**
– – ossis temporalis A02.1.06.078 **13**
– colica splenica A13.2.01.011 **100**
– costalis
– – pulmonis A06.5.01.006 **60**
– – scapulae A02.4.01.002 **18**
– diaphragmatica
– – cordis A12.1.00.004 **75**
– – hepatis A05.8.01.002 **54**
– – pulmonis A06.5.01.010 **60**
– – splenica A13.2.01.007 **100**
– distalis dentis A05.1.03.041 **48**
– dorsales digitorum A01.2.07.033 **5**, A01.2.08.042 **6**
– dorsalis ossis sacri A02.2.05.013 **17**
– externa ossis
– – frontalis A02.1.03.003 **10**
– – parietalis A02.1.02.007 **9**
– gastrica A13.2.01.010 **100**
– – splenica A13.2.01.010 **100**
– glutea ossis ilii A02.5.01.116 **21**
– inferior
– – cordis A12.1.00.004 **75**
– – linguae A05.1.04.007 **49**
– – partis petrosae ossis temporalis A02.1.06.040 **12**
– inferolateralis prostatae A09.3.08.009 **69**
– infratemporalis
– – alaris majoris ossis sphenoidalis A02.1.05.027 **11**
– – corporis maxillae A02.1.12.013 **14**
– interlobaris pulmonis A06.5.01.011 **60**
– interna ossis
– – frontalis A02.1.03.015 **10**
– – parietalis A02.1.02.002 **9**
– intervertebralis A02.2.01.003 **16**
– intestinalis uteri A09.1.03.006 **65**
– labialis dentis A05.1.03.037 **48**
– lateralis
– – fibulae A02.5.07.007 **23**
– – ossis zygomatici A02.1.14.002 **15**
– – ovarii A09.1.01.004 **65**
– – radii A02.4.05.010 **20**
– – testis A09.3.01.004 **67**
– – tibiae A02.5.06.016 **23**
– lingualis dentis A05.1.03.038 **48**
– lunata acetabuli A02.5.01.006 **21**
– malleolaris
– – lateralis tali A02.5.10.013 **24**
– – medialis tali A02.5.10.015 **24**
– maxillaris
– – alaris majoris ossis sphenoidalis A02.1.05.029 **11**
– – ossis palatini A02.1.13.004 **14**
– medialis
– – cartilaginis arytenoideae A06.2.04.010 **58**
– – et inferior hemispherii cerebri A14.1.09.201 **125**
– – fibulae A02.5.07.008 **23**
– – ovarii A09.1.01.003 **65**
– – testis A09.3.01.005 **67**
– – tibiae A02.5.06.013 **23**
– – ulnae A02.4.06.010 **20**
– mediastinalis pulmonis A06.5.01.008 **60**
– mesialis dentis A05.1.03.040 **48**
– nasalis
– – corporis maxillae A02.1.12.017 **14**
– – laminae horizontalis ossis palatini A02.1.13.014 **15**
– – ossis palatini A02.1.13.003 **14**
– occlusalis dentis A05.1.03.034 **48**
– orbitalis
– – alaris majoris ossis sphenoidalis A02.1.05.030 **11**
– – corporis maxillae A02.1.12.003 **14**
– – ossis
– – – frontalis A02.1.03.023 **10**
– – – zygomatici A02.1.14.004 **15**
– palatina/alis A02.1.13.015 **15**
– – dentis A05.1.03.039 **48**
– – laminae horizontalis ossis palatini A02.1.13.015 **15**
– palmares digitorum A01.2.07.032 **5**
– pancreatica splenica A13.2.01.012 **100**
– patellaris femoris A02.5.04.027 **22**
– pelvica ossis sacri A02.2.05.009 **17**
– plantares digitorum A01.2.08.041 **6**
– poplitea femoris A02.5.04.018 **22**
– posterior
– – cartilaginis arytenoideae A06.2.04.011 **58**
– – corneae A15.2.02.017 **144**
– – corporis pancreatis A05.9.01.008 **56**
– – fibulae A02.5.07.009 **23**
– – glandulae suprarenalis A11.5.00.003 **74**
– – humeri A02.4.04.013 **19**
– – iridis A15.2.03.024 **145**
– – lentis A15.2.05.011 **146**
– – palpebrae A15.2.07.029 **147**
– – partis petrosae ossis temporalis A02.1.06.031 **12**
– – prostatae A09.3.08.008 **69**
– – radii A02.4.05.009 **20**
– – renis A08.1.01.007 **63**
– – scapulae A02.4.01.004 **18**
– – tibiae A02.5.06.014 **23**
– – ulnae A02.4.06.009 **20**
– – uteri A09.1.03.006 **65**
– pulmonalis dextra/sinistra cordis A12.1.00.005 **75**
– renalis
– – glandulae suprarenalis A11.5.00.004 **74**
– – splenica A13.2.01.009 **100**
– sacropelvica ossis ilii A02.5.01.120 **21**
– sternocostalis cordis A12.1.00.003 **75**
– superior tali A02.5.10.012 **24**
– superolateralis hemispherii cerebri A14.1.09.101 **124**
– symphysialis A02.5.01.304 **21**
– temporalis
– – alaris majoris ossis sphenoidalis A02.1.05.026 **11**
– – ossis
– – – frontalis A02.1.03.011 **10**
– – – zygomatici A02.1.14.003 **15**
– – partis squamosae ossis temporalis A02.1.06.065 **13**
– urethralis A09.4.01.006 **69**
– vesicalis uteri A09.1.03.008 **65**
– vestibularis dentis A05.1.03.035 **48**
– visceralis
– – hepatis A05.8.01.012 **54**
– – splenica A13.2.01.008 **100**
Falx
– cerebelli A14.1.01.106 **104**
– cerebri A14.1.01.103 **104**
– inguinalis A04.5.01.020 **38**
Fascia/e
– abdominis A04.5.02.001 **38**
– – parietalis A04.5.02.006 **38**
– – visceralis A04.5.02.002 **38**
– antebrachii A04.6.03.008 **41**
– axillaris A04.6.03.002 **41**
– brachii A04.6.03.005 **41**
– buccopharyngea/is A04.1.04.010 **35**, A05.3.01.116 **51**
– capitis et colli A04.0.00.032 **33**
– cervicalis A04.2.05.001 **35**
– clavipectoralis A04.4.01.018 **37**
– clitoridis A09.2.02.007 **67**
– colli A04.2.05.001 **35**
– cremasterica A09.3.04.004 **68**
– cribrosa A04.7.03.020 **43**
– cruris A04.7.03.021 **43**
– deltoidea A04.6.03.004 **41**
– diaphragmatica A04.4.02.017 **38**
– dorsalis
– – manus A04.6.03.009 **41**
– – pedis A04.7.03.030 **44**
– endoabdominalis A04.5.02.006 **38**
– endopelvina A04.5.03.007 **39**
– endothoracica A04.4.01.020 **37**, **62**
– extraperitonealis
– – abdominis A04.5.02.004 **38**
– – pelvis A04.5.03.005 **39**
– extraserosalis A04.0.00.035 **33**
– iliaca A04.5.02.007 **39**, A04.7.03.009 **43**
– iliopsoas A04.5.02.007 **39**
– inferior diaphragmatis pelvis A04.5.03.020 **39**
– infraspinata A04.6.02.009 **40**
– investiens/tes A04.0.00.039 **34**
– – abdominis A04.5.02.015 **39**

– – intermediae abdominis A04.5.02.017 **39**
– – perinei superficialis A09.5.02.002 **71**
– – profunda abdominis A04.5.02.016 **39**
– – superficialis abdominis A04.5.02.018 **39**
– lata A04.7.03.002 **43**
– masseterica A04.1.04.011 **35**
– membrorum A04.0.00.037 **34**
– musculares bulbi A15.2.07.008 **147**
– musculi
– – piriformis A04.5.03.011 **39**
– – quadrati lumborum A04.3.02.504 **37**
– musculorum A04.0.00.038 **34**
– nuchae A04.3.01.017 **36**
– obturatoria A04.5.03.009 **39**
– parietalis A04.0.00.034 **33**
– – thoracis A04.4.01.020 **37, 62**
– parotidea A04.1.04.012 **35**
– pectoralis A04.4.01.017 **37**
– pelvica A04.5.03.001 **39**
– pelvis A04.5.03.001 **39**
– – parietalis A04.5.03.007 **39**
– – visceralis A04.5.03.002 **39**
– penis A09.4.01.026 **69**
– perinei A09.5.02.002 **71**
– pharyngobasilaris A05.3.01.027 **50**
– phrenicopleuralis A07.1.02.019 **62**
– precaecocolica A05.7.02.010 **53**
– presacralis A04.5.03.018 **39**
– propria
– – musculi A04.0.00.040 **34**
– – organi
– – – abdominis A04.5.02.003 **38, 39**
– – – pelvis A04.5.03.003 **39**
– rectoprostatica A04.5.03.004 **39**
– rectosacralis A04.5.03.019 **39**
– rectovaginalis A04.5.03.004 **39**
– renalis A08.1.01.010 **63**
– spermatica
– – externa A09.3.04.002 **68**
– – interna A09.3.04.005 **68**
– superior diaphragmatis pelvis A04.5.03.012 **39**
– supraspinata A04.6.02.007 **40**
– temporalis A04.1.04.013 **35**
– thoracica A04.4.01.019 **37**
– thoracolumbalis A04.3.02.501 **37**
– transversalis A04.5.02.011 **39**
– trunci A04.0.00.033 **33**
– umbilicalis A04.5.02.014 **39**
– visceralis A04.0.00.036 **33**
Fasciculus/i A14.1.00.012 **104**
– anterior m. palatopharyngei A05.2.01.106 **50, 51**
– arcuatus A14.1.09.557 **131**
– atrioventricularis A12.1.06.005 **77**
– ciliaris partis palpebralis m. orbicularis oculi palpebralis A04.1.03.015 **34**
– cuneatus A14.1.02.244 **107**, A14.1.04.016 **109**, A14.1.04.108 **109**
– gracilis A14.1.02.243 **107**, A14.1.04.018 **109**, A14.1.04.107 **109**
– interfascicularis A14.1.02.242 **107**
– lateralis A14.2.03.021 **138**
– – plexus brachialis A14.2.03.021 **138**
– lenticularis [H2] A14.1.08.664 **122**, A14.1.09.521 **130**
– longitudinalis/es
– – dorsalis A14.1.04.114 **109**, A14.1.05.305 **112**, A14.1.06.211 **116**, A14.1.08.946 **124**
– – inferior A14.1.09.556 **131**
– – lig. cruciformis atlantis A03.2.04.005 **27**
– – medialis A14.1.04.113 **109**, A14.1.05.304 **112**, A14.1.06.209 **116**
– – posterior A14.1.04.114 **109**, A14.1.05.305 **112**, A14.1.06.211 **116**, A14.1.08.946 **124**
– – superior A14.1.09.557 **131**
– mammillotegmentalis A14.1.08.953 **124**
– mammillothalamicus A14.1.08.671 **122**, A14.1.08.954 **124**
– medialis
– – plexus brachialis A14.2.03.022 **138**
– – telencephali A14.1.08.955 **124**
– occipitales
– – horizontales A14.1.09.566 **131**
– – verticales A14.1.09.563 **131**
– occipitofrontalis
– – inferior A14.1.09.561 **131**
– – superior A14.1.09.562 **131**
– peduncularis A14.1.09.427 **129**
– plexus brachialis A14.2.03.009 **138**
– posterior
– – m. palatopharyngei A05.2.01.107 **50**
– – plexus brachialis A14.2.03.023 **138**
– proprius
– – anterior A14.1.02.203 **107**
– – lateralis A14.1.02.216 **107**
– – posterior A14.1.02.240 **107**
– retroflexus A14.1.08.502 **121**
– semilunaris A14.1.02.242 **107**
– septomarginalis A14.1.02.241 **107**
– subcallosus A14.1.09.562 **131**
– subthalamicus A14.1.08.677 **122**, A14.1.09.522 **130**
– sulcomarginalis A14.1.02.204 **107**
– thalamicus [H1] A14.1.08.679 **123**, A14.1.09.523 **130**
– transversi aponeurosis plantaris A04.7.03.032 **44**
– uncinatus
– – cerebri A14.1.09.560 **131**
– – cerebelli A14.1.07.420 **120**
– vasculares medullae renalis A08.1.01.024 **63**
Fastigium A14.1.05.714 **115**
Fauces A05.2.01.001 **50**
Femur A01.1.00.035 **2**, A02.5.04.001 **22**
Fenestra
– cochleae A15.3.02.015 **149**
– vestibuli A15.3.02.009 **149**
Fibra/e A14.1.00.015 **104**
– anuloolivares A14.1.05.327 **113**
– arcuatae
– – cerebri A14.1.09.554 **131**
– – externae
– – – anteriores A14.1.04.009 **108, 109**
– – – posteriores A14.1.04.121 **109**
– – internae A14.1.04.109 **109**
– associationis A14.1.00.016 **104**
– – breves telencephali A14.1.09.559 **131**
– – longae telencephali A14.1.09.558 **131**
– – telencephali A14.1.09.553 **131**
– caudales A14.1.09.565 **131**
– cerebelloolivares A14.1.05.328 **113, 116**
– circulares m. ciliaris A15.2.03.018 **145**
– commissurales telencephali A14.1.09.569 **131**
– commissuralis A14.1.00.017 **104**
– corporis callosi A14.1.09.570 **131**
– corticomesencephalicae A14.1.06.223 **117**
– corticonucleares
– – bulbi A14.1.04.104 **109**
– – capsulae internae A14.1.09.530 **130**
– – mesencephali A14.1.06.202 **116**
– – pontis A14.1.05.105 **112**
– corticopontinae A14.1.05.107 **112**
– corticoreticulares A14.1.04.105 **109**, A14.1.05.106 **112**, A14.1.06.110 **116**, A14.1.09.533 **130**
– corticorubrales A14.1.09.534 **130**
– corticospinales A14.1.04.103 **109**, A14.1.05.104 **112**, A14.1.06.103 **116**, A14.1.09.535 **130**
– corticotectales A14.1.09.546 **131**
– corticothalamicae A14.1.09.549 **131**
– corticothalamici A14.1.09.536 **130**
– cuneatae A14.1.09.567 **131**
– cuneocerebellares A14.1.04.133 **110**
– cuneospinales A14.1.02.245 **108**
– frontopontinae A14.1.06.106 **116**

– geniculocalcarinae A14.1.09.542 **130**
– geniculotemporales A14.1.09.545 **131**
– gracilispinales A14.1.02.246 **108**
– horizontales
– – cuneatae occipitales A14.1.09.567 **131**
– – linguales occipitales A14.1.09.568 **131**
– hypothalamospinales A14.1.02.233 **107**, A14.1.04.126 **109**, A14.1.06.203 **116**
– intercrurales anuli inguinalis superficialis A04.5.01.016 **38**
– intrathalamicae A14.1.08.669 **122**
– laterales A14.1.09.564 **131**
– lentis A15.2.05.005 **146**
– linguales A14.1.09.568 **131**
– longitudinales m. ciliaris A15.2.03.016 **145**
– medulloreticulospinales A14.1.04.130 **110**
– meridionales m. ciliaris A15.2.03.015 **144**
– obliquae m. sphincter pyloricus A05.5.01.025 **52**
– occipitopontinae A14.1.06.107 **116**, A14.1.09.540 **130**
– occipitotectales A14.1.09.541 **130**
– olivospinales A14.1.02.213 **107**, A14.1.02.223 **107**
– paraventriculohypophysiales A14.1.08.951 **124**
– parietopontinae A14.1.06.108 **116**, A14.1.09.537 **130**
– periventriculares A14.1.08.674 **122**, A14.1.08.957 **124**
– pontis
– – longitudinales A14.1.05.103 **112**
– – transversae A14.1.05.109 **112**
– pontocerebellares A14.1.05.110 **112**
– postcommissurales columnae fornicis A14.1.09.257 **127**
– precommissurales columnae fornicis A14.1.09.256 **127**
– pretectoolivares A14.1.05.306 **113, 116**
– projectionis A14.1.00.018 **104**
– radiales m. ciliaris A15.2.03.017 **145**
– reticulospinales A14.1.02.208 **107**
– rubroolivares A14.1.05.326 **113, 116**
– spinobulbares A14.1.04.144 **110, 113**
– spinocuneatae A14.1.02.247 **108**
– spinograciles A14.1.02.248 **108**
– spinohypothalamicae A14.1.04.143 **110, 113, 116**
– spinomesencephalicae A14.1.04.140 **110, 113, 116**
– spinoolivares A14.1.04.145 **110, 113**
– spinoperiaqueductales A14.1.04.142 **110, 113, 116**
– spinoreticulares A14.1.04.139 **110, 113, 116**
– spinotectales A14.1.04.141 **110, 113, 116**
– spinothalamicae A14.1.04.138 **110, 113, 116**
– striae terminalis A14.1.08.948 **124**
– supraopticohypophysiales A14.1.08.952 **124**
– tectoolivares A14.1.05.307 **113, 117**
– tectopontinae A14.1.05.108 **112**
– tectoreticulares A14.1.05.308 **113**
– temporopontinae A14.1.06.109 **116**, A14.1.09.548 **131**
– thalamoparietales A14.1.09.538 **130**
– verticales
– – caudale occipitales A14.1.09.565 **131**
– – laterales occipitales A14.1.09.564 **131**
– zonulares A15.2.05.016 **146**
Fibrocartilago interpubica A03.6.02.002 **30**
Fibula A02.5.07.001 **23**
Fibularis A01.0.00.041 **1**
Filum/a
– olfactoria A14.2.01.005 **133**
– pars spinalis A14.1.02.005 **105**
– radicularia A14.2.00.028 **133**
– terminale A14.1.01.401 **105**
Fimbria/e
– hippocampi A14.1.09.239 **127**, A14.1.09.332 **128**
– ovarica A09.1.02.005 **65**
– tubae uterinae A09.1.02.004 **65**
Fissura/e
– ansoparamedianis A14.1.07.211 **119**
– anterior inferior cerebelli A14.1.07.218 **119**
– antitragohelicina A15.3.01.026 **148**
– cerebelli A14.1.07.002 **118**
– choroidea ventriculi lateralis A14.1.09.278 **127**
– horizontalis
– – cerebelli A14.1.07.209 **119**
– – pulmonis dextri A06.5.01.022 **60**
– intercruralis cerebelli A14.1.07.209 **119**
– intrabiventralis A14.1.07.218 **119**
– intraculminalis A14.1.07.114 **119**
– intratonsillaris A05.2.01.013 **50**
– ligamenti
– – teretis A05.8.01.014 **54**
– – venosi A05.8.01.010 **54**
– longitudinalis cerebri A14.1.09.007 **124**
– lunogracilis A14.1.07.211 **119**
– mediana anterior medullae
– – oblongatae A14.1.04.001 **108**
– – spinalis A14.1.02.007 **105**
– obliqua pulmonis A06.5.01.021 **60**
– occlusalis A05.1.03.017 **48**
– orbitalis
– – inferior A02.1.00.084 **9**
– – superior A02.1.00.083 **9**, A02.1.05.023 **11**
– petrooccipitalis A02.1.00.047 **8**
– petrosquamosa A02.1.06.075 **13**
– petrotympanica A02.1.06.074 **13**
– portalis
– – dextra A05.8.01.036 **55**
– – principalis A05.8.01.035 **55**
– post clivalis A14.1.07.205 **119**
– postcentralis cerebelli A14.1.07.111 **119**
– posterior superior cerebelli A14.1.07.205 **119**
– posterolateralis cerebelli A14.1.07.223 **119**
– postlingualis A14.1.07.104 **119**
– postpyramidalis cerebelli A14.1.07.220 **119**
– prebiventralis A14.1.07.214 **119**
– precentralis cerebelli A14.1.07.104 **119**
– preclivalis A14.1.07.119 **119**
– preculminalis A14.1.07.111 **119**
– prepyramidalis cerebelli A14.1.07.214 **119**
– prima cerebelli A14.1.07.119 **119**
– pterygomaxillaris A02.1.00.026 **8**
– secunda cerebelli A14.1.07.220 **119**
– sphenopetrosa A02.1.00.046 **8**
– tonsillaris A05.2.01.013 **50**
– transversa cerebri A14.1.09.008 **124**
– tympanomastoidea A02.1.06.077 **13**
– tympanosquamosa A02.1.06.076 **13**
– umbilicalis A05.8.01.034 **55**
Flexio A03.0.00.058 **26**
Flexor A01.0.00.045 **1**
Flexura/e
– anorectalis A05.7.05.002 **54**
– coli
– – dextra A05.7.03.003 **53**
– – hepatica A05.7.03.003 **53**
– – sinistra A05.7.03.005 **53**
– – splenica A05.7.03.005 **53**
– duodeni
– – inferior A05.6.02.006 **52**
– – superior A05.6.02.004 **52**
– duodenojejunalis A05.6.02.009 **52**
– inferior lateralis recti A05.7.04.006 **54**
– inferodextra lateralis recti A05.7.04.006 **54**

– intermedia lateralis recti
A05.7.04.005 **54**
– intermediosinistra lateralis recti
A05.7.04.005 **54**
– laterales recti A05.7.04.003 **53**
– perinealis A05.7.05.002 **54**
– sacralis recti A05.7.04.002 **53**
– superior lateralis recti
A05.7.04.004 **54**
– superodextra lateralis recti
A05.7.04.004 **54**
Flocculus [H X] A14.1.07.304 **119**
Flumina pilorum
A16.0.00.025 **154**
Folium/a
– cerebelli A14.1.07.003 **118**
– intergeniculatum
A14.1.08.807 **123**
– vermis [VII A] A14.1.07.206 **119**
Folliculus/i
– ovarici vesiculosi
A09.1.01.013 **65**
– pili A16.0.00.023 **154**
Fonticulus/i
– anterior A02.1.00.028 **8**
– anterolateralis A02.1.00.030 **8**
– cranii A02.1.00.027 **8**
– mastoideus A02.1.00.031 **8**
– posterior A02.1.00.029 **8**
– posterolateralis A02.1.00.031 **8**
– sphenoidalis A02.1.00.030 **8**
Foramen/ina
– alveolaria corporis maxillae
A02.1.12.014 **14**
– apicis dentis A05.1.03.050 **48**
– caecum A02.1.03.018 **10**
– – linguae A05.1.04.020 **49**
– – medullae oblongatae
A14.1.04.002 **108**
– costotransversarium
A03.3.04.010 **28**
– cribrosa A02.1.07.003 **13**
– epiploicum A10.1.02.403 **72**
– ethmoidale
– – anterius A02.1.00.079 **9**
– – posterius A02.1.00.080 **9**
– incisiva A02.1.00.062 **9, 14**
– infraorbitale A02.1.12.008 **14**
– interventriculare
A14.1.08.411 **120, 127**
– intervertebrale A02.2.01.008 **16**
– intervertebralia A02.2.05.011 **17**
– ischiadicum
– – majus A03.6.03.008 **30**
– – minus A03.6.03.009 **30**
– jugulare A02.1.00.054 **8**
– lacerum A02.1.00.055 **8**
– magnum A02.1.04.002 **10**
– mandibulae A02.1.15.028 **15**
– mastoideum A02.1.06.008 **12**
– mentale A02.1.15.007 **15**
– nasalia A02.1.10.003 **14**
– nervosa A15.3.03.033 **151**
– nutricium A02.0.00.041 **7**
– obturatum A02.5.01.008 **21**
– omentale A10.1.02.403 **72**
– ovale A02.1.05.036 **11**
– – cordis A12.1.01.007 **76**
– palatina minora A02.1.00.059 **9**,
A02.1.13.016 **15**
– palatinum majus A02.1.00.058 **9**
– papillaria renalis
A08.1.01.031 **63**
– parietale A02.1.02.019 **10**
– petrosum A02.1.05.039 **11**
– rotundum A02.1.05.035 **11**
– sacralia
– – anteriora A02.2.05.012 **17**
– – posteriora A02.2.05.015 **17**
– singulare A15.3.03.052 **152**
– sphenopalatinum
A02.1.00.097 **9**
– spinosum A02.1.05.038 **11**
– stylomastoideum
A02.1.06.048 **13**
– thyroideum A06.2.02.012 **58**
– transversarium vertebrae
cervicales A02.2.02.003 **16**
– venae cavae A04.4.02.014 **38**
– venarum minimarum
A12.1.01.004 **76**
– venosum A02.1.05.037 **11**
– vertebrale A02.2.01.011 **16**
– zygomaticofaciale
A02.1.14.010 **15**
– zygomaticoorbitale
A02.1.14.009 **15**
– zygomaticotemporale
A02.1.14.011 **15**
Forceps
– frontalis A14.1.09.250 **127**
– major A14.1.09.251 **127**
– minor A14.1.09.250 **127**
– occipitalis A14.1.09.251 **127**
Formatio reticularis
A14.1.00.021 **104**
– spinalis A14.1.02.140 **106**
– tegmentum
– – mesencephali
A14.1.06.327 **117**
– – pontis A14.1.05.403 **113**
Fornix A14.1.08.949 **124**,
A14.1.09.255 **127**
– conjunctivae
– – inferior A15.2.07.053 **147**
– – superior A15.2.07.052 **147**
– gastricus A05.5.01.010 **51**
– pharyngis A05.3.01.004 **50**
– sacci lacrimalis
A15.2.07.069 **148**
– vaginae A09.1.04.002 **66**
Fossa A02.0.00.034 **7**
– acetabuli A02.5.01.004 **21**
– antihelica A15.3.01.028 **148**
– articularis A03.0.00.023 **25**
– axillaris A01.2.03.010 **4**
– canina A02.1.12.009 **14**,
A05.1.03.061 **49**
– cerebellaris A02.1.04.037 **11**
– cerebralis A02.1.04.036 **11**
– condylaris A02.1.04.017 **10**
– coronoidea A02.4.04.025 **19**
– cranii
– – anterior A02.1.00.048 **8**
– – media A02.1.00.049 **8**
– – posterior A02.1.00.050 **8**
– cubitalis A01.2.07.010 **4**
– digastrica A02.1.15.009 **15**
– epigastrica A01.2.04.003 **4**
– glandulae lacrimalis
A02.1.03.026 **10**
– hyaloidea A15.2.06.011 **146**
– hypophysialis A02.1.05.009 **11**
– iliaca A02.5.01.115 **21**
– incisiva A02.1.00.060 **9**
– incudis A15.3.02.025 **149**
– infraclavicularis A01.2.03.003 **4**
– infraspinata A02.4.01.008 **18**
– infratemporalis A02.1.00.024 **8**
– inguinalis
– – lateralis A10.1.02.435 **73**
– – medialis A10.1.02.432 **73**
– intercondylaris A02.5.04.028 **22**
– interpeduncularis
A14.1.06.001 **115**
– ischioanalis A09.5.04.001 **71**
– jugularis A02.1.06.041 **12**
– lateralis cerebri
A14.1.09.009 **124**
– malleoli lateralis
A02.5.07.016 **23**
– mandibularis A02.1.06.071 **13**
– navicularis urethrae
A09.4.02.022 **70**
– occlusalis A05.1.03.018 **48**
– olecrani A02.4.04.024 **19**
– ovalis A12.1.01.005 **76**
– ovarica ♀ A10.1.02.510 **73**
– pararectalis A10.1.02.514 **73**
– paravesicalis A10.1.02.502 **73**
– poplitea A01.2.08.013 **5**
– pterygoidea A02.1.05.046 **12**
– pterygopalatina A02.1.00.025 **8**
– radialis A02.4.04.026 **19**
– retromolaris A02.1.15.023 **15**
– rhomboidea A14.1.05.702 **115**
– sacci lacrimalis A02.1.00.082 **9**
– scaphoidea A02.1.05.047 **12**
– subarcuata A02.1.06.034 **12**
– subscapularis A02.4.01.003 **18**
– supraclavicularis
– – major A01.2.02.011 **3**
– – minor A01.2.02.008 **3**
– supraspinata A02.4.01.007 **18**
– supratonsillaris A05.2.01.010 **50**
– supravesicalis A10.1.02.430 **73**
– temporalis A02.1.00.022 **8**
– tonsillaris A05.2.01.009 **50**
– triangularis auriculae
A15.3.01.010 **148**
– trochanterica A02.5.04.006 **22**
– vesicae biliaris felleae
A05.8.01.013 **54**
– vestibuli vaginae
A09.2.01.012 **66**
Fossula/e
– fenestrae
– – cochleae A15.3.02.016 **149**
– – vestibuli A15.3.02.010 **149**
– petrosa A02.1.06.050 **13**
– tonsillae/res
– – palatini A05.2.01.014 **50, 100**
– – pharyngealis A05.3.01.007 **50,
100**

Fovea
– articularis capitis radii
A02.4.05.003 **19**
– capitis femoris A02.5.04.003 **22**
– centralis A15.2.04.022 **145**
– costalis
– – inferior A02.2.03.003 **17**
– – processus transversi
A02.2.03.004 **17**
– – superior A02.2.03.002 **17**
– dentis atlantis A02.2.02.106 **16**
– distalis atlantis A05.1.03.063 **49**
– inferior sulci limitantis
A14.1.05.726 **115**
– mesialis dentis A05.1.03.062 **49**
– oblonga cartilaginis arytenoideae
A06.2.04.008 **58**
– pterygoidea A02.1.15.038 **16**
– sublingualis A02.1.15.014 **15**
– submandibularis A02.1.15.015 **15**
– superior sulci limitantis
A14.1.05.725 **115**
– triangularis cartilaginis
arytenoideae A06.2.04.009 **58**
– trochlearis A02.1.03.025 **10**
Foveola/e A15.2.04.023 **145**
– coccygea A01.2.05.004 **4**
– gastricae A05.5.01.032 **52**
– granulares A02.1.00.039 **8**
– suprameatalis A02.1.06.069 **13**
– suprameatica A02.1.06.069 **13**
Frenulum
– clitoridis A09.2.01.010 **66**
– labii
– – inferioris A05.1.01.011 **47**
– – superioris A05.1.01.010 **47**
– labiorum pudendi
A09.2.01.008 **66**
– linguae A05.1.04.012 **49**
– ostii ilealis A05.7.02.004 **53**
– preputii A09.4.01.012 **69**
– veli A14.1.05.005 **112**
– – medullaris superioris
A14.1.05.720 **115**,
A14.1.06.010 **115**
Frons A02.1.00.013 **8**
Frontalis A01.0.00.015 **1**
Fundus
– gastricus A05.5.01.009 **51**
– meatus acustici interni
A15.3.03.046 **151**
– uteri A09.1.03.002 **65**
– vesicae A08.3.01.004 **64**
– – biliaris/felleae
A05.8.02.002 **56**
Funiculus/i A14.1.00.010 **104**
– anterior medullae spinalis
A14.1.02.202 **107**
– lateralis medullae
– – oblongatae A14.1.04.007 **108**
– – spinalis A14.1.02.215 **107**
– medullae spinalis
A14.1.02.013 **105**
– posterior medullae spinalis
A14.1.02.239 **107**
– separans A14.1.05.711 **115**
– spermaticus A09.3.04.001 **68**

G

Galea aponeurotica
A04.1.03.007 **34**
Ganglion/ia A14.2.00.002 **132**
– aorticorenalia A14.3.03.028 **143**
– autonomicum A14.2.00.008 **132**
– cardiaca A14.3.03.014 **143**
– cervicale
– – inferioris A14.3.01.019 **141**
– – medium A14.3.01.016 **141**
– – superius A14.3.01.009 **141**
– cervicothoracicum
A14.3.01.020 **141**
– ciliare A14.3.02.003 **142**
– cochleare A14.2.01.134 **136**
– coeliaca A14.3.03.027 **143**
– craniospinale sensorium
A14.2.00.005 **132**
– geniculatum A14.2.01.116 **135**
– geniculi A14.2.01.116 **135**
– impar A14.3.01.037 **142**
– inferius
– – n. glossopharyngei
A14.2.01.137 **136**
– – n. vagi A14.2.01.157 **136**
– intermedia A14.3.01.008 **141**
– lumbalia A14.3.01.033 **142**
– mesentericum
– – inferius A14.3.03.037 **143**
– – superius A14.3.03.030 **143**
– oticum A14.3.02.014 **142**
– parasympathicum
A14.2.00.012 **132**
– pelvica A14.3.02.017 **142**
– phrenica A14.3.03.020 **143**
– pterygopalatinum
A14.3.02.006 **142**
– renalia A14.3.03.033 **143**
– sacralia A14.3.01.035 **142**
– sensorium nervi
– – cranialis A14.2.00.007 **132**
– – spinalis A14.2.00.006 **132**
– spirale cochleae
A14.2.01.134 **136**,
A15.3.03.125 **153**
– stellatum A14.3.01.020 **141**
– sublinguale A14.3.02.011 **142**
– submandibulare
A14.3.02.009 **142**
– superius
– – n. glossopharyngei
A14.2.01.136 **136**
– – n. vagi A14.2.01.154 **136**
– sympathicum A14.2.00.011 **132**
– terminale A14.2.01.003 **133**
– thoracica A14.3.01.024 **141**
– thoracicum splanchnicum
A14.3.01.029 **141**
– trigeminale A14.2.01.014 **133**
– trunci sympathici
A14.3.01.003 **141**
– tympanicum A14.2.01.139 **136**
– vertebrale A14.3.01.017 **141**
– vestibulare A14.2.01.123 **135**
Gaster A05.5.01.001 **51**
Gemma gustatoria
A15.4.00.002 **153**
Geniculum A14.2.01.100 **135**
– canalis nervi facialis
A02.1.06.010 **12**
– nervi faciales A14.2.01.100 **135**
Genu A01.1.00.036 **2**,
A14.1.09.243 **127**
– capsulae internae
A14.1.09.529 **130**
– corporis callosi A14.1.09.243 **127**
– nervi facialis A14.1.05.314 **113**
Gingiva A03.1.03.003 **26**,
A05.1.01.108 **47**
Ginglymus A03.0.00.046 **25**
Glabella A02.1.03.006 **10**
Glandula/e
– areolares A16.0.02.013 **155**
– bronchiales A06.4.02.030 **60**
– buccales A05.1.02.015 **47**
– bulbourethralis A09.3.09.001 **69**
– cervicales A09.1.03.020 **66**
– ciliares A15.2.07.043 **147**
– conjunctivales A15.2.07.055 **147**
– cutis A16.0.00.028 **154**
– ductus
– – biliaris A05.8.02.019 **56**
– – choledochi A05.8.02.019 **56**
– duodenales A05.6.02.017 **53**
– endocrinae A11.0.00.000 **74**
– gastricae A05.5.01.033 **52**
– intestini/intestinales
– – crassi A05.7.01.008 **53**
– – tenuis A05.6.01.012 **52**
– labiales A05.1.02.014 **47**
– lacrimalis/es A15.2.07.057 **148**
– – accessoriae A15.2.07.061 **148**
– laryngeales A06.2.09.020 **59**
– linguales A05.1.02.018 **47**
– mammaria A16.0.02.006 **154**
– molares A05.1.02.016 **47**
– nasales A06.1.02.020 **57**
– oesophageae A05.4.01.017 **51**
– olfactoriae A15.1.00.003 **144**
– oris A05.1.02.001 **47**
– palatinae A05.1.02.017 **47**
– parathyroidea/e A11.4.00.001 **74**
– – accessoriae A11.4.00.004 **74**
– – inferior A11.4.00.003 **74**
– – superior A11.4.00.002 **74**
– parotidea A05.1.02.003 **47**
– – accessoria A05.1.02.006 **47**
– pharyngeales A05.3.01.030 **51**
– pinealis A11.2.00.001 **74, 120**
– pituitaria A11.1.00.001 **74**
– preputiales A09.4.01.028 **70**
– salivariae
– – majores A05.1.02.002 **47**
– – minores A05.1.02.013 **47**
– sebacea A16.0.00.030 **154**
– sebaceae A15.2.07.044 **147**
– seminalis A09.3.06.001 **68**
– sublingualis A05.1.02.008 **47**
– submandibularis
A05.1.02.011 **47**
– sudorifera A16.0.00.029 **154**
– suprarenalis/es A11.5.00.001 **74**
– – accessoriae A11.5.00.011 **74**
– tarsales A15.2.07.042 **147**
– thyroidea/e A11.3.00.001 **74**
– – accessoriae A11.3.00.005 **74**
– tracheales A06.3.01.011 **59**

– tubariae A15.3.02.084 **151**
– urethrales A09.2.03.013 **67**, A09.4.02.025 **70**
– uterinae A09.1.03.028 **66**
– vesiculosa A09.3.06.001 **68**
– vestibulares minores A09.2.01.017 **67**
– vestibularis major A09.2.01.016 **67**
Glans
– clitoridis A09.2.02.004 **67**
– penis A09.4.01.007 **69**
Globus pallidus
– lateralis A14.1.09.509 **130**
– medialis A14.1.09.511 **130**
Glomus/era
– aortica A12.2.04.003 **79**
– caroticum A12.2.04.007 **79**
– choroideum A14.1.01.308 **105**, A14.1.09.283 **127**
– coccygeum A12.2.12.011 **87**
– jugulare A12.3.05.003 **93**
Glottis A06.2.09.012 **59**
Gomphosis A03.0.00.006 **25**, A03.1.03.001 **26**
Gonion A02.1.00.021 **8**
Granulationes arachnoideae A14.1.01.205 **105**
Gyrus/i
– angularis A14.1.09.124 **125**
– breves insulae A14.1.09.152 **125**
– cerebri A14.1.09.004 **124**
– cinguli A14.1.09.231 **126**
– dentatus A14.1.09.237 **127**, A14.1.09.339 **128**
– fasciolaris A14.1.09.233 **126**
– frontalis
– – inferior A14.1.09.113 **125**
– – medialis A14.1.09.207 **126**
– – medius A14.1.09.118 **125**
– – superior A14.1.09.121 **125**
– insulae A14.1.09.150 **125**
– lingualis A14.1.09.226 **126**
– longus insulae A14.1.09.151 **125**
– occipitotemporalis
– – lateralis A14.1.09.227 **126**
– – medialis A14.1.09.228 **126**
– olfactorius
– – lateralis A14.1.09.220 **126**
– – medialis A14.1.09.221 **126**
– orbitales A14.1.09.216 **126**
– paracentralis
– – anterior A14.1.09.210 **126**
– – posterior A14.1.09.222 **126**
– parahippocampalis A14.1.09.234 **126**
– paraolfactorii A14.1.09.214 **126**
– paraterminalis A14.1.09.212 **126**
– postcentralis A14.1.09.128 **125**
– precentralis A14.1.09.119 **125**
– rectus A14.1.09.218 **126**
– supramarginalis A14.1.09.131 **125**
– temporalis/es
– – inferior A14.1.09.148 **125–126**
– – medius A14.1.09.146 **125**
– – superior A14.1.09.138 **125**
– – transversus/ii A14.1.09.140 **125**
– – – anterior A14.1.09.141 **125**
– – – posterior A14.1.09.142 **125**

H

Habenula A14.1.08.003 **120**
Haema A12.0.00.009 **75**
Hallux A01.2.08.036 **6**
Hamulus
– lacrimalis A02.1.09.004 **14**
– laminae spiralis A15.3.03.034 **151**
– ossis hamati A02.4.08.013 **20**
– pterygoideus A02.1.05.051 **12**
Haustra coli A05.7.03.009 **53**
Helicotrema A15.3.03.044 **151**
Helix A15.3.01.005 **148**
Hemispherium
– cerebelli [H II – H X] A14.1.07.004 **118**
– cerebri A14.1.09.002 **124**
Hepar A05.8.01.001 **54**
Hiatus
– adductorius A04.7.03.008 **43**
– aorticus A04.4.02.010 **38**
– canalis nervi petrosi
– – majoris A02.1.06.024 **12**
– – minoris A02.1.06.026 **12**
– maxillaris A02.1.12.021 **14**
– oesophageus A04.4.02.011 **38**
– sacralis A02.2.05.020 **17**
– saphenus A04.7.03.016 **43**
– semilunaris A02.1.07.018 **13**, A06.1.02.028 **57**
– urogenitalis A04.5.04.010 **40**
Hilum
– glandulae suprarenalis A11.5.00.009 **74**
– lienale A13.2.01.017 **100**
– nodi lymphoidei A13.2.03.004 **100**
– nuclei
– – dentati A14.1.07.408 **120**
– – olivaris inferioris A14.1.04.224 **110**
– ovarii A09.1.01.002 **65**
– pulmonis A06.5.01.015 **60**
– renale A08.1.01.004 **63**
– splenicum A13.2.01.017 **100**
Hippocampus A14.1.09.321 **128**
– proprius A14.1.09.327 **128**
Hirci A16.0.00.021 **154**
Horizontalis A01.0.00.002 **1**
Humerus A02.4.04.001 **19**
Humor
– aquosus A15.2.06.002 **146**
– vitreus A15.2.06.014 **146**
Hymen A09.1.04.008 **66**
Hypochondrium A01.2.04.002 **4**
Hypodermis A16.0.03.001 **155**
Hypogastrium A01.2.04.007 **4**
Hyponychium A16.0.01.011 **154**
Hypophysis A11.1.00.001 **74**
– pharyngealis A05.3.01.005 **50**
Hypothalamus A14.1.08.401 **120**, A14.1.08.901 **123**
Hypothenar A01.2.07.024 **5**

I

Ileum A05.6.04.001 **53**
Ilium A02.5.01.101 **21**
Impressio/nes
– cardiaca
– – faciei diaphragmaticae hepatis A05.8.01.004 **54**
– – pulmonis A06.5.01.009 **60**
– colica hepatis A05.8.01.021 **55**
– digitatae A02.1.00.040 **8**
– duodenalis hepatis A05.8.01.020 **55**
– gastrica hepatis A05.8.01.019 **54**
– gyrorum A02.1.00.040 **8**
– ligamenti costoclavicularis A02.4.02.004 **19**
– oesophageale hepatis A05.8.01.018 **54**
– renalis hepatis A05.8.01.022 **55**
– suprarenalis hepatis A05.8.01.023 **55**
– trigeminalis A02.1.06.028 **12**
Incisura/e A02.0.00.033 **7**
– acetabuli A02.5.01.005 **21**
– angularis gastricae A05.5.01.006 **51**
– anterior auriculae A15.3.01.018 **148**
– apicis cordis A12.1.00.008 **76**
– cardiaca pulmonis sinistri A06.5.01.013 **60**
– cardialis A05.5.01.011 **52**
– cartilaginis meatus acustici A15.3.01.050 **149**
– clavicularis A02.3.03.003 **18**
– costales A02.3.03.008 **18**
– ethmoidalis A02.1.03.028 **10**
– fibularis A02.5.06.023 **23**
– frontalis/foramen frontale A02.1.03.010 **10**
– interarytenoidea A06.2.09.006 **59**
– intertragica A15.3.01.019 **148**
– ischiadica
– – major A02.5.01.009 **21**
– – minor A02.5.01.206 **21**
– jugularis ossis
– – occipitalis A02.1.04.019 **10**
– – sterni A02.3.03.004 **18**
– – temporale A02.1.06.039 **12**, A02.1.06.045 **13**
– lacrimalis A02.1.12.026 **14**
– ligamenti teretis A05.8.01.025 **55**
– mandibulae A02.1.15.034 **15**
– mastoidea A02.1.06.005 **12**
– nasalis A02.1.12.010 **14**
– pancreatis A05.9.01.004 **56**
– parietalis A02.1.06.063 **13**
– preoccipitalis A14.1.09.109 **125**
– pterygoidea A02.1.05.045 **12**
– radialis A02.4.06.005 **20**
– scapulae A02.4.01.015 **19**
– sphenopalatina A02.1.13.005 **14**
– supraorbitalis/foramen supraorbitale A02.1.03.009 **10**
– tentorii A14.1.01.105 **104**

– terminalis auricularis
A15.3.01.025 **148**
– thyroidea
– – inferior A06.2.02.006 **58**
– – superior A06.2.02.005 **58**
– trochlearis A02.4.06.006 **20**
– tympanica A02.1.06.059 **13**,
A15.3.01.047 **149**
– ulnaris A02.4.05.019 **20**
– vertebralis
– – inferior A02.2.01.010 **16**
– – superior A02.2.01.009 **16**
Inclinatio pelvis A02.5.02.022 **22**
Incus A15.3.02.038 **150**
Index A01.2.07.028 **5**
Indusium griseum
A14.1.09.246 **127**
Inferior A01.0.00.018 **1**
Infundibulum A11.1.00.007 **74, 120**
– ethmoidale A02.1.07.017 **13**,
A06.1.02.027 **57**
– hypophysis A11.1.00.007 **74, 120**
– tubae uterinae A09.1.02.003 **65**
– vesicae biliaris/felleae
A05.8.02.003 **56**
Inguen A01.2.04.006 **4**
Inion A02.1.00.018 **8**
Insertio A04.0.00.003 **33**
– partis superficialis musculi
sphincteris ani externi
A04.5.04.019 **40**
Insula/e
– lobus A14.1.09.149 **125**
– olfactoriae A14.1.09.428 **129**
– pancreaticae A05.9.01.019 **56, 74**
Integumentum commune
A16.0.00.001 **154**
Intermedius A01.0.00.008 **1**
Internus A01.0.00.031 **1**
Intersectio/nes
– tendinea/e A04.0.00.046 **34**,
A04.5.01.002 **38**
Intestinum
– crassum A05.7.01.001 **53**
– tenue A05.6.01.001 **52**
Intumescentia
– cervicalis A14.1.02.002 **105**
– lumbosacralis A14.1.02.003 **105**
– tympanica A14.2.01.139 **136**
Iris A15.2.03.020 **145**
Ischium A02.5.01.201 **21**
Isocortex A14.1.09.307 **128**
Isthmus
– aortae A12.2.04.002 **79**
– cartilaginis auricularis
A15.3.01.024 **148**
– faucium A05.2.01.002 **50**
– glandulae thyroideae
A11.3.00.003 **74**
– gyri cinguli A14.1.09.232 **126**
– prostatae A09.3.08.016 **69**
– tubae
– – auditivae/auditoriae
A15.3.02.076 **150**
– – uterinae A09.1.02.007 **65**
– uteri A09.1.03.012 **65**

J

Jejunum A05.6.03.001 **53**
Jugum/a
– alveolaria
– – mandibulae A02.1.15.021 **15**
– – maxillae A02.1.12.040 **14**
– cerebralia A02.1.00.040 **8**
– sphenoidale A02.1.05.003 **11**
Junctio anorectalis
A05.7.05.003 **54**
Junctura/e A03.0.00.000 **25**,
A03.0.00.001 **25**
– cartilaginea/e A03.0.00.015 **25**
– – cranii A03.1.04.001 **27**
– cinguli
– – pectoralis A03.5.00.002 **28**
– – pelvic/i A03.4.00.001 **28**,
A03.6.00.002 **30**
– columnae vertebralis
A03.2.00.001 **27**
– cranii A03.1.00.001 **26**
– fibrosa/e A03.0.00.004 **25**
– – cranii A03.1.00.002 **26**
– membri
– – inferioris liberi
A03.6.04.001 **30**
– – superioris liberi
A03.5.00.001 **28**
– – – liberi A03.5.05.001 **29**
– ossea A03.0.00.019 **25**
– ossium A03.0.00.002 **25**
– synovialis A03.0.00.020 **25**
– thoracis A03.3.00.001 **28**

K

Kyphosis
– sacralis A02.2.00.004 **16**
– thoracica A02.2.00.003 **16**

L

Labium/a
– anterius ostii uteri
A09.1.03.016 **66**
– externum cristae iliacae
A02.5.01.107 **21**
– inferius/oris A05.1.01.009 **47**
– internum cristae iliacae
A02.5.01.110 **21**
– laterale
– – lineae asperae
A02.5.04.014 **22**
– – sulci intertubercularis
A02.4.04.008 **19**
– limbi
– – tympanicum laminae spiralis
ossei A15.3.03.105 **152**
– – vestibulare laminae spiralis
ossei A15.3.03.106 **153**
– majus pudendi A09.2.01.003 **66**
– mediale
– – lineae asperae
A02.5.04.015 **22**
– – sulci intertubercularis
A02.4.04.009 **19**
– minus pudendi A09.2.01.007 **66**
– oris A05.1.01.005 **47**
– posterius ostii uteri
A09.1.03.017 **66**
– superius A05.1.01.006 **47**
Labrum
– acetabuli A03.6.07.008 **30**
– articulare A03.0.00.025 **25**
– glenoidale scapulae
A03.5.08.002 **29**
– ileocaecale A05.7.02.006 **53**
– ileocolicum A05.7.02.005 **53**
– inferius ostii ilealis
A05.7.02.006 **53**
– superius ostii ilealis
A05.7.02.005 **53**
Labyrinthus
– cochlearis A15.3.03.091 **152**
– corticis renalis A08.1.01.016 **63**
– ethmoidalis A02.1.07.007 **13**
– membranaceus
A15.3.03.059 **152**
– osseus A15.3.03.003 **151**
– vestibularis A15.3.03.062 **152**
Lacertus
– fibrosus A04.6.02.016 **40**
– musculi recti lateralis bulbi
A15.2.07.014 **147**
Lacuna/e
– laterales A12.3.05.110 **94**
– musculorum retroinguinalis
A04.7.03.010 **43**
– urethrales A09.2.03.014 **67**,
A09.4.02.024 **70**
– vasorum retroinguinalis
A04.7.03.011 **43**
Lacus lacrimalis A15.2.07.063 **148**
Lambda A02.1.00.017 **8**
Lamella
– anterior nuclei olivaris principalis
A14.1.04.222 **110**
– lateralis nuclei olivaris principalis
A14.1.04.223 **110**
– posterior nuclei olivaris
principalis A14.1.04.221 **110**
– tympanica A15.3.03.032 **151**
– vestibularis A15.3.03.031 **151**
Lamina/e A14.1.00.008 **104**
– affixa A14.1.09.276 **127**
– anterior
– – fasciae thoracolumbalis
A04.3.02.504 **37**
– – vaginae musculi recti
abdominis A04.5.01.004 **38**
– arcus vertebrae A02.2.01.007 **16**
– basalis
– – choroideae A15.2.03.007 **144**
– – corporis ciliaris
A15.2.03.019 **145**
– basilaris ductus cochlearis
A15.3.03.102 **152**
– cartilaginis
– – cricoideae A06.2.03.003 **58**
– – thyroideae dextra/sinistra
A06.2.02.004 **58**
– choroidocapillaris
A15.2.03.006 **144**
– colliculi superioris
– – I A14.1.06.606 **118**
– – II A14.1.06.607 **118**
– – III A14.1.06.608 **118**

- - IV A14.1.06.609 **118**
- - V A14.1.06.610 **118**
- - VI A14.1.06.611 **118**
- - VII A14.1.06.612 **118**
- cribrosa
- - ossis ethmoidalis A02.1.07.002 **13**
- - sclerae A15.2.02.011 **144**
- dextra/sinistra cartilaginis thyroideae A06.2.02.004 **58**
- epiphysialis A02.0.00.020 **7**
- episcleralis A15.2.02.008 **144**
- externa calvariae A02.1.00.034 **8**
- fusca sclerae A15.2.02.010 **144**
- granularis
- - externa isocorticis [Lamina II] A14.1.09.310 **128**
- - interna isocorticis [Lamina IV] A14.1.09.312 **128**
- horizontalis ossis palatini A02.1.13.013 **15**
- interna calvariae A02.1.00.037 **8**
- lateralis
- - cartilagis tubae auditivae A15.3.02.081 **150**
- - processi pterygoideus ossis sphenoidalis A02.1.05.043 **12**
- limitans
- - anterior corneae A15.2.02.019 **144**
- - posterior corneae A15.2.02.021 **144**
- media asciae thoracolumbalis A04.3.02.503 **37**
- medialis
- - cartilagis tubae auditivae A15.3.02.080 **150**
- - processi pterygoideus ossis sphenoidalis A02.1.05.044 **12**
- medullaris
- - accessoria corporis striati A14.1.09.513 **130**
- - externa corporis striati A14.1.09.508 **130**
- - interna corporis striati A14.1.09.510 **130**
- - lateralis
- - - corporis striati A14.1.09.508 **130**
- - - thalami A14.1.08.660 **122**
- - medialis
- - - corporis striati A14.1.09.510 **130**
- - - thalami A14.1.08.661 **122**
- membranacea tubae auditivae A15.3.02.082 **150**
- modioli cochleae A15.3.03.040 **151**
- molecularis isocorticis [Lamina I] A14.1.09.309 **128**
- multiformis isocorticis [Lamina VI] A14.1.09.314 **128**
- muscularis mucosae
- - gastricae A05.5.01.029 **52**
- - intestini
- - - crassi A05.7.01.007 **53**
- - - tenuis A05.6.01.010 **52**
- - oesophageae A05.4.01.016 **51**
- orbitalis ossis ethmoidalis A02.1.07.011 **13**
- parietalis
- - pericardii A12.1.08.006 **78**
- - tunicae vaginalis testis A09.3.01.009 **67**
- perpendicularis ossis
- - ethmoidalis A02.1.07.006 **13**
- - palatini A02.1.13.002 **14**
- posterior
- - fasciae
- - - temporalis
- - - - profunda A04.1.04.015 **35**
- - - - superficialis A04.1.04.014 **35**
- - - thoracolumbalis A04.3.02.502 **37**
- - vaginae musculi recti abdominis A04.5.01.005 **38**
- pretrachealis fasciae cervicalis A04.2.05.004 **35**
- prevertebralis fasciae cervicalis A04.2.05.006 **36**
- profunda
- - fasciae
- - - temporalis A04.1.04.015 **35**
- - - thoracolumbalis A04.3.02.504 **37**
- - m. levatoris palpebrae superioris A15.2.07.022 **147**
- pyramidalis
- - externa isocorticis [Lamina III] A14.1.09.311 **128**
- - interna isocorticis [Lamina V] A14.1.09.313 **128**
- quadrigemina A14.1.06.011 **115, 118**
- septi pellucidi A14.1.09.264 **127**
- spinalis/es
- - I A14.1.02.117 **106**
- - II A14.1.02.119 **106**
- - III et IV A14.1.02.121 **106**
- - V A14.1.02.122 **106**
- - VI A14.1.02.124 **106**
- - VII A14.1.02.131 **106**
- - VII–IX A14.1.02.104 **106**
- - X A14.1.02.302 **108**
- spiralis
- - ossea A15.3.03.029 **151**
- - secundaria A15.3.03.035 **151**
- superficialis
- - fasciae
- - - cervicalis A04.2.05.002 **35**
- - - temporalis A04.1.04.014 **35**
- - - thoracolumbalis A04.3.02.502 **37**
- - m. levatoris palpebrae superioris A15.2.07.021 **147**
- suprachoroidea A15.2.03.003 **144**
- tecti A14.1.06.011 **115, 118**
- terminalis A14.1.08.419 **121, 127**
- tragi A15.3.01.051 **149**
- vasculosa A15.2.03.005 **144**
- visceralis
- - pericardii A12.1.08.007 **78**
- - tunicae vaginalis testis A09.3.01.010 **67**

Lanugo A16.0.00.015 **154**
Larynx A06.2.01.001 **58**
Lateralis A01.0.00.010 **1**
Latus A01.2.04.004 **4**
Lemniscus A14.1.00.014 **104**
- lateralis A14.1.05.317 **113**, A14.1.06.204 **116**, A14.1.08.670 **122**
- medialis A14.1.04.111 **109, 112**, A14.1.06.207 **116**, A14.1.08.672 **122**
- spinalis A14.1.04.137 **110, 113**, A14.1.06.215 **116**, A14.1.08.676 **122**
- trigeminalis A14.1.05.310 **113**, A14.1.06.208 **116**, A14.1.08.680 **123**

Lens A15.2.05.001 **146**
Leptomeninx A14.1.01.003 **104**
Lien A13.2.01.001 **100**
Ligamentum/a A03.0.00.034 **25**
- acromioclaviculare A03.5.03.002 **28**
- alaria A03.2.04.002 **27**
- anococcygeum A04.5.04.016 **40, 71**
- anulare
- - radii A03.5.09.007 **29**
- - stapediale A15.3.02.060 **150**
- anularia tracheales A06.3.01.006 **59**
- apicis dentis A03.2.04.003 **27**
- arcuatum
- - laterale A04.4.02.007 **38**
- - mediale A04.4.02.006 **38**
- - medianum A04.4.02.005 **38**
- arteriosum (Ductus arteriosus) A12.2.01.202 **78**
- atlantooccipitale
- - anterius A03.1.08.003 **27**
- - laterale A03.1.08.005 **27**
- auriculare/aria A15.3.01.032 **148**
- - anterius A15.3.01.033 **148**
- - posterius A15.3.01.035 **148**
- - superius A15.3.01.034 **148**
- bifurcatum A03.6.10.511 **31**
- calcaneocuboideum A03.6.10.513 **31**
- - dorsale A03.6.10.515 **31**
- - plantare A03.6.10.518 **31**
- calcaneofibulare A03.6.10.011 **31**
- calcaneonaviculare A03.6.10.512 **31**
- - plantare A03.6.10.203 **31**
- capitis
- - costae
- - - intraarticulare A03.3.04.004 **28**
- - - radiatum A03.3.04.003 **28**
- - femoris A03.6.07.010 **30**
- - fibulae
- - - anterius A03.6.09.002 **31**
- - - posterius A03.6.09.003 **31**
- capsularia A03.0.00.036 **25**
- cardinale A09.1.03.031 **66**
- carpi radiatum A03.5.11.103 **29**
- carpometacarpalia
- - dorsalia A03.5.11.302 **29**
- - palmaria A03.5.11.303 **29**

– ceratocricoideum A06.2.03.008 **58**
– collaterale/ia
– – articulationis
– – – interphalangeae
– – – – manus A03.5.11.602 **30**
– – – – pedis A03.6.10.902 **32**
– – – metacarpophalangeae A03.5.11.502 **30**
– – – metatarsophalangeae A03.6.10.802 **32**
– – carpi
– – – radiale A03.5.11.008 **29**
– – – ulnare A03.5.11.007 **29**
– – fibulare A03.6.08.011 **30**
– – laterale articulationis talocruralis A03.6.10.008 **31**
– – mediale articulationis talocruralis A03.6.10.003 **31**
– – radiale A03.5.09.006 **29**
– – tibiale A03.6.08.012 **31**
– – ulnare A03.5.09.005 **29**
– conoideum A03.5.03.006 **28**
– coracoacromiale A03.5.01.002 **28**
– coracoclaviculare A03.5.03.004 **28**
– coracohumerale A03.5.08.004 **29**
– coronarium hepatis A10.1.02.302 **72**
– costoclaviculare A03.5.04.005 **29**
– costotransversarium A03.3.04.006 **28**
– – laterale A03.3.04.008 **28**
– – superius A03.3.04.007 **28**
– costoxiphoidea A03.3.05.005 **28**
– cricoarytenoideum A06.2.04.016 **58**
– cricopharyngeum A06.2.04.017 **58**
– cricothyroideum medianum A06.2.03.009 **58**
– cricotracheale A06.2.03.010 **58**
– cruciatum
– – anterius A03.6.08.007 **30**
– – posterius A03.6.08.008 **30**
– cruciforme atlantis A03.2.04.004 **27**
– cuboideonaviculare
– – dorsale A03.6.10.510 **31**
– – plantare A03.6.10.520 **31**
– cuneocuboideum
– – dorsale A03.6.10.509 **31**
– – interosseum A03.6.10.504 **31**
– – plantare A03.6.10.522 **31**
– cuneometatarsalia interossea A03.6.10.604 **32**
– cuneonavicularia
– – dorsalia A03.6.10.514 **31**
– – plantaria A03.6.10.519 **31**
– deltoideum A03.6.10.003 **31**
– denticulatum A14.1.01.310 **105**
– epididymidis
– – inferius A09.3.01.012 **67**
– – superius A09.3.01.011 **67**
– extracapsularia A03.0.00.037 **25**
– extraperitoneale
– – abdominis A04.5.02.005 **38**
– – pelvis A04.5.03.006 **39**
– falciforme hepatis A10.1.02.303 **72**
– flava A03.2.01.003 **27**
– fundiforme
– – clitoridis ♀ A04.5.02.023 **39, 67, 70**
– – penis ♂ A04.5.02.023 **39, 67, 70**
– gastrocolicum A10.1.02.205 **72**
– gastrolienale A10.1.02.203 **72**
– gastrophrenicum A10.1.02.202 **72**
– gastrosplenicum A10.1.02.203 **72**
– glenohumeralia A03.5.08.003 **29**
– hepatis A10.1.02.301 **72**
– hepatocolicum A10.1.02.106 **72**
– hepatoduodenale A10.1.02.105 **72**
– hepatoesophageale A10.1.02.103 **72**
– hepatogastricum A10.1.02.104 **72**
– hepatophrenicum A10.1.02.102 **72**
– hepatorenale A10.1.02.306 **72**
– hyoepiglotticum A06.2.07.006 **59**
– iliofemorale A03.6.07.003 **30**
– iliolumbale A03.2.07.002 **27**
– incudis
– – posterius A15.3.02.058 **150**
– – superius A15.3.02.057 **150**
– inguinale A04.5.01.009 **38**
– intercarpalia
– – dorsalia A03.5.11.104 **29**
– – interossea A03.5.11.106 **29**
– – palmaria A03.5.11.105 **29**
– interclaviculare A03.5.04.006 **29**
– intercuneiformia
– – dorsalia A03.6.10.508 **31**
– – interossea A03.6.10.505 **31**
– – plantaria A03.6.10.521 **31**
– interfoveolare A04.5.02.012 **39**
– interspinalia A03.2.01.002 **27**
– intertransversaria A03.2.01.004 **27**
– intracapsularia A03.0.00.035 **25**
– ischiofemorale A03.6.07.006 **30**
– lacunare A04.5.01.010 **38**
– laterale
– – articulationis temporomandibularis A03.1.07.003 **27**
– – puboprostaticum ♂ A04.5.03.015 **39**
– – pubovesicale ♀ A04.5.03.015 **39**
– – vesicae A04.5.03.016 **39**
– latum uteri ♀ A10.1.02.505 **73**
– lienorenale A10.1.02.207 **72**
– longitudinale
– – anterius A03.2.01.007 **27**
– – posterius A03.2.01.008 **27**
– lumbocostale A03.3.04.009 **28**
– mallei
– – anterius A15.3.02.054 **150**
– – laterale A15.3.02.056 **150**
– – superius A15.3.02.055 **150**
– mediale
– – articulationis temporomandibularis A03.1.07.004 **27**
– – puboprostaticum ♂ A04.5.03.013 **39**
– – pubovesicale ♀ A04.5.03.013 **39**
– meniscofemorale
– – anterius A03.6.08.003 **30**
– – posterius A03.6.08.004 **30**
– metacarpale transversum
– – profundum A03.5.11.504 **30**
– – superficiale A04.6.03.011 **41**
– metacarpalia
– – dorsalia A03.5.11.402 **29**
– – interossea A03.5.11.404 **29**
– – palmaria A03.5.11.403 **29**
– metatarsale transversum
– – profundum A03.6.10.804 **32**
– – superficiale A04.7.03.033 **44**
– metatarsalia
– – dorsalia A03.6.10.703 **32**
– – interossea A03.6.10.702 **32**
– – plantaria A03.6.10.704 **32**
– nuchae A03.2.01.006 **27**
– ossiculorum auditus/auditorium A15.3.02.053 **150**
– ovarii proprium A09.1.01.017 **65**
– palmaria
– – articulationis
– – – interphalangeae manus A03.5.11.603 **30**
– – – metacarpophalangeae A03.5.11.503 **30**
– palpebrale
– – laterale A15.2.07.040 **147**
– – mediale A15.2.07.041 **147**
– pancreaticocolicum A10.1.02.209 **72**
– pancreaticosplenicum A10.1.02.208 **72**
– patellae A03.6.08.015 **31**
– pectineum A04.5.01.011 **38**
– phrenicocolicum A10.1.02.211 **72**
– phrenicooesophagealis A04.4.02.012 **38**
– phrenicosplenicum A10.1.02.206 **72**
– pisohamatum A03.5.11.108 **29**
– pisometacarpale A03.5.11.109 **29**
– plantare longum A03.6.10.517 **31**
– plantaria
– – articulationis
– – – interphalangeae pedis A03.6.10.903 **32**
– – – metatarsophalangeae A03.6.10.803 **32**
– popliteum
– – arcuatum A03.6.08.014 **31**
– – obliquum A03.6.08.013 **31**
– pterygospinale A03.1.01.002 **26**
– pubicum
– – inferius A03.6.02.004 **30**
– – superius A03.6.02.003 **30**
– pubocervicale A09.1.03.030 **66**

– pubofemorale A03.6.07.007 **30**
– puboprostaticum A04.5.03.015 **39**
– pubovesicale A04.5.03.013 **39**
– pulmonale A07.1.02.017 **62**
– quadratum A03.5.09.008 **29**
– radiocarpale
– – dorsale A03.5.11.003 **29**
– – palmare A03.5.11.004 **29**
– recti laterale A05.7.04.016 **54**
– rectouterinum A09.1.03.032 **66**
– reflexum A04.5.01.012 **38**
– sacrococcygeum
– – anterius A03.2.08.004 **28**
– – dorsale
– – – profundum A03.2.08.003 **28**
– – – superficiale A03.2.08.002 **27**
– – laterale A03.2.08.005 **28**
– – posterius
– – – profundum A03.2.08.003 **28**
– – – superficiale A03.2.08.002 **27**
– – ventrale A03.2.08.004 **28**
– sacroiliacum
– – anterius A03.6.03.002 **30**
– – interosseum A03.6.03.003 **30**
– – posterius A03.6.03.004 **30**
– sacrospinale A03.6.03.007 **30**
– sacrotuberale A03.6.03.005 **30**
– sphenomandibulare A03.1.07.007 **27**
– spirale ductus cochlearis A15.3.03.099 **152**
– splenocolicum A10.1.02.210 **72**
– splenorenale A10.1.02.207 **72**
– sternoclaviculare
– – anterius A03.5.04.003 **29**
– – posterius A03.5.04.004 **29**
– sternocostale intraarticulare A03.3.05.002 **28**
– sternocostalia radiata A03.3.05.003 **28**
– sternopericardiaca A12.1.08.003 **78**
– stylohyoideum A03.1.01.003 **26**
– stylomandibulare A03.1.07.008 **27**
– supraspinale A03.2.01.005 **27**
– suspensoria mammaria A16.0.02.015 **155**
– suspensorium
– – axillae A04.6.03.003 **41**
– – bulbi A15.2.07.005 **147**
– – clitoridis ♀ A04.5.02.019 **39, 67, 69**
– – duodeni A05.6.02.011 **52**
– – glandulae thyroideae A04.2.05.005 **36**
– – ovarii ♀ A09.1.01.018 **65, 73**
– – penis ♂ A04.5.02.019 **39, 67, 69**
– talocalcaneum
– – interosseum A03.6.10.503 **31**
– – laterale A03.6.10.102 **31**
– – mediale A03.6.10.103 **31**
– – posterius A03.6.10.104 **31**
– talofibulare
– – anterius A03.6.10.009 **31**
– – posterius A03.6.10.010 **31**
– talonaviculare A03.6.10.507 **31**
– tarsi A03.6.10.501 **31**
– – dorsalia A03.6.10.506 **31**
– – interossea A03.6.10.502 **31**
– – plantaria A03.6.10.516 **31**
– tarsometatarsalia
– – dorsalia A03.6.10.602 **31**
– – plantaria A03.6.10.603 **32**
– teres
– – hepatis A05.8.01.015 **54, 98**
– – uteri A09.1.03.029 **66**
– thyroepiglotticum A06.2.07.005 **59**
– thyrohyoideum
– – laterale A06.2.02.017 **58**
– – medianum A06.2.02.014 **58**
– tibiofibulare
– – anterius A03.6.05.003 **30**
– – posterius A03.6.05.004 **30**
– trachealia A06.3.01.006 **59**
– transversa columnae vertebralis A03.2.01.009 **27**
– transversum
– – acetabuli A03.6.07.009 **30**
– – atlantis A03.2.04.006 **27**
– – cervicis A09.1.03.031 **66**
– – genus A03.6.08.006 **30**
– – humeri A03.5.08.005 **29**
– – perinei ♂ A09.5.03.003 **71**
– – scapulae
– – – inferius A03.5.01.004 **28**
– – – superius A03.5.01.003 **28**
– trapezoideum A03.5.03.005 **28**
– triangulare
– – dextrum hepatis A10.1.02.304 **72**
– – sinistrum hepatis A10.1.02.305 **72**
– ulnocarpale
– – dorsale A03.5.11.005 **29**
– – palmare A03.5.11.006 **29**
– umbilicale medianum A08.3.01.007 **64**
– uteroovaricum A09.1.01.017 **65**
– venae cavae sinistrae A12.3.01.008 **91**
– venosum A05.8.01.011 **54, 98**
– vestibulare A06.2.09.023 **59**
– vocale A06.2.09.025 **59**
Limbus
– acetabuli A02.5.01.003 **21**
– anterior palpebrae A15.2.07.035 **147**
– corneae A15.2.02.014 **144**
– fossae ovalis A12.1.01.006 **76**
– laminae spiralis ossei A15.3.03.104 **152**
– posterior palpebrae A15.2.07.036 **147**
– sphenoidalis A02.1.05.004 **11**
– spiralis A15.3.03.104 **152**
Limen
– insulae A14.1.09.155 **125**
– nasi A06.1.02.010 **57**
Linea/e A02.0.00.032 **7**
– alba A04.5.01.022 **38**
– anocutanea A05.7.05.008 **54**
– arcuata
– – ilii A02.5.01.105 **21**
– – vaginae musculi recti abdominis A04.5.01.006 **38**
– aspera A02.5.04.013 **22**
– axillaris
– – anterior A01.2.00.017 **3**
– – media A01.2.00.018 **3**
– – posterior A01.2.00.019 **3**
– distractiones A16.0.00.008 **154**
– epiphysialis A02.0.00.021 **7**
– glutea
– – anterior A02.5.01.117 **21**
– – inferior A02.5.01.119 **21**
– – posterior A02.5.01.118 **21**
– intercondylaris A02.5.04.029 **23**
– intermedia cristae iliacae A02.5.01.109 **21**
– intertrochanterica A02.5.04.009 **22**
– mammillaris A01.2.00.016 **3**
– mediana
– – anterior A01.2.00.012 **3**
– – posterior A01.2.00.022 **3**
– medioclavicularis A01.2.00.015 **3**
– musculi solei A02.5.06.015 **23**
– mylohyoidea A02.1.15.012 **15**
– nuchalis
– – inferior A02.1.04.026 **11**
– – superior A02.1.04.025 **11**
– – suprema A02.1.04.024 **11**
– obliqua
– – cartilaginis thyroideae A06.2.02.009 **58**
– – mandibulae A02.1.15.008 **15**
– parasternalis A01.2.00.014 **3**
– paravertebralis A01.2.00.021 **3**
– pectinata canalis analis A05.7.05.009 **54**
– pectinea femoris A02.5.04.016 **22**
– scapularis A01.2.00.020 **3**
– semilunaris A04.5.01.025 **38**
– sternalis A01.2.00.013 **3**
– supracondylaris
– – lateralis A02.5.04.020 **22**
– – medialis A02.5.04.019 **22**
– temporalis A02.1.03.013 **10**
– – inferior ossis parietalis A02.1.02.009 **9**
– – ossis frontalis A02.1.03.013 **10**
– – superior ossis parietalis A02.1.02.008 **9**
– terminalis A02.5.02.007 **22**
– – pelvis A02.5.02.007 **22**
– transversae A02.2.05.010 **17**
– – ossis sacri A02.2.05.010 **17**
– trapezoidea A02.4.02.011 **19**
Lingua A05.1.04.001 **49**
Lingula
– cerebelli [I] A14.1.07.103 **118**
– mandibulae A02.1.15.029 **15**
– pulmonis sinistri A06.5.01.018 **60**
– sphenoidalis A02.1.05.013 **11**
Liquor cerebrospinalis A14.1.01.203 **105**
Lobulus/i A06.5.02.027 **61**
– ansiformis cerebelli [H VII A] A14.1.07.207 **119**

– anteromedialis prostatae A09.3.08.014 **69**
– auriculae A15.3.01.003 **148**
– biventer [H VIII] A14.1.07.216 **119**
– centralis cerebelli [II et III] A14.1.07.105 **119**
– epididymidis A09.3.02.003 **68**
– glandulae
– – mammariae A16.0.02.009 **154**
– – thyroideae A11.3.00.009 **74**
– gracilis [H VII B] A14.1.07.213 **119**
– hepatis A05.8.01.056 **55**
– inferolateralis prostatae A09.3.08.012 **69**
– inferoposterior prostatae A09.3.08.011 **69**
– paracentralis A14.1.09.209 **126**
– parafloccularis dorsalis [H VIII B] A14.1.07.219 **119**
– paramedianus [H VII B] A14.1.07.213 **119**
– parietalis
– – inferior A14.1.09.125 **125**
– – superior A14.1.09.130 **125**
– pulmonis A06.5.02.027 **61**
– quadrangularis
– – anterior cerebelli [H IV et V] A14.1.07.116 **119**
– – posterior cerebelli [H VI] A14.1.07.204 **119**
– semilunares cerebelli A14.1.07.207 **119**
– semilunaris
– – inferior cerebelli A14.1.07.210 **119**
– – superior cerebelli A14.1.07.208 **119**
– simplex cerebelli [H VI et VI] A14.1.07.202 **119**
– superomedialis prostatae A09.3.08.013 **69**
– testis A09.3.01.020 **67**
– thymi/ci A13.1.02.003 **100**, A13.1.02.006 **100**
Lobus/i
– anterior hypophysis A11.1.00.002 **74**
– caudatus hepatis A05.8.01.030 **55**, A05.8.01.043 **55**, A05.8.01.044 **55**
– cerebelli
– – anterior A14.1.07.102 **118**
– – posterior A14.1.07.201 **119**
– cerebri A14.1.09.005 **124**
– flocculonodularis A14.1.07.301 **119**
– frontalis A14.1.09.110 **125, 126**
– glandulae
– – mammariae A16.0.02.008 **154**
– – thyroideae A11.3.00.002 **74**
– hepatis
– – dexter A05.8.01.026 **55**
– – sinister A05.8.01.027 **55**
– inferior pulmonis A06.5.01.020 **60**
– insularis A14.1.09.149 **125**
– limbicus A14.1.09.230 **126**
– medius A09.3.08.015 **69**
– – prostatae A09.3.08.015 **69**
– – pulmonis dextri A06.5.01.019 **60**
– nervosus neurohypophysis A11.1.00.008 **74, 120**
– occipitalis A14.1.09.132 **125, 126**
– parietalis A14.1.09.123 **125, 126**
– posterior hypophysis A11.1.00.006 **74, 120, 124**
– prostatae dexter et sinister A09.3.08.010 **69**
– pyramidalis glandulae thyroideae A11.3.00.004 **74**
– quadratus hepatis A05.8.01.029 **55**
– renales A08.1.01.014 **63**
– superior pulmonis A06.5.01.017 **60**
– – dextri A06.5.02.002 **60**
– – sinistri A06.5.02.015 **61**
– temporalis A14.1.09.136 **125, 126**
– thymi A13.1.02.002 **100**
Locus caeruleus A14.1.05.706 **115**
Longitudinalis A01.0.00.028 **1**
Lordosis
– cervicis A02.2.00.006 **16**
– colli A02.2.00.006 **16**
– lumbalis A02.2.00.007 **16**
Luminalis A01.0.00.032 **1**
Lunula/e A16.0.01.005 **154**
– unguis A16.0.01.005 **154**
– valvularum semilunarium valvae
– – aortae A12.1.04.017 **77**
– – trunci pulmonalis A12.1.02.015 **77**
Lympha A12.0.00.043 **75**
Lymphonodus A13.2.03.001 **100**

M

Macula/e A15.3.03.082 **152**
– cribrosa/e A15.3.03.011 **151**
– – inferior A15.3.03.014 **151**
– – media A15.3.03.013 **151**
– – superior A15.3.03.012 **151**
– lutea A15.2.04.021 **145**
– sacculi A15.3.03.084 **152**
– utriculi A15.3.03.083 **152**
– utriculosaccularis A15.3.03.082 **152**
Malleolus
– lateralis A02.5.07.014 **23**
– medialis A02.5.06.020 **23**
Malleus A15.3.02.043 **150**
Mamma A16.0.02.001 **154**
– accessoria A16.0.02.003 **154**
Mammillae dentes A05.1.03.059 **49**
Mandibula A02.1.15.001 **15**
Manubrium
– mallei A15.3.02.044 **150**
– sterni A02.3.03.002 **18**
Manus A01.1.00.025 **2**
Margo
– acetabuli A02.5.01.003 **21**
– anterior
– – corporis pancreatis A05.9.01.011 **56**
– – fibulae A02.5.07.011 **23**
– – pulmonis A06.5.01.012 **60**
– – radii A02.4.05.013 **20**
– – testis A09.3.01.006 **67**
– – tibiae A02.5.06.017 **23**
– – ulnae A02.4.06.012 **20**
– arcuatus hiatus saphenus A04.7.03.017 **43**
– ciliaris iridis A15.2.03.022 **145**
– dexter cordis A12.1.00.006 **76**
– falciformis hiatus saphenus A04.7.03.017 **43**
– fibularis pedis A01.2.08.026 **5**
– frontalis
– – alaris majoris ossis sphenoidalis A02.1.05.032 **11**
– – ossis parietalis A02.1.02.014 **10**
– gingivalis A05.1.01.109 **47**
– incisalis dentis A05.1.03.046 **48**
– inferior
– – corporis pancreatis A05.9.01.012 **56**
– – hepatis A05.8.01.024 **55**
– – pulmonis A06.5.01.014 **60**
– – splenica A13.2.01.015 **100**
– inferolateralis hemispherii cerebri A14.1.09.012 **124**
– inferomedialis hemispherii cerebri A14.1.09.011 **124**
– infraorbitalis A02.1.00.072 **9**
– – corporis maxillae A02.1.12.006 **14**
– interosseus
– – fibulae A02.5.07.012 **23**
– – radii A02.4.05.012 **20**
– – tibiae A02.5.06.019 **23**
– – ulnae A02.4.06.011 **20**
– lacrimalis corporis maxillae A02.1.12.020 **14**
– lambdoideus ossis occipitalis A02.1.04.012 **10**
– lateralis A01.2.07.015 **5**, A02.1.00.073 **9**, A02.4.01.013 **19**, A02.4.04.018 **19**, A08.1.01.002 **63**, A16.0.01.007 **154**
– – antebrachii A01.2.07.015 **5**
– – humeri A02.4.04.018 **19**
– – orbitae A02.1.00.073 **9**
– – pedis A01.2.08.026 **5**
– – renis A08.1.01.002 **63**
– – scapulae A02.4.01.013 **19**
– – unguis A16.0.01.007 **154**
– liber
– – ovarii A09.1.01.005 **65**
– – unguis A16.0.01.008 **154**
– linguae A05.1.04.009 **49**
– mastoideus ossis occipitalis A02.1.04.011 **10**
– medialis
– – antebrochii A01.2.07.016 **5**
– – glandulae suprarenalis A11.5.00.006 **74**
– – humeri A02.4.04.015 **19**
– – orbitae A02.1.00.074 **9**
– – pedis A01.2.08.027 **5**
– – renis A08.1.01.003 **63**

- – scapulae A02.4.01.012 **18**
- – tibiae A02.5.06.018 **23**
– mesovaricus ovarii A09.1.01.006 **65**
– nasalis ossis frontalis A02.1.03.021 **10**
– occipitalis ossis
- – parietalis A02.1.02.011 **9**
- – temporalis A02.1.06.003 **12**
– occultus unguis A16.0.01.006 **154**
– orbitalis A02.1.00.070 **9**
– parietalis
- – alaris majoris ossis sphenoidalis A02.1.05.033 **11**
- – ossis frontalis A02.1.03.012 **10**
- – partis squamosae ossis temporalis A02.1.06.062 **13**
– posterior
- – fibulae A02.5.07.013 **23**
- – partis petrosae ossis temporalis A02.1.06.037 **12**
- – radii A02.4.05.014 **20**
- – testis A09.3.01.007 **67**
- – ulnae A02.4.06.013 **20**
– pupillaris iridis A15.2.03.021 **145**
– radialis antebrachii A01.2.07.015 **5**
– sagittalis ossis parietalis A02.1.02.013 **10**
– sphenoidalis
- – ossis frontalis A02.1.03.027 **10**
- – partis squamosae ossis temporalis A02.1.06.064 **13**
– squamosus A02.1.02.012 **9**, A02.1.05.034 **11**
- – alaris majoris ossis sphenoidalis A02.1.05.034 **11**
- – ossis parietalis A02.1.02.012 **9**
– superior
- – corporis pancreatis A05.9.01.010 **56**
- – glandulae suprarenalis A11.5.00.005 **74**
- – hemispherii cerebri A14.1.09.010 **124**
- – partis petrosae ossis temporalis A02.1.06.029 **12**
- – scapulae A02.4.01.014 **19**
- – splenica A13.2.01.016 **100**
– supraorbitalis A02.1.00.071 **9**
- – ossis frontalis A02.1.03.008 **10**
– tibialis pedis A01.2.08.027 **5**
– ulnaris A01.2.07.016 **5**
– uteri A09.1.03.005 **65**
– zygomaticus alaris majoris ossis sphenoidalis A02.1.05.031 **11**
Massa lateralis atlantis A02.2.02.102 **16**
Matrix unguis A16.0.01.002 **154**
Maxilla A02.1.12.001 **14**
Meatus
– acusticus
- – externus A02.1.06.055 **13**, A15.3.01.045 **149**
- – – cartilagineus A15.3.01.048 **149**
- – internus A02.1.06.033 **12, 151**
– nasi
- – communis A02.1.00.093 **9**, A06.1.02.031 **57**
- – inferior A02.1.00.091 **9**, A06.1.02.029 **57**
- – medius A02.1.00.090 **9**, A06.1.02.024 **57**
- – superior A02.1.00.089 **9**, A06.1.02.023 **57**
– nasopharyngeus A02.1.00.095 **9**, A06.1.02.032 **57**
Medialis A01.0.00.009 **1**
Medianus A01.0.00.003 **1**
Mediastinum A07.1.02.101 **62**
– anterius A07.1.02.104 **62**
– inferius A07.1.02.103 **62**
– medium A07.1.02.105 **62**
– posterius A07.1.02.106 **62**
– superius A07.1.02.102 **62**
– testis A09.3.01.018 **67**
Medius A01.0.00.025 **1**
Medulla
– glandulae suprarenalis A11.5.00.008 **74**
– nodi lymphoidei A13.2.03.006 **101**
– oblongata A14.1.03.003 **108**
– ossium A13.1.01.001 **100**
- – flava A02.0.00.039 **7**
- – rubra A02.0.00.040 **7**
– ovarii A09.1.01.012 **65**
– renalis A08.1.01.020 **63**
– spinalis A14.1.02.001 **105**
– thymi A13.1.02.005 **100**
Membrana
– atlantooccipitalis
- – anterior A03.1.08.002 **27**
- – posterior A03.1.08.004 **27**
– bronchopericardiaca A12.1.08.004 **78**
– fibroelastica laryngis A06.2.09.021 **59**
– fibrosa A03.0.00.027 **25**
– intercostalis
- – externa A03.3.01.002 **28, 37**
- – interna A03.3.01.003 **28, 37**
– interossea A03.0.00.007 **25**
- – antebrachii A03.5.06.002 **29**
- – cruris A03.6.05.002 **30**
– obturatoria A03.6.01.002 **30**
– perinei A09.5.03.002 **71**
– pupillaris A15.2.03.036 **145**
– quadrangularis A06.2.09.022 **59**
– reticularis organi spiralis A15.3.03.122 **153**
– spiralis A15.3.03.100 **152**
– stapedialis A15.3.02.059 **150**
– statoconiorum A15.3.03.085 **152**
– sterni A03.3.05.004 **28**
– suprapleuralis A07.1.02.018 **62**
– synovialis A03.0.00.028 **25**
- – inferior articulationis temporomandibularis A03.1.07.006 **27**
- – superior articulationis temporomandibularis A03.1.07.005 **27**
– tectoria A03.2.04.007 **27**
- – ducti cochlearis A15.3.03.108 **153**
– thyrohyoidea A06.2.02.013 **58**
– tympanica A15.3.01.052 **149**
- – secundaria A15.3.02.019 **149**
– vestibularis A15.3.03.094 **152**
– vitrea A15.2.06.012 **146**
Membrum
– inferius A01.1.00.031 **2**
– superius A01.1.00.019 **2**
Meninges A14.1.01.001 **104**
Meniscus
– articularis A03.0.00.033 **25**
– lateralis A03.6.08.002 **30**
– medialis A03.6.08.005 **30**
Mentum A01.1.00.011 **2**
Meridiani bulbi oculi A15.2.01.005 **144**
Mesencephalon A14.1.03.005 **108, 115**
Mesenterium A10.1.02.007 **72**
Mesoappendix A10.1.02.014 **72**
Mesocolon A10.1.02.009 **72**
– ascendens A10.1.02.011 **72**
– descendens A10.1.02.012 **72**
– sigmoideum A10.1.02.013 **72**
– transversum A10.1.02.010 **72**
Mesocortex A14.1.09.306 **128**
Mesometrium ♀ A10.1.02.506 **73**
Mesosalpinx ♀ A10.1.02.507 **73**
Mesotendineum A04.8.01.008 **44**
Mesovarium ♀ A10.1.02.508 **73**
Metacarpus A01.1.00.027 **2**
Metaphysis A02.0.00.022 **7**
Metatarsus A01.1.00.043 **2**
Metathalamus A14.1.08.301 **120**, A14.1.08.801 **123**
Metencephalon A14.1.03.004 **108**
Modiolus
– anguli oris A04.1.03.035 **34**
– cochleae A15.3.03.038 **151**
Mons pubis A09.2.01.002 **66**
Musculus/i A04.0.00.000 **33**
– abdominis A04.5.00.001 **38**
– abductor A04.0.00.020 **33**
- – digiti minimi
- – – manus A04.6.02.062 **41**
- – – pedis A04.7.02.063 **43**
- – hallucis A04.7.02.056 **43**
- – metatarsi quinti A04.7.02.064 **43**
- – pollicis
- – – brevis A04.6.02.054 **41**
- – – longus A04.6.02.049 **41**
– adductor A04.0.00.021 **33**
- – brevis A04.7.02.027 **42**
- – hallucis A04.7.02.060 **43**
- – longus A04.7.02.026 **42**
- – magnus A04.7.02.028 **42**
- – minimus A04.7.02.029 **42**
- – pollicis A04.6.02.059 **41**
– anconeus A04.6.02.023 **40**
– anoperinealis A05.7.04.014 **54**
– anorectoperineales A05.7.04.012 **54**
– antitragicus A15.3.01.042 **149**
– arrector pili A16.0.00.024 **154**
– articularis
- – cubiti A04.6.02.024 **40**

– – genus A04.7.02.024 **42**
– arytenoideus
– – obliquus A06.2.08.010 **59**
– – transversus A06.2.08.012 **59**
– auriculares A15.3.01.036 **148**
– auricularis
– – anterior A04.1.03.020 **34**
– – posterior A04.1.03.022 **34**
– – superior A04.1.03.021 **34**
– biceps A04.0.00.012 **33**
– – brachii A04.6.02.013 **40**
– – femoris A04.7.02.032 **42**
– bipennatus A04.0.00.016 **33**
– biventer A04.0.00.011 **33**
– brachialis A04.6.02.018 **40**
– brachioradialis A04.6.02.039 **41**
– bronchooesophageus
A05.4.01.012 **51**
– buccinator A04.1.03.036 **35**
– bulbospongiosus
A09.5.02.005 **71**
– capitis A04.1.00.001 **34**
– ceratocricoideus
A06.2.08.005 **59**
– ceratoglossus A05.1.04.104 **49**
– cervicis A04.2.00.001 **35**
– chondroglossus A05.1.04.103 **49**
– ciliaris A15.2.03.014 **144**
– coccygeus A04.5.04.011 **40**
– colli A04.2.00.001 **35**
– compressor urethrae ♀
A09.5.03.005 **71**
– constrictor pharyngis
– – inferior A05.3.01.111 **51**
– – medius A05.3.01.108 **51**
– – superior A05.3.01.103 **51**
– coracobrachialis
A04.6.02.017 **40**
– corrugator supercilii
A04.1.03.018 **34**
– cremaster ♂ A09.3.04.003 **68**,
A04.5.01.018 **38**
– cricoarytenoideus
– – lateralis A06.2.08.006 **59**
– – posterior A06.2.08.004 **59**
– cricopharyngeus A05.3.01.113 **51**
– cricothyroideus A06.2.08.001 **59**
– cutaneus A04.0.00.019 **33**
– dartos A09.4.03.005 **70**
– deltoideus A04.6.02.002 **40**
– depressor
– – anguli oris A04.1.03.026 **34**
– – labii inferioris A04.1.03.033 **34**
– – septi nasi A04.1.03.012 **34**
– – supercilii A04.1.03.019 **34**
– detrusor vesicae
A08.3.01.014 **64**
– digastricus A04.2.03.002 **35**
– dilatator A04.0.00.029 **33**
– – pupillae A15.2.03.030 **145**
– dorsi A04.3.00.001 **36**
– – proprii A04.3.02.001 **36**
– epicranius A04.1.03.002 **34**
– erector spinae A04.3.02.002 **36**
– extensor A04.0.00.024 **33**
– – carpi
– – – radialis
– – – – brevis A04.6.02.041 **41**
– – – – longus A04.6.02.040 **41**
– – – ulnaris A04.6.02.045 **41**
– – digiti minimi A04.6.02.044 **41**
– – digitorum A04.6.02.042 **41**
– – – brevis A04.7.02.055 **43**
– – – longus A04.7.02.038 **42**
– – hallucis
– – – brevis A04.7.02.054 **43**
– – – longus A04.7.02.040 **42**
– – indicis A04.6.02.052 **41**
– – pollicis
– – – brevis A04.6.02.050 **41**
– – – longus A04.6.02.051 **41**
– externi bulbi oculi
A04.1.01.001 **34, 147**
– faciei A04.1.03.001 **34**
– fibularis
– – brevis A04.7.02.042 **42**
– – longus A04.7.02.041 **42**
– – tertius A04.7.02.039 **42**
– flexor A04.0.00.023 **33**
– – accessorius A04.7.02.068 **43**
– – carpi
– – – radialis A04.6.02.028 **41**
– – – ulnaris A04.6.02.030 **41**
– – digiti minimi brevis
– – – manus A04.6.02.063 **41**
– – – pedis A04.7.02.066 **43**
– – digitorum
– – – brevis A04.7.02.067 **43**
– – – longus A04.7.02.052 **43**
– – – profundus A04.6.02.036 **41**
– – – superficialis A04.6.02.033 **41**
– – hallucis
– – – brevis A04.7.02.057 **43**
– – – longus A04.7.02.053 **43**
– – pollicis
– – – brevis A04.6.02.055 **41**
– – – longus A04.6.02.037 **41**
– fusiformis A04.0.00.006 **33**
– gastrocnemius A04.7.02.044 **43**
– gemellus
– – inferior A04.7.02.014 **42**
– – superior A04.7.02.013 **42**
– genioglossus A05.1.04.101 **49**
– geniohyoideus A04.2.03.007 **35**
– gluteus
– – maximus A04.7.02.006 **42**
– – medius A04.7.02.007 **42**
– – minimus A04.7.02.008 **42**
– gracilis A04.7.02.030 **42**
– helicis
– – major A15.3.01.037 **148**
– – minor A15.3.01.038 **148**
– hyoglossus A05.1.04.102 **49**
– iliacus A04.7.02.003 **42**
– iliococcygeus A04.5.04.008 **40**
– iliocostalis A04.3.02.005 **36**
– – cervicis/colli A04.3.02.009 **36**
– – lumborum A04.3.02.006 **36**
– iliopsoas A04.7.02.002 **42**
– incisurae terminalis auriculae
A15.3.01.040 **148**
– infrahyoidei A04.2.04.001 **35**
– infraspinatus A04.6.02.008 **40**
– intercostales
– – externi A04.4.01.012 **37**
– – interni A04.4.01.013 **37**
– – intimi A04.4.01.014 **37**
– interossei
– – dorsales
– – – manus A04.6.02.066 **41**
– – – pedis A04.7.02.070 **43**
– – palmares A04.6.02.067 **41**
– – plantares A04.7.02.071 **43**
– interspinales A04.3.02.301 **37**
– – cervicis/colli A04.3.02.304 **37**
– – lumborum A04.3.02.302 **37**
– – thoracis A04.3.02.303 **37**
– intertransversarii
– – anteriores cervicis/colli
A04.3.01.012 **36**
– – dorsi proprii A04.3.02.401 **37**
– – laterales lumborum
A04.3.01.014 **36**
– – mediales lumborum
A04.3.02.402 **37**
– – posteriores
– – – laterales cervicis/colli
A04.3.01.013 **36**
– – – mediales cervicis/colli
A04.3.02.404 **37**
– – thoracis A04.3.02.403 **37**
– ischiocavernosus
A09.5.02.004 **71**
– ischiococcygeus A04.5.04.011 **40**
– laryngis A04.2.07.001 **36, 59**
– latissimus dorsi A04.3.01.006 **36**
– levator/es
– – anguli oris A04.1.03.034 **34**
– – ani A04.5.04.002 **39**
– – costarum A04.4.01.009 **37**
– – – breves A04.4.01.011 **37**
– – – longi A04.4.01.010 **37**
– – glandulae thyroideae
A04.2.04.008 **35**
– – labii superioris
A04.1.03.031 **34**
– – – alaeque nasi A04.1.03.032 **34**
– – palpebrae superioris
A15.2.07.020 **147**
– – prostatae ♂ A04.5.04.005 **39, 69**
– – scapulae A04.3.01.009 **36**
– – veli palatini A05.2.01.102 **50**
– linguae A04.1.05.001 **35, 49**
– longissimus A04.3.02.010 **36**
– – capitis A04.3.02.014 **36**
– – cervicis/colli A04.3.02.013 **36**
– – thoracis A04.3.02.011 **36**
– longitudinalis
– – inferior linguae
A05.1.04.107 **49**
– – superior linguae
A05.1.04.106 **49**
– longus
– – capitis A04.2.01.003 **35**
– – cervicis/colli A04.2.01.002 **35**
– lumbricales
– – manus A04.6.02.065 **41**
– – pedis A04.7.02.069 **43**
– masseter A04.1.04.002 **35**
– masticatorii A04.1.04.001 **35**
– membri
– – inferioris A04.7.00.001 **42**
– – superioris A04.6.00.001 **40**
– mentalis A04.1.03.037 **35**
– multifidus/i
– – cervicis/colli A04.3.02.205 **37**

– – lumborum A04.3.02.203 **37**
– – thoracis A04.3.02.204 **37**
– multipennatus A04.0.00.017 **33**
– mylohyoideus A04.2.03.006 **35**
– nasalis A04.1.03.009 **34**
– obliquus
– – auriculae A15.3.01.044 **149**
– – capitis
– – – inferior A04.2.02.007 **35**
– – – superior A04.2.02.006 **35**
– – externus abdominis A04.5.01.008 **38**
– – inferior bulbi A15.2.07.019 **147**
– – internus abdominis A04.5.01.017 **38**
– – superior bulbi A15.2.07.016 **147**
– obturatorius
– – externus A04.7.02.031 **42**
– – internus A04.7.02.012 **42**
– occipitofrontalis A04.1.03.003 **34**
– omohyoideus A04.2.04.003 **35**
– opponens A04.0.00.027 **33**
– – digiti minimi
– – – manus A04.6.02.064 **41**
– – – pedis A04.7.02.065 **43**
– – pollicis A04.6.02.058 **41**
– orbicularis A04.0.00.018 **33**
– – oculi A04.1.03.013 **34**
– – oris A04.1.03.023 **34**
– orbitalis A15.2.07.009 **147**
– ossiculorum auditus/auditorium A04.1.02.001 **34, 150**
– palati mollis et faucium A04.1.06.001 **35, 50**
– palatoglossus A05.1.04.110 **49, 50**
– palatopharyngeus A05.2.01.105 **50, 51**
– palmaris
– – brevis A04.6.02.053 **41**
– – longus A04.6.02.029 **41**
– papillaris/es cordis A12.1.00.022 **76**
– – anterior ventriculi
– – – dextri A12.1.02.017 **77**
– – – sinistri A12.1.04.007 **77**
– – posterior ventriculi
– – – dextri A12.1.02.018 **77**
– – – sinistri A12.1.04.008 **77**
– – septalis ventriculi dextri A12.1.02.019 **77**
– pectinati atrii
– – dextri A12.1.01.008 **76**
– – sinistri A12.1.03.003 **77**
– pectineus A04.7.02.025 **42**
– pectoralis
– – major A04.4.01.002 **37**
– – minor A04.4.01.006 **37**
– pennatus A04.0.00.016 **33**
– perinei A04.5.05.001 **40, 71**
– peroneus
– – brevis A04.7.02.042 **42**
– – longus A04.7.02.041 **42**
– – tertius A04.7.02.039 **42**
– pharyngis A04.2.06.001 **36, 51**
– piriformis A04.7.02.011 **42**
– plantaris A04.7.02.049 **43**
– planus A04.0.00.007 **33**
– pleurooesophageus A05.4.01.013 **51**
– popliteus A04.7.02.050 **43**
– procerus A04.1.03.008 **34**
– pronator A04.0.00.025 **33**
– – quadratus A04.6.02.038 **41**
– – teres A04.6.02.025 **40**
– psoas
– – major A04.7.02.004 **42**
– – minor A04.7.02.005 **42**
– pterygoideus
– – lateralis A04.1.04.006 **35**
– – medialis A04.1.04.009 **35**
– puboanalis A04.5.04.006 **39**
– pubococcygeus A04.5.04.003 **39**
– puboperineales A04.5.04.004 **39**
– puboprostaticus A04.5.04.005 **39, 69**
– puborectalis A04.5.04.007 **40**
– pubovaginalis ♀ A04.5.04.005 **39, 69**
– pubovesicalis A04.5.03.014 **39**, A08.3.01.020 **64**
– pyramidalis A04.5.01.007 **38**
– – auriculae A15.3.01.041 **148**
– quadratus A04.0.00.010 **33**
– – femoris A04.7.02.015 **42**
– – lumborum A04.5.01.027 **38**
– – plantae A04.7.02.068 **43**
– quadriceps A04.0.00.014 **33**
– – femoris A04.7.02.017 **42**
– rectococcygeus A05.7.04.011 **54**
– rectoperinealis A05.7.04.013 **54**
– rectourethralis/es A05.7.04.012 **54**
– – inferior A05.7.04.014 **54**
– – superior A05.7.04.013 **54**
– rectouterinus A09.1.03.026 **66**
– rectovesicalis A04.5.03.017 **39, 54, 64**
– rectus A04.0.00.008 **33**
– – abdominis A04.5.01.001 **38**
– – capitis
– – – anterior A04.2.02.002 **35**
– – – lateralis A04.2.02.003 **35**
– – – posterior
– – – – major A04.2.02.004 **35**
– – – – minor A04.2.02.005 **35**
– – femoris A04.7.02.018 **42**
– – inferior bulbi A15.2.07.011 **147**
– – lateralis bulbi A15.2.07.013 **147**
– – medialis bulbi A15.2.07.012 **147**
– – superior bulbi A15.2.07.010 **147**
– regionis
– – analis A09.5.00.003 **71**
– – urogenitalis A09.5.00.004 **71**
– rhomboideus
– – major A04.3.01.007 **36**
– – minor A04.3.01.008 **36**
– risorius A04.1.03.028 **34**
– rotator A04.0.00.022 **33**
– rotatores A04.3.02.210 **37**
– – cervicis/colli A04.3.02.213 **37**
– – lumborum A04.3.02.211 **37**
– – thoracis A04.3.02.212 **37**
– salpingopharyngeus A05.3.01.115 **51**
– sartorius A04.7.02.016 **42**
– scalenus
– – anterior A04.2.01.004 **35**
– – medius A04.2.01.005 **35**
– – minimus A04.2.01.007 **35**
– – posterior A04.2.01.006 **35**
– semimembranosus A04.7.02.036 **42**
– semipennatus A04.0.00.015 **33**
– semispinalis A04.3.02.206 **37**
– – capitis A04.3.02.209 **37**
– – cervicis/colli A04.3.02.208 **37**
– – thoracis A04.3.02.207 **37**
– semitendinosus A04.7.02.035 **42**
– serratus
– – anterior A04.4.01.008 **37**
– – posterior
– – – inferior A04.3.01.010 **36**
– – – superior A04.3.01.011 **36**
– soleus A04.7.02.047 **43**
– sphincter A04.0.00.028 **33**
– – ampullae hepatopancreatica A05.8.02.018 **56**
– – ani
– – – externus A04.5.04.012 **40, 54, 71**
– – – internus A05.7.05.011 **54**
– – ductus
– – – biliaris/choledochi A05.8.02.014 **56**
– – – pancreatici A05.9.01.016 **56**
– – inferior ductus choledochi A05.8.02.016 **56**
– – palatopharyngeus A05.2.01.107 **50**
– – pupillae A15.2.03.029 **145**
– – pyloricus A05.5.01.024 **52**
– – superior A05.8.02.015 **56**
– – – ductus choledochi A05.8.02.015 **56**
– – supracollicularis A09.4.02.013 **70**
– – urethrae
– – – externus ♀ A09.2.03.006 **67, 71**
– – – externus ♂ A09.4.02.016 **70**, A09.4.02.017 **71**
– – – internus A09.4.02.013 **70**
– – urethrovaginalis ♀ A09.5.03.006 **71**
– spinalis A04.3.02.015 **36**
– – capitis A04.3.02.018 **36**
– – cervicis/colli A04.3.02.017 **36**
– – thoracis A04.3.02.016 **36**
– spinotransversales A04.3.02.101 **36**
– splenius A04.3.02.102 **36**
– – capitis A04.3.02.103 **37**
– – cervicis/colli A04.3.02.104 **37**
– stapedius A15.3.02.062 **150**
– sternalis A04.4.01.001 **37**
– sternocleidomastoideus A04.2.01.008 **35**
– sternohyoideus A04.2.04.002 **35**
– sternothyroideus A04.2.04.006 **35**

– styloglossus A05.1.04.105 **49**
– stylohyoideus A04.2.03.005 **35**
– stylopharyngeus A05.3.01.114 **51**
– subclavius A04.4.01.007 **37**
– subcostales A04.4.01.015 **37**
– suboccipitales A04.2.02.001 **35**
– subscapularis A04.6.02.012 **40**
– supinator A04.0.00.026 **33**, A04.6.02.048 **41**
– suprahyoidei A04.2.03.001 **35**
– supraspinatus A04.6.02.006 **40**
– suspensorius duodeni A05.6.02.011 **52**
– tarsalis
– – inferior A15.2.07.046 **147**
– – superior A15.2.07.045 **147**
– temporalis A04.1.04.005 **35**
– temporoparietalis A04.1.03.006 **34**
– tensor
– – fasciae latae A04.7.02.010 **42**
– – tympani A15.3.02.061 **150**
– – veli palatini A05.2.01.103 **50**
– teres
– – major A04.6.02.011 **40**
– – minor A04.6.02.010 **40**
– thoracis A04.4.00.001 **37**
– thyroarytenoideus A06.2.08.008 **59**
– thyrohyoideus A04.2.04.007 **35**
– thyropharyngeus A05.3.01.112 **51**
– tibialis
– – anterior A04.7.02.037 **42**
– – posterior A04.7.02.051 **43**
– trachealis A06.3.01.005 **59**
– tragicus A15.3.01.039 **148**
– transversospinales A04.3.02.201 **37**
– transversus
– – abdominis A04.5.01.019 **38**
– – auriculae A15.3.01.043 **149**
– – linguae A05.1.04.108 **49**
– – menti A04.1.03.027 **34**
– – nuchae A04.3.01.005 **36**
– – perinei
– – – profundus ♂ A09.5.03.004 **71**
– – – superficialis A09.5.02.003 **71**
– – thoracis A04.4.01.016 **37**
– trapezius A04.3.01.001 **36**
– triangularis A04.0.00.009 **33**
– triceps A04.0.00.013 **33**
– – brachii A04.6.02.019 **40**
– – surae A04.7.02.043 **43**
– trigoni vesicae A08.3.01.011 **64**
– – profundus A08.3.01.013 **64**
– – superficialis A08.3.01.012 **64**
– unipennatus A04.0.00.015 **33**
– uvulae A05.2.01.104 **50**
– vastus
– – intermedius A04.7.02.022 **42**
– – lateralis A04.7.02.021 **42**
– – medialis A04.7.02.023 **42**
– verticalis linguae A05.1.04.109 **49**
– vesicoprostaticus ♂ A08.3.01.021 **64, 69**
– vesicovaginalis ♀ A08.3.01.021 **64, 69**
– vocalis A06.2.08.007 **59**
– zygomaticus
– – major A04.1.03.029 **34**
– – minor A04.1.03.030 **34**
Myelencephalon A14.1.03.003 **108**
Myocardium A12.1.06.001 **77**
Myometrium A09.1.03.025 **66**

N

Nares A06.1.02.002 **57**
Nasion A02.1.00.015 **8**
Nasus A01.1.00.009 **2**, A06.1.01.001 **57**
Nates A01.1.00.033 **2**
Neocerebellum A14.1.07.012 **118**
Neocortex A14.1.09.304 **128**
Nephros A08.1.01.001 **63**
Nervus/i A14.2.00.013 **132**
– abducens [VI] A14.2.01.098 **135**
– accessorius [XI] A14.2.01.184 **137**
– alveolares superiores A14.2.01.049 **134**
– alveolaris inferior A14.2.01.089 **135**
– ampullaris
– – anterior A14.2.01.128 **135**
– – lateralis A14.2.01.129 **136**
– – posterior A14.2.01.131 **136**
– anales
– – inferiores A14.2.07.038 **140**
– – superiores A14.3.03.051 **143**
– anococcygeus A14.2.07.045 **140**
– auriculares/is
– – anteriores A14.2.01.079 **134**
– – magnus A14.2.02.018 **137**
– – posterior A14.2.01.102 **135**
– auriculotemporalis A14.2.01.074 **134**
– autonomicus A14.2.00.039 **133**
– axillaris A14.2.03.059 **139**
– buccalis A14.2.01.073 **134**
– canalis pterygoidei A14.3.02.007 **142**
– cardiacus cervicalis
– – inferior A14.3.01.022 **141**
– – medius A14.3.01.018 **141**
– – superior A14.3.01.015 **141**
– carotici externi A14.3.01.013 **141**
– caroticotympanici A14.2.01.142 **136, 142**
– caroticus internus A14.3.01.011 **141**
– cavernosi
– – clitoridis ♀ A14.3.03.056 **143**
– – penis ♂ A14.3.03.056 **143**
– cervicales [C1–C8] A14.2.02.002 **137**
– ciliares breves A14.3.02.005 **142**
– ciliares longi A14.2.01.027 **134**
– clunium
– – inferiores A14.2.07.034 **140**
– – medii A14.2.06.006 **139**
– – superiores A14.2.05.006 **139**
– coccygeus A14.2.07.043 **140**
– cochlearis A14.2.01.133 **136**
– craniales A14.2.01.001 **133**
– cranialis A14.2.00.038 **133**
– curvaturae minoris
– – anterior A14.2.01.176 **136**
– – posterior A14.2.01.181 **137**
– cutaneus
– – antebrachii
– – – lateralis A14.2.03.026 **138**
– – – medialis A14.2.03.028 **138**
– – – posterior A14.2.03.052 **138**
– – brachii
– – – lateralis
– – – – inferior A14.2.03.051 **138**
– – – – superior A14.2.03.061 **139**
– – – medialis A14.2.03.027 **138**
– – – posterior A14.2.03.050 **138**
– – dorsalis
– – – intermedius A14.2.07.053 **140**
– – – lateralis A14.2.07.063 **141**
– – – medialis A14.2.07.052 **140**
– – femoris
– – – lateralis A14.2.07.011 **140**
– – – posterior A14.2.07.033 **140**
– – perforans A14.2.07.036 **140**
– – surae
– – – lateralis A14.2.07.048 **140**
– – – medialis A14.2.07.061 **141**
– digitales
– – dorsales
– – – manus A14.2.03.043 **138**, A14.2.03.058 **139**
– – – pedis A14.2.07.054 **140**, A14.2.07.057 **140**
– – palmares
– – – communes A14.2.03.038 **138**, A14.2.03.046 **138**
– – – proprii A14.2.03.039 **138**, A14.2.03.047 **138**
– – plantares
– – – communes A14.2.07.067 **141**, A14.2.07.071 **141**
– – – proprii A14.2.07.068 **141**, A14.2.07.072 **141**
– dorsalis
– – clitoridis ♀ A14.2.07.042 **140**
– – penis ♂ A14.2.07.042 **140**
– – scapulae A14.2.03.011 **138**
– ethmoidalis
– – anterior A14.2.01.030 **134**
– – posterior A14.2.01.028 **134**
– facialis [VII] A14.2.01.099 **135**
– femoralis A14.2.07.020 **140**
– fibularis
– – communis A14.2.07.047 **140**
– – profundus A14.2.07.055 **140**
– – superficialis A14.2.07.050 **140**
– frontalis A14.2.01.020 **133**
– genitofemoralis A14.2.07.008 **139**
– glossopharyngeus [IX] A14.2.01.135 **136**
– gluteus
– – inferior A14.2.07.032 **140**
– – superior A14.2.07.031 **140**
– hypogastricus A14.3.03.047 **143**
– hypoglossus [XII] A14.2.01.191 **137**

– iliohypogastricus A14.2.07.003 **139**
– ilioinguinalis A14.2.07.006 **139**
– iliopubicus A14.2.07.003 **139**
– infraorbitalis A14.2.01.059 **134**
– infratrochlearis A14.2.01.035 **134**
– intercostales A14.2.04.006 **139**
– intercostobrachiales A14.2.04.012 **139**
– intermedius A14.2.01.115 **135**
– interosseus
– – antebrachii
– – – anterior A14.2.03.034 **138**
– – – posterior A14.2.03.055 **138**
– – cruris A14.2.07.060 **141**
– ischiadicus A14.2.07.046 **140**
– jugularis A14.3.01.010 **141**
– labiales
– – anteriores ♀ A14.2.07.007 **139**
– – posteriores ♀ A14.2.07.040 **140**
– lacrimalis A14.2.01.018 **133**
– laryngeus
– – recurrens A14.2.01.166 **136**
– – superior A14.2.01.160 **136**
– lingualis A14.2.01.081 **135**
– lumbales [L1–L5] A14.2.05.001 **139**
– mandibularis [Vc] A14.2.01.064 **134**
– massetericus A14.2.01.070 **134**
– maxillaris [Vb] A14.2.01.037 **134**
– meatus acustici externi A14.2.01.075 **134**
– medianus A14.2.03.031 **138**
– mentalis A14.2.01.094 **135**
– mixtus A14.2.00.023 **133**
– motorius A14.2.00.021 **133**
– musculi
– – obturatorii interni A14.2.07.028 **140**
– – piriformis A14.2.07.029 **140**
– – pterygoideus medialis A14.2.01.066 **134**
– – quadrati femoris A14.2.07.030 **140**
– – tensoris
– – – tympani A14.2.01.069 **134**
– – – veli palatini A14.2.01.068 **134**
– musculocutaneus A14.2.03.024 **138**
– mylohyoideus A14.2.01.090 **135**
– nasociliaris A14.2.01.025 **133**
– nasopalatinus A14.2.01.043 **134**
– obturatorius A14.2.07.012 **140**
– – accessorius A14.2.07.019 **140**
– occipitalis
– – major A14.2.02.008 **137**
– – minor A14.2.02.017 **137**
– – tertius A14.2.02.009 **137**
– oculomotorius [III] A14.2.01.007 **133**
– olfactorius [I] A14.2.01.004 **133**
– ophthalmicus [Va] A14.2.01.016 **133**
– opticus [II] A15.2.04.024 **145**, A14.2.01.006 **133**
– palatini minores A14.2.01.047 **134**
– palatinus major A14.2.01.045 **134**
– pectoralis
– – lateralis A14.2.03.018 **138**
– – medialis A14.2.03.017 **138**
– perineales A14.2.07.039 **140**
– peroneus
– – communis A14.2.07.047 **140**
– – profundus A14.2.07.055 **140**
– – superficialis A14.2.07.050 **140**
– petrosus
– – major A14.2.01.117 **135, 142**
– – minor A14.2.01.149 **136, 142**
– – profundus A14.3.02.008 **142**
– pharyngeus A14.2.01.044 **134**
– phrenici accessorii A14.2.02.031 **137**
– phrenicus A14.2.02.028 **137**
– pinealis A14.3.01.012 **141**
– plantaris
– – lateralis A14.2.07.069 **141**
– – medialis A14.2.07.066 **141**
– presacralis A14.3.03.046 **143**
– pterygoideus
– – lateralis A14.2.01.072 **134**
– – medialis A14.2.01.066 **134**
– pudendus A14.2.07.037 **140**
– radialis A14.2.03.049 **138**
– rectales inferiores A14.2.07.038 **140**
– saccularis A14.2.01.132 **136**
– sacrales et nervus coccygeus [S1–S5, Co] A14.2.06.001 **139**
– saphenus A14.2.07.023 **140**
– scrotales ♂
– – anteriores A14.2.07.007 **139**
– – posteriores A14.2.07.040 **140**
– sensorius A14.2.00.022 **133**
– spinales A14.2.02.001 **137**
– spinalis A14.2.00.027 **133**
– spinosus A14.2.01.065 **134**
– splanchnici
– – lumbales A14.3.01.034 **142**
– – pelvici A14.3.02.018 **142**
– – sacrales A14.3.01.036 **142**
– splanchnicus
– – imus A14.3.01.032 **142**
– – major A14.3.01.028 **141**
– – minor A14.3.01.030 **141**
– stapedius A14.2.01.101 **135**
– subclavius A14.2.03.013 **138**
– subcostalis A14.2.04.016 **139**
– sublingualis A14.2.01.085 **135**
– suboccipitalis A14.2.02.007 **137**
– subscapulares A14.2.03.015 **138**
– supraclaviculares A14.2.02.024 **137**
– – intermedii A14.2.02.026 **137**
– – laterales A14.2.02.027 **137**
– – mediales A14.2.02.025 **137**
– supraorbitalis A14.2.01.021 **133**
– suprascapularis A14.2.03.014 **138**
– supratrochlearis A14.2.01.024 **133**
– suralis A14.2.07.062 **141**
– temporales profundi A14.2.01.071 **134**
– terminalis [0] A14.2.01.002 **133**
– thoracici [T1–T12] A14.2.04.001 **139**
– thoracicus longus A14.2.03.012 **138**
– thoracodorsalis A14.2.03.016 **138**
– tibialis A14.2.07.058 **141**
– transversus cervicalis/colli A14.2.02.021 **137**
– trigeminus [V] A14.2.01.012 **133**
– trochlearis [IV] A14.2.01.011 **133**
– tympanicus A14.2.01.138 **136**
– ulnaris A14.2.03.040 **138**
– utricularis A14.2.01.127 **135**
– utriculoampullaris A14.2.01.126 **135**
– vaginales ♀ A14.3.03.053 **143**
– vagus [X] A14.2.01.153 **136**
– vasorum A14.2.00.045 **133**
– vertebralis A14.3.01.023 **141**
– vestibularis A14.2.01.122 **135**
– vestibulocochlearis [VIII] A14.2.01.121 **135**
– zygomaticus A14.2.01.056 **134**
Neurocranium A02.1.00.007 **8**
Neurofibra/e A13.0.00.001 **104**
– afferentes A14.2.00.017 **132**
– autonomicae A14.2.00.020 **132**
– efferentes A14.2.00.018 **132**
– postganglionicae A14.2.00.010 **132**
– preganglionicae A14.2.00.009 **132**
– somaticae A14.2.00.019 **132**
– tangentiales isocorticis A14.1.09.320 **128**
Neuroglia A14.0.00.005 **104**
Neurohypophysis A11.1.00.006 **74, 120, 124**
Neuron A14.0.00.002 **104**
Nodulus/i
– lymphoidei
– – aggregati
– – – appendicis vermiformis A05.7.02.009 **53, 101**
– – – intestini tenuis A05.6.01.014 **52, 101**
– – lienales A13.2.01.021 **100**
– – pharyngeales A05.3.01.009 **50, 100**
– – solitarii intestini tenuis A05.6.01.013 **52, 101**
– – splenici A13.2.01.021 **100**
– – tonsillae lingualis A05.1.04.023 **49, 100**
– valvularum semilunarium valvae
– – aortae A12.1.04.016 **77**
– – trunci pulmonalis A12.1.02.014 **77**
– vermis [X] A14.1.07.302 **119**
Nodus/i
– atrioventricularis A12.1.06.004 **77**
– lymphoidei/aticus/lymphonodus A13.2.03.001 **100**
– – abdominis A13.3.03.001 **102**

– – – parietales A13.3.03.002 **102**
– – – viscerales A13.3.03.014 **102**
– – accessorii A13.3.00.037 **101**
– – anorectales A13.3.04.030 **103**
– – anterior jugulodigastrici A13.3.00.031 **101**
– – anteriores juguloomohyoidei A13.3.00.035 **101**
– – aortici laterales A13.3.03.004 **102**
– – arcus venae azygos A13.3.02.009 **102**
– – appendiculares A13.3.03.039 **102**
– – axillares A13.3.01.002 **101**
– – axillarum
– – – anteriores A13.3.01.006 **101**
– – – apicales A13.3.01.003 **101**
– – – centrales A13.3.01.007 **101**
– – – laterales A13.3.01.004 **101**
– – – posteriores A13.3.01.005 **101**
– – brachiales A13.3.01.010 **101**
– – brachiocephalici A13.3.02.007 **102**
– – bronchopulmonales A13.3.02.015 **102**
– – buccinatorius A13.3.00.010 **101**
– – capitis et colli A13.3.00.001 **101**
– – cavales laterales A13.3.03.009 **102**
– – cervicales
– – – anteriores A13.3.00.017 **101**
– – – – profundi A13.3.00.019 **101**
– – – – superficiales A13.3.00.018 **101**
– – – laterales A13.3.00.026 **101**
– – – – profundi
– – – – – inferiores A13.3.00.032 **101**
– – – – – superiores A13.3.00.028 **101**
– – – – superficiales A13.3.00.027 **101**
– – coeliaci A13.3.03.015 **102**
– – colici
– – – dextri A13.3.03.042 **103**
– – – medii A13.3.03.042 **103**
– – – sinistri A13.3.03.042 **103**
– – colli
– – – anteriores A13.3.00.017 **101**
– – – laterales A13.3.00.026 **101**
– – cubitales A13.3.01.011 **101**
– – cysticus A13.3.03.031 **102**
– – deltopectorales A13.3.01.009 **101**
– – epigastrici inferiores A13.3.03.013 **102**
– – faciales A13.3.00.009 **101**
– – fibularis A13.3.05.016 **103**
– – foraminalis A13.3.03.032 **102**
– – gastrici dextri/sinistri A13.3.03.016 **102**
– – gastroomentales dextri/sinistri A13.3.03.018 **102**
– – gluteales A13.3.04.019 **103**
– – – inferiores A13.3.04.021 **103**
– – – superiores A13.3.04.020 **103**
– – hepatici A13.3.03.030 **102**
– – humerales A13.3.01.004 **101**
– – ileocolici A13.3.03.036 **102**
– – iliaci
– – – communes A13.3.04.003 **103**
– – – – intermedii A13.3.04.005 **103**
– – – – laterales A13.3.04.006 **103**
– – – – mediales A13.3.04.004 **103**
– – – externi A13.3.04.009 **103**
– – – – intermedii A13.3.04.011 **103**
– – – – laterales A13.3.04.012 **103**
– – – – mediales A13.3.04.010 **103**
– – – interni A13.3.04.018 **103**
– – inferiores A13.3.03.025 **102**
– – infraauriculares A13.3.00.007 **101**
– – infraclaviculares A13.3.01.009 **101**
– – infrahyoidei A13.3.00.020 **101**
– – inguinales A13.3.05.002 **103**
– – – profundi A13.3.05.007 **103**
– – – – distalis A13.3.05.010 **103**
– – – – intermedius A13.3.05.009 **103**
– – – – proximalis A13.3.05.008 **103**
– – – superficiales A13.3.05.003 **103**
– – – – inferiores A13.3.05.006 **103**
– – – – superolaterales A13.3.05.005 **103**
– – – – superomediales A13.3.05.004 **103**
– – intercostales A13.3.02.004 **102**
– – interiliaci A13.3.04.016 **103**
– – interpectorales A13.3.01.008 **101**
– – intraglandulares A13.3.00.008 **101**
– – intrapulmonales A13.3.02.016 **102**
– – jugulodigastricus A13.3.00.029 **101**
– – juguloomohyoideus A13.3.00.033 **101**
– – juxtaintestinales A13.3.03.034 **102**
– – juxtaoesophageales A13.3.02.017 **102**
– – lacunaris vasculorum
– – – intermedius A13.3.04.014 **103**
– – – lateralis A13.3.04.015 **103**
– – – medialis A13.3.04.013 **103**
– – lateralis
– – – jugulodigastrici A13.3.00.030 **101**
– – – juguloomohyoidei A13.3.00.034 **101**
– – lienales A13.3.03.026 **102**
– – ligamenti arteriosi A13.3.02.008 **102**
– – linguales A13.3.00.014 **101**
– – lumbales
– – – dextri A13.3.03.008 **102**
– – – intermedii A13.3.03.007 **102**
– – – sinistri A13.3.03.003 **102**
– – malaris A13.3.00.012 **101**
– – mandibularis A13.3.00.013 **101**
– – mastoidei A13.3.00.003 **101**
– – membri
– – – inferioris A13.3.05.001 **103**
– – – superioris A13.3.01.001 **101**
– – mesenterici
– – – inferiores A13.3.03.043 **103**
– – – superiores A13.3.03.033 **102**
– – mesocolici A13.3.03.040 **103**
– – nasolabialis A13.3.00.011 **101**
– – obturatorii A13.3.04.017 **103**
– – occipitales A13.3.00.002 **101**
– – pancreatici A13.3.03.023 **102**
– – pancreaticoduodenales A13.3.03.027 **102**
– – – inferiores A13.3.03.029 **102**
– – – superiores A13.3.03.028 **102**
– – paracolici A13.3.03.041 **103**
– – paramammarii A13.3.02.002 **102**
– – pararectales A13.3.04.030 **103**
– – parasternales A13.3.02.003 **102**
– – paratracheales A13.3.00.024 **101**, A13.3.02.011 **102**
– – parauterini ♀ A13.3.04.028 **103**
– – paravaginales ♀ A13.3.04.029 **103**
– – paravesicales A13.3.04.024 **103**
– – parietales A13.3.03.002 **102**, A13.3.04.002 **103**
– – parotidei
– – – profundi A13.3.00.005 **101**
– – – superficiales A13.3.00.004 **101**
– – pectorales A13.3.01.006 **101**
– – pelvis A13.3.04.001 **103**
– – – parietales A13.3.04.002 **103**
– – – viscerales A13.3.04.023 **103**
– – pericardiaci laterales A13.3.02.010 **102**
– – phrenici
– – – inferiores A13.3.03.012 **102**
– – – superiores A13.3.02.005 **102**
– – poplitei A13.3.05.011 **103**
– – – profundi A13.3.05.013 **103**
– – – superficiales A13.3.05.012 **103**
– – postaortici A13.3.03.006 **102**
– – postcavales A13.3.03.011 **102**
– – postvesicales A13.3.04.026 **103**
– – preaortici A13.3.03.005 **102**
– – precaecales A13.3.03.037 **102**
– – precavales A13.3.03.010 **102**
– – prelaryngei A13.3.00.021 **101**
– – prepericardiaci A13.3.02.006 **102**
– – pretracheales A13.3.00.023 **101**
– – prevertebrales A13.3.02.018 **102**
– – prevesicales A13.3.04.025 **103**

- – profundi membri superioris A13.3.01.014 **102**
- – promontorii A13.3.04.008 **103**
- – pylorici A13.3.03.019 **102**
- – rectales superiores A13.3.03.045 **103**
- – regionales A12.4.02.001 **99, 101**
- – retroaortici A13.3.03.006 **102**
- – retrocaecales A13.3.03.038 **102**
- – retrocavales A13.3.03.011 **102**
- – retropharyngeales A13.3.00.038 **101**
- – retropharyngei A13.3.00.025 **101**
- – retropylorici A13.3.03.022 **102**
- – retrovesicales A13.3.04.026 **103**
- – sacrales A13.3.04.022 **103**
- – sigmoidei A13.3.03.044 **103**
- – splenici A13.3.03.026 **102**
- – subaortici A13.3.04.007 **103**
- – submandibulares A13.3.00.016 **101**
- – submentales A13.3.00.015 **101**
- – subpylorici A13.3.03.021 **102**
- – subscapulares A13.3.01.005 **101**
- – superficiales membri superioris A13.3.01.013 **102**
- – superiores A13.3.03.024 **102**
- – – centrales A13.3.03.035 **102**
- – supraclaviculares A13.3.00.036 **101**
- – suprapyloricus A13.3.03.020 **102**
- – supratrochleares A13.3.01.012 **101**
- – thoracis A13.3.02.001 **102**
- – thyroidei A13.3.00.022 **101**
- – tibialis
- – – anterior A13.3.05.014 **103**
- – – posterior A13.3.05.015 **103**
- – tracheobronchiales A13.3.02.012 **102**
- – – inferiores A13.3.02.014 **102**
- – – superiores A13.3.02.013 **102**
- – vesicales laterales A13.3.04.027 **103**
- – viscerales A13.3.03.014 **102**, A13.3.04.023 **103**

Norma
- basalis A02.1.00.006 **8**
- facialis A02.1.00.002 **8**
- frontalis A02.1.00.002 **8**
- inferior A02.1.00.006 **8**
- lateralis A02.1.00.005 **8**
- occipitalis A02.1.00.004 **8**
- superior A02.1.00.003 **8**
- verticalis A02.1.00.003 **8**

Nucleus/i A14.1.00.003 **104**
- accessorius/i
- – lateralis tractus optici A14.1.06.316 **117**
- – medialis tractus optici A14.1.06.317 **117**
- – nervi oculomotorii A14.1.06.303 **117**
- – posterior tractus optici A14.1.06.315 **117**
- – tractus optici A14.1.06.314 **117**
- accumbens A14.1.09.440 **129**
- ambiguus A14.1.04.253 **111**
- amygdalae
- – basalis
- – – lateralis A14.1.09.407 **129**
- – – medialis A14.1.09.408 **129**
- – centralis A14.1.09.409 **129**
- – corticalis A14.1.09.410 **129**
- – interstitialis A14.1.09.411 **129**
- – lateralis A14.1.09.412 **129**
- – medialis A14.1.09.413 **129**
- ansae lenticularis A14.1.08.919 **123**
- anterior/es
- – corporis trapezoidei A14.1.05.422 **114**
- – hypothalami A14.1.08.903 **123**
- – lemnisci lateralis A14.1.05.434 **114**
- – medullae spinalis A14.1.02.106 **106**
- – pontis A14.1.05.203 **112**
- – thalami A14.1.08.603 **121**
- – ventrolateralis thalami A14.1.08.650 **122**
- anterodorsalis thalami A14.1.08.604 **121**
- anterolateralis
- – medullae spinalis A14.1.02.105 **106**
- – nuclei principalis nervi trigemini A14.1.05.408 **114**
- anteromedialis
- – accessorii nervi oculomotorii A14.1.06.305 **117**
- – medullae spinalis A14.1.02.107 **106**
- – thalami A14.1.08.605 **121**
- anteroventralis A14.1.08.606 **121**
- – thalami A14.1.08.606 **121**
- arcuatus A14.1.04.256 **111**, A14.1.08.923 **123**
- autonomici A14.1.06.304 **117**
- basales et structurae pertinentes A14.1.09.501 **130**
- basalis
- – telencephali A14.1.09.418 **129**
- – ventralis medialis thalami A14.1.08.645 **122**
- basilaris internus medullae spinalis A14.1.02.126 **106**
- caeruleus A14.1.05.436 **114**
- campi
- – dorsalis subthalamici [H1] A14.1.08.705 **123**
- – medialis subthalamici [H] A14.1.08.704 **123**
- – perizonalis subthalamici [H, H1, H2] A14.1.08.703 **123**
- – ventralis subthalamici [H2] A14.1.08.706 **123**
- caudatus A14.1.09.502 **130**
- centralis
- – colliculi inferioris A14.1.06.603 **118**
- – lateralis thalami A14.1.08.616 **121**
- – medialis thalami A14.1.08.617 **121**
- – medullae spinalis A14.1.02.111 **106**
- centromedianus thalami A14.1.08.618 **121**
- cerebelli A14.1.07.406 **120**
- cervicalis
- – lateralis A14.1.02.127 **106**
- – medialis A14.1.02.128 **106**
- cochleares
- – in medulla oblongata A14.1.04.247 **111**
- – in tegmento ponti A14.1.05.430 **114**
- cochlearis
- – anterior A14.1.04.249 **111**
- – posterior A14.1.04.248 **111**
- colliculi inferioris A14.1.06.602 **118**
- commissurae posterioris A14.1.06.309 **117**
- commissuralis A14.1.04.232 **111**
- – nervi vagi A14.1.04.252 **111**
- – rhomboidalis A14.1.08.633 **122**
- corporis
- – geniculati medialis A14.1.08.808 **123**
- – trapezoidei A14.1.05.421 **114**
- cuneatus A14.1.04.206 **110**
- – accessorius A14.1.04.209 **110**
- cuneiformis A14.1.06.334 **117, 118**
- dentatus A14.1.07.407 **120**
- dorsales thalami A14.1.08.607 **121**
- dorsalis
- – accessorii nervi pculomotorii A14.1.06.306 **117**
- – corporis geniculati
- – – lateralis A14.1.08.802 **123**
- – – medialis A14.1.08.810 **123**
- – hypothalami A14.1.08.921 **123**
- – lateralis A14.1.08.608 **121**
- – – thalami A14.1.08.608 **121**
- – nervi vagi A14.1.04.229 **110**
- – thoracici A14.1.02.135 **106**
- dorsomedialis
- – hypothalamicae
- – – dorsalis A14.1.08.917 **123**
- – – intermediae A14.1.08.922 **123**
- emboliformis A14.1.07.409 **120**
- endolemniscalis A14.1.04.259 **111**
- endopeduncularis A14.1.08.918 **123**
- externus colliculi inferioris A14.1.06.604 **118**
- fastigii A14.1.07.411 **120**
- gelatinosus solitarius A14.1.04.233 **111**
- gigantocellularis A14.1.04.302 **111**
- – anterior A14.1.04.304 **111**
- globosus A14.1.07.410 **120**
- gracilis A14.1.04.202 **110**

– habenularis
– – lateralis A14.1.08.503 **121**
– – medialis A14.1.08.504 **121**
– infundibularis A14.1.08.923 **123**
– intercalatus A14.1.04.264 **111**
– interfascicularis
– – nervi hypoglossi A14.1.04.306 **111**
– – tegmentalis A14.1.06.331 **117**
– intermediolateralis medullae spinalis A14.1.02.133 **106**
– intermediomedialis medullae spinalis A14.1.02.137 **106**
– intermedius
– – lemnisci lateralis A14.1.05.433 **114**
– – solitarius A14.1.04.234 **111**
– interpeduncularis A14.1.06.313 **117**
– interpositus
– – anterior A14.1.07.409 **120**
– – posterior A14.1.07.410 **120**
– interstitialis/es A14.1.06.307 **117**
– – fasciculi longitudinalis medialis A14.1.05.438 **114**
– – hypothalami anteriores A14.1.08.905 **123**
– – solitarius A14.1.04.235 **111**
– intralaminares thalami A14.1.08.615 **121**
– lacrimalis A14.1.05.414 **114**
– lateral/ises A14.1.05.420 **114**
– – accessorii tracti optici A14.1.06.316 **117**
– – cerebelli A14.1.07.407 **120**
– – colliculi inferioris A14.1.06.604 **118**
– – corporis trapezoidei A14.1.05.423 **114**
– – pontis A14.1.05.204 **112**
– – posterior thalami A14.1.08.609 **121**
– lemnisci lateralis A14.1.05.431 **114**
– lentiformis A14.1.09.506 **130**
– lentis A15.2.05.004 **146**
– limitans A14.1.08.635 **122**
– linearis
– – inferioris A14.1.06.402 **117**
– – intermedius A14.1.06.403 **118**
– – superior A14.1.06.404 **118**
– mammillaris
– – lateralis A14.1.08.935 **124**
– – medialis A14.1.08.936 **124**
– marginalis
– – corporis restiformis A14.1.04.246 **111**
– – medullae spinalis A14.1.02.117 **106**
– mediales A14.1.05.419 **114**
– – thalami A14.1.08.621 **121**
– medialis A14.1.06.317 **117**
– – accessorii tracti optici A14.1.02.141 **106**
– – anterior medullae spinalis A14.1.02.141 **106**
– – cerebelli A14.1.07.411 **120**
– – corporis trapezoidei A14.1.05.424 **114**
– – magnocellularis corporis geniculati medialis A14.1.08.811 **123**
– – solitarius A14.1.04.236 **111**
– mediani thalami A14.1.08.627 **122**
– medianus pontis A14.1.05.205 **112**
– mediodorsalis thalami A14.1.08.622 **122**
– medioventralis A14.1.08.626 **122**
– mesencephalicus nervi trigemini A14.1.05.409 **114, 117**
– motorius nervi trigemini A14.1.05.410 **114**
– nervi
– – abducentis A14.1.05.411 **114**
– – accessorii A14.1.02.112 **106**
– – cranialis A14.1.00.004 **104**
– – facialis A14.1.05.412 **114**
– – hypoglossi A14.1.04.227 **110**
– – oculomotorii A14.1.06.302 **117**
– – phrenici A14.1.02.113 **106**
– – pudendi A14.1.02.139 **106**
– – trochlearis A14.1.06.319 **117**
– olfactorius anterior A14.1.09.416 **129**
– olivaris/es
– – accessorius
– – – medialis A14.1.04.226 **110**
– – – posterior A14.1.04.225 **110**
– – inferiores A14.1.04.219 **110**
– – principalis A14.1.04.220 **110**
– – superior A14.1.05.415 **114**
– – – lateralis A14.1.05.416 **114**
– – – medialis A14.1.05.417 **114**
– originis A14.1.00.005 **104**
– parabigeminalis A14.1.06.320 **117**
– parabrachialis/es A14.1.05.439 **114**
– – lateralis A14.1.05.441 **114**
– – medialis A14.1.05.446 **114**
– paracentralis thalami A14.1.08.619 **121**
– paracommissuralis solitarius A14.1.04.237 **111**
– parafascicularis thalami A14.1.08.620 **121**
– paragigantocellularis
– – lateralis A14.1.04.305 **111**
– – posterior A14.1.04.313 **112**
– paralemniscalis A14.1.05.504 **114**
– paramedianus
– – pontis A14.1.05.206 **112**
– – posterior A14.1.04.228 **110**
– paranigralis A14.1.06.333 **117**
– parapeduncularis A14.1.06.702 **118**
– parasolitarius A14.1.04.231 **111**
– parasympathici sacrales A14.1.02.138 **106**
– parataenialis A14.1.08.628 **122**
– paraventricularis/es
– – anterior thalami A14.1.08.630 **122**
– – hypothalami A14.1.08.909 **123**
– – posterior thalami A14.1.08.631 **122**
– – thalami A14.1.08.629 **122**
– peduncularis pontis A14.1.05.207 **112**
– pericentralis colliculi inferioris A14.1.06.605 **118**
– pericuneatus
– – lateralis A14.1.04.261 **111**
– – medialis A14.1.04.260 **111**
– perifornicalis A14.1.08.931 **124**
– perihypoglossales A14.1.04.262 **111**
– periolivares A14.1.05.418 **114**
– periolivarum
– – laterales A14.1.05.420 **114**
– – mediales A14.1.05.419 **114**
– peripeduncularis A14.1.06.322 **117**
– peritrigeminalis A14.1.04.266 **111**
– periventricularis A14.1.08.924 **123**
– – posterior A14.1.08.925 **123**
– – ventralis A14.1.08.904 **123**
– pigmentosus parabrachialis A14.1.06.332 **117**
– pontis A14.1.05.202 **112**
– pontobulbaris A14.1.04.267 **111**
– posterior
– – accessorii tracti optici A14.1.06.315 **117**
– – funiculi lateralis A14.1.02.129 **106**
– – – medullae spinalis A14.1.02.129 **106**
– – hypothalami A14.1.08.939 **124**
– – lateralis pontis A14.1.05.209 **112**
– – lemnisci lateralis A14.1.05.432 **114**
– – medialis pontis A14.1.05.210 **112**
– – nervi vagi A14.1.04.229 **110**
– – pontis A14.1.05.208 **112**
– – thalami A14.1.08.636 **122**
– – ventrolateralis thalami A14.1.08.651 **122**
– posteriores thalami A14.1.08.634 **122**
– posterolateralis medullae spinalis A14.1.02.108 **106**
– posteromedialis
– – medullae spinalis A14.1.02.110 **106**
– – nuclei principalis nervi trigemini A14.1.05.407 **114**
– precommissuralis centralis A14.1.06.308 **117**
– precuneatus accessorius A14.1.04.210 **110**
– pregeniculatus A14.1.08.806 **123**
– premammillaris
– – dorsalis A14.1.08.934 **124**
– – ventralis A14.1.08.938 **124**
– preopticus
– – lateralis A14.1.08.906 **123**
– – medialis A14.1.08.907 **123**
– – medianus A14.1.08.908 **123**

– – periventricularis A14.1.08.910 **123**
– prepositus A14.1.04.265 **111**
– pretectales A14.1.08.506 **121**
– pretectalis
– – anterior A14.1.08.507 **121**
– – olivaris A14.1.08.509 **121**
– – posterior A14.1.08.510 **121**
– principalis
– – nervi trigemini A14.1.05.406 **113**
– – ventralis medialis thalami A14.1.08.646 **122**
– proprius medullae spinalis A14.1.02.121 **106**
– pulposus A03.2.02.005 **27**
– pulvinares A14.1.08.610 **121**
– pulvinaris
– – anterior A14.1.08.611 **121**
– – inferior A14.1.08.612 **121**
– – lateralis A14.1.08.613 **121**
– – medialis A14.1.08.614 **121**
– raphes
– – magnus A14.1.04.321 **112, 115**
– – medianus A14.1.05.603 **115**
– – in basilari ponti A14.1.04.318 **112**
– – in medulla oblongata A14.1.04.257 **111**
– – in mesencephale A14.1.06.401 **117**
– – in tegmento ponti A14.1.05.402 **113**, A14.1.05.601 **115**
– – obscurus A14.1.04.319 **112**
– – pallidus A14.1.04.320 **112**
– – pontis A14.1.05.602 **115**
– – posterior
– – – pontis A14.1.05.604 **115**
– – – – mesencephali A14.1.05.604 **117**
– reticularis/es
– – centralis A14.1.04.314 **112**
– – in medulla oblongata A14.1.04.301 **111**
– – in mesencephale A14.1.06.701 **118**
– – in tegmento pontis A14.1.05.501 **114**
– – intermedius A14.1.04.307 **111**
– – lateralis A14.1.04.308 **111**
– – medialis A14.1.04.317 **112**
– – paramedianus A14.1.05.505 **115**
– – parvocellularis A14.1.04.312 **112**
– – pontis
– – – caudalis A14.1.05.502 **114**
– – – rostralis A14.1.05.503 **114**
– – tegmenti pontis A14.1.05.211 **112**, A14.1.05.506 **115**
– – thalami A14.1.08.638 **122**
– retroambiguus A14.1.04.254 **111**
– retrobulbaris [A8] A14.1.09.607 **131**
– retrofacialis A14.1.04.218 **110**
– retroposterolateralis medullae spinalis A14.1.02.109 **106**
– retrotrigeminalis A14.1.04.217 **110**
– reuniens A14.1.08.632 **122**
– ruber A14.1.06.323 **117**
– saguli A14.1.06.328 **117**
– salivatorius
– – inferior A14.1.04.255 **111**
– – superior A14.1.05.413 **114**
– semilunaris A14.1.08.923 **123**
– septalis/es A14.1.09.266 **127**
– – dorsalis A14.1.09.267 **127**, A14.1.09.444 **129**
– – lateralis A14.1.09.268 **127**, A14.1.09.445 **129**
– – medialis A14.1.09.269 **127**, A14.1.09.446 **129**
– – precommissuralis A14.1.09.265 **127**
– septofimbrialis A14.1.09.270 **127**, A14.1.09.447 **129**
– solitarius
– – anterior A14.1.04.240 **111**
– – anterolateralis A14.1.04.241 **111**
– – posterior A14.1.04.238 **111**
– – posterolateralis A14.1.04.239 **111**
– spinalis nervi trigemini A14.1.04.211 **110**, A14.1.05.404 **113**
– striae
– – diagonalis A14.1.09.425 **129**
– – terminalis A14.1.09.419 **129**
– subbrachialis A14.1.06.329 **117**
– subcaeruleus A14.1.05.437 **114**
– subcuneiformis A14.1.06.335 **117, 118**
– subhypoglossalis A14.1.04.263 **111**
– submedialis thalami A14.1.08.647 **122**
– subparabrachialis A14.1.05.440 **114**
– subthalamicus A14.1.08.702 **123**
– suprachiasmaticus A14.1.08.911 **123**
– suprageniculatus A14.1.08.637 **122**
– supralemniscalis A14.1.05.450 **114**
– supramammillaris A14.1.08.937 **124**
– supraopticus A14.1.08.912 **123**
– supraspinalis A14.1.04.268 **111**
– tegmentalis/es
– – anteriores
– – – mesencephali A14.1.06.330 **117**
– – – ponti A14.1.05.435 **114**
– – pedunculopontinus A14.1.06.336 **117, 118**
– – posterior A14.1.05.449 **114**
– – posterolateralis A14.1.06.318 **117**
– terminationis A14.1.00.006 **104**
– thalami
– – medioventralis A14.1.08.626 **122**
– – posterior A14.1.08.636 **122**
– thoracicus posterior A14.1.02.135 **106**
– tractus
– – olfactorii lateralis A14.1.09.414 **129**
– – optici A14.1.08.508 **121**
– – solitarii A14.1.04.230 **111**
– triangularis A14.1.09.271 **127**
– – septi A14.1.09.448 **129**
– tuberales laterales A14.1.08.927 **123**, A14.1.08.930 **124**
– tuberomammillaris A14.1.08.932 **124**
– ventrales
– – laterales thalami A14.1.08.649 **122**
– – mediales thalami A14.1.08.644 **122**
– – thalami A14.1.08.639 **122**
– ventralis A14.1.08.809 **123**
– – anterior thalami A14.1.08.652 **122**
– – corporis geniculati
– – – lateralis A14.1.08.806 **123**
– – – medialis A14.1.08.809 **123**
– – intermedius thalami A14.1.08.655 **122**
– – posterior
– – – inferior thalami A14.1.08.648 **122**
– – – internus thalami A14.1.08.657 **122**
– – posterolateralis thalami A14.1.08.641 **122**, A14.1.08.656 **122**
– – posteromedialis thalami A14.1.08.642 **122**
– ventrobasales thalami A14.1.08.640 **122**
– ventromedialis hypothalami A14.1.08.928 **124**
– ventroposterior parvocellularis thalami A14.1.08.658 **122**
– vestibulares
– – in medulla oblongata A14.1.04.242 **111**
– – in tegmento ponti A14.1.05.425 **114**
– vestibularis
– – inferior A14.1.04.243 **111**
– – lateralis A14.1.05.427 **114**
– – medialis
– – – in medulla oblongata A14.1.04.245 **111**
– – – in tegmento ponti A14.1.05.426 **114**
– – superior A14.1.05.429 **114**
– visceralis/es A14.1.06.304 **117**
– – anteromedialis A14.1.06.305 **117**
– – dorsalis A14.1.06.306 **117**

O

Obex A14.1.04.021 **109**, A14.1.05.723 **115**
Occipitalis A01.0.00.016 **1**

Occiput A01.1.00.003 **2**, A02.1.00.014 **8**
Oculus A01.1.00.007 **2**, A15.2.00.001 **144**
Oesophagus A05.4.01.001 **51**
Olecranon A02.4.06.002 **20**
Oliva A14.1.04.008 **108**
Omentum
– majus A10.1.02.201 **72**
– minus A10.1.02.101 **72**
Operculum
– frontale A14.1.09.112 **125**
– parietale A14.1.09.126 **125**
– temporale A14.1.09.139 **125**
Opisthion A02.1.04.004 **10**
Oppositio A03.0.00.062 **26**
Ora serrata retinae A15.2.04.006 **145**
Orbiculus ciliaris A15.2.03.013 **144**
Orbita A02.1.00.067 **9**
Orchis A09.3.01.001 **67**
Organum/a
– genitalia
– – feminina
– – – externa A09.2.00.001 **66, 71**
– – – interna A09.1.00.001 **65**
– – masculina
– – – externa A09.4.00.001 **69, 71**
– – – interna A09.3.00.001 **67**
– gustatorium A15.4.00.001 **153**
– gustus A15.4.00.001 **153**
– juxtaorale A05.1.01.016 **47**
– lymphoidea
– – primaria A13.1.00.001 **100**
– – secundaria A13.2.00.001 **100**
– olfactorium A15.1.00.001 **144**
– olfactus A15.1.00.001 **144**
– sensuum A15.0.00.000 **144**
– spirale A15.3.03.121 **153**
– subcommissurale A14.1.08.511 **121**
– subfornicale A14.1.08.412 **121, 127**, A14.1.09.449 **129**
– vasculosum laminae terminalis A14.1.08.940 **124, 127**
– vestibulocochleare A15.3.03.002 **151**
– vomeronasale A06.1.02.008 **57**
Os/oris A01.1.00.010 **2**, A05.1.00.001 **47**
Os/sa A02.0.00.000 **7**
– breve A02.0.00.012 **7**
– capitatum A02.4.08.011 **20**
– carpi/alia A02.4.08.001 **20**
– centrale A02.4.08.002 **20**
– coccygis A02.2.06.001 **17**
– coxae A02.5.01.001 **21**
– cranii A02.1.01.001 **9**
– cuboideum A02.5.16.001 **24**
– cuneiforme
– – intermedium A02.5.14.001 **24**
– – laterale A02.5.15.001 **24**
– – mediale A02.5.13.001 **24**
– digitorum
– – manus A02.4.10.001 **20**
– – pedis A02.5.18.001 **24**
– ethmoidale A02.1.07.001 **13**
– femoris A02.5.04.001 **22**
– frontale A02.1.03.001 **10**
– hamatum A02.4.08.012 **20**
– hyoideum A02.1.16.001 **16**
– ilium A02.5.01.101 **21**
– incisivum A02.1.12.031 **14**
– interparietale A02.1.04.013 **10**
– irregulare A02.0.00.014 **7**
– ischii A02.5.01.201 **21**
– lacrimale A02.1.09.001 **13**
– longum A02.0.00.011 **7**
– lunatum A02.4.08.005 **20**
– manus A02.4.07.001 **20**
– membri
– – inferioris A02.5.00.001 **21**
– – superioris A02.4.00.001 **18**
– metacarpi/alia [I–V] A02.4.09.001 **20**
– metatarsi/alia [I–V] A02.5.17.001 **24**
– nasale A02.1.10.001 **14**
– naviculare A02.5.12.001 **24**
– occipitale A02.1.04.001 **10**
– palatinum A02.1.13.001 **14**
– parietale A02.1.02.001 **9**
– pedis A02.5.08.001 **23**
– pisiforme A02.4.08.007 **20**
– planum A02.0.00.013 **7**
– pneumaticum A02.0.00.015 **7**
– pubis A02.5.01.301 **21**
– sacrum [vertebrae sacrales I–V] A02.2.05.001 **17, 21**
– scaphoideum A02.4.08.003 **20**
– sesamoidea
– – manus A02.4.11.001 **21**
– – pedis A02.5.19.001 **24**
– sesamoideum A02.0.00.016 **7**
– sphenoidale A02.1.05.001 **11**
– suprasternalia A02.3.03.009 **18**
– suturale A02.1.00.043 **8**
– tarsi/alia A02.5.09.001 **23**
– temporale A02.1.06.001 **12**
– trapezium A02.4.08.008 **20**
– trapezoideum A02.4.08.010 **20**
– trigonum A02.5.10.021 **24**
– triquetrum A02.4.08.006 **20**
– zygomaticum A02.1.14.001 **15**
Ossicula auditus/oria A02.1.17.001 **16, 149**
Ostium/a
– abdominale tubae uterinae A09.1.02.002 **65**
– anatomicum uteri internum A09.1.03.009 **65**
– aortae A12.1.04.010 **77**
– appendicis vermiformis A05.7.02.008 **53**
– atrioventriculare
– – dextrum A12.1.02.002 **76**
– – sinistrum A12.1.04.002 **77**
– canalis nasolacrimalis A02.1.00.092 **9**
– cardiacum A05.5.01.008 **51**
– histologicum uteri internum A09.1.03.013 **65**
– ileale A05.7.02.003 **53**
– pharyngeum tubae auditivae/oriae A05.3.01.011 **50**, A15.3.02.085 **151**
– pyloricum A05.5.01.018 **52**
– sinus coronarii A12.1.01.009 **76**
– trunci pulmonalis A12.1.02.009 **76**
– tympanicum tubae auditivae/oriae A15.3.02.074 **150**
– ureteris A08.3.01.026 **64**
– urethrae
– – externum A09.2.03.005 **67**, A09.4.02.030 **70**
– – internum A08.3.01.027 **64, 67, 70**
– – – accipiens A09.2.03.001 **67**, A09.4.02.001 **70**
– – – evacuans A09.2.03.002 **67**, A09.4.02.002 **70**
– uteri A09.1.03.015 **66**
– uterinum tubae uterinae A09.1.02.009 **65**
– vaginae A09.2.01.015 **67**
– venae cavae
– – inferioris A12.1.01.010 **76**
– – superioris A12.1.01.011 **76**
– venarum pulmonalium A12.1.03.004 **77**
Ovarium A09.1.01.001 **65**

P

Pachymeninx A14.1.01.002 **104**
Palatum A05.1.01.102 **47**
– durum A05.1.01.103 **47**
– molle A05.1.01.104 **47**, A05.2.01.003 **50**
– osseum A02.1.00.056 **9**
Paleocerebellum A14.1.07.011 **118**
Paleocortex A14.1.09.303 **128**
Pallidum A14.1.09.518 **130**
– dorsale A14.1.09.519 **130**
– ventrale A14.1.09.438 **129–130**
Pallium A14.1.09.003 **124**
Palma A01.1.00.028 **2**, A01.2.07.022 **5**
Palmaris A01.0.00.043 **1**
Palpebra/e A15.2.07.024 **147**
– inferior A15.2.07.026 **147**
– superior A15.2.07.025 **147**
Pancreas A05.9.01.001 **56**
– accessorium A05.9.01.018 **56**
Panniculus adiposus
– telae subcutaneae A16.0.03.002 **155**
– – abdominis A04.5.02.024 **39**
Papilla/e
– dentis A05.1.03.054 **48**
– dermis A16.0.00.012 **154**
– ductus parotidei A05.1.01.017 **47**
– duodeni
– – major A05.6.02.015 **53**
– – minor A05.6.02.016 **53**
– filiformes A05.1.04.014 **49**
– foliatae A05.1.04.017 **49**
– fungiformes A05.1.04.015 **49**
– gingivalis A05.1.01.110 **47**
– ilealis A05.7.02.002 **53**
– incisiva A05.1.01.107 **47**
– interdentalis A05.1.01.110 **47**
– lacrimalis A15.2.07.064 **148**
– linguales A05.1.04.013 **49**
– mammaria A16.0.02.004 **154**
– renalis A08.1.01.027 **63**

- vallatae A05.1.04.016 **49**
Paracervix A09.1.03.022 **66**
Paradidymis A09.3.03.001 **68**
Paraflocculus ventralis [H IX] A14.1.07.222 **119**
Paraganglia sympathica A14.3.01.078 **142**
Parametrium A09.1.03.021 **66**
Parasubiculum A14.1.09.322 **128**
Parenchyma
- glandulae thyroideae A11.3.00.008 **74**
- prostatae A09.3.08.018 **69**
- testis A09.3.01.021 **68**
Paries
- anterior
- - gastricae A05.5.01.002 **51**
- - vaginae A09.1.04.006 **66**
- caroticus cavi tympani A15.3.02.031 **149**
- externus ductus cochlearis A15.3.03.095 **152**
- inferior orbitae A02.1.00.076 **9**
- jugularis cavi tympani A15.3.02.006 **149**
- labyrinthicus cavi tympani A15.3.02.008 **149**
- lateralis orbitae A02.1.00.077 **9**
- mastoideus cavi tympani A15.3.02.020 **149**
- medialis orbitae A02.1.00.078 **9**
- membranaceus
- - trachealis A06.3.01.007 **59**
- - cavi tympani A15.3.02.032 **149**
- posterior
- - gastricae A05.5.01.003 **51**
- - vaginae A09.1.04.007 **66**
- superior orbitae A02.1.00.075 **9**
- tegmentalis cavi tympani A15.3.02.003 **149**
- tympanicus ductus cochlearis A15.3.03.100 **152**
- vestibularis ductus cochlearis A15.3.03.094 **152**
Paroophoron A09.1.06.001 **66**
Pars/tes
- abdominalis
- - aortae A12.2.12.001 **87**
- - ductus thoracici A12.4.01.011 **99**
- - m. pectoralis majoris A04.4.01.005 **37**
- - oesophageae A05.4.01.006 **51**
- - plexus visceralis et ganglii visceralis A14.3.03.018 **143**
- - ureteris A08.2.01.002 **64**
- acromialis A04.6.02.004 **40**
- - m. deltoidei A04.6.02.004 **40**
- alaris A04.1.03.011 **34**
- - m. nasalis A04.1.03.011 **34**
- alpha A14.1.04.303 **111**
- - nuclei gigantocellularis A14.1.04.303 **111**
- alveolaris A02.1.15.016 **15**
- - mandibulae A02.1.15.016 **15**
- anterior
- - commissurae anterioris A14.1.09.253 **127, 131**
- - culminis A14.1.07.113 **119**
- - faciei diaphragmaticae hepatis A05.8.01.005 **54**
- - fornicis vaginae A09.1.04.003 **66**
- - linguae A05.1.04.005 **49**
- - lobuli
- - - centralis cerebelli A14.1.07.106 **119**
- - - quadrangularis anterioris cerebelli A14.1.07.117 **119**
- - nuclei
- - - cochlearis anterior A14.1.04.250 **111**
- - - parabrachialis lateralis A14.1.05.445 **114**
- anularis vaginae fibrosae digitorum
- - manus A04.8.04.016 **45**
- - pedis A04.8.06.015 **46**
- aryepiglottica m. arytenoidei obliqui A06.2.08.011 **59**
- ascendens A04.3.01.004 **36**, A05.6.02.008 **52**
- - aortae A12.2.03.001 **79**
- - duodeni A05.6.02.008 **52**
- atlantica a. vertebralis A12.2.08.009 **84**
- autonomica systematis nervosi peripherici A14.3.00.001 **141**
- basalis A12.2.01.115 **78**, A12.2.01.216 **79**
- - aa. lobariis inferioris pulmonis sinistri A12.2.01.216 **79**
- - aa. lobarium inferiorium pulmonis dextri A12.2.01.115 **78**
- - telencephali A14.1.09.401 **129**
- basilaris
- - ossis occipitalis A02.1.04.005 **10**
- - pontis A14.1.05.101 **112**
- buccopharyngea m. constrictoris pharyngis superioris A05.3.01.105 **51**
- caeca retinae A15.2.04.003 **145**
- canalis n. optici A15.2.04.026 **145**
- cardiaca gastricae A05.5.01.007 **51**
- cartilaginea A02.0.00.005 **7**
- - septi nasi A06.1.02.006 **57**
- - tubae auditivae A15.3.02.078 **150**
- caudalis nuclei spinalis nervi trigemini A14.1.04.212 **110**
- cavernosa a. carotis internae A12.2.06.007 **81**
- centralis
- - nuclei
- - - cuneati A14.1.04.207 **110**
- - - gracilis A14.1.04.203 **110**
- - systemae nervosi A14.1.00.001 **104**
- - ventriculi lateralis A14.1.09.274 **127**
- ceratopharyngea m. constrictoris pharyngis medii A05.3.01.110 **51**
- cerebralis a. carotis internae A12.2.06.015 **81**
- cervicalis
- - a. carotis internae A12.2.06.002 **81**
- - a. vertebralis A12.2.08.004 **84**
- - ductus thoracici A12.4.01.009 **99**
- - medullae spinalis A14.1.02.014 **105**
- - oesophageae A05.4.01.002 **51**
- - tracheae A06.3.01.002 **59**
- cervicis vesicae m. detrusoris vesicae A08.3.01.016 **64**
- chondropharyngea m. constrictoris pharyngis medii A05.3.01.109 **51**
- ciliaris retinae A15.2.04.004 **145**
- clavicularis
- - m. deltoidei A04.6.02.003 **40**
- - m. pectoralis majoris A04.4.01.003 **37**
- coccygea medullae spinalis A14.1.02.018 **105**
- coeliacoduodenalis m. suspensorii duodeni A05.6.02.013 **52**
- colli
- - ductus thoracici A12.4.01.009 **99**
- - oesophageae A05.4.01.002 **51**
- - tracheae A06.3.01.002 **59**
- - vesicae m. detrusoris vesicae A08.3.01.016 **64**
- compacta
- - nuclei tegmentalis pedunculopontinus A14.1.06.337 **117, 118**
- - substantiae nigrae A14.1.06.112 **116**
- copularis lobuli paramediani [H VIII A] A14.1.07.217 **119**
- corneoscleralis sclerae A15.2.02.005 **144**
- corporis humani A01.1.00.000 **??**
- costalis
- - diaphragmatis A04.4.02.008 **38**
- - pleurae parietalis A07.1.02.007 **62**
- cranialis partis parasympathici divisionis autonomici systematis nervosi A14.3.02.002 **142**
- craniocervicalis plexus visceralis et ganglii visceralis A14.3.03.002 **142**
- cricopharyngea m. constrictoris pharyngis inferioris A05.3.01.113 **51**
- cruciformis vaginae fibrosae digitorum
- - manus A04.8.04.017 **45**
- - pedis A04.8.06.016 **46**
- cuneiformis vomeris A02.1.11.005 **14**
- cupularis recessi epitympanici A15.3.02.005 **149**
- descendens
- - aortae A12.2.10.001 **86**
- - duodeni A05.6.02.005 **52**

– – lig. iliofemoralis A03.6.07.005 **30**
– – m. trapezii A04.3.01.002 **36**
– dextra faciei diaphragmaticae hepatis A05.8.01.006 **54**
– diaphragmatica pleurae parietalis A07.1.02.008 **62**
– dissipata nuclei tegmentalis pedunculopontinus A14.1.06.338 **117, 118**
– distalis
– – adenohypophysis A11.1.00.005 **74**
– – prostatae A09.3.08.005 **68**
– – urethrae prosticae A09.4.02.006 **70**
– dorsalis/es/ium
– – alaris lobuli centralis cerebelli [H III] A14.1.07.110 **119**
– – culminis [V] A14.1.07.115 **119**
– – lobuli
– – – centralis cerebelli [III] A14.1.07.107 **119**
– – – quadrangularis anterioris cerebelli [H V] A14.1.07.118 **119**
– – mm. intertransversarii laterales lumborum A04.3.01.015 **36**
– – m. trapezii ascendens A04.3.01.004 **36**
– – nuclei
– – – commissurae posterioris A14.1.06.312 **117**
– – – reticularis centralis A14.1.04.315 **112**
– dorsolateralis nuclei supraoptici A14.1.08.913 **123**
– dorsomedialis nuclei
– – rubri A14.1.06.326 **117**
– – supraoptici A14.1.08.914 **123**
– duralis fili terminalis A14.1.01.402 **105**
– extraocularis
– – a. centralis retinae A12.2.06.025 **81**
– – v. centralis retinae A12.3.06.112 **95**
– fasciae iliopsoaticae A04.5.02.009 **39**
– flaccida membranae tympanicae A15.3.01.053 **149**
– funicularis ductus deferentis A09.3.05.003 **68**
– gastrocnemialis compartimenti cruris posterioris A04.7.01.007 **42**
– glossopharyngea m. constrictoris pharyngis superioris A05.3.01.107 **51**
– hepatis
– – dextra A05.8.01.045 **55**
– – sinistra A05.8.01.037 **55**
– horizontalis
– – a. cerebri medii A12.2.07.047 **83**
– – duodeni A05.6.02.007 **52**
– iliaca fasciae iliopsoaticae A04.5.02.009 **39**
– inferior
– – alaris lobuli centralis cerebelli A14.1.07.109 **119**
– – duodeni A05.6.02.007 **52**
– – ganglionis vestibularis A14.2.01.130 **136**
– – v. lingularis A12.3.02.310 **92**
– infraclavicularis plexus brachialis A14.2.03.020 **138**
– infralobaris v. posterior lobi superioris pulmonis dextri A12.3.02.109 **91**
– inguinalis ductus deferentis A09.3.05.004 **68**
– insularis a. cerebri medii A12.2.07.053 **83**
– intercartilaginea rimae glottidis A06.2.09.016 **59**
– intermedia
– – adenohypophysis A11.1.00.004 **74**
– – uretrae A09.4.02.017 **70**
– intermembranacea rimae glottidis A06.2.09.015 **59**
– interpolaris nuclei spinalis nervi trigemini A14.1.04.216 **110**
– intersegmentali v. apicalis lobi superioris pulmonis dextri A12.3.02.104 **91**
– intersegmentalis
– – v. anterioris lobi superioris pulmonis
– – – dextri A12.3.02.107 **91**
– – – sinistri A12.3.02.307 **92**
– – v. apicoposterioris lobi superioris pulmonis sinistri A12.3.02.304 **92**
– – v. basalis anterioris lobi inferioris pulmonis
– – – dextri A12.3.02.209 **92**
– – – sinistri A12.3.02.409 **92**
– – v. superioris lobi inferioris pulmonis
– – – dextri A12.3.02.204 **92**
– – – sinistri A12.3.02.404 **92**
– interstitiali nuclei commissurae posterioris A14.1.06.311 **117**
– intracranialis
– – a. vertebralis A12.2.08.010 **84**
– – n. optici A15.2.04.025 **145**
– intralaminaris n. optici intraocularis A15.2.04.030 **145**
– intralobaris (intersegmentalis) v. posterior lobi superioris pulmonis dextri A12.3.02.110 **91**
– intramuralis
– – ureteris A08.2.01.004 **64**
– – urethrae ♀ A09.2.03.003 **67**
– – urethrae ♂ A09.4.02.003 **70**
– intraocularis
– – a. centralis retinae A12.2.06.026 **81, 146**
– – n. optici A15.2.04.028 **145**
– – v. centralis retinae A11.3.06.113 **95, 146**
– intrasegmentalis
– – v. anterioris lobi superioris pulmonis
– – – dextri A12.3.02.106 **91**
– – – sinistri A12.3.02.306 **92**
– – v. apicalis lobi superioris pulmonis dextri A12.3.02.103 **91**
– – v. apicoposterioris lobi superioris pulmonis sinistri A12.3.02.303 **92**
– – v. basalis anterioris lobi inferioris pulmonis
– – – dextri A12.3.02.208 **92**
– – – sinistri A12.3.02.408 **92**
– – v. superioris lobi inferioris pulmonis
– – – dextri A12.3.02.203 **92**
– – – sinistri A12.3.02.403 **92**
– iridica retinae A15.2.04.005 **145**
– labialis m. orbicularis oris A04.1.03.025 **34**
– laryngea pharyngis A05.3.01.023 **50**
– lateralis
– – arci pedis longitudinalis A01.2.08.029 **5**
– – compartimenti antebrachii posterioris A04.6.01.008 **40**
– – fornicis vaginae A09.1.04.005 **66**
– – globi pallidi medialis A14.1.09.512 **130**
– – lobuli biventralis A14.1.07.217 **119**
– – nuclei
– – – accumbens A14.1.09.441 **129**
– – – parabrachialis
– – – – lateralis A14.1.05.442 **114**
– – – – medialis A14.1.05.448 **114**
– – ossis
– – – occipitalis A02.1.04.009 **10**
– – – sacri A02.2.05.006 **17**
– – substantiae nigrae A14.1.06.113 **116**
– – v. lobi medii pulmonis dextri A12.3.02.112 **91**
– libera membri
– – inferioris A02.5.03.001 **22**
– – superioris A02.4.03.001 **19**
– lumbalis
– – diaphragmatis A04.4.02.002 **38**
– – m. iliocostalis lumborum A04.3.02.007 **36**
– – m. longissimi thoracis A04.3.02.012 **36**
– – medullae spinalis A14.1.02.016 **105**
– magnocellularis
– – medialis nuclei mediodorsalis A14.1.08.624 **122**
– – nuclei
– – – mediodorsalis thalami A14.1.08.624 **122**
– – – reticularis lateralis A14.1.04.309 **112**
– – – rubri A14.1.06.324 **117**
– – – ventralis anterior thalami A14.1.08.653 **122**
– – – vestibularis inferioris A14.1.04.244 **111**
– marginalis m. orbicularis oris A04.1.03.024 **34**
– medialis

– – arci pedis longitudinalis A01.2.08.030 **5**
– – globi pallidi A14.1.09.514 **130**
– – lobuli biventralis A14.1.07.219 **119**
– – nuclei
– – – accumbens A14.1.09.442 **129**
– – – parabrachialis
– – – – lateralis A14.1.05.443 **114**
– – – – medialis A14.1.05.447 **114**
– – v. lobi medii pulmonis dextri A12.3.02.113 **91**
– mediastinalis pleurae parietalis A07.1.02.009 **62**
– membranacea A02.0.00.006 **7**
– – septi
– – – interventricularis A12.1.00.015 **76**
– – – nasi A06.1.02.005 **57**
– – urethrae A09.4.02.017 **70**
– mobilis septi nasi A06.1.01.009 **57**
– muscularis septi interventricularis A12.1.00.014 **76**
– mylopharyngea m. constrictoris pharyngis superioris A05.3.01.106 **51**
– nasalis
– – ossis frontalis A02.1.03.019 **10**
– – pharyngis A05.3.01.003 **50**
– nervosa neurohypophysis A11.1.00.008 **74, 120**
– nonstratificata m. detrusoris vesicae A08.3.01.015 **64**
– obliqua A06.2.08.003 **59**
– – m. cricothyroidei A06.2.08.003 **59**
– occlusa a. umbilicalis A12.2.15.025 **89**
– olfactoria tunicae mucosae nasi A06.1.02.019 **57**, A15.1.00.002 **144**
– opercularis A14.1.09.116 **125**
– optica retinae A15.2.04.007 **145**
– oralis pharyngis A05.3.01.019 **50**
– orbitalis
– – glandulae lacrimalis A15.2.07.058 **148**
– – gyrus frontalis inferior A14.1.09.114 **125**
– – m. orbicularis oculi A04.1.03.017 **34**
– – n. optici A15.2.04.027 **145**
– – ossis frontalis A02.1.03.022 **10**
– ossea A02.0.00.001 **7**
– – septi nasi A06.1.02.007 **57**
– – tubae auditivae A15.3.02.075 **150**
– palpebralis
– – glandulae lacrimalis A15.2.07.059 **148**
– – m. orbicularis oculi A04.1.03.014 **34**
– paralaminaris nuclei mediodorsalis thalami A14.1.08.625 **122**
– parasympathica divisionis autonomici systematis nervosi A14.3.02.001 **142**
– parvocellularis A14.1.04.310 **112**, A14.1.05.428 **114**, A14.1.06.325 **117**
– – lateralis nuclei mediodorsalis thalami A14.1.08.623 **122**
– – nuclei
– – – reticularis lateralis A14.1.04.310 **112**
– – – rubri A14.1.06.325 **117**
– – – ventralis posteromedialis thalami A14.1.08.643 **122**
– – – vestibularis lateralis A14.1.05.428 **114**
– patens a. umbilicalis A12.2.15.021 **89**
– pelvica
– – ductus deferentis A09.3.05.005 **68**
– – partis parasympathici divisionis autonomici systematis nervosi A14.3.02.016 **142**
– – plexus visceralis et ganglii visceralis A14.3.03.045 **143**
– – ureteris A08.2.01.003 **64**
– peripherica A14.2.00.001 **132**
– petrosa
– – a. carotis internae A12.2.06.004 **81**
– – ossis temporalis A02.1.06.002 **12**
– phrenicocoeliaca m. suspensorii duodeni A05.6.02.012 **52**
– pialis fili terminalis A14.1.01.403 **105**
– postcommunicalis
– – a. cerebri
– – – anterioris A12.2.07.033 **83**
– – – posterioris A12.2.07.088 **84**
– posterior
– – commissurae anterioris A14.1.09.254 **127, 131**
– – culminis A14.1.07.115 **119**
– – faciei diaphragmaticae hepatis A05.8.01.007 **54**
– – fornicis vaginae A09.1.04.004 **66**
– – funiculi lateralis medullae spinalis A14.1.02.229 **107**
– – hepatis A05.8.01.043 **55**
– – linguae A05.1.04.006 **49**
– – lobuli
– – – centralis cerebelli A14.1.07.107 **119**
– – – quadrangularis anterioris cerebelli A14.1.07.118 **119**
– – nuclei
– – – cochlearis anterior A14.1.04.251 **111**
– – – parabrachialis lateralis A14.1.05.444 **114**
– posteromedialis nuclei rubri A14.1.06.326 **117**
– postlaminaris n. optici intraocularis A15.2.04.029 **145**
– postsulcalis linguae A05.1.04.006 **49**
– precommunicalis a. cerebri
– – anterioris A12.2.07.023 **82**
– – posterioris A12.2.07.083 **84**
– prelaminaris n. optici intraocularis A15.2.04.031 **145**
– preprostatica A09.4.02.003 **70**
– presulcalis linguae A05.1.04.005 **49**
– prevertebralis a. vertebralis A12.2.08.003 **84**
– principalis nuclei ventralis anterior thalami A14.1.08.654 **122**
– profunda
– – compartimenti
– – – antebrachii anterioris A04.6.01.006 **40**
– – – cruris posterioris A04.7.01.008 **42**
– – glandulae parotidis A05.1.02.005 **47**
– – m. masseterica A04.1.04.004 **35**
– – m. sphincteris ani externus A04.5.04.015 **40, 54**
– – partis palpebralis m. orbicularis oculi A04.1.03.016 **34**
– prostatica A09.4.02.004 **70**
– proximalis
– – prostatae A09.3.08.003 **68**
– – urethrae prosticae A09.4.02.005 **70**
– psoatica fasciae iliopsoaticae A04.5.02.008 **39**
– pterygopharyngea m. constrictoris pharyngis superioris A05.3.01.104 **51**
– pylorica gastricae A05.5.01.014 **52**
– radialis compartimenti antebrachii posteriori A04.6.01.008 **40**
– recta m. cricothyroidei A06.2.08.002 **59**
– respiratoria tunicae mucosae nasi A06.1.02.018 **57**
– reticularis substantiae nigrae A14.1.06.114 **116**
– retrolentiformis A14.1.09.539 **130**
– retrorubralis substantiae nigrae A14.1.06.115 **116**
– rostralis nuclei
– – cuneati A14.1.04.208 **110**
– – gracilis A14.1.04.204 **110**
– sacralis medullae spinalis A14.1.02.017 **105**
– scrotalis ductus deferentis A09.3.05.002 **68**
– solealis ompartimenti cruris posterioris A04.7.01.008 **42**
– sphenoidalis a. cerebri medii A12.2.07.047 **83**
– spinalis
– – fili terminalis A14.1.02.005 **105**
– – m. deltoidei A04.6.02.005 **40**
– – n. accessorius A14.2.01.186 **137**
– spongiosa A09.4.02.021 **70**
– squamosa ossis temporalis A02.1.06.061 **13**
– sternalis diaphragmatis A04.4.02.009 **38**
– sternocostalis m. pectoralis majoris A04.4.01.004 **37**

- subcutanea m. sphincteris ani externus A04.5.04.013 **40, 54**
- sublenticularis amygdalae A14.1.09.420 **129**
- sublentiformis apsulae internae A14.1.09.544 **131**
- subtrigeminalis nuclei reticularis lateralis A14.1.04.311 **112**
- superficialis
- – compartimenti
- – – antebrachii anterioris A04.6.01.005 **40**
- – – cruris posterioris A04.7.01.007 **42**
- – glandulae parotidis A05.1.02.004 **47**
- – m. masseterica A04.1.04.311 **112**
- – m. sphincteris ani externus A04.5.04.014 **40, 54**
- superior
- – alaris lobuli centralis cerebelli A14.1.07.110 **119**
- – duodeni A05.6.02.002 **52**
- – faciei diaphragmaticae hepatis A05.8.01.003 **54**
- – ganglionis vestibularis A14.2.01.125 **135**
- – v. lingularis A12.3.02.309 **92**
- supraclavicularis plexus brachialis A14.2.03.010 **138**
- sympathica divisionis autonomici systematis nervosi A14.3.01.001 **141**
- tecta duodeni A05.6.02.010 **52**
- tensa membranae tympanicae A15.3.01.054 **149**
- terminalis A05.6.04.002 **53**
- thoracica A05.4.01.003 **51**, A06.3.01.003 **59**, A12.4.01.010 **99**, A14.1.02.015 **105**, A14.3.03.011 **143**
- – aortae A12.2.11.001 **86**
- – ductus thoracici A12.4.01.010 **99**
- – medullae spinalis A14.1.02.015 **105**
- – m. iliocostalis lumborum A04.3.02.008 **36**
- – oesophageae A05.4.01.003 **51**
- – plexus visceralis et ganglii visceralis A14.3.03.010 **143**
- – tracheae A06.3.01.003 **59**
- thyroepiglottica m. thyroarytenoidei A06.2.08.009 **59**
- thyropharyngea m. constrictoris pharyngis inferioris A05.3.01.112 **51**
- tibiocalcanea lig. collateralis medialis articulationis talocruralis A03.6.10.005 **31**
- tibionavicularis lig. collateralis medialis articulationis talocruralis A03.6.10.004 **31**
- tibiotalaris
- – anterior lig. collateralis medialis articulationis talocruralis A03.6.10.006 **31**
- – posterior lig. collateralis medialis articulationis talocruralis A03.6.10.007 **31**
- transversa
- – lig. iliofemoralis A03.6.07.004 **30**
- – m. nasalis A04.1.03.010 **34**
- – m. trapezii A04.3.01.003 **36**
- – r. sinistri v. portae hepatis A12.3.12.006 **98**
- transversaria a. vertebralis A12.2.08.004 **84**
- triangularis A14.1.09.115 **125**
- tricipitalis compartimenti cruris posterioris A04.7.01.007 **42**
- tuberalis adenohypophysis A11.1.00.003 **74**
- tympanica ossis temporalis A02.1.06.052 **13**
- umbilicalis r. sinistri v. portae hepatis A12.3.12.008 **98**
- uterina tubariae A09.1.02.008 **65**
- uvealis sclerae A15.2.02.006 **144**
- vagalis n. accessorius A14.2.01.185 **137**
- ventralis/es/ium A14.1.04.316 **112**, A14.1.06.310 **117**
- – alaris lobuli centralis cerebelli [H II] A14.1.07.109 **119**
- – culminis [IV] A14.1.07.113 **119**
- – lobuli
- – – centralis cerebelli [II] A14.1.07.106 **119**
- – – quadrangularis anterioris cerebelli [H IV] A14.1.07.117 **119**
- – mm. intertransversarii laterales lumborum A04.3.01.016 **36**
- – nuclei
- – – commissurae posterioris A14.1.06.310 **117**
- – – reticularis centralis A14.1.04.316 **112**
- ventromedialis nuclei supraoptici A14.1.08.915 **123**
- vertebralis faciei costalis pulmonis A06.5.01.007 **60**

Patella A02.5.05.001 **23**

Pecten
- analis A05.7.05.010 **54**
- ossis pubis A02.5.01.308 **21**

Pectus A01.1.00.015 **2**

Pediculus arcus vertebrae A02.2.01.006 **16**

Pedunculus/i
- cerebellares A14.1.07.412 **120**
- cerebellaris
- – inferior A14.1.04.013 **109**, A14.1.07.413 **120**
- – medius A14.1.05.003 **112**, A14.1.07.416 **120**
- – superior A14.1.05.006 **112**, A14.1.06.009 **115**, A14.1.06.216 **116**, A14.1.07.417 **120**, A14.1.08.678 **122**
- cerebri A14.1.06.004 **115–116**
- flocculi A14.1.07.303 **119**
- olfactorius A14.1.09.430 **129**

Pelvis A01.1.00.017 **2**, A02.5.02.001 **22**
- major A02.5.02.005 **22**
- minor A02.5.02.006 **22**
- renalis A08.1.05.001 **64**

Penicilli A13.2.01.020 **100**

Penis A09.4.01.001 **69**

Pericardium A12.1.08.001 **78**
- fibrosum A12.1.08.002 **78**
- serosum A12.1.08.005 **78**

Perichondrium A02.0.00.008 **7**

Pericranium A02.1.00.011 **8**

Perikaryon A14.0.00.003 **104**

Perilympha A15.3.03.056 **152**

Perimetrium A09.1.03.023 **66**

Perimysium A04.0.00.042 **34**

Perineum A09.5.00.001 **71**

Perineurium A14.2.00.015 **132**

Periodontium A03.1.03.002 **26**, A05.1.03.058 **49**
- insertionis A03.1.03.005 **26**
- protectionis A03.1.03.004 **26**

Perionyx A16.0.01.009 **154**

Periorbita A15.2.07.002 **147**

Periosteum A02.0.00.007 **7**
- externum cranii A02.1.00.011 **8**

Periphericus/alis A01.0.00.038 **1**

Peritoneum A10.1.02.002 **72**
- parietale A10.1.02.005 **72**
- urogenitale A10.1.02.501 **73**
- viscerale A10.1.02.006 **72**

Peronealis A01.0.00.041 **1**

Pes A01.1.00.040 **2**
- hippocampi A14.1.09.323 **128**

Petiolus epiglottidis A06.2.07.003 **58**

Phalanx/ges A02.4.10.001 **20**, A02.5.18.001 **24**
- distalis
- – manus A02.4.10.004 **21**
- – pedis A02.5.18.004 **24**
- media
- – manus A02.4.10.003 **20**
- – pedis A02.5.18.003 **24**
- proximalis
- – manus A02.4.10.002 **20**
- – pedis A02.5.18.002 **24**

Pharynx A05.3.01.001 **50**

Philtrum A05.1.01.007 **47**

Pia mater A14.1.01.301 **105**
- cranialis A14.1.01.302 **105**
- encephali A14.1.01.302 **105**
- spinalis A14.1.01.309 **105**

Pili A16.0.00.014 **154**

Planta A01.1.00.044 **2**, A01.2.08.025 **5**

Plantaris A01.0.00.044 **1**

Planum/a
- coronalia A01.2.00.001 **3**
- frontalia A01.2.00.001 **3**
- horizontalia A01.2.00.002 **3**
- interspinale A01.2.00.011 **3**
- intertuberculare A01.2.00.010 **3**
- medianum A01.2.00.004 **3**

- occipitale A02.1.04.027 **11**
- paramediana A01.2.00.005 **3**
- sagittalia A01.2.00.003 **3**
- subcostale A01.2.00.008 **3**
- supracristale A01.2.00.009 **3**
- temporale A14.1.09.143 **125**
- transpyloricum A01.2.00.007 **3**
- transversalia A01.2.00.006 **3**

Platysma A04.2.01.001 **35**

Pleura A07.1.02.001 **62**
- parietalis A07.1.02.005 **62**
- pulmonalis A07.1.02.002 **62**
- visceralis A07.1.02.002 **62**

Plexus
- nervosus/orum
- – aorticus
- – – abdominalis A14.3.03.018 **143**
- – – thoracicus A14.3.03.011 **143**
- – autonomicus brachialis A14.3.03.008 **143**
- – cardiacus A14.3.03.012 **143**
- – caroticus
- – – communis A14.3.03.003 **142**
- – – externus A14.3.03.006 **143**
- – – internus A14.3.03.004 **142**
- – cavernosus A14.3.03.005 **142**
- – cervicalis A14.2.02.012 **137**
- – – posterior A14.2.02.010 **137**
- – coeliacus A14.3.03.020 **143**
- – deferentialis ♂ A14.3.03.053 **143**
- – dentalis
- – – inferior A14.2.01.091 **135**
- – – superior A14.2.01.053 **134**
- – entericus A14.3.03.038 **143**
- – femoralis A14.3.03.043 **143**
- – gastrici A14.3.03.023 **143**
- – hepaticus A14.3.03.021 **143**
- – hypogastricus
- – – inferior A14.3.03.047 **143**
- – – superior A14.3.03.045 **143**
- – iliacus A14.3.03.042 **143**
- – intermesentericus A14.3.03.030 **143**
- – intraparotideus A14.2.01.108 **135**
- – lienalis A14.3.03.022 **143**
- – lumbalis posterior A14.2.05.007 **139**
- – mesentericus
- – – inferior A14.3.03.035 **143**
- – – superior A14.3.03.028 **143**
- – myentericus A14.3.03.040 **143**
- – oesophageus A14.3.03.015 **143**
- – ovaricus ♀ A14.3.03.034 **143**
- – pancreaticus A14.3.03.024 **143**
- – pelvicus A14.3.03.047 **143**
- – periarterialis A14.2.00.044 **133**
- – prostaticus ♂ A14.3.03.051 **143**
- – pulmonalis A14.3.03.015 **143**
- – rectalis
- – – inferior A14.3.03.049 **143**
- – – medius A14.3.03.048 **143**
- – – superior A14.3.03.037 **143**
- – renalis A14.3.03.031 **143**
- – spinalium A14.2.00.037 **133**
- – splenicus A14.3.03.022 **143**
- – subclavius A14.3.03.007 **143**
- – submucosus A14.3.03.041 **143**
- – subserosus A14.3.03.039 **143**
- – suprarenalis A14.3.03.025 **143**
- – testicularis ♂ A14.3.03.034 **143**
- – uretericus A14.3.03.033 **143**
- – uterovaginalis ♀ A14.3.03.051 **143**
- – vascularis A14.2.00.043 **133**
- – vertebralis A14.3.03.009 **143**
- – vesicalis A14.3.03.054 **143**
- – visceralis/es A14.2.00.042 **133**
- vasculosus A12.0.00.010 **75**
- venosus A12.0.00.011 **75**
- – pampiniformis A12.3.09.015 **97**
- – areolaris A12.3.08.013 **96**
- – basilaris A12.3.05.106 **93**
- – canalis nervi hypoglossi A12.3.05.306 **94**
- – caroticus internus A12.3.05.308 **94**
- – foraminis ovalis A12.3.05.307 **94**
- – pharyngeus A12.3.05.006 **93**
- – prostaticus ♂ A12.3.10.013 **97**
- – pterygoideus A12.3.05.036 **93**
- – rectalis A12.3.10.010 **97**
- – sacralis A12.3.10.009 **97**
- – suboccipitalis A12.3.04.016 **92**
- – thyroideus impar A12.3.04.003 **92**
- – uterinus ♀ A12.3.10.016 **97**
- – vaginalis ♀ A12.3.10.017 **97**
- – vertebralis
- – – externus
- – – – anterior A12.3.07.019 **96**
- – – – posterior A12.3.07.020 **96**
- – – internus
- – – – anterior A12.3.07.021 **96**
- – – – posterior A12.3.07.026 **96**
- – vesicalis A12.3.10.012 **97**

Plica/e
- alares plicae synovialis infrapatellaris A03.6.08.010 **30**
- anterior faucium A05.2.01.005 **50**
- aryepiglottica A06.2.09.003 **59**
- caecales A10.1.02.423 **73**
- caecalis vascularis A10.1.02.419 **73**
- chordae tympani A15.3.02.066 **150**
- ciliares A15.2.03.012 **144**
- circulares intestini tenuis A05.6.01.007 **52**
- duodenalis
- – inferior A10.1.02.412 **73**
- – superior A10.1.02.410 **73**
- duodenojejunalis A10.1.02.410 **72**
- duodenomesocolica A10.1.02.412 **73**
- epigastrica A10.1.02.434 **73**
- fimbriata linguae A05.1.04.008 **49**
- gastricae A05.5.01.028 **52**
- gastropancreatica A10.1.02.408 **72**
- glossoepiglottica
- – lateralis A05.3.01.022 **50**
- – mediana A05.3.01.021 **50**
- hepatopancreatica A10.1.02.409 **72**
- ileocaecalis A10.1.02.421 **73**
- incudialis A15.3.02.071 **150**
- interarytenoidea rimae glottidis A06.2.09.017 **59**
- interureterica A08.3.01.025 **64**
- iridis A15.2.03.027 **145**
- lacrimalis A15.2.07.071 **148**
- longitudinalis duodeni A05.6.02.014 **53**
- mallearis
- – anterior A15.3.01.055 **149**, A15.3.02.065 **150**
- – posterior A15.3.01.056 **149**, A15.3.02.064 **150**
- mucosae vesicae biliaris A05.8.02.010 **56**
- nervi laryngei superioris A05.3.01.025 **50**
- palatinae transversae A05.1.01.106 **47**
- palmatae canalis cervicis uteri A09.1.03.019 **66**
- palpebronasalis A15.2.07.028 **147**
- paraduodenalis A10.1.02.414 **73**
- posterior faucium A05.2.01.007 **50**
- presplenica A10.1.02.204 **72**
- rectouterina ♀ A10.1.02.511 **73**
- salpingopalatina A05.3.01.014 **50**
- salpingopharyngea A05.3.01.013 **50**
- semilunares coli A05.7.03.008 **53**
- semilunaris
- – faucium A05.2.01.008 **50**
- – conjunctivae A15.2.07.048 **147**
- spiralis A05.8.02.012 **56**
- stapedialis A15.3.02.072 **150**
- sublingualis A05.1.01.113 **47**
- synovialis/es A03.0.00.029 **25**
- – infrapatellaris A03.6.08.009 **30**
- transversae recti A05.7.04.007 **54**
- triangularis A05.2.01.006 **50**
- tubariae A09.1.02.014 **65**
- umbilicalis
- – lateralis A10.1.02.434 **73**
- – medialis A10.1.02.431 **73**
- – mediana A10.1.02.429 **73**
- venae cavae sinistrae A12.1.08.010 **78**
- vesicalis transversa A10.1.02.503 **73**
- vestibularis A06.2.09.008 **59**
- villosae gastricae A05.5.01.031 **52**
- vocalis A06.2.09.013 **59**

Pollex A01.2.07.027 **5**

Polus

– anterior
– – bulbi oculi A15.2.01.002 **144**
– – lentis A15.2.05.008 **146**
– frontalis A14.1.09.111 **125**
– inferior
– – renis A08.1.01.009 **63**
– – testis A09.3.01.003 **67**
– occipitalis A14.1.09.133 **125**
– posterior
– – bulbi oculi A15.2.01.003 **144**
– – lentis A15.2.05.009 **146**
– superior
– – renis A08.1.01.008 **63**
– – testis A09.3.01.002 **67**
– temporalis A14.1.09.137 **125**
Pons/tes A14.1.03.010 **108, 112**
– et cerebellum A14.1.03.004 **108**
– grisei caudatolenticulares A14.1.09.525 **130**
Pontocerebellum A14.1.07.009 **118**
Poples A01.1.00.037 **2**
Porta hepatis A05.8.01.016 **54**
Portio
– supravaginalis cervicis A09.1.03.011 **65**
– vaginalis cervicis A09.1.03.014 **66**
Porus
– acusticus
– – externus A02.1.06.054 **13**, A15.3.01.046 **149**
– – internus A02.1.06.032 **12, 151**
– gustatorius A15.4.00.003 **153**
Posterior A01.0.00.012 **1**
Precuneus A14.1.09.223 **126**
Premaxilla A02.1.12.031 **14**
Preputium
– clitoridis A09.2.01.009 **66**
– penis A09.4.01.011 **69**
Presubiculum A14.1.09.325 **128**
Primarium A02.0.00.044 **7**
Processus A02.0.00.028 **7**
– accessorius vertebrae lumbalis A02.2.04.002 **17**
– alveolaris maxillae A02.1.12.035 **14**
– anterior mallei A15.3.02.048 **150**
– articularis
– – inferior vertebrae A02.2.01.016 **16**
– – superior
– – – ossis sacri A02.2.05.005 **17**
– – – vertebrae A02.2.01.014 **16**
– axillaris A16.0.02.007 **154**
– calcaneus cuboidei A02.5.16.004 **24**
– caudatus lobi caudati hepatis A05.8.01.032 **55**
– ciliares A15.2.03.011 **144**
– clinoideus
– – anterior A02.1.05.022 **11**
– – medius A02.1.05.008 **11**
– – posterior A02.1.05.011 **11**
– cochleariformis A15.3.02.018 **149**
– condylaris mandibulae A02.1.15.035 **16**
– coracoideus A02.4.01.023 **19**
– coronoideus
– – mandibulae A02.1.15.032 **15**
– – ulnae A02.4.06.003 **20**
– costalis A02.2.04.003 **17**
– costiformis vertebrae lumbalis A02.2.04.003 **17**
– ethmoidalis conchae nasalis inferioris A02.1.08.004 **13**
– falciformis lig. sacrotuberalis A03.6.03.006 **30**
– frontalis
– – maxillae A02.1.12.024 **14**
– – ossis zygomatici A02.1.14.006 **15**
– intrajugularis A02.1.04.021 **11**, A02.1.06.046 **13**
– jugularis A02.1.04.020 **11**
– lacrimalis conchae nasalis inferioris A02.1.08.002 **13**
– lateralis
– – cartilaginis septi nasi A06.1.01.014 **57**
– – mallei A15.3.02.047 **150**
– – mammae A16.0.02.007 **154**
– – tali A02.5.10.014 **24**
– – tuberis calcanei A02.5.11.004 **24**
– lenticularis incudis A15.3.02.041 **150**
– mamillaris vertebrae lumbalis A02.2.04.004 **17**
– mammillaris A02.2.04.004 **17**
– mastoideus A02.1.06.004 **12**
– maxillaris conchae nasalis inferioris A02.1.08.003 **13**
– medialis tuberis calcanei A02.5.11.003 **24**
– muscularis artilaginis arytenoideae A06.2.04.013 **58**
– orbitalis ossis palatini A02.1.13.011 **15**
– palatinus maxillae A02.1.12.029 **14**
– papillaris lobi caudati hepatis A05.8.01.031 **55**
– paramastoideus A02.1.04.035 **11**
– posterior
– – cartilaginis septi nasi A06.1.01.015 **57**
– – tali A02.5.10.016 **24**
– pterygoideus ossis sphenoidalis A02.1.05.042 **12**
– pterygospinosus A02.1.05.054 **12**
– pyramidalis ossis palatini A02.1.13.007 **15**
– sphenoidalis
– – cartilago septi nasi A06.1.01.015 **57**
– – ossis palatini A02.1.13.012 **15**
– spinosus vertebrae A02.2.01.012 **16**
– styloideus
– – ossis
– – – metacarpi tertii [III] A02.4.09.005 **20**
– – – temporale A02.1.06.047 **13**
– – radii A02.4.05.015 **20**
– – ulnae A02.4.06.017 **20**
– supracondylaris A02.4.04.017 **19**
– temporalis ossis zygomatici A02.1.14.005 **15**
– transversus vertebrae A02.2.01.013 **16**
– uncinatus
– – ossis ethmoidalis A02.1.07.016 **13**
– – pancreatis A05.9.01.003 **56**
– – vertebrae
– – – cervicales A02.2.02.002 **16**
– – – thoracicae primae A02.2.03.005 **17**
– vaginalis ossis sphenoidalis A02.1.05.048 **12**
– vertebrae lumbalis costalis A02.2.04.003 **17**
– vocalis cartilaginis arytenoideae A06.2.04.005 **58**
– xiphoideus A02.3.03.007 **18**
– zygomaticus
– – maxillae A02.1.12.028 **14**
– – ossis
– – – frontalis A02.1.03.014 **10**
– – – temporalis A02.1.06.067 **13**
Profundus A01.0.00.034 **1**
Prominentia
– canalis
– – facialis A15.3.02.023 **149**
– – semicircularis lateralis A15.3.02.022 **149**
– laryngea A06.2.02.003 **58**
– mallearis A15.3.01.057 **149**
– spiralis ductus cochlearis A15.3.03.097 **152**
– styloidea A15.3.02.007 **149**
Promontorium
– ossis sacri A02.2.05.003 **17**
– tympani A15.3.02.011 **149**
Pronatio A03.0.00.060 **26**
Prosencephalon A14.1.03.006 **108**
Prostata A09.3.08.001 **68**
Protuberantia
– mentalis A02.1.15.005 **15**
– occipitalis
– – externa A02.1.04.022 **11**
– – interna A02.1.04.029 **11**
Proximalis A01.0.00.035 **1**
Pterion A02.1.00.019 **8**
Pubes A16.0.00.022 **154**
Pubis A02.5.01.301 **21**
Pudendum femininum A09.2.01.001 **66**
Pulmo/nes A06.5.01.001 **60**
– dexter A06.5.01.002 **60**
– dexter, lobus
– – inferior A06.5.02.009 **61**
– – medius A06.5.02.006 **61**
– – superior A06.5.02.002 **60**
– sinister A06.5.01.003 **60**
– sinister, lobus
– – inferior A06.5.02.020 **61**
– – superior A06.5.02.015 **61**
Pulpa
– alba A13.2.01.006 **100**
– coronalis A05.1.03.052 **48**
– dentis A05.1.03.051 **48**
– lienalis A13.2.01.004 **100**
– radicularis A05.1.03.053 **48**
– rubra A13.2.01.005 **100**

– splenica A13.2.01.004 **100**
Pulvinar thalami A14.1.08.104 **120**
Punctum
– fixum A04.0.00.004 **33**
– lacrimale A15.2.07.065 **148**
– mobile A04.0.00.005 **33**
Pupilla A15.2.03.028 **145**
Putamen A14.1.09.507 **130**
Pylorus A05.5.01.017 **52**
Pyramides renales
A08.1.01.029 **63**
Pyramis
– bulbi A14.1.04.003 **108**
– medullae oblongatae
A14.1.04.003 **108**
– vermis [VIII] A14.1.07.215 **119**
– vestibuli A15.3.03.008 **151**

R

Radialis A01.0.00.039 **1**
Radiatio
– acustica A14.1.08.662 **122**,
A14.1.09.545 **131**
– anterior thalami
A14.1.08.666 **122**
– centralis thalami
A14.1.08.667 **122**
– corporis callosi A14.1.09.249 **127**
– inferior thalami
A14.1.08.668 **122**
– optica A14.1.08.673 **122**,
A14.1.09.542 **130**,
A14.1.09.547 **131**
– posterior thalami
A14.1.08.675 **122**
– thalami
– – anterior A14.1.09.527 **130**
– – centralis A14.1.09.532 **130**
– thalamica posterior
A14.1.09.543 **131**
Radius/i A02.4.05.001 **19**
– lentiium A15.2.05.014 **146**
– medullares renis
A08.1.01.018 **63**
Radix/ces
– accessoria A05.1.03.070 **49**
– anterior A14.2.00.029 **133**
– buccalis A05.1.03.064 **49**
– clinica dentis A05.1.03.033 **48**
– cranialis n. accessorius
A14.2.01.185 **137**
– dentis A05.1.03.031 **48**
– distalis dentis A05.1.03.067 **49**
– inferior ansae cervicalis
A14.2.02.015 **137**
– intermedia ganglii
pterygopalatini
A14.2.01.117 **135, 142**
– lateralis
– – nervi mediani
A14.2.03.033 **138**
– – tractus optici A14.1.08.405 **120**
– linguae A05.1.04.003 **49**
– medialis
– – nervi mediani
A14.2.03.032 **138**
– – tractus optici A14.1.08.406 **120**
– mesenterii A10.1.02.008 **72**
– mesialis A05.1.03.066 **49**
– mesiobuccalis A05.1.03.068 **49**
– mesiolingualis A05.1.03.069 **49**
– motoria
– – m. spinalis A14.2.00.029 **133**
– – n. trigemini A14.2.01.015 **133**
– nasi A06.1.01.002 **57**
– nasociliaris ganglii ciliaris
A14.2.01.026 **134, 142**
– oculomotoria ganglii ciliaris
A14.2.01.010 **133, 142**
– palatinalis dentis
A05.1.03.065 **49**
– parasympathica ganglii/orum
– – ciliaris A14.2.01.010 **133, 142**
– – otici A14.2.01.149 **136, 142**
– – pelvicorum A14.3.02.018 **142**
– – pterygopalatini
A14.2.01.117 **135, 142**
– – sublingualis A14.3.02.012 **142**
– – submandibularis
A14.2.01.118 **135, 142**
– penis A09.4.01.002 **69**
– plexus brachialis
A14.2.03.002 **137**
– posterior A14.2.00.030 **133**
– pulmonis A06.5.01.016 **60**
– sensoria
– – ganglii
– – – ciliaris A14.2.01.026 **134, 142**
– – – otici A14.2.01.067 **134, 142**
– – – pterygopalatini
A14.2.01.039 **134, 142**
– – – sublingualis
A14.2.01.088 **135, 142**
– – – submandibularis
A14.2.01.087 **135, 142**,
A14.2.01.088 **135**
– – gangliorum pelvicorum
A14.3.02.020 **142**
– – n. spinalis A14.2.00.030 **133**
– – n. trigemini A14.2.01.013 **133**
– spinalis A14.2.01.186 **137**
– – n. accessorius A14.2.01.186 **137**
– superior ansae cervicalis
A14.2.02.014 **137**
– sympathica
– – ganglii
– – – ciliaris A14.3.02.004 **142**
– – – otici A14.3.02.015 **142**
– – – pterygopalatini
A14.3.02.008 **142**
– – – sublingualis
A14.3.02.013 **142**,
A14.3.03.005 **142**
– – – submandibularis
A14.3.02.011 **142**
– – gangliorum pelvicorum
A14.3.02.019 **142**
Ramis/i
Rami arteriarum succedant
Rami ductorum vide paginam 210
Rami nervorum vide paginam 210
Rami ossum vide paginam 213
Rami subendocardiales vide paginam 213
Rami sulcorum vide paginam 213
Rami venarum vide paginam 213
Ramus/i (arteriae/arum)
– accessorius a. meningea media
A12.2.05.062 **80**
– acetabularis
– – a. circumflexae femoris
medialis A12.2.16.024 **90**
– – a. obturatoriae
A12.2.15.010 **89**
– acromialis
– – a. suprascapularis
A12.2.08.052 **85**
– – a. thoracoacromialis
A12.2.09.006 **85**
– anastomoticus cum
– – a. lacrimali a. meningea media
A12.2.05.068 **81**
– – a. meningea media a. lacrimalis
A12.2.06.028 **82**
– anterior/es A12.3.02.105 **91**
– – a. centralis posteromedialis a.
communicantis posterioris
A12.2.07.070 **83**
– – a. obturatoriae A12.2.15.011 **89**
– – a. pancreaticoduodenalis
inferioris A12.2.12.055 **88**
– – a. recurrentis ulnaris
A12.2.09.043 **86**
– – a. suprarenalis inferioris
A12.2.12.078 **88**
– articularis/esa. descendentis
genus A12.2.16.019 **90**
– ascendens
– – a. circumflexae femoris
– – – lateralis A12.2.16.028 **90**
– – – medialis A12.2.16.025 **90**
– – a. epigastricae inferioris
A12.2.16.009 **90**
– – a. segmentalis
– – – anterior pulmonis sinistri
A12.2.01.206 **78**
– – – anterioris pulmonis dextri
A12.2.01.105 **78**
– – – posterior pulmonis sinistri
A12.2.01.209 **78**
– – – posterioris pulmonis dextri
A12.2.01.108 **78**
– – r. superficialis a. transversa colli
A12.2.08.055 **85**
– atrialis/es
– – a. coronariae
– – – dextrae A12.2.03.105 **79**
– – – sinistrae A12.2.03.214 **79**
– – anastomoticus a. coronariae
sinistrae A12.2.03.207 **79**
– – intermedius a. coronariae
– – – dextrae A12.2.03.107 **79**
– – – sinistrae A12.2.03.210 **79**
– atrioventriculares a. coronariae
– – dextrae A12.2.03.102 **79**
– – sinistrae A12.2.03.208 **79**
– auricularis/es
– – anteriores a. temporalis
superficialis A12.2.05.048 **80**
– – a. auricularis posterioris
A12.2.05.042 **80**
– – a. occipitalis A12.2.05.032 **80**
– basalis tentorii partis cavernosae
a. carotis internae
A12.2.06.008 **81**
– bronchiales

– – a. thoracicae internae A12.2.08.032 **85**
– – partis thoracicae aortae A12.2.11.002 **86**
– calcanei
– – a. ficularis A12.2.16.075 **91**
– – a. tibialis posterioris A12.2.16.059 **91**
– – r. malleolaris lateralis a. fibularis A12.2.16.075 **91**
– calcarinus a. occipitalis medialis A12.2.07.102 **84**
– capsulares
– – a. intrarenalium A08.1.03.009 **63**
– – a. renalis A12.2.12.076 **88**
– carpalis
– – dorsalis
– – – a. radialis A12.2.09.032 **86**
– – – a. ulnaris A12.2.09.053 **86**
– – palmaris
– – – a. radialis A12.2.09.030 **86**
– – – a. ulnaris A12.2.09.054 **86**
– caudae nuclei caudati a. choroideae anterioris A12.2.07.012 **82**
– chiasmaticus/i
– – a. choroideae anterioris A12.2.07.005 **82**
– – a. communicantis posterioris A12.2.07.072 **83**
– choroideus/i
– – posteriores
– – – laterales a. cerebri posterioris A12.2.07.092 **84**
– – – mediales a. cerebri posterioris A12.2.07.091 **84**
– – ventriculi
– – – lateralis a. choroideae anterioris A12.2.07.002 **82**
– – – quarti a. inferioris posterioris cerebelli A12.2.08.015 **84**
– – – tertii a. choroideae anterioris A12.2.07.003 **82**
– cingularis a. callosomarginalis A12.2.07.041 **83**
– circumflexus
– – a. coronariae sinistrae A12.2.03.206 **79**
– – fibularis a. tibialis posterioris A12.2.16.056 **90**
– – peronealis a. tibialis posterioris A12.2.16.056 **90**
– clavicularis a. thoracoacromialis A12.2.09.008 **85**
– clivales partis cerebralis a. carotis internae A12.2.06.021 **81**
– cochlearis a. vestibulocochlearis A15.3.03.132 **153**
– coeliaci trunci vagalis posterioris A14.2.01.182 **137**
– colicus a. ileocolicae A12.2.12.064 **88**
– collateralis
– – a. intercostalis posterioris A12.2.11.017 **87**
– coni arteriosi
– – a. coronariae
– – – dextrae A12.2.03.103 **79**
– – – sinistrae A12.2.03.203 **79**
– corporis
– – amygdaloidei a. choroideae anterioris A12.2.07.015 **82**
– – callosi dorsalis a. occipitalis medialis A12.2.07.099 **84**
– – geniculati lateralis a. choroideae anterioris A12.2.07.007 **82**
– corticales
– – inferiores a. cerebri medii A12.2.07.055 **83**
– – superiores a. cerebri medii A12.2.07.061 **83**
– costalis lateralis a. thoracicae internae A12.2.08.038 **85**
– cricothyroideus a. thyroideae superioris A12.2.05.006 **80**
– cruris
– – cerebri a. choroideae anterioris A12.2.07.021 **82**
– – posterioris capsulae internae a. choroideae anterioris A12.2.07.009 **82**
– cutaneus
– – lateralis
– – – a. intercostalis posterioris A12.2.11.018 **87**
– – – r. dorsalis a. intercostalis posterioris A12.2.11.010 **86**
– – medialis r. dorsalis a. intercostalis posterioris A12.2.11.009 **86**
– deltoideus
– – a. profundae brachii A12.2.09.022 **86**
– – a. thoracoacromialis A12.2.09.009 **85**
– dentales
– – a. alveolaris
– – – inferioris A12.2.05.057 **80**
– – – superiorts posterioris A12.2.05.076 **81**
– – a. infraorbitalis A12.2.05.080 **81**
– descendens
– – a. circumflexae femoris
– – – lateralis A12.2.16.029 **90**
– – – medialis A12.2.16.026 **90**
– – a. occipitalis A12.2.05.036 **80**
– – a. segmentalis
– – – anterior pulmonis sinistri A12.2.01.207 **78**
– – – anterioris pulmonis dextri A12.2.01.106 **78**
– – – posterior pulmonis sinistri A12.2.01.210 **78**
– – – posterioris pulmonis dextri A12.2.01.109 **78**
– – r. superficialis a. transversa colli A12.2.08.056 **85**
– dexter a. hepaticae A12.2.12.030 **87**
– dorsalis/es
– – a. intercostalis posterioris A12.2.11.008 **86**
– – a. lumbalis A12.2.12.005 **87**
– – a. subcostalis A12.2.11.021 **87**
– – – secundae A12.2.08.064 **85**
– – linguae a. lingualis A12.2.05.017 **80**
– duodenales a. pancreaticoduodenalis superioris
– – anterioris A12.2.12.027 **87**
– – posterioris A12.2.12.020 **87**
– epididymales a. testicularis ♂ A12.2.12.088 **88**
– frontalis
– – a. meningea media A12.2.05.063 **81**
– – a. temporalis superficialis A12.2.05.051 **80**
– – anteromedialis a. callosomarginalis A12.2.07.038 **83**
– – intermediomedialis a. callosomarginalis A12.2.07.039 **83**
– – posteromedialis a. callosomarginalis A12.2.07.040 **83**
– ganglionares trigeminales partis cavernosae a. carotis internae A12.2.06.013 **81**
– gastrici a. gastroomentalis
– – dextrae A12.2.12.023 **87**
– – sinistrae A12.2.12.048 **88**
– genus capsulae internae a. choroideae anterioris A12.2.07.008 **82**
– gingivales
– – a. facialis A12.2.05.024 **80**
– – a. thyroideae inferioris A12.2.08.045 **85**
– – anterior a. thyroideae superioris A12.2.05.007 **80**
– – lateralis a. thyroideae superioris A12.2.05.009 **80**
– – posterior a. thyroideae superioris A12.2.05.008 **80**
– globi pallidi a. choroideae anterioris A12.2.07.011 **82**
– gyri angularis a. cerebri medii A12.2.07.060 **83**
– helicini a. uterinae ♀ A12.2.15.030 **89**
– hippocampi a. choroideae anterioris A12.2.07.013 **82**
– hypothalamicus a. communicantis posterioris A12.2.07.077 **83**
– ilealis a. ileocolicae A12.2.12.063 **88**
– iliacus a. iliolumbalis A12.2.15.005 **89**
– inferior/es r. profundi a. gluteae superioris A12.2.15.017 **89**
– infrahyoideus a. thyroideae superioris A12.2.05.003 **79**
– inguinales a. pudendae externae profundae A12.2.16.016 **90**
– intercostales anteriores a. thoracicae internae A12.2.08.039 **85**
– intermedius a. hepaticae A12.2.12.039 **88**
– interventriculares septales a. coronariae
– – dextrae A12.2.03.109 **79**
– – sinistrae A12.2.03.205 **79**

– interventricularis
– – anterior a. coronariae sinistrae A12.2.03.202 **79**
– – posterior a. coronariae dextrae A12.2.03.108 **79**
– labiales
– – anteriores a. pudendae externae profundae ♀ A12.2.16.015 **90**
– – posteriores a. perinealis ♀ A12.2.15.041 **89**
– lateralis/es A12.2.07.075 **83**, A12.2.08.023 **84**, A12.3.12.009 **98**
– – a. coronariae sinistrae A12.2.03.204 **79**
– – a. pontis A12.2.08.023 **84**
– – a. superioris cerebelli A12.2.08.028 **85**
– – a. tuberis cinerei A12.2.07.075 **83**
– – nasi a. facialis A12.2.05.028 **80**
– lienales a. splenicae A12.2.12.051 **88**
– lumbalis a. iliolumbalis A12.2.15.003 **89**
– malleolares
– – laterales a. fibularis A12.2.16.074 **91**
– – mediales a. tibialis posterioris A12.2.16.057 **91**
– mammarii
– – laterales
– – – a. thoracicae lateralis A12.2.09.012 **85**
– – – r. cutaneus lateralis a. intercostalis posterioris A12.2.11.019 **87**
– – medialesrr. perforantium a. thoracicae internae A12.2.08.037 **85**
– marginalis
– – dexter a. coronariae dextrae A12.2.03.106 **79**
– – sinister a. coronariae sinistrae A12.2.03.209 **79**
– – tentorii partis cavernosae a. carotis internae A12.2.06.009 **81**
– mastoideus A12.2.05.031 **80**
– – a. occipitalis A12.2.05.031 **80**
– – a. tympanicae posterioris A12.2.05.040 **80**
– medialis/es A14.2.01.023 **133**
– – a. pontis A12.2.08.022 **84**
– – a. superioris cerebelli A12.2.08.026 **85**
– – a. tuberis cinerei A12.2.07.074 **83**
– mediastinales
– – a. thoracicae internae A12.2.08.030 **85**
– – partis thoracicae aortae A12.2.11.005 **86**
– medullares
– – laterales a. vertebralis A12.2.08.018 **84**
– – mediales a. vertebralis A12.2.08.017 **84**
– meningeus/i
– – a. occipitalis A12.2.05.035 **80**
– – a. vertebralis A12.2.08.011 **84**
– – anterior a. ethmoidalis anterioris A12.2.06.040 **82**
– – partis
– – – cavernosae a. carotis internae A12.2.06.010 **81**
– – – cerebralis a. carotis internae A12.2.06.022 **81**
– – recurrens a. ophthalmicae A12.2.06.030 **82**
– mentalis/es a. alveolaris inferioris A12.2.05.059 **80**
– muscularis/es a. vertebralis A12.2.08.008 **84**
– mylohyoideus a. alveolaris inferioris A12.2.05.060 **80**
– nasales anteriores laterales a. ethmoidalis anterioris A12.2.06.042 **82**
– nervi oculomotorii a. communicantis posterioris A12.2.07.079 **83**
– nervorum partis cavernosae a. carotis internae A12.2.06.014 **81**
– nodi
– – atrioventricularis a. coronariae
– – – dextrae A12.2.03.110 **79**
– – – sinistrae A12.2.03.213 **79**
– – sinuatrialis a. coronariae
– – – dextrae A12.2.03.104 **79**
– – – sinistrae A12.2.03.212 **79**
– nuclei rubri a. choroideae anterioris A12.2.07.020 **82**
– nucleorum
– – hypothalami a. choroideae anterioris A12.2.07.017 **82**
– – thalami a. choroideae anterioris A12.2.07.018 **82**
– obturatorius r. pubici a. epigastricae inferioris A12.2.16.005 **90**
– occipitalis/es A12.2.05.043 **80**, A14.2.01.103 **135**
– – a. auricularis posterioris A12.2.05.043 **80**
– – a. occipitalis A12.2.05.034 **80**
– occipitotemporalis a. occipitalis medialis A12.2.07.103 **84**
– oesophagei/ales A14.2.01.168 **136**
– – a. gastricae sinistrae A12.2.12.014 **87**
– – a. thyroideae inferioris A12.2.08.047 **85**
– – partis thoracicae aortae A12.2.11.003 **86**
– omentales a. gastroomentalis
– – dextrae A12.2.12.024 **87**
– – sinistrae A12.2.12.049 **88**
– ovaricus a. uterinae ♀ A12.2.15.033 **89**
– palmaris
– – profundus a. ulnaris A12.2.09.055 **86**
– – superficialis a. radialis A12.2.09.031 **86**
– pancreatici
– – a. pancreaticoduodenalis superioris
– – – anterioris A12.2.12.026 **87**
– – – posterioris A12.2.12.019 **87**
– – a. splenicae A12.2.12.041 **88**
– paracentrales A12.2.07.042 **83**
– parietalis
– – a. meningea media A12.2.05.065 **81**
– – a. occipitalis medialis A12.2.07.100 **84**
– – a. temporalis superficialis A12.2.05.052 **80**
– parietooccipitalis/es
– – a. occipitalis medialis A12.2.07.101 **84**
– – a. pericallosa A12.2.07.045 **83**
– parotideus/ei A12.2.05.044 **80**, A12.2.05.046 **80**
– – a. auricularis posterioris A12.2.05.044 **80**
– – a. temporalis superficialis A12.2.05.046 **80**
– partis retrolentiformis capsulae internae a. choroideae anterioris A12.2.07.010 **82**
– pectorales a. thoracoacromialis A12.2.09.010 **85**
– pedunculares a. cerebri posterioris A12.2.07.093 **84**
– perforans/tes
– – a. fibularis A12.2.16.072 **91**
– – a. interosseae posterioris A12.2.09.051 **86**
– – a. metatarsalis plantaris A12.2.16.067 **91**
– – a. thoracicae internae A12.2.08.036 **85**
– – arci palmaris profundi A12.2.09.040 **86**
– – partis thoracicae aortae A12.2.11.004 **86**
– peridentales
– – a. alveolaris
– – – inferioris A12.2.05.058 **80**
– – – superioris posterioris A12.2.05.077 **81**
– – a. infraorbitalis A12.2.05.081 **81**
– petrosus a. meningea media A12.2.05.066 **81**
– pharyngeus/ei/eales
– – a. canalis pterygoidei A12.2.05.083 **81**
– – a. palatinae descendentis A12.2.05.087 **81**
– – a. pharyngeae ascendentis A12.2.05.012 **80**
– – a. thyroideae inferioris A12.2.08.046 **85**
– postcentralis r. spinalis r. dorsalis a. intercostalis posterioris A12.2.11.012 **87**
– posterior/is
– – a. centralis posteromedialis a. communicantis posterioris A12.2.07.071 **83**
– – a. obturatoriae A12.2.15.012 **89**

– – a. pancreaticoduodenalis inferioris A12.2.12.056 **88**
– – a. recurrentis ulnaris A12.2.09.044 **86**
– – a. suprarenalis inferioris A12.2.12.083 **88**
– posterolateralis dexter a. coronariae dextrae A12.2.03.111 **79**
– precuneales a. pericallosa A12.2.07.044 **83**
– prelaminaris r. spinalis r. dorsalis a. intercostalis posterioris A12.2.11.013 **87**
– profundus
– – a. circumflexae femoris medialis A12.2.16.023 **90**
– – a. gluteae superioris A12.2.15.015 **89**
– – a. plantaris medialis A12.2.16.062 **91**
– – a. transversa colli A12.2.08.057 **85**
– prostatici
– – a. rectalis mediae ♂ A12.2.15.037 **89**
– – a. vesicalis inferioris ♂ A12.2.15.028 **89**
– pterygoidei a. temporalis profundae posterioris A12.2.05.073 **81**
– pubicus
– – a. epigastricae inferioris A12.2.16.004 **90**
– – a. obturatoriae A12.2.15.009 **89**
– radiculares rr.spinalium a. vertebralis A12.2.08.006 **84**
– sacrales laterales a. sacralis medianae A12.2.12.010 **87**
– saphenus a. descendentis genus A12.2.16.018 **90**
– scrotales
– – anteriores a. pudendae externae profundae ♂ A12.2.16.015 **90**
– – posteriores a. perinealis ♂ A12.2.15.041 **89**
– septales
– – anteriores a. ethmoidalis anterioris A12.2.06.041 **82**
– – posteriores a. sphenopalatinae A12.2.05.090 **81**
– septi nasi a. labialis superioris A12.2.05.027 **80**
– sinister a. hepaticae A12.2.12.035 **87**
– sinus cavernosi partis cavernosae a. carotis internae A12.2.06.011 **81**
– spinalis/es
– – a. cervicalis ascendentis A12.2.08.050 **85**
– – a. iliolumbalis A12.2.15.004 **89**
– – a. intercostalis posterioris secundae A12.2.08.065 **85**
– – a. lumbalis A12.2.12.006 **87**
– – a. sacralis lateralis A12.2.15.007 **89**
– – a. subcostalis A12.2.11.022 **87**
– – a. vertebralis A12.2.08.005 **84**
– – r. dorsalis a. intercostalis posterioris A12.2.11.011 **87**
– splenici a. splenicae A12.2.12.051 **88**
– stapedius a. tympanicae posterioris A12.2.05.041 **80**
– sternales a. thoracicae internae A12.2.08.035 **85**
– sternocleidomastoideus/i
– – a. occipitalis A12.2.05.033 **80**
– – a. thyroideae superioris A12.2.05.004 **80**
– striati
– – distales laterales aa. centralium anterolateralium A12.2.07.050 **83**
– – proximales laterales aa. centralium anterolateralium A12.2.07.049 **83**
– subscapulares a. axillaris A12.2.09.003 **85**
– substantiae
– – nigrae a. choroideae anterioris A12.2.07.019 **82**
– – perforatae anterioris a. choroideae anterioris A12.2.07.004 **82**
– superficialis
– – a. circumflexae femoris medialis A12.2.16.022 **90**
– – a. gluteae superioris A12.2.15.014 **89**
– – a. plantaris medialis A12.2.16.063 **91**
– – a. transversa colli A12.2.08.054 **85**
– superior/es r. profundi a. gluteae superioris A12.2.15.016 **89**
– suprahyoideus a. lingualis A12.2.05.016 **80**
– temporalis/es A14.2.01.109 **135**
– – anterior/es
– – – a. cerebri medii A12.2.07.056 **83**
– – – a. occipitalis lateralis A12.2.07.095 **84**
– – intermedii a. occipitalis lateralis A12.2.07.096 **84**
– – medius/i
– – – a. cerebri medii A12.2.07.057 **83**
– – – a. occipitalis lateralis A12.2.07.096 **84**
– – posterior/es
– – – a. cerebri medii A12.2.07.058 **83**
– – – a. occipitalis lateralis A12.2.07.097 **84**
– temporooccipitalis a. cerebri medii A12.2.07.059 **83**
– terminales
– – inferiores a. cerebri medii A12.2.07.055 **83**
– – superiores a. cerebri medii A12.2.07.061 **83**
– thymici a. thoracicae internae A12.2.08.031 **85**
– tonsillae cerebelli a. inferioris posterioris cerebelli A12.2.08.014 **84**
– tonsillaris a. facialis A12.2.05.022 **80**
– tracheales A12.2.08.033 **85**, A12.2.08.048 **85**, A14.2.01.167 **136**
– – a. thoracicae internae A12.2.08.033 **85**
– – a. thyroideae inferioris A12.2.08.048 **85**
– tractus optici a. choroideae anterioris A12.2.07.006 **82**
– transversus a. circumflexae femoris lateralis A12.2.16.030 **90**
– tubarius/i
– – a. ovaricae ♀ A12.2.12.088 **88**
– – a. uterinae ♀ A12.2.15.034 **89**
– tuberis cinerei a. choroideae anterioris A12.2.07.016 **82**
– uncales a. choroideae anterioris A12.2.07.014 **82**
– ureterici
– – a. ovaricae ♀ A12.2.12.087 **88**
– – a. suprarenalis inferioris A12.2.12.085 **88**
– – a. testicularis ♂ A12.2.12.087 **88**
– – a. umbilicalis A12.2.15.023 **89**
– vaginales
– – a. rectalis mediae ♀ A12.2.15.037 **89**
– – a. uterinae ♀ A12.2.15.031 **89**
– vestibularis posterior a. vestibulocochlearis A15.3.03.131 **153**
Ramus/i (ducti/orum)
– anterior ducti hepatici dextri A05.8.01.063 **56**
– lateralis ducti hepatici sinistri A05.8.01.066 **56**
– medialis ducti hepatici sinistri A05.8.01.067 **56**
– posterior ducti hepatici dextri A05.8.01.064 **56**
Ramus/i (nervi/orum)
– ad ganglion ciliare n. oculomotorii A14.2.01.010 **133, 142**
– anterior/es A12.3.02.105 **91**
– – n. auricularis magnus A14.2.02.020 **137**
– – n. cervicalium A14.2.02.011 **137**
– – n. cutanei antebrachii medialis A14.2.03.029 **138**
– – n. lumbalium A14.2.05.008 **139**
– – n. obturatorii A14.2.07.013 **140**
– – n. sacralium et n. coccygei A14.2.06.007 **139**
– – n. spinalis A14.2.00.034
– – n. thoracicorum A14.2.04.006 **139**
– articularis/es
– – n. mixti A14.2.00.025 **133**
– – r. posterioris n. obturatorii A14.2.07.018 **140**

– auricularis/es
– – n. auricularis posterioris A14.2.01.104 **135**
– – n. vagi A14.2.01.156 **136**
– autonomicus nervi autonomici A14.2.00.040 **133**
– bronchiales n. vagi A14.2.01.171 **136**
– buccales n. facialis A14.2.01.111 **135**
– calcanei
– – laterales n. suralis A14.2.07.064 **141**
– – mediales n. tibialis A14.2.07.065 **141**
– cardiaci
– – cervicales
– – – inferiores n. vagi A14.2.01.165 **136**
– – – superiores n. vagi A14.2.01.164 **136**
– – thoracici
– – – ganglionum thoracicorum A14.3.01.025 **141**
– – – n. vagi A14.2.01.170 **136**
– cervicalis n. facialis A14.2.01.114 **135**
– collateralis n. intercostalis A14.2.04.008 **139**
– colli n. facialis A14.2.01.114 **135**
– communicans/tes
– – albus nervorum spinalium A14.3.01.007 **141**
– – cochlearis n. vestibularis A14.2.01.124 **135**
– – cum
– – – chorda tympani A14.2.01.152 **136**
– – – ganglio ciliari A14.2.01.026 **134, 142**
– – – n. auriculotemporali A14.2.01.151 **136**
– – – n. faciali A14.2.01.078 **134**
– – – n. glossopharyngeo A14.2.01.107 **135**, A14.2.01.143 **136**
– – – n. hypoglosso A14.2.01.083 **135**
– – – n. laryngeo recurrente A14.2.01.163 **136**
– – – n. ulnari A14.2.03.037 **138**
– – – n. vago A14.2.01.120 **135**
– – – n. zygomatico A14.2.01.019 **133**
– – – plexu tympanico A14.2.01.119 **135**
– – – ramo
– – – – auriculare nervi vagi A14.2.01.143 **136**
– – – – meningeo A14.2.01.150 **136**
– – fibularis A14.2.07.049 **140**
– – ganglionis vestibularis cum n. cochleari A14.2.01.124 **135**
– – griseus nervorum spinalium A14.3.01.006 **141**
– – n. auriculotemporalis cum n. faciali A14.2.01.078 **134**
– – n. facialis cum n. glossopharyngeo A14.2.01.107 **135**
– – n. fibularis communis cum n. cutaneo surae mediali A14.2.07.049 **140**
– – n. glossopharyngei cum
– – – chorda tympani A14.2.01.152 **136**
– – – n. auriculotemporali A14.2.01.151 **136**
– – – r. meningeo n. vagi A14.2.01.150 **136**
– – n. intermedii cum
– – – n. vago A14.2.01.120 **135**
– – – plexu tympanico A14.2.01.119 **135**
– – n. interossei antebrachii anterior cum n. ulnari A14.2.03.037 **138**
– – n. lacrimalis cum n. zygomatico A14.2.01.019 **133**
– – n. lingualis cum n. hypoglosso A14.2.01.083 **135**
– – n. nasociliaris cum ganglio ciliari A14.2.01.026 **134, 142**
– – n. peronei communis cum n. cutaneo surae mediali A14.2.07.049 **140**
– – n. radialis cum n. ulnari A14.2.03.057 **139**
– – n. spinalis A14.2.00.033 **133**
– – n. spinalium A14.3.01.005 **141**
– – n. vagi cum n. glossopharyngeo A14.2.01.143 **136**
– – peroneus A14.2.07.049 **140**
– – plexi tympanici cum r. auriculari n. vagi A14.2.01.143 **136**
– – r. laryngeo interni cum n. laryngeo recurrente A14.2.01.163 **136**
– – ulnaris A14.2.03.057 **139**
– cutaneus/i
– – anterior/es
– – – abdominalis A14.2.04.015 **139**
– – – – n. intercostalis A14.2.04.015 **139**
– – – n. femoralis A14.2.07.022 **140**
– – – n. iliohypogastrici A14.2.07.005 **139**
– – – pectoralis n. intercostalis A14.2.04.013 **139**
– – cruris mediales n. sapheni A14.2.07.025 **140**
– – lateralis
– – – abdominalis n. intercostalis A14.2.04.011 **139**
– – – n. iliohypogastrici A14.2.07.004 **139**
– – – pectoralis n. intercostalis A14.2.04.009 **139**
– – n. mixti A14.2.00.024 **133**
– – n. obturatorii A14.2.07.014 **140**
– – posterior
– – – n. sacralis et n. coccygei A14.2.06.005 **139**
– – – r. dorsalis n. cervicalis A14.2.02.006 **137**
– – – r. posterioris n.
– – – – lumbalis A14.2.05.005 **139**
– – – – thoracici A14.2.04.005 **139**
– – r. anterioris n. obturatorii A14.2.07.014 **140**
– digastricus n. facialis A14.2.01.105 **135**
– dorsalis/es
– – n. cervicalium A14.2.02.003 **137**
– – n. lumbalium A14.2.05.002 **139**
– – n. sacralium et n. coccygei A14.2.06.002 **139**
– – n. thoracicorum A14.2.04.002 **139**
– – n. ulnaris A14.2.03.042 **138**
– externus
– – n. accessorius A14.2.01.189 **137**
– – n. laryngei superioris A14.2.01.161 **136**
– femoralis n. genitofemoralis A14.2.07.010 **140**
– ganglionares
– – ad ganglioni
– – – otio A14.2.01.067 **134, 142**
– – – pterygopalatino A14.2.01.039 **134, 142**
– – – sublinguali A14.2.01.088 **135, 142**
– – – submandibulari A14.2.01.087 **135**
– – n. lingualis ad ganglion
– – – sublinguale A14.2.01.088 **135, 142**
– – – submandibulare A14.2.01.087 **135**
– – n. mandibularis ad ganglion
– – – submandibulare A14.2.01.088 **135, 142**
– – – oticum A14.2.01.067 **134, 142**
– – n. maxillaris ad ganglion pterygopalatinum A14.2.01.039 **134, 142**
– gastrici
– – anteriores trunci vagalis anterioris A14.2.01.175 **136**
– – posteriores trunci vagalis posterioris A14.2.01.180 **137**
– genitalis n. genitofemoralis A14.2.07.009 **140**
– gingivales
– – inferiores A14.2.01.093 **135**
– – n. mentalis A14.2.01.097 **135**
– – superiores A14.2.01.055 **134**
– hepatici trunci vagalis anterioris A14.2.01.177 **136**
– inferior/es
– – n. oculomotorii A14.2.01.009 **133**
– – n. transversus colli A14.2.02.023 **137**
– infrapatellaris n. sapheni A14.2.07.024 **140**
– interganglionares trunci sympathetici A14.3.01.004 **141**
– internus

– – n. accessorius A14.2.01.188 **137**
– – n. laryngei superioris A14.2.01.162 **136**
– isthmi faucium n. lingualis A14.2.01.082 **135**
– labiales
– – n. mentalis A14.2.01.096 **135**
– – superiores n. infraorbitalis A14.2.01.063 **134**
– laryngopharyngei ganglionis cervicalis superioris A14.3.01.014 **141**
– lateralis/es
– – n. sacralis et n. coccygei A14.2.06.004 **139**
– – n. supraorbitalis A14.2.01.022 **133**
– – – medialis A14.2.01.023 **133**
– – r. dorsalis n. cervicalis A14.2.02.005 **137**
– – r. posterioris
– – – n. lumbalis A14.2.05.004 **139**
– – – n. thoracici A14.2.04.004 **139**
– lingualis/es
– – n. facialis A14.2.01.112 **135**
– – n. glossopharyngei A14.2.01.148 **136**
– – n. hypoglossi A14.2.01.192 **137**
– – n. lingualis A14.2.01.086 **135**
– mammarii
– – laterales n. intercostalis A14.2.04.010 **139**
– – mediales n. intercostalis A14.2.04.014 **139**
– marginalis mandibularis n. facialis A14.2.01.113 **135**
– medialis/es A14.2.01.023 **133**
– – n. sacralis aut n. coccygei A14.2.06.003 **139**
– – r. posterioris
– – – n. lumbalis A14.2.05.003 **139**
– – – n. thoracici A14.2.04.003 **139**
– membranae tympani n. auriculotemporalis A14.2.01.076 **134**
– meningeus/i
– – anterior
– – – n. ethmoidalis posterioris A14.2.01.029 **134**
– – – n. mandibularis A14.2.01.065 **134**
– – – n. maxillaris A14.2.01.038 **134**
– – – n. spinalis A14.2.00.032 **133**
– – – n. vagi A14.2.01.155 **136**
– – recurrens n. ophthalmici A14.2.01.017 **133**
– mentalis/es n. mentalis A14.2.01.095 **135**
– muscularis/es
– – n. accessorius A14.2.01.190 **137**
– – n. axillaris A14.2.03.060 **139**
– – n. femoralis A14.2.07.021 **140**
– – n. fibularis
– – – profundus A14.2.07.056 **140**
– – – superficialis A14.2.07.051 **140**
– – n. intercostalis A14.2.04.007 **139**
– – n. interossei antebrachii anterior A14.2.03.035 **138**
– – n. musculocutanei A14.2.03.025 **138**
– – n. perinealium A14.2.07.041 **140**
– – n. radialis A14.2.03.053 **138**
– – n. spinalis A14.2.00.026 **133**
– – n. tibialis A14.2.07.059 **141**
– – n. ulnaris A14.2.03.041 **138**
– – partis supraclavicularis plexus brachialis A14.2.03.019 **138**
– – r. anterioris n. obturatorii A14.2.07.015 **140**
– – r. posterioris n. obturatorii A14.2.07.017 **140**
– musculi stylopharyngei n. glossopharyngei A14.2.01.145 **136**
– n. alveolarium superiorium
– – anteriores A14.2.01.052 **134**
– – medius A14.2.01.051 **134**
– – posteriores A14.2.01.050 **134**
– n. oculomotorii ad ganglio ciliari A14.2.01.010 **133, 142**
– nasales
– – n. ethmoidalis anterioris A14.2.01.034 **134**
– – – n. infraorbitalis A14.2.01.061 **134**
– – interni
– – – laterales n. ethmoidalis anterioris A14.2.01.032 **134**
– – – mediales n. ethmoidalis anterioris A14.2.01.033 **134**
– – – n. ethmoidalis anterioris A14.2.01.031 **134**
– – – n. infraorbitalis A14.2.01.062 **134**
– – posteriores
– – – inferiores n. palatinus major A14.2.01.046 **134**
– – – superiores
– – – – laterales n. maxillaris A14.2.01.041 **134**
– – – – mediales n. maxillaris A14.2.01.042 **134**
– occipitalis/es n. auricularis posterioris ganglionum thoracicorum A14.3.01.027 **141**
– omentales a. gastroomentalis n. maxillaris A14.2.01.040 **134**
– palmaris
– – n. interossei antebrachii anterior A14.2.03.036 **138**
– – n. ulnaris A14.2.03.044 **138**
– palpebrales
– – inferiores n. infraorbitalis A14.2.01.060 **134**
– – n. infratrochlearis A14.2.01.036 **134**
– parotideus n. auriculotemporalis A14.2.01.077 **134**
– pericardiacus/i n. phrenici A14.2.02.029 **137**
– perineales n. cutanei femoris posterioris A14.2.07.035 **140**
– pharyngeus/ei/eales
– – n. glossopharyngei A14.2.01.144 **136**
– – n. laryngei recurrentis A14.2.01.169 **136**
– – n. vagi A14.2.01.158 **136**
– phrenicoabdominales n. phrenici A14.2.02.030 **137**
– plexi nervosi
– – dentales
– – – inferiores A14.2.01.092 **135**
– – – superiores A14.2.01.054 **134**
– – gingivales
– – – inferiores A14.2.01.093 **135**
– – – superiores A14.2.01.055 **134**
– posterior/is
– – n. auricularis magnus A14.2.02.019 **137**
– – n. cervicalium A14.2.02.003 **137**
– – n. cutanei antebrachii medialis A14.2.03.030 **138**
– – n. lumbalium A14.2.05.002 **139**
– – n. obturatorii A14.2.07.016 **140**
– – n. sacralium et n. coccygei A14.2.06.002 **139**
– – n. spinalis A14.2.00.035 **133**
– – n. thoracicorum A14.2.04.002 **139**
– profundus
– – n. plantaris lateralis A14.2.07.073 **141**
– – n. radialis A14.2.03.054 **138**
– – n. ulnaris A14.2.03.048 **138**
– pulmonales A14.3.03.017 **143**
– – plexus nervosi pulmonalis A14.3.03.016 **143**
– – thoracici ganglionum thoracicorum A14.3.01.026 **141**
– pyloricus trunci vagalis anterioris A14.2.01.178 **136**
– recurrens A14.2.00.032 **133**
– renalis/es
– – n. splanchnici minoris A14.3.01.031 **141**
– – n. vagi A14.2.01.183 **137**
– sinus carotici n. glossopharyngei A14.2.01.146 **136**
– stylohyoideus n. facialis A14.2.01.106 **135**
– superficialis
– – n. plantaris lateralis A14.2.07.070 **141**
– – n. radialis A14.2.03.056 **138**
– – n. ulnaris A14.2.03.045 **138**
– superior/es
– – n. oculomotorii A14.2.01.008 **133**
– – n. transversus colli A14.2.02.022 **137**
– temporalis/es A14.2.01.109 **135**
– – n. facialis A14.2.01.109 **135**
– – superficiales n. auriculotemporalis A14.2.01.080 **135**
– tentorius n. ophthalmici A14.2.01.017 **133**

– thyrohyoideus ansae cervicalis A14.2.02.016 **137**
– tonsillaris/es A12.2.05.022 **80**
– – n. glossopharyngei A14.2.01.147 **136**
– – n. palatini minores A14.2.01.048 **134**
– tracheales
– – n. laryngei recurrentis A14.2.01.167 **136**
– tubarius plexi tympanici A14.2.01.141 **136**
– ventrales
– – n. cervicalium A14.2.02.011 **137**
– – n. lumbalium A14.2.05.008 **139**
– – n. sacralium et n. coccygei A14.2.06.007 **139**
– – n. thoracicorum A14.2.04.006 **139**
– zygomatici n. facialis A14.2.01.110 **135**
– zygomaticofacialis n. zygomatici A14.2.01.058 **134**
– zygomaticotemporalis n. zygomatici A14.2.01.057 **134**
Ramus/i (ossis/um)
– inferior ossis pubis A02.5.01.313 **22**
– ischiopubicus A02.5.01.007 **21**
– mandibulae A02.1.15.024 **15**
– ossis ischii A02.5.01.203 **21**
– superior ossis pubis A02.5.01.306 **21**
Ramus/i (subendocardiales)
– subendocardiales fasciculi atrioventricularis A12.1.06.008 **77**
Ramus/i (sulci/orum)
– anterior sulci lateralis cerebri A14.1.09.107 **125**
– ascendens sulci lateralis cerebri A14.1.09.106 **124**
– marginalis sulci cinguli A14.1.09.204 **126**
– posterior sulci lateralis cerebri A14.1.09.105 **124**
Ramus/i (venae/arum)
– anterior/es A12.3.02.105 **91**
– – r. dextri v. portae hepatis A12.3.12.003 **98**
– – v. pulmonalis
– – – dextrae superioris A12.3.02.105 **91**
– – – sinistrae superioris A12.3.02.305 **92**
– apicalis v. pulmonalis dextrae superioris A12.3.02.102 **91**
– apicoposterior v. pulmonalis sinistrae superioris A12.3.02.302 **92**
– basalis anterior
– – v. basalis superioris lobi inferioris pulmonis dextri A12.3.02.207 **92**
– – v. pulmonalis sinistri inferioris A12.3.02.407 **92**
– dexter v. portae hepatis A12.3.12.002 **98**
– dorsalis v. intercostalis posterioris A12.3.07.015 **96**
– laterales r. sinistri v. portae hepatis A12.3.12.009 **98**
– lingularis v. pulmonalis sinistrae superioris A12.3.02.308 **92**
– lobi
– – caudati r. sinistri v. portae hepatis A12.3.12.007 **98**
– – medii v. pulmonalis dextrae superioris A12.3.02.111 **91**
– – mediales r. sinistri v. portae hepatis A12.3.12.011
– parotidei v. facialis A12.3.05.028 **93**
– posterior
– – r. dextri v. portae hepatis A12.3.12.004 **98**
– – v. pulmonalis dextrae superioris A12.3.02.108 **91**
– pubicus v. obturatoria accessoria A12.3.10.026 **97**
– sinister v. portae hepatis A12.3.12.005 **98**
– spinalis v. intercostalis posterioris A12.3.07.017 **96**
– superior v. pulmonalis
– – – dextrae inferioris A12.3.02.202 **92**
– – – sinistri inferioris A12.3.02.402 **92**
Raphe
– medullae oblongatae A14.1.04.122 **109**
– musculi iliococcygei A04.5.04.018 **40**
– palati A05.1.01.105 **47**
– penis A09.4.01.013 **69**
– perinei A09.5.00.002 **71**
– pharyngis A05.3.01.101 **51**
– pontis A14.1.05.303 **112**
– pterygomandibularis A05.3.01.102 **51**
– scroti A09.4.03.002 **70**
Recessus
– anterior membranae tympanicae A15.3.02.068 **150**
– articularis A03.0.00.038 **25**
– cochlearis A15.3.03.010 **151**
– costodiaphragmaticus A07.1.02.013 **62**
– costomediastinalis A07.1.02.014 **62**
– duodenalis
– – inferior A10.1.02.413 **73**
– – superior A10.1.02.411 **73**
– ellipticus A15.3.03.005 **151**
– epitympanicus A15.3.02.004 **149**
– hepatorenalis recessi subhepatici A10.1.02.427 **73**
– ileocaecalis
– – inferior A10.1.02.420 **73**
– – superior A10.1.02.418 **73**
– inferior bursae omentalis A10.1.02.406 **72**
– infundibuli/aris A14.1.08.417 **121**
– intersigmoideus A10.1.02.417 **73**
– lateralis ventriculi quarti A14.1.05.717 **115**
– lienalis bursae omentalis A10.1.02.407 **72**
– membranae tympanicae A15.3.02.067 **150**
– paraduodenalis A10.1.02.415 **73**
– pharyngeus A05.3.01.017 **50**
– phrenicomediastinalis A07.1.02.015 **62**
– pinealis A14.1.08.415 **121**
– piriformis A05.3.01.024 **50**
– pleurales A07.1.02.012 **62**
– posterior membranae tympanicae A15.3.02.070 **150**
– retrocaecalis A10.1.02.422 **73**
– retroduodenalis A10.1.02.416 **73**
– sacciformis articulationis
– – cubiti A03.5.09.009 **29**
– – radioulnaris distalis A03.5.10.003 **29**
– saccularis A15.3.03.009 **151**
– sphenoethmoidalis A02.1.00.094 **9**, A06.1.02.022 **57**
– sphericus A15.3.03.009 **151**
– splenicus A10.1.02.407 **72**
– subhepaticus A10.1.02.426 **73**
– subphrenicus A10.1.02.425 **73**
– subpopliteus A04.8.05.024 **45**
– superior
– – bursae omentalis A10.1.02.405 **72**
– – membranae tympanicae A15.3.02.069 **150**
– supraopticus A14.1.08.418 **121**
– suprapinealis A14.1.08.413 **121**
– utriculi/aris A15.3.03.064 **152**
– – labyrinthi membranacei A15.3.03.064 **152**
– – labyrinthi ossei A15.3.03.005 **151**
– vertebromediastinalis A07.1.02.016 **62**
Recessus, fossae et plicae A10.1.02.401 **72**
Rectum A05.7.04.001 **53**
Regio/nes
– abdominales A01.2.04.001 **4**
– analis A01.2.06.002 **4**
– antebrachialis A01.2.07.012 **4**
– – anterior A01.2.07.013 **4**
– – posterior A01.2.07.014 **5**
– antebrachii
– – anterior A01.2.07.013 **4**
– – posterior A01.2.07.014 **5**
– auricularis A01.2.01.006 **3**
– axillaris A01.2.03.009 **4**
– brachialis A01.2.07.003 **4**
– – anterior A01.2.07.004 **4**
– – posterior A01.2.07.007 **4**
– brachii
– – anterior A01.2.07.004 **4**
– – posterior A01.2.07.007 **4**
– buccalis A01.2.01.013 **3**
– calcanea A01.2.08.023 **5**
– capitis A01.2.01.001 **3**
– carpalis A01.2.07.018 **5**
– – anterior A01.2.07.019 **5**

– – posterior A01.2.07.020 **5**
– cervicais/les A01.2.02.001 **3**
– – anterior A01.2.02.002 **3**
– – lateralis A01.2.02.009 **3**
– – posterior A01.2.02.012 **4**
– colli posterior A01.2.02.012 **4**
– cornus ammonis I–IV
A14.1.09.328 **128**,
A14.1.09.329 **128**,
A14.1.09.330 **128**,
A14.1.09.331 **128**
– coxae A01.2.08.005 **5**
– cruris A01.2.08.014 **5**
– – anterior A01.2.08.015 **5**
– – posterior A01.2.08.016 **5**
– cubitalis A01.2.07.008 **4**
– – anterior A01.2.07.009 **4**
– – posterior A01.2.07.011 **4**
– deltoidea A01.2.07.002 **4**
– dorsalis/es A01.2.05.001 **4**
– – manus A01.2.07.021 **5**
– – pedis A01.2.08.024 **5**
– dorsi A01.2.05.001 **4**
– epigastrica A01.2.04.003 **4**
– facialis A01.2.01.008 **3**
– femoris A01.2.08.006 **5**
– – anterior A01.2.08.007 **5**
– – posterior A01.2.08.009 **5**
– frontalis A01.2.01.002 **3**
– genus A01.2.08.010 **5**
– – anterior A01.2.08.011 **5**
– – posterior A01.2.08.012 **5**
– glutealis A01.2.08.002 **5**
– hippocampi proprii I–IV
A14.1.09.328 **128**,
A14.1.09.329 **128**,
A14.1.09.330 **128**,
A14.1.09.331 **128**
– hypochondriaca A01.2.04.002 **4**
– inframammaria A01.2.03.008 **4**
– infraorbitalis A01.2.01.012 **3**
– infrascapularis A01.2.05.007 **4**
– inguinalis A01.2.04.006 **4**
– interfascicularis medullae renalis
A08.1.01.025 **63**
– lateralis A01.2.04.004 **4**
– lumbalis A01.2.05.008 **4**
– mammaria A01.2.03.007 **4**
– manus A01.2.07.017 **5**
– mastoidea A01.2.01.007 **3**
– membri
– – inferioris A01.2.08.001 **5**
– – superioris A01.2.07.001 **4**
– mentalis A01.2.01.020 **3**
– metacarpalis A01.2.07.025 **5**
– metatarsalis A01.2.08.034 **6**
– nasalis A01.2.01.016 **3**
– occipitalis A01.2.01.004 **3**
– oralis A01.2.01.018 **3**
– orbitalis A01.2.01.010 **3**
– palmaris A01.2.07.022 **5**
– parietalis A01.2.01.003 **3**
– parotideomasseterica
A01.2.01.014 **3**
– pectoralis A01.2.03.005 **4**
– – lateralis A01.2.03.006 **4**
– pedis A01.2.08.022 **5**
– perinealis A01.2.06.001 **4**
– plantaris A01.2.08.025 **5**
– presternalis A01.2.03.002 **4**
– pubica A01.2.04.007 **4**
– retromalleolaris
– – lateralis A01.2.08.020 **5**
– – medialis A01.2.08.021 **5**
– sacralis A01.2.05.003 **4**
– scapularis A01.2.05.005 **4**
– sternocleidomastoidea
A01.2.02.007 **3**
– surae A01.2.08.017 **5**
– talocruralis
– – anterior A01.2.08.018 **5**
– – posterior A01.2.08.019 **5**
– tarsalis A01.2.08.033 **6**
– temporalis A01.2.01.005 **3**
– thoracicae anteriores et laterales
A01.2.03.001 **4**
– umbilicalis A01.2.04.005 **4**
– urogenitalis A01.2.06.003 **4**
– vertebralis A01.2.05.002 **4**
– zygomatica A01.2.01.015 **3**
Ren A08.1.01.001 **63**
Repositio A03.0.00.063 **26**
Rete
– acromiale a. thoracoacromialis
A12.2.09.007 **85**
– arteriosum A12.0.00.012 **75**
– articulare
– – cubiti A12.2.09.045 **86**
– – genus A12.2.16.040 **90**
– calcaneum A12.2.16.076 **91**
– carpale dorsale A12.2.09.033 **86**
– lymphocapillare
A12.0.00.045 **75**
– malleolare
– – laterale A12.2.16.047 **90**
– – mediale A12.2.16.058 **91**
– mirabile A12.0.00.013 **75**
– patellare A12.2.16.041 **90**
– testis A09.3.01.024 **68**
– vasculosum articulare
A12.0.00.014 **75**
– venosum A12.0.00.015 **75**
– – dorsale
– – – manus A12.3.08.023 **96**
– – – pedis A12.3.11.011 **98**
– – plantare A12.3.11.015 **98**
Reticulum trabeculare sclerae
A15.2.02.004 **144**
Retina A15.2.04.002 **145**
Retinaculum/a
– caudale A16.0.00.006 **154**
– cutis A16.0.00.005 **154**
– – mammae A16.0.02.015 **155**
– musculorum
– – extensorum A04.6.03.010 **41**
– – – inferius pedis
A04.7.03.027 **43**
– – – manus A04.6.03.010 **41**
– – – superius pedis
A04.7.03.025 **43**
– – fibularium
– – – inferius A04.7.03.029 **44**
– – – superius A04.7.03.028 **44**
– – flexorum A04.6.03.013 **41**,
A04.7.03.026 **43**
– – – manus A04.6.03.013 **41**
– – – pedis A04.7.03.026 **43**
– – peroneorum
– – – inferius A04.7.03.029 **44**
– – – superius A04.7.03.028 **44**
– patellae
– – laterale A03.6.08.017 **31**
– – mediale A03.6.08.016 **31**
Rhombencephalon
A14.1.03.002 **108**
Rima
– glottidis A06.2.09.014 **59**
– oris A05.1.01.004 **47**
– palpebrarum A15.2.07.030 **147**
– pudendi A09.2.01.006 **66**
– vestibuli A06.2.09.009 **59**
– vocalis A06.2.09.014 **59**
Rivus lacrimalis A15.2.07.062 **148**
Rostralis A01.0.00.021 **1**
Rostrum
– corporis callosi A14.1.09.242 **127**
– sphenoidale A02.1.05.015 **11**
Rotatio
– externa A03.0.00.055 **25**
– interna A03.0.00.056 **26**
– lateralis A03.0.00.055 **25**
– medialis A03.0.00.056 **26**
Rugae A05.8.02.010 **56**
– palatinae A05.1.01.106 **47**
– vaginales A09.1.04.012 **66**
– vesicae biliaris A05.8.02.010 **56**

S

Sacculus
– laryngis A06.2.09.011 **59**
– vestibularis A15.3.03.065 **152**
Saccus
– conjunctivalis A15.2.07.054 **147**
– endolymphaticus
A15.3.03.080 **152**
– lacrimalis A15.2.07.068 **148**
– profundus perinei
A09.5.03.001 **71**
– subcutaneus perinei
A09.5.01.001 **71**
Sagittalis A01.0.00.005 **1**
Sagulum A14.1.06.328 **117**
Salpinx A09.1.02.001 **65**
Sanguis A12.0.00.009 **75**
Scala
– media A15.3.03.092 **152**
– tympani A15.3.03.045 **151**
– vestibuli A15.3.03.043 **151**
Scapha A15.3.01.012 **148**
Scapula A02.4.01.001 **18**
Schindylesis A03.0.00.014 **25**
Sclera A15.2.02.002 **144**
Scoliosis A02.2.00.008 **16**
Scrotum A09.4.03.001 **70**
Secundarium A02.0.00.045 **7**
Segmentatio hepatis: lobi, partes, divisiones et segmenta
A05.8.01.033 **55**
Segmentum/a
– a. cerebri
– – anterioris
– – – A1 A12.2.07.023 **82**
– – – A2 A12.2.07.033 **83**
– – medii
– – – M1 A12.2.07.047 **83**

- - - M2 A12.2.07.053 **83**, A12.2.07.055 **83**, A12.2.07.061 **83**
- - posterioris
- - - P1 A12.2.07.083 **84**
- - - P2 A12.2.07.088 **84**
- - - P3 A12.2.07.094 **84**
- - - P4 A12.2.07.098 **84**
- anterius A15.2.01.009 **144**
- - bulbi oculi A15.2.01.009 **144**
- - inferius renis A08.1.02.004 **63**
- - laterale
- - - dextrum hepatis A05.8.01.050 **55**
- - - sinistrum hepatis A05.8.01.040 **55**
- - mediale dextrum hepatis A05.8.01.047 **55**
- - pulmonis
- - - dextri [S III] A06.5.02.005 **61**
- - - sinistri [S III] A06.5.02.017 **61**
- - superius renis A08.1.02.003 **63**
- apicale pulmonis dextri [S I] A06.5.02.003 **61**
- apicoposterius pulmonis sinistri [S I + II] A06.5.02.016 **61**
- basale
- - anterius
- - - pulmonis
- - - - dextri [S VIII] A06.5.02.012 **61**
- - - - sinistri [S VIII] A06.5.02.023 **61**
- - laterale
- - - pulmonis
- - - - dextri [S IX] A06.5.02.013 **61**
- - - - sinistri [S IX] A06.5.02.024 **61**
- - mediale
- - - pulmonis
- - - - dextri A06.5.02.011 **61**
- - - - sinistri A06.5.02.022 **61**
- - posterius
- - - pulmonis
- - - - dextri [S X] A06.5.02.014 **61**
- - - - sinistri [S X] A06.5.02.025 **61**
- bronchopulmonalia A06.5.02.001 **60**
- cardiacum
- - pulmonis
- - - dextri [S VII] A06.5.02.011 **61**
- - - sinistri [S VII] A06.5.02.022 **61**
- cervicalia [1–8] A14.1.02.014 **105**
- coccygea [1–3] A14.1.02.018 **105**
- hepatis
- - I A05.8.01.044 **55**
- - II A05.8.01.039 **55**
- - III A05.8.01.040 **55**
- - IV A05.8.01.042 **55**
- - V A05.8.01.047 **55**
- - VI A05.8.01.050 **55**
- - VII A05.8.01.051 **55**
- - VIII A05.8.01.048 **55**
- inferius renis A08.1.02.005 **63**
- laterale pulmonis dextri [S IV] A06.5.02.007 **61**
- lingulare
- - inferius pulmonis sinistri [S V] A06.5.02.019 **61**
- - superius pulmonis sinistri [S IV] A06.5.02.018 **61**
- lumbalia [1–5] A14.1.02.016 **105**
- mediale
- - pulmonis dextri [S V] A06.5.02.008 **61**
- - sinistrum hepatis A05.8.01.042 **55**
- posterius
- - bulbi oculi A15.2.01.010 **144**
- - hepatis A05.8.01.044 **55**
- - laterale
- - - dextrum hepatis A05.8.01.051 **55**
- - - sinistrum hepatis A05.8.01.039 **55**
- - mediale dextrum hepatis A05.8.01.048 **55**
- - pulmonis dextri [S II] A06.5.02.004 **61**
- - renis A08.1.02.006 **63**
- renalia A08.1.02.001 **63**
- sacralia [1–5] A14.1.02.017 **105**
- superius
- - pulmonis
- - - dextri [S VI] A06.5.02.010 **61**
- - - sinistri [S VI] A06.5.02.021 **61**
- - renis A08.1.02.002 **63**
- thoracica [1–12] A14.1.02.015 **105**
Sella turcica A02.1.05.006 **11**
Semicanalis
- musculi tensoris tympani A02.1.06.018 **12**
- tubae auditivae/auditoriae A02.1.06.019 **12**
Septula testis A09.3.01.019 **67**
Septum/a
- atrioventriculare A12.1.00.016 **76**
- canalis musculotubarii A02.1.06.020 **12**
- cervicale intermedium A14.1.01.311 **105**
- cochleae A15.3.03.037 **151**
- corporum cavernosorum A09.2.02.006 **67**
- femorale A04.7.03.015 **43**
- glandis penis A09.4.01.009 **69**
- interalveolaria
- - mandibulae A02.1.15.018 **15**
- - maxillae A02.1.12.038 **14**
- interatriale A12.1.00.019 **76**
- intermusculare A04.3.02.004 **36**
- - brachii
- - - laterale A04.6.03.007 **41**
- - - mediale A04.6.03.006 **41**
- - cruris
- - - anterius A04.7.03.022 **43**
- - - posterius A04.7.03.023 **43**
- - femoris
- - - laterale A04.7.03.004 **43**
- - - mediale A04.7.03.005 **43**
- - m. erectoris spinae A04.3.02.004 **36**
- - vastoadductorium A04.7.03.007 **43**
- interradicularia
- - mandibulae A02.1.15.020 **15**
- - maxillae A02.1.12.039 **14**
- interventriculare A12.1.00.013 **76**
- linguae A05.1.04.024 **49**
- medianum posterius medullae spinalis A14.1.02.009 **105**
- nasi A06.1.02.004 **57**
- - osseum A02.1.00.087 **9**
- orbitale A15.2.07.003 **147**
- pellucidum A14.1.09.262 **127**
- penis A09.4.01.019 **69**
- rectovaginale ♀ A04.5.03.004 **39**
- rectovesicale ♂ A04.5.03.004 **39**
- scroti A09.4.03.004 **70**
- sinuum
- - frontalium A02.1.03.031 **10**
- - sphenoidalium A02.1.05.017 **11**
Sinciput A01.1.00.002 **2**
Sinister A01.0.00.007 **1**
Sinus
- anales A05.7.05.006 **54**
- aortae A12.2.03.002 **79**
- caroticus A12.2.04.008 **79**, A12.2.06.003 **81**
- cavernosus A12.3.05.116 **94**
- coronarius A12.3.01.002 **91**
- durae matris A12.3.05.101 **93**
- epididymidis A09.3.01.013 **67**
- frontalis A02.1.03.029 **10**, A06.1.03.004 **57**
- intercavernosus
- - anterior A12.3.05.117 **94**
- - posterior A12.3.05.118 **94**
- lactiferi A16.0.02.011 **154**
- lienalis A13.2.01.019 **100**
- marginalis A12.3.05.104 **93**
- maxillaris A02.1.12.023 **14**, A06.1.03.002 **57**
- obliquus pericardii A12.1.07.002 **78**
- occipitalis A12.3.05.105 **93**
- paranasales A06.1.03.001 **57**
- petrosquamosus A12.3.05.107 **93**
- petrosus
- - inferior A12.3.05.113 **94**
- - superior A12.3.05.115 **94**
- posterior cavi tympani A15.3.02.026 **149**
- prostaticus A09.4.02.010 **70**
- rectus A12.3.05.112 **94**
- renalis A08.1.01.005 **63**
- sagittalis
- - inferior A12.3.05.111 **94**
- - superior A12.3.05.109 **93**
- sigmoideus A12.3.05.108 **93**
- sphenoidalis A02.1.05.016 **11**, A06.1.03.003 **57**
- sphenoparietalis A12.3.05.119 **94**
- splenicus A13.2.01.019 **100**

– tarsi A02.5.11.009 **24**
– tonsillaris A05.2.01.009 **50**
– transversus A12.3.05.102 **93**
– – pericardii A12.1.07.001 **77**
– trunci pulmonalis A12.2.01.002 **78**
– tympani A15.3.02.014 **149**
– venarum cavarum A12.1.01.012 **76**
– venosus A12.0.00.016 **75**
– – sclerae A12.3.06.109 **95, 144**
Siphon caroticum A12.2.06.023 **81**
Skeleton
– appendiculare A02.0.00.010 **7**
– axiale A02.0.00.009 **7**
– thoracis A02.3.00.001 **17**
Spatium/a
– anguli iridocornealis A15.2.03.033 **145**
– endolymphaticum A15.3.03.060 **152**
– epidurale A14.1.01.110 **104**, A14.1.01.112 **104**
– episclerale A15.2.07.006 **147**
– extradurale A14.1.01.110 **104**
– extraperitoneale A10.1.01.001 **72**
– intercostale A02.3.04.007 **18**
– interossea
– – metacarpi A03.5.11.405 **30**
– – metatarsi A03.6.10.705 **32**
– intervaginale subarachnoidale n. optici A15.2.04.034 **146**
– lateropharyngeum A05.3.01.119 **51**
– leptomeningeum A14.1.01.202 **104**
– – n. optici A15.2.04.034 **146**
– parapharyngeum A05.3.01.119 **51**
– perichoroideum A15.2.03.004 **144**
– peridurale A14.1.01.112 **104**
– perilymphaticum A15.3.03.055 **152**
– peripharyngeum A05.3.01.117 **51**
– pharyngeum laterale A05.3.01.119 **51**
– profundum perinei A09.5.03.001 **71**
– retroinguinale A10.1.01.004 **72**
– retroperitoneale A10.1.01.002 **72**
– retropharyngeum A05.3.01.118 **51**
– retropubicum A10.1.01.003 **72**
– retrozonulare A15.2.06.007 **146**
– subarachnoideum A14.1.01.202 **104**
– subdurale A14.1.01.109 **104**
– superficiale perinei A09.5.02.001 **71**
– suprasternale A04.2.05.003 **35**
– zonularia A15.2.05.017 **146**
Sphincter urethrae internus A09.2.03.009 **67**
Spina/e
– geni
– – inferior A02.1.15.011 **15**
– – superior A02.1.15.010 **15**
– helicis A15.3.01.007 **148**
– iliaca
– – anterior
– – – inferior A02.5.01.112 **21**
– – – superior A02.5.01.111 **21**
– – posterior
– – – inferior A02.5.01.114 **21**
– – – superior A02.5.01.113 **21**
– ischiadica A02.5.01.205 **21**
– mentalis
– – inferior A02.1.15.011 **15**
– – superior A02.1.15.010 **15**
– nasalis A02.1.03.020 **10**
– – anterior corporis maxillae A02.1.12.011 **14**
– – ossis frontalis A02.1.03.020 **10**
– – posterior laminae horizontalis ossis palatini A02.1.13.017 **15**
– ossis sphenoidalis A02.1.05.040 **11**
– palatinae A02.1.12.033 **14**
– scapulae A02.4.01.005 **18**
– suprameatalis A02.1.06.070 **13**
– suprameatica A02.1.06.070 **13**
– trochlearis A02.1.03.024 **10**
– tympanica
– – major A02.1.06.056 **13**
– – minor A02.1.06.057 **13**
Spinocerebellum A14.1.07.008 **118**
Splen A13.2.01.001 **100**
– accessorius A13.2.01.022 **100**
Splenium corporis callosi A14.1.09.245 **127**
Squama
– frontalis A02.1.03.002 **10**
– occipitalis A02.1.04.010 **10**
Stapes A15.3.02.033 **149**
Statoconium A15.3.03.086 **152**
Sternum A02.3.03.001 **18**
Stratum/a
– circulare
– – m. detrusoris vesicae A08.3.01.018 **64**
– – tunicae muscularis
– – – coli A05.7.03.017 **53**
– – – gastricae A05.5.01.023 **52**
– – – intestini tenuis A05.6.01.006 **52**
– – – recti A05.7.04.015 **54**
– – – urethrae A09.2.03.008 **67**
– – – – prosticae A09.4.02.012 **70**
– cornus ammonis A14.1.09.334 **128**
– externum longitudinale cervicis vesicae A08.3.01.017 **64**
– fibrosum
– – capsulae articularis A03.0.00.027 **25**
– – panniculi adiposi telae subcutaneae A16.0.03.004 **155**
– – vagina tendinis A04.8.01.006 **44**
– ganglionicum retinae A15.2.04.016 **145**
– granulare gyri dentati A14.1.09.342 **128**
– granulosum corticis cerebelli A14.1.07.403 **119**
– griseum
– – intermedium colliculi superioris A14.1.06.609 **118**
– – profundum colliculi superioris A14.1.06.611 **118**
– – superficiale colliculi superioris A14.1.06.607 **118**
– gyri dentati A14.1.09.340 **128**
– helicoidale
– – brevis gradus tunicae muscularis intestini tenuis A05.6.01.006 **52**
– – longi gradus tunicae muscularis intestini tenuis A05.6.01.005 **52**
– hippocampi moleculare et substratum lacunosum A14.1.09.335 **128**
– internum longitudinale cervicis vesicae A08.3.01.019 **64**
– isocorticis A14.1.09.308 **128**
– koniocellulare nuclei dorsalis corporis geniculati lateralis A14.1.08.803 **123**
– limitans
– – externum retinae A15.2.04.011 **145**
– – internum retinae A15.2.04.018 **145**
– longitudinale
– – externum m. detrusoris vesicae A08.3.01.017 **64**
– – internum m. detrusoris vesicae A08.3.01.019 **64**
– – tunicae muscularis
– – – coli A05.7.03.012 **53**
– – – gastricae A05.5.01.022 **52**
– – – intestini tenuis A05.6.01.005 **52**
– – – recti A05.7.04.010 **54**
– – – urethrae A09.2.03.010 **67**
– – – – intermediae A09.4.02.019 **70**
– – – – prosticae A09.4.02.014 **70**
– – – – spongiosa A09.4.02.028 **70**
– magnocellularia nuclei dorsalis corporis geniculati lateralis A14.1.08.804 **123**
– medullare
– – intermedium colliculi superioris A14.1.06.610 **118**
– – profundum colliculi superioris A14.1.06.612 **118**
– membranosum
– – telae subcutaneae A16.0.03.005 **155**
– – – abdominis A04.5.02.022 **39**
– – – perinei A09.5.00.007 **71**
– moleculare
– – corticis cerebelli A14.1.07.405 **119**
– – et substratum lacunosum hippocampi A14.1.09.335 **128**
– – gyri dentati A14.1.09.341 **128**
– multiforme gyri dentati A16.0.03.003 **155**
– musculosum panniculi adiposi telae subcutaneae A16.0.03.003 **155**

– nervosum retinae A15.2.04.009 **145**
– neurofibrarum retinae A15.2.04.017 **145**
– nucleare
– – externum retinae A15.2.04.012 **145**
– – internum retinae A15.2.04.014 **145**
– opticum colliculi superioris A14.1.06.608 **118**
– oriens hippocampi A14.1.09.336 **128**
– papillare dermis A16.0.00.011 **154**
– parvocellularia nuclei dorsalis corporis geniculati lateralis A14.1.08.805 **123**
– pigmentosum retinae A15.2.04.008 **145**
– plexiforme
– – externum retinae A15.2.04.013 **145**
– – internum retinae A15.2.04.015 **145**
– purkinjense corticis cerebelli A14.1.07.404 **119**
– pyramidale hippocampi A14.1.09.337 **128**
– radiatum hippocampi A14.1.09.338 **128**
– reticulare dermis A16.0.00.013 **154**
– segmentorum externorum et internorum retinae A15.2.04.010 **145**
– synoviale
– – capsulae articularis A03.0.00.028 **25**
– – vagina tendinis A04.8.01.007 **44**
– zonale colliculi superioris A14.1.06.606 **118**
Stria/e A14.1.00.020 **104**
– canina A05.1.03.060 **49**
– cochlearis
– – anterior A14.1.05.319 **113**
– – intermedia A14.1.05.320 **113**
– – posterior A14.1.05.321 **113**
– diagonalis A14.1.09.422 **129**
– externa medullae renalis A08.1.01.022 **63**
– interna medullae renalis A08.1.01.023 **63**
– laminae
– – granularis
– – – externae isocorticis A14.1.09.316 **128**
– – – internae isocorticis A14.1.09.317 **128**
– – molecularis isocorticis A14.1.09.315 **128**
– – pyramidalis internae isocorticis A14.1.09.319 **128**
– longitudinalis
– – lateralis A14.1.09.247 **127**
– – medialis A14.1.09.248 **127**
– mallearis A15.3.01.058 **149**
– medullares ventriculi quarti A14.1.05.318 **113**, A14.1.05.707 **115**
– medullaris thalami A14.1.08.106 **120, 121**
– occipitalis laminae granularis internae isocorticis A14.1.09.318 **128**
– olfactoria/e A14.1.09.434 **129**
– – lateralis A14.1.09.436 **129**
– – medialis A14.1.09.435 **129**
– terminalis A14.1.09.275 **127**
– vascularis ductus cochlearis A15.3.03.096 **152**
Striatum A14.1.09.516 **130**
– dorsale A14.1.09.517 **130**
– ventrale A14.1.09.439 **129–130**
Striola A15.3.03.087 **152**
Stroma A11.3.00.007 **74**
– ganglii A14.2.00.004 **132**
– glandulae thyroideae A11.3.00.007 **74**
– iridis A15.2.03.031 **145**
– ovarii A09.1.01.010 **65**
– vitreum A15.2.06.013 **146**
Structurae
– centrales medullae spinalis A14.1.02.301 **108**
– oculi accessoriae A15.2.07.001 **147**
Subiculum A14.1.09.326 **128**
– promontorii tympani A15.3.02.013 **149**
Subnucleus
– gelatinosus nuclei spinalis nervi trigemini A14.1.04.214 **110**
– magnocellularis nuclei spinalis nervi trigemini A14.1.04.215 **110**
– oralis nuclei spinalis nervi trigemini A14.1.05.405 **113**
– rostrodorsalis nuclei gracilis A14.1.04.205 **110**
– zonalis nuclei spinalis nervi trigemini A14.1.04.213 **110**
Substantia
– alba A14.1.00.009 **104**, A14.1.06.201 **116**
– – hypothalami A14.1.08.945 **124**
– – medullae
– – – oblongatae A14.1.04.101 **109**
– – – spinalis A14.1.02.024 **106**, A14.1.02.201 **107**
– – partis basilaris pontis A14.1.05.102 **112**
– – tegmenti
– – – mesencephali A14.1.06.201 **116**
– – – pontis A14.1.05.302 **112**
– – thalami A14.1.08.659 **122**
– basalis telencephali A14.1.09.417 **129**
– compacta A02.0.00.003 **7**
– corticalis A02.0.00.002 **7**
– gelatinosa A14.1.02.119 **106**
– – centralis medullae spinalis A14.1.02.025 **106**
– – cornu posterioris medullae spinalis A14.1.02.119 **106**
– grisea A14.1.00.002 **104**
– – centralis A14.1.06.321 **117**
– – medullae
– – – oblongatae A14.1.04.201 **110**
– – – spinalis A14.1.02.020 **106**
– – partis basilaris pontis A14.1.05.201 **112**
– – tegmenti
– – – mesencephali A14.1.06.301 **117**
– – – pontis A14.1.05.401 **113**
– – thalami A14.1.08.602 **121**
– innominata A14.1.09.426 **129**
– intermedia
– – centralis medullae spinalis A14.1.02.134 **106**
– – lateralis medullae spinalis A14.1.02.136 **106**
– lentis A15.2.05.002 **146**
– muscularis prostatae A09.3.08.020 **69**
– nigra A14.1.06.111 **116**
– perforata
– – anterior A14.1.09.437 **129**
– – posterior A14.1.06.002 **115**
– – rostralis A14.1.09.437 **129**
– propria
– – corneae A15.2.02.020 **144**
– – sclerae A15.2.02.009 **144**
– spongiosa A02.0.00.004 **7**
– trabecularis A02.0.00.004 **7**
– visceralis secundaria medullae spinalis A14.1.02.125 **106**
Subthalamus A14.1.08.201 **120**, A14.1.08.701 **123**
Sulcus/i A02.0.00.035 **7**
– ampullaris A15.3.03.089 **152**
– anterolateralis medullae
– – oblongatae A14.1.04.005 **108**
– – spinalis A14.1.02.010 **105**
– arteriae
– – meningeae mediae A02.1.02.005 **9**
– – occipitalis A02.1.06.007 **12**
– – subclaviae A02.3.02.016 **18**
– – temporalis mediae A02.1.06.066 **13**
– – vertebralis A02.2.02.109 **17**
– arteriosi A02.1.00.042 **8**, A02.1.02.006 **9**
– basilaris A14.1.05.002 **112**
– bicipitalis
– – lateralis A01.2.07.005 **4**
– – medialis A01.2.07.006 **4**
– – radialis A01.2.07.005 **4**
– – ulnaris A01.2.07.006 **4**
– bulbopontinus A14.1.05.001 **112**
– calcanei A02.5.11.008 **24**
– calcarinus A14.1.09.225 **126**
– caninus A05.1.03.060 **49**
– caroticus A02.1.05.012 **11**
– carpi A02.4.08.014 **20**
– centralis
– – cerebri A14.1.09.103 **124, 126**
– – insulae A14.1.09.153 **125**
– cerebri A14.1.09.006 **124**
– cinguli A14.1.09.203 **126**
– circularis insulae A14.1.09.154 **125**

– collateralis A14.1.09.206 **126, 127**
– coronarius A12.1.00.011 **76**
– corporis callosi A14.1.09.202 **126**
– costae A02.3.02.011 **18**
– cruris helicis A15.3.01.027 **148**
– cutis A16.0.00.003 **154**
– ethmoidalis A02.1.10.002 **14**
– fimbriodentatus A14.1.09.238 **127**
– frontalis
– – inferior A14.1.09.117 **125**
– – superior A14.1.09.122 **125**
– gingivalis A05.1.01.111 **47**
– glutealis A01.2.08.004 **5**
– habenularis A14.1.08.004 **120**
– hamuli pterygoidei A02.1.05.052 **12**
– hippocampalis A14.1.09.236 **126**
– hypothalamicus A14.1.08.422 **121**
– infraorbitalis A02.1.12.005 **14**
– infrapalpebralis A01.2.01.011 **3**
– interlobares cerebri A14.1.09.102 **124, 125**
– intermammarius A16.0.02.002 **154**
– intermedius posterior medullae spinalis A14.1.02.012 **105**
– intersphinctericus analis A05.7.05.012 **54**
– intertubercularis A02.4.04.007 **19**
– interventricularis
– – anterior A12.1.00.009 **76**
– – posterior A12.1.00.010 **76**
– intraparietalis A14.1.09.127 **125**
– lacrimalis A02.1.00.081 **9**
– – ossis lacrimalis A02.1.09.003 **14**
– – ossis maxillae A02.1.12.018 **14**
– lateralis
– – cerebri A14.1.09.104 **124**
– – mesencephali A14.1.06.006 **115**
– limitans A14.1.05.724 **115**
– lunatus A14.1.09.134 **125**
– malleolaris A02.5.06.021 **23**, A02.5.07.017 **23**
– marginalis A14.1.09.204 **126**
– medianus
– – linguae A05.1.04.018 **49**
– – posterior
– – – medullae
– – – – oblongatae A14.1.04.020 **109**
– – – – spinalis A14.1.02.008 **105**
– – ventriculi quarti A14.1.05.703 **115**
– mentolabialis A01.2.01.019 **3**
– musculi subclavii A02.4.02.006 **19**
– mylohyoideus A02.1.15.031 **15**
– nasolabialis A01.2.01.017 **3**
– nervi
– – oculomotorii A14.1.06.003 **115**
– – petrosi
– – – majoris A02.1.06.025 **12**
– – – minoris A02.1.06.027 **12**
– – radialis A02.4.04.014 **19**
– – spinalis A02.2.02.007 **16**
– – ulnaris A02.4.04.028 **19**
– obturatorius A02.5.01.310 **22**
– occipitalis transversus A14.1.09.135 **125**
– occipitotemporalis A14.1.09.229 **126**
– olfactorius A06.1.02.011 **57**, A14.1.09.219 **126**
– orbitales A14.1.09.217 **126**
– palatini A02.1.12.034 **14**
– palatinus major A02.1.12.022 **14**, A02.1.13.006 **15**
– palatovaginalis A02.1.05.049 **12**
– paracentralis A14.1.09.208 **126**
– paracolici A10.1.02.424 **73**
– paraolfactorii A14.1.09.215 **126**
– parietooccipitalis A14.1.09.108 **125, 126**
– popliteus A02.5.04.026 **22**
– postcentralis A14.1.09.129 **125**
– posterior auriculae A15.3.01.022 **148**
– posterolateralis medullae
– – oblongatae A14.1.04.012 **108**
– – spinalis A14.1.02.011 **105**
– precentralis A14.1.09.120 **125**
– prechiasmaticus A02.1.05.005 **11**
– preolivaris A14.1.04.006 **108**
– promontorii tympani A15.3.02.012 **149**
– pulmonalis A02.3.04.005 **18**
– retroolivaris A14.1.04.010 **108**
– rhinalis A14.1.09.240 **127**
– sclerae A15.2.02.003 **144**
– sinus
– – marginalis A02.1.04.034 **11**
– – occipitalis A02.1.04.033 **11**
– – petrosi
– – – inferioris A02.1.00.052 **8**, A02.1.04.008 **10**, A02.1.06.038 **12**
– – – superioris A02.1.06.030 **12**
– – sagittalis superioris A02.1.00.038 **8**, A02.1.02.004 **9**, A02.1.03.017 **10**
– – sigmoidei A02.1.02.003 **9**, A02.1.04.032 **11**, A02.1.06.006 **12**
– – transversi A02.1.04.031 **11**
– spiralis
– – externus A15.3.03.124 **153**
– – internus A15.3.03.123 **153**
– subparietalis A14.1.09.205 **126**
– supraacetabularis A02.5.01.103 **21**
– suprapalpebralis A01.2.01.009 **3**
– tali A02.5.10.009 **24**
– temporalis
– – inferior A14.1.09.147 **125–126**
– – superior A14.1.09.145 **125**
– – transversus A14.1.09.144 **125**
– tendinis musculi
– – fibularis longi A02.5.11.013 **24**, A02.5.16.002 **24**
– – flexoris hallucis longi A02.5.10.017 **24**, A02.5.11.007 **24**
– – peronei longi A02.5.11.013 **24**, A02.5.16.002 **24**
– tendinum musculorum extensorum A02.4.05.018 **20**
– terminalis
– – cordis A12.1.01.013 **76**
– – linguae A05.1.04.019 **49**
– tubae auditivae/auditoriae A02.1.05.041 **12**
– tympanicus A02.1.06.058 **13**
– venae
– – cavae A05.8.01.009 **54**
– – subclaviae A02.3.02.017 **18**
– venosi A02.1.00.041 **8**
– vomeris A02.1.11.003 **14**
– vomerovaginalis A02.1.05.050 **12**
Supercilium/a A15.2.07.023 **147**, A16.0.00.017 **154**
Superficialis A01.0.00.033 **1**
Superior A01.0.00.017 **1**
Supinatio A03.0.00.061 **26**
Sura A01.1.00.039 **2**
Sustentaculum tali A02.5.11.006 **24**
Sutura/e A03.0.00.008 **25**
– coronalis A03.1.02.002 **26**
– cranii A03.1.02.001 **26**
– denticulata A03.0.00.013 **25**
– ethmoidolacrimalis A03.1.02.020 **26**
– ethmoidomaxillaris A03.1.02.019 **26**
– frontalis persistens A02.1.03.007 **10, 26**
– frontoethmoidalis A03.1.02.014 **26**
– frontolacrimalis A03.1.02.016 **26**
– frontomaxillaris A03.1.02.015 **26**
– frontonasalis A03.1.02.013 **26**
– frontozygomatica A03.1.02.017 **26**
– incisiva A02.1.12.032 **14**
– infraorbitalis A02.1.12.012 **14**
– intermaxillaris A03.1.02.029 **26**
– internasalis A03.1.02.025 **26**
– lacrimoconchalis A03.1.02.028 **26**
– lacrimomaxillaris A03.1.02.027 **26**
– lambdoidea A03.1.02.004 **26**
– limbosa A03.0.00.011 **25**
– metopica A02.1.03.007 **10, 26**
– nasomaxillaris A03.1.02.026 **26**
– occipitomastoidea A03.1.02.005 **26**
– palatina
– – mediana A03.1.02.032 **26**
– – transversa A03.1.02.033 **26**
– palatoethmoidalis A03.1.02.031 **26**
– palatomaxillaris A03.1.02.030 **26**
– parietomastoidea A03.1.02.011 **26**
– plana A03.0.00.009 **25**

- sagittalis A03.1.02.003 **26**
- serrata A03.0.00.012 **25**
- sphenoethmoidalis A03.1.02.007 **26**
- sphenofrontalis A03.1.02.006 **26**
- sphenomaxillaris A03.1.02.023 **26**
- sphenoparietalis A03.1.02.009 **26**
- sphenosquamosa A03.1.02.008 **26**
- sphenovomeralis A03.1.02.021 **26**
- sphenozygomatica A03.1.02.022 **26**
- squamomastoidea A03.1.02.012 **26**
- squamosa A03.0.00.010 **25**, A03.1.02.010 **26**
- temporozygomatica A03.1.02.024 **26**
- zygomaticomaxillaris A02.1.12.012 **14**, A03.1.02.018 **26**

Symphysis A03.0.00.017 **25**
- intervertebralis A03.2.02.002 **27**
- mandibulae A02.1.15.004 **15**
- manubriosternalis A03.3.02.006 **28**
- pubica A03.6.02.001 **30**
- xiphosternalis A03.3.02.005 **28**

Synapsis A14.0.00.004 **104**
Synarthrosis A03.0.00.003 **25**
Synchondrosis/es A03.0.00.016 **25**
- columnae vertebralis A03.2.02.001 **27**
- costae primae A03.3.02.003 **28**
- costosternalis A03.3.02.002 **28**
- cranii A03.1.05.001 **27**
- intraoccipitalis
- - anterior A03.1.05.007 **27**
- - posterior A03.1.05.006 **27**
- manubriosternalis A03.3.02.007 **28**
- petrooccipitalis A03.1.05.004 **27**
- sphenoethmoidalis A03.1.05.008 **27**
- sphenooccipitalis A03.1.05.002 **27**
- sphenopetrosa A03.1.05.003 **27**
- sternales A03.3.02.004 **28**
- thoracis A03.3.02.001 **28**

Syndesmosis/es A03.0.00.005 **25**
- cinguli
- - membri superioris A03.5.01.001 **28**
- - pectoralis A03.5.01.001 **28**
- - pelvici A03.6.01.001 **30**
- columnae vertebralis A03.2.01.001 **27**
- cranii A03.1.01.001 **26**
- dentoalveolaris A03.1.03.001 **26**
- radioulnaris A03.5.06.001 **29**
- thoracis A03.3.01.001 **28**
- tibiofibularis A03.6.05.001 **30**
- tympanostapedialis A15.3.02.052 **150**

Synostosis A03.0.00.019 **25**
Synovia A03.0.00.031 **25**
Systema/ta
- articulare A03.0.00.000 **25**
- cardiovasculare A12.0.00.000 **75**
- conducente cordis A12.1.06.002 **77**
- digestorium A05.0.00.000 **47**
- genitale
- - femininum A09.0.00.001 **65**
- - masculinum A09.0.00.002 **65**
- genitalia A09.0.00.000 **65**
- lymphoideum A13.0.00.000 **100**
- musculare A04.0.00.000 **33**
- nervosum A14.0.00.000 **104**
- - centrale A14.1.00.001 **104**
- - periphericum A14.2.00.001 **132**
- respiratorium A06.0.00.000 **57**
- skeletale A02.0.00.000 **7**
- urinarium A08.0.00.000 **63**

T

Taenia/e
- choroidea A14.1.09.277 **127**
- cinerea A14.1.05.712 **115**
- coli A05.7.03.013 **53**
- fornicis A14.1.09.261 **127**
- libera A05.7.03.016 **53**
- mesocolica A05.7.03.014 **53**
- omentalis A05.7.03.015 **53**
- thalami A14.1.08.105 **120–121**

Talus A02.5.10.001 **23**
Tapetum A14.1.09.252 **127**
Tarsus A01.1.00.041 **2**
- inferior A15.2.07.039 **147**
- superior A15.2.07.038 **147, 154**

Tectum mesencephali A14.1.06.601 **118**
Tegmen
- tympani A02.1.06.022 **12**
- ventriculi quarti A14.1.05.713 **115**

Tegmentum
- mesencephali A14.1.06.007 **115–116**
- pontis A14.1.05.301 **112**

Tela
- choroidea ventriculi
- - quarti A14.1.01.303 **105**, A14.1.05.716 **115**
- - tertii A14.1.01.305 **105, 121**
- subcutanea A16.0.03.001 **155**
- - abdominis A04.5.02.021 **39**
- - penis A09.4.01.027 **70**
- - perinei A09.5.00.006 **71**
- submucosa A05.3.01.028 **51**
- - bronchi A06.4.02.028 **60**
- - gastricae A05.5.01.026 **52**
- - intestini
- - - crassi A05.7.01.005 **53**
- - - tenuis A05.6.01.008 **52**
- - oesophageae A05.4.01.014 **51**
- - pharyngea A05.3.01.028 **51**
- - vesicae A08.3.01.022 **64**
- subserosa
- - gastricae A05.5.01.020 **52**
- - hepatis A05.8.01.053 **55**
- - intestini
- - - crassi A05.7.01.003 **53**
- - - tenuis A05.6.01.003 **52**
- - oesophageae A05.4.01.008 **51**
- - pericardii A12.1.08.009 **78**
- - peritonei A10.1.02.004 **72**
- - pleurae
- - - parietalis A07.1.02.011 **62**
- - - visceralis A07.1.02.004 **62**
- - testis A09.3.01.015 **67**
- - tubae uterinae A09.1.02.011 **65**
- - uteri A09.1.03.024 **66**
- - vesicae A08.3.01.009 **64**
- - - biliaris A05.8.02.007 **56**

Telencephalon A14.1.03.008 **108**, A14.1.09.001 **124**
Tempora A01.1.00.004 **2**
Tendo A04.0.00.044 **34**
- calcaneus A04.7.02.048 **43**
- conjunctivus A04.5.01.020 **38**
- cricooesophageus A05.4.01.011 **51**
- infundibuli A12.1.00.028 **76**
- intermedius A04.0.00.045 **34**
- musculi pubococcygei A04.5.04.017 **40**
- valvulae venae cavae inferioris A12.1.00.029 **76**

Tentorium cerebelli A14.1.01.104 **104**
Terminationes nervorum A16.0.00.031 **154**
Testis A09.3.01.001 **67**
Textus connectivus laxus
- abdominis A04.5.02.020 **39**
- telae subcutaneae A16.0.03.006 **155**

Thalamus A14.1.08.101 **120**, A14.1.08.601 **121**
Thenar A01.2.07.023 **5**
Thorax A01.1.00.014 **2**
Thymus A13.1.02.001 **100**
Tibia A02.5.06.001 **23**
Tibialis A01.0.00.042 **1**
Tonsilla
- cerebelli A14.1.07.222 **119**
- lingualis A05.1.04.022 **49, 100**
- palatina A05.2.01.011 **50, 100**
- pharyngea A05.3.01.006 **50, 100**
- pharyngealis A05.3.01.006 **50, 100**
- tubaria A05.3.01.016 **50, 100**

Toruli tactiles A16.0.00.007 **154**
Torus
- levatorius A05.3.01.015 **50**
- mandibularis A02.1.15.013 **15**
- palatinus A02.1.00.063 **9**
- tubarius A05.3.01.012 **50**

Trabecula/e A13.2.03.003 **100**
- arachnoideae A14.1.01.206 **105**
- carneae
- - cordis A12.1.00.020 **76**
- - ventriculi
- - - dextri A12.1.02.021 **77**
- - - sinistri A12.1.04.011 **77**
- corporis spongiosi A09.4.01.021 **69**
- corporum cavernosorum A09.4.01.020 **69**
- nodi lymphoidei A13.2.03.003 **100**
- septomarginalis A12.1.02.020 **77**

– splenicae A13.2.01.003 **100**
Trachea A06.3.01.001 **59**
Tractus A14.1.00.011 **104**
– anterolaterales A14.1.04.137 **110**, **113**, A14.1.06.215 **116**
– bulboreticulospinalis A14.1.02.221 **107**
– – lateralis A14.1.04.129 **109**
– caeruleospinalis A14.1.02.232 **107**
– corticopontinus A14.1.06.105 **116**
– corticospinalis
– – anterior A14.1.02.205 **107**
– – lateralis A14.1.02.219 **107**
– fastigiospinalis A14.1.02.217 **107**
– frontopontinus A14.1.09.528 **130**
– habenulointerpeduncularis A14.1.08.502 **121**
– hypothalamohypophysialis A14.1.08.950 **124**
– hypothalamospinalis A14.1.05.329 **113**
– iliopubicus A04.5.02.013 **39**
– iliotibialis A04.7.03.003 **43**
– interpositospinalis A14.1.02.218 **107**
– interstitiospinalis A14.1.02.210 **107**, A14.1.04.127 **109**, A14.1.05.330 **113**
– mesencephalicus nervi trigemini A14.1.05.313 **113**, A14.1.06.210 **116**
– olfactorius A14.1.09.431 **129**
– olivocerebellaris A14.1.04.118 **109**
– olivocochlearis A14.1.05.316 **113**
– opticus A14.1.08.404 **120**
– paraventriculohypophysialis A14.1.08.956 **124**
– pontoreticulospinalis A14.1.02.209 **107**
– – anterior A14.1.05.322 **113**
– posterolateralis A14.1.02.228 **107**
– pyramidalis A14.1.04.102 **109**, A14.1.06.102 **116**
– raphespinalis
– – anterior A14.1.02.212 **107**, A14.1.04.123 **109**
– – lateralis A14.1.02.234 **107**, A14.1.04.128 **109**
– reticulospinalis anterior A14.1.04.124 **109**
– retinohypothalamicus A14.1.08.960 **124**
– rubrobulbaris A14.1.04.134 **110**
– rubronuclearis A14.1.06.212 **116**
– rubroolivaris A14.1.04.135 **110**, A14.1.06.214 **116**
– rubropontinus A14.1.05.331 **113**
– rubrospinalis A14.1.02.220 **107**, A14.1.04.136 **110**, A14.1.05.332 **113**, A14.1.06.213 **116**
– solitariospinalis A14.1.02.235 **107**
– solitarius A14.1.04.120 **109**
– spinalis nervi trigemini A14.1.04.115 **109**, A14.1.05.309 **113**
– spinocerebellaris
– – anterior A14.1.02.226 **107**, A14.1.04.125 **109**, A14.1.05.323 **113**
– – posterior A14.1.02.227 **107**, A14.1.04.132 **110**
– spinocervicalis A14.1.02.236 **107**
– spinoolivaris A14.1.02.230 **107**, A14.1.04.117 **109**
– spinoreticularis A14.1.02.231 **107**
– spinotectalis A14.1.02.224 **107**
– spinothalamicus
– – anterior A14.1.02.214 **107**
– – lateralis A14.1.02.225 **107**
– spinovestibularis A14.1.02.237 **107**, A14.1.04.146 **110**
– spiralis foraminosus A15.3.03.054 **152**
– supraopticohypophysialis A14.1.08.958 **124**
– tectobulbaris A14.1.04.147 **110**, A14.1.05.333 **113**, A14.1.06.218 **116**
– – lateralis A14.1.06.206 **116**
– tectopontinus A14.1.05.334 **113**, A14.1.06.205 **116**, A14.1.06.219 **116**
– tectospinalis A14.1.02.211 **107**, A14.1.04.112 **109, 113, 116**
– tegmentalis centralis A14.1.05.325 **113, 116**
– trigeminospinalis A14.1.02.238 **107**
– trigeminothalamicus A14.1.05.310 **113**
– – anterior A14.1.05.311 **113**
– – posterior A14.1.05.312 **113**
– vestibulospinalis
– – lateralis A14.1.02.206 **107**, A14.1.04.131 **110**
– – medialis A14.1.02.207 **107**
Tragus/i A15.3.01.017 **148**, A16.0.00.019 **154**
Transversalis A01.0.00.027 **1**
Transversus A01.0.00.026 **1**
Trigonum
– auscultationis A01.2.05.006 **4**
– caroticum A01.2.02.004 **3**
– cervicale/colli
– – anterius A01.2.02.002 **3**
– – posterius A01.2.02.009 **3**
– clavipectorale A01.2.03.004 **4**
– collaterale A14.1.09.280 **127**
– cystohepaticum A10.1.02.428 **73**
– deltopectorale A01.2.03.004 **4**
– femorale A04.7.03.013 **43**
– femoris A01.2.08.008 **5**
– fibrosum
– – dextrum cordis A12.1.00.025 **76**
– – sinistrum cordis A12.1.00.026 **76**
– habenulare A14.1.08.005 **120**
– inguinale A10.1.02.433 **73**
– lemnisci lateralis A14.1.06.008 **115**
– lumbale
– – inferius A01.2.05.009 **4**
– – superius A01.2.05.010 **4**
– lumbocostale A04.4.02.016 **38**
– musculare A01.2.02.005 **3**
– nervi
– – hypoglossi A14.1.05.708 **115**
– – vagi A14.1.05.709 **115**
– nodi sinuatrialis A12.1.00.030 **76**
– olfactorium A14.1.09.432 **129**
– omoclaviculare A01.2.02.010 **3**
– omotracheale A01.2.02.005 **3**
– parietale laterale pelvis ♀ A10.1.02.509 **73**
– retromolare A02.1.15.022 **15**
– sternocostale A04.4.02.015 **38**
– submandibulare A01.2.02.003 **3**
– submentale A01.2.02.006 **3**
– vagale A14.1.05.709 **115**
– vesicae A08.3.01.024 **64**
Trochanter
– major A02.5.04.005 **22**
– minor A02.5.04.007 **22**
– tertius A02.5.04.008 **22**
Trochlea A15.2.07.017 **147**
– fibularis A02.5.11.014 **24**
– humeri A02.4.04.023 **19**
– muscularis A04.0.00.049 **34**
– musculi obliqui superioris bulbi A15.2.07.017 **147**
– peronealis A02.5.11.014 **24**
– phalangis
– – manus A02.4.10.009 **21**
– – pedis A02.5.18.009 **24**
– tali A02.5.10.011 **24**
Truncus/i A01.1.00.013 **2**
– brachiocephalicus A12.2.04.004 **79**
– bronchomediastinalis A12.4.01.005 **99**
– coeliacus A12.2.12.012 **87**
– corporis callosi A14.1.09.244 **127**
– costocervicalis A12.2.08.059 **85**
– encephali A14.1.03.009 **108**
– et ductus lymphatici A12.4.01.001 **99**
– inferior plexus brachialis A14.2.03.006 **138**
– intestinales A12.4.01.014 **99**
– jugularis A12.4.01.002 **99**
– linguofacialis A12.2.05.014 **80**
– lumbalis A12.4.01.013 **99**
– lumbosacralis A14.2.07.026 **140**
– lymphaticus
– – bronchomediastinalis A12.4.01.005 **99**
– – intestinales A12.4.01.014 **99**
– – jugularis A12.4.01.002 **99**
– – lumbalis A12.4.01.013 **99**
– – subclavius A12.4.01.003 **99**
– medius plexus brachialis A14.2.03.005 **137**
– nervi
– – accessorii A14.2.01.187 **137**
– – spinalis A14.2.00.031 **133**
– plexus brachialis A14.2.03.003 **137**

– pulmonalis A12.2.01.001 **78**
– subclavius A12.4.01.003 **99**
– superior plexus brachialis A14.2.03.004 **137**
– sympathicus A14.3.01.002 **141**
– thyrocervicalis A12.2.08.042 **85**
– vagalis
– – anterior A14.2.01.174 **136**
– – posterior A14.2.01.179 **137**
Tuba
– auditiva/auditoria A15.3.02.073 **150**
– uterina A09.1.02.001 **65**
Tuber A02.0.00.024 **7**
– calcanei A02.5.11.002 **24**
– cinereum A14.1.08.408 **120**
– frontale A02.1.03.004 **10**
– ischiadicum A02.5.01.204 **21**
– maxillae A02.1.12.016 **14**
– omentale
– – hepatis A05.8.01.017 **54**
– – pancreatis A05.9.01.013 **56**
– parietale A02.1.02.010 **9**
– vermis [VII B] A14.1.07.212 **119**
Tuberculum/a A02.0.00.025 **7**, A05.1.01.008 **47**
– adductorium femoris A02.5.04.023 **22**
– anomale dentis A05.1.03.071 **49**
– anterior calcanei A02.5.11.005 **24**
– anterius
– – atlantis A02.2.02.107 **16**
– – thalami A14.1.08.102 **120**
– – vertebrae cervicalis A02.2.02.004 **16**
– areolae A16.0.02.014 **155**
– articulare ossis temporalis A02.1.06.073 **13**
– auriculare A15.3.01.020 **148**
– calcanei A02.5.11.005 **24**
– caroticum A02.2.02.005 **16**
– conoideum A02.4.02.010 **19**
– corniculatum A06.2.05.002 **58**, A06.2.09.004 **59**
– costae A02.3.02.008 **18**
– cuneatum A14.1.04.017 **109**
– cuneiforme A06.2.06.002 **58**, A06.2.09.005 **59**
– deltoideum A02.4.01.006 **18**
– dentis A05.1.03.013 **48**
– dorsale A02.4.05.017 **20**
– epiglotticum A06.2.07.004 **58**
– gracile A14.1.04.019 **109**
– iliacum A02.5.01.108 **21**
– infraglenoidale A02.4.01.021 **19**
– intercondylare
– – laterale A02.5.06.010 **23**
– – mediale A02.5.06.009 **23**
– intervenosum A12.1.01.014 **76**
– jugulare A02.1.04.018 **10**
– labii superioris A05.1.01.008 **47**
– laterale tali A02.5.10.018 **24**
– majus A02.4.04.005 **19**
– marginale A02.1.14.008 **15**
– mediale tali A02.5.10.019 **24**
– mentale A02.1.15.006 **15**
– minus A02.4.04.006 **19**
– molare A05.1.03.073 **49**
– musculi scaleni anterioris A02.3.02.015 **18**
– obturatorium
– – anterius A02.5.01.311 **22**
– – posterius A02.5.01.312 **22**
– olfactorium A14.1.09.433 **129**
– orbitale A02.1.14.007 **15**
– ossis
– – scaphoidei A02.4.08.004 **20**
– – trapezii A02.4.08.009 **20**
– paramolare A05.1.03.072 **49**
– pharyngeum A02.1.04.007 **10**
– posterius
– – atlantis A02.2.02.111 **17**
– – vertebrae cervicalis A02.2.02.006 **16**
– pubicum A02.5.01.303 **21**
– quadratum A02.5.04.011 **22**
– sellae A02.1.05.007 **11**
– supraglenoidale A02.4.01.020 **19**
– supratragicum A15.3.01.023 **148**
– thyroideum
– – inferius A06.2.02.008 **58**
– – superius A06.2.02.007 **58**
– trigeminale A14.1.04.015 **109**
Tuberositas A02.0.00.026 **7**
– deltoidea A02.4.04.020 **19**
– glutea A02.5.04.017 **22**
– iliaca A02.5.01.122 **21**
– ligamenti coracoclavicularis A02.4.02.009 **19**
– masseterica A02.1.15.026 **15**
– musculi serrati anterioris A02.3.02.019 **18**
– ossis
– – cuboidei A02.5.16.003 **24**
– – metatarsi
– – – primi [I] A02.5.17.005 **24**
– – – quinti [V] A02.5.17.006 **24**
– – navicularis A02.5.12.002 **24**
– – sacri A02.2.05.008 **17**
– phalangis distalis
– – manus A02.4.10.005 **21**
– – pedis A02.5.18.005 **24**
– pronatoria A02.4.05.011 **20**
– pterygoidea A02.1.15.027 **15**
– radii A02.4.05.007 **20**
– tibiae A02.5.06.012 **23**
– ulnae A02.4.06.004 **20**
Tubuli seminiferi
– contorti A09.3.01.022 **68**
– recti A09.3.01.023 **68**
Tunica
– adventitia
– – ductus deferentis A09.3.05.008 **68**
– – glandulae vesiculosae A09.3.06.002 **68**
– – oesophageae A05.4.01.009 **51**
– – pelvis renalis A08.1.05.009 **64**
– – ureteris A08.2.01.005 **64**
– albuginea
– – corporis spongiosi A09.4.01.018 **69**
– – corporum cavernosorum A09.4.01.017 **69**
– – ovarii A09.1.01.009 **65**
– – testis A09.3.01.016 **67**
– conjunctiva A15.2.07.047 **147**
– – bulbi A15.2.07.050 **147**
– – palpebrarum A15.2.07.051 **147**
– dartos A09.4.03.003 **70**
– externa A12.0.00.017 **75**
– fibromusculocartilaginea bronchi A06.4.02.027 **60**
– fibrosa
– – bulbi A15.2.02.001 **144**
– – hepatis A05.8.01.054 **55**
– – splenica A13.2.01.002 **100**
– interna bulbi A15.2.04.001 **145**
– intima A12.0.00.018 **75**
– media A12.0.00.019 **75**
– mucosa
– – bronchi A06.4.02.029 **60**
– – cavitatis tympanicae A15.3.02.063 **150**
– – ductus deferentis A09.3.05.010 **68**
– – gastricae A05.5.01.027 **52**
– – glandulae vesiculosae A09.3.06.004 **68**
– – intestini
– – – crassi A05.7.01.006 **53**
– – – tenuis A05.6.01.009 **52**
– – laryngis A06.2.09.019 **59**
– – linguae A05.1.04.011 **49**
– – nasi A06.1.02.017 **57**
– – oesophageae A05.4.01.015 **51**
– – oris A05.1.01.002 **47**
– – pelvis renalis A08.1.05.011 **64**
– – pharyngea A05.3.01.029 **51**
– – tracheae A06.3.01.010 **59**
– – tubae
– – – auditivae A15.3.02.083 **151**
– – – uterinae A09.1.02.013 **65**
– – ureteris A08.2.01.007 **64**
– – urethrae A09.2.03.012 **67**
– – – intermediae A09.4.02.020 **70**
– – – prosticae A09.4.02.015 **70**
– – – spongiosa A09.4.02.029 **70**
– – uteri A09.1.03.027 **66**
– – vaginae A09.1.04.011 **66**
– – vesicae A08.3.01.023 **64**
– – – biliaris A05.8.02.009 **56**
– muscularis
– – coli A05.7.03.011 **53**
– – ductus deferentis A09.3.05.009 **68**
– – gastricae A05.5.01.021 **52**
– – glandulae vesiculosae A09.3.06.003 **68**
– – intestini
– – – crassi A05.7.01.004 **53**
– – – tenuis A05.6.01.004 **52**
– – oesophageae A05.4.01.010 **51**
– – pelvis renalis A08.1.05.010 **64**
– – pharyngis A04.2.06.001 **36, 51**
– – recti A05.7.04.009 **54**
– – tubae uterinae A09.1.02.012 **65**
– – ureteris A08.2.01.006 **64**
– – urethrae A09.2.03.007 **67**
– – – intermediae A09.4.02.018 **70**
– – – prosticae A09.4.02.011 **70**
– – – spongiosa A09.4.02.027 **70**
– – uteri A09.1.03.025 **66**
– – vaginae A09.1.04.010 **66**
– – vesicae A08.3.01.010 **64**

– – – biliaris A05.8.02.008 **56**
– serosa
– – gastricae A05.5.01.019 **52**
– – hepatis A05.8.01.052 **55**
– – intestini
– – – crassi A05.7.01.002 **53**
– – – tenuis A05.6.01.002 **52**
– – oesophageae A05.4.01.007 **51**
– – pericardii A12.1.08.008 **78**
– – peritonei A10.1.02.003 **72**
– – pleurae
– – – parietalis A07.1.02.010 **62**
– – – visceralis A07.1.02.003 **62**
– – splenica A13.2.01.018 **100**
– – testis A09.3.01.014 **67**
– – tubae uterinae A09.1.02.010 **65**
– – uteri A09.1.03.023 **66**
– – vesicae A08.3.01.008 **64**
– – – biliaris A05.8.02.006 **56**
– spongiosa
– – urethrae A09.2.03.011 **67**
– – vaginae A09.1.04.017 **66**
– vaginalis testis A09.3.01.008 **67**
– vasculosa A09.3.01.017 **67**
– – bulbi A15.2.03.001 **144**
– – testis A09.3.01.017 **67**
Typus
– ampullaris A08.1.05.008 **64**
– – pelvis renalis A08.1.05.008 **64**
– dendriticus A08.1.05.002 **64**
– – pelvis renalis A08.1.05.002 **64**

U

Ulna A02.4.06.001 **20**
Ulnaris A01.0.00.040 **1**
Umbilicus A01.2.04.005 **4**
Umbo membranae tympanicae A15.3.01.059 **149**
Uncus A14.1.09.235 **126**
– corporis vertebrae
– – cervicales A02.2.02.002 **16**
– – thoracicae primae A02.2.03.005 **17**
Unguis A16.0.01.001 **154**
Ureter A08.2.01.001 **64**
Urethra
– feminina A08.4.01.001 **64, 67**
– masculina A08.5.01.001 **64, 70**
Uterus A09.1.03.001 **65**
Utriculus
– prostaticus A09.4.02.009 **70**
– – vestibularis A15.3.03.063 **152**
Uvula
– palatina A05.2.01.004 **50**
– vermis [IX] A14.1.07.221 **119**
– vesicae A08.3.01.006 **64**

V

Vagina/e A09.1.04.001 **66**
– bulbi A15.2.07.004 **147**
– carotica A04.2.05.007 **36**
– communis tendinum musculorum
– – fibularium A04.8.06.011 **46**
– – flexorum manus A04.8.04.007 **44**
– – peroneorum A04.8.06.011 **46**
– externa n. optici A15.2.04.032 **145**
– fibrosa A04.8.01.006 **44**
– fibrosae digitorum
– – manus A04.8.04.015 **45**
– – pedis A04.8.06.014 **46**
– interna n. optici A15.2.04.033 **146**
– musculi recti abdominis A04.5.01.003 **38**
– plantaris tendinis musculi
– – fibularis longi A04.8.06.012 **46**
– – peronei longi A04.8.06.012 **46**
– processus styloidei A02.1.06.060 **13**
– synoviales digitorum
– – manus A04.8.04.018 **45**
– – pedis A04.8.06.017 **46**
– synovialis A03.0.00.040 **25, 34,** A04.8.01.007 **44**
– tendinis/ium A04.8.01.005 **44**
– – carpales A04.8.04.003 **44**
– – – dorsales A04.8.04.008 **44**
– – – palmares A04.8.04.004 **44**
– – digitorum pedis A04.8.06.013 **46**
– – et bursae A04.8.00.001 **44**
– – membri
– – – inferioris A04.8.06.001 **45**
– – – superioris A04.8.04.001 **44**
– – intertubercularis A04.8.04.002 **44**
– – musculi/orum
– – – abductoris longi et extensoris pollicis brevis A04.8.04.009 **44**
– – – extensoris/orum
– – – – carpi
– – – – – radialium A04.8.04.010 **44**
– – – – – ulnaris A04.8.04.014 **45**
– – – – digiti minimi brevis A04.8.04.013 **45**
– – – – digitorum
– – – – – et extensoris indicis A04.8.04.012 **44**
– – – – – longi A04.8.06.005 **45**
– – – – hallucis longi A04.8.06.004 **45**
– – – – pollicis longi A04.8.04.011 **44**
– – – flexoris
– – – – carpi radialis A04.8.04.006 **44**
– – – – digitorum longi A04.8.06.007 **45**
– – – – hallucis longi A04.8.06.009 **46**
– – – – pollicis longi A04.8.04.005 **44**
– – – obliqui superioris bulbi A15.2.07.018 **147**
– – – tibialis
– – – – anterioris A04.8.06.003 **45**
– – – – posterioris A04.8.06.008 **45**
– – tarsales
– – – anteriores A04.8.06.002 **45**
– – – fibulares A04.8.06.010 **46**
– – – tibiales A04.8.06.006 **45**
Vallecula
– cerebelli A14.1.07.005 **118**
– epiglottica A05.3.01.020 **50**
Vallum unguis A16.0.01.003 **154**
Valva A12.0.00.020 **75**
– aortae A12.1.04.012 **77**
– atrioventricularis
– – dextra A12.1.02.003 **76**
– – sinistra A12.1.04.003 **77**
– mitralis A12.1.04.003 **77**
– tricuspidalis A12.1.02.003 **76**
– trunci pulmonalis A12.1.02.010 **76**
Valvula/e A12.0.00.021 **75**
– anales A05.7.05.005 **54**
– coronaria
– – dextrae valvae aortae A12.1.04.013 **77**
– – sinistra valvae aortae A12.1.04.014 **77**
– foraminis ovalis A12.1.03.005 **77**
– fossae navicularis A09.4.02.023 **70**
– lymphatica A12.0.00.042 **75**
– non coronaria valvae aortae A12.1.04.015 **77**
– semilunaris
– – anterior valvae trunci pulmonalis A12.1.02.013 **77**
– – dextrae valvae
– – – aortae A12.1.04.013 **77**
– – – trunci pulmonalis A12.1.02.011 **77**
– – posterior valvae aortae A12.1.04.015 **77**
– – sinistra valvae
– – – aortae A12.1.04.014 **77**
– – – trunci pulmonalis A12.1.02.012 **77**
– sinus coronarii A12.1.01.016 **76**
– venae cavae inferioris A12.1.01.015 **76**
– venosa A12.0.00.023 **75**
Vas/a
– anastomoticum A12.0.00.024 **75**
– capillare A12.0.00.025 **75**
– collaterale A12.0.00.026 **75**
– lymphaticum A12.0.00.038 **75**
– – profundum A12.0.00.040 **75**
– – superficiale A12.0.00.039 **75**
– lymphocapillare A12.0.00.044 **75**
– nervorum A12.0.00.029 **75**
– prominens ductus cochlearis A15.3.03.098 **152**
– recta renis A08.1.03.008 **63**
– sanguinea
– – auris internae A15.3.03.126 **153**
– – choroideae A15.2.03.008 **144**
– – intrapulmonalia A06.5.01.023 **60**
– – retinae A15.2.04.035 **146**
– sanguineum A12.0.00.001 **75**
– sinusoideum A12.0.00.027 **75**
– spirale A15.3.03.103 **152**
– vasorum A12.0.00.028 **75**
Velum

- medullare
- - inferius A14.1.05.721 **115**
- - superius A14.1.05.007 **112**, A14.1.05.719 **115**
- palatinum A05.1.01.104 **47**, A05.2.01.003 **50**
Vena/e A12.0.00.030 **75**, A12.3.00.001 **91**
- anastomotica
- - inferior A12.3.06.010 **94**
- - superior A12.3.06.012 **94**
- angularis A12.3.05.019 **93**
- anterior
- - lobi superioris pulmonis
- - - dextri A12.3.02.105 **91**
- - - sinistri A12.3.02.305 **92**
- - septi pellucidi A12.3.06.031 **94**
- anteriores cerebri A12.3.06.019 **94**
- apicalis lobi superioris pulmonis dextri A12.3.02.102 **91**
- apicoposterior lobi superioris pulmonis sinistri A12.3.02.302 **92**
- appendicularis A12.3.12.025 **99**
- aqueductus
- - cochleae A12.3.05.004 **93**, A15.3.03.136 **153**
- - vestibuli A15.3.03.134 **153**
- arcuatae renis A08.1.04.003 **63**
- articulares A12.3.05.042 **93**
- atriales
- - dextrae A12.3.01.014 **91**
- - sinistrae A12.3.01.016 **91**
- auricularis/es
- - anteriores A12.3.05.040 **93**
- - posterior A12.3.05.046 **93**
- axillaris A12.3.08.005 **96**
- azygos A12.3.07.001 **95**
- basalis A12.3.06.018 **94**
- - anterior lobi inferioris pulmonis
- - - dextri A12.3.02.207 **92**
- - - sinistri A12.3.02.407 **92**
- - communis lobi inferioris pulmonis
- - - dextri A12.3.02.205 **92**
- - - sinistri A12.3.02.405 **92**
- - inferior lobi inferioris pulmonis
- - - dextri A12.3.02.210 **92**
- - - sinistri A12.3.02.410 **92**
- - superior lobi inferioris pulmonis
- - - dextri A12.3.02.206 **92**
- - - sinistri A12.3.02.406 **92**
- basilica A12.3.08.018 **96**
- - antebrachii A12.3.08.022 **96**
- basivertebrales A12.3.07.022 **96**
- brachiales A12.3.08.029 **96**
- brachiocephalica A12.3.04.001 **92**
- bronchiales A12.3.04.009 **92**, A12.3.07.007 **95**
- bulbi
- - penis ♂ A12.3.10.023 **97**
- - vestibuli ♀ A12.3.10.023 **97**
- canalis pterygoidei A12.3.05.039 **93**
- capsulares A12.3.09.010 **97**
- cardiaca
- - magna A12.3.01.003 **91**
- - media A12.3.01.009 **91**
- - parva A12.3.01.010 **91**
- cardiacae
- - anteriores A12.3.01.012 **91**
- - minimae A12.3.01.013 **91**
- cava
- - inferior A12.3.09.001 **96**
- - superior A12.3.03.001 **92**
- cavernosae A09.4.01.025 **69**
- - penis A09.4.01.025 **69**
- centralis/es
- - glandulae suprarenalis A11.5.00.010 **74**
- - hepatis A05.8.01.059 **55**
- - retinae A12.3.06.111 **95**
- - retinae, pars intraocularis A12.3.06.113 **95, 146**
- cephalica A12.3.08.015 **96**
- - accessoria A12.3.08.017 **96**
- - antebrachii A12.3.08.021 **96**
- cerebelli A12.3.06.056 **95**
- cervicalis profunda A12.3.04.017 **92**
- choroidea
- - inferior A12.3.06.025 **94**
- - superior A12.3.06.029 **94**
- ciliares A12.3.06.107 **95**
- - anteriores A12.3.06.108 **95**
- circumflexa/e
- - femoris
- - - laterales A12.3.11.026 **98**
- - - mediales A12.3.11.025 **98**
- - humeri
- - - anterior A12.3.08.010 **96**
- - - posterior A12.3.08.009 **96**
- - ilium
- - - profunda A12.3.10.027 **97**
- - - superficialis A12.3.11.005 **98**
- - scapulae A12.3.08.007 **96**
- cisternae cerebellomedullaris A12.3.06.055 **95**
- colica
- - dextra A12.3.12.026 **99**
- - media A12.3.12.027 **99**
- - sinistra A12.3.12.033 **99**
- colli profunda A12.3.04.017 **92**
- columnae vertebralis A12.3.07.018 **96**
- comitans A12.0.00.031 **75**
- - nervi hypoglossi A12.3.05.011 **93**
- conjunctivales A12.3.06.116 **95**
- cordis A12.3.01.001 **91**
- - anteriores A12.3.01.012 **91**
- - magna A12.3.01.003 **91**
- - media A12.3.01.009 **91**
- - minimae A12.3.01.013 **91**
- - parva A12.3.01.010 **91**
- corticales radiatae renis A08.1.04.004 **63**
- cutanea A12.0.00.032 **75**
- cystica A12.3.12.012 **98**
- digitales
- - dorsales pedis A12.3.11.014 **98**
- - palmares A12.3.08.027 **96**
- - plantares A12.3.11.018 **98**
- diploica/e A12.3.05.201 **94**
- - frontalis A12.3.05.202 **94**
- - occipitalis A12.3.05.205 **94**
- - temporalis
- - - anterior A12.3.05.203 **94**
- - - posterior A12.3.05.204 **94**
- directae laterales A12.3.06.036 **95**
- - ventriculi lateralis A12.3.06.036 **95**
- dorsalis/es
- - corporis callosi A12.3.06.037 **95**
- - linguae A12.3.05.010 **93**
- - profunda
- - - clitoridis ♀ A12.3.10.014 **97**
- - - penis ♂ A12.3.10.014 **97**
- - superficiales
- - - clitoridis ♀ A12.3.11.008 **98**
- - - penis ♂ A12.3.11.008 **98**
- - v. intercostalis posterioris A12.3.07.015 **96**
- ductuum semicircularium A15.3.03.135 **153**
- emissaria/e A12.0.00.033 **75**, A12.3.06.001 **94**
- - condylaris A12.3.05.304 **94**
- - mastoidea A12.3.05.303 **94**
- - occipitalis A12.3.05.305 **94**
- - parietalis A12.3.05.302 **94**
- encephali
- epigastrica/e
- - inferior A12.3.10.025 **97**
- - superficialis A12.3.11.006 **98**
- - superiores A12.3.04.019 **92**
- episclerales A12.3.06.114 **95**
- ethmoidales A12.3.06.104 **95**
- facialis A12.3.05.018 **93**
- femoralis A12.3.11.023 **98**
- fenestrae cochleae A15.3.03.143 **153**
- fibulares A12.3.11.033 **98**
- frontales A12.3.06.005 **94**
- gastrica/e
- - breves A12.3.12.030 **99**
- - dextra A12.3.12.016 **98**
- - sinistra A12.3.12.015 **98**
- gastroepiploica
- - dextra A12.3.12.021 **99**
- - sinistra A12.3.12.031 **99**
- gastroomentalis
- - dextra A12.3.12.021 **99**
- - sinistra A12.3.12.031 **99**
- geniculares A12.3.11.030 **98**
- gluteae
- - inferiores A12.3.10.006 **97**
- - superiores A12.3.10.005 **97**
- gyri olfactorii A12.3.06.023 **94**
- hemiazygos A12.3.07.004 **95**
- - accessoria A12.3.07.005 **95**
- hepatica/e A12.3.09.005 **97**
- - dextra A12.3.09.006 **97**
- - intermedia A12.3.09.007 **97**
- - sinistra A12.3.09.008 **97**
- ileales A12.3.12.020 **99**
- ileocolica A12.3.12.024 **99**
- iliaca
- - communis A12.3.10.001 **97**
- - externa A12.3.10.024 **97**
- - interna A12.3.10.004 **97**
- iliolumbalis A12.3.10.003 **97**
- inferior vermis A12.3.06.058 **95**

– inferiores
– – cerebelli A12.3.06.060 **95**
– – cerebri A12.3.06.013 **94**
– insulares A12.3.06.021 **94**
– intercapitulares
– – manus A12.3.08.024 **96**
– – pedis A12.3.11.019 **98**
– intercollicularis A12.3.06.041 **95**
– intercostalis/es
– – anteriores A12.3.04.022 **92**
– – posteriores A12.3.07.014 **96**
– – superior
– – – dextra A12.3.07.003 **95**
– – – sinistra A12.3.04.024 **92**
– – suprema A12.3.04.023 **92**
– interlobares renis A08.1.04.002 **63**
– interlobulares
– – hepatis A05.8.01.058 **55**
– – renis A08.1.04.004 **63**
– internae cerebri A12.3.06.028 **94**
– interosseae
– – anteriores A12.3.08.032 **96**
– – posteriores A12.3.08.033 **96**
– interpedunculares A12.3.06.040 **95**
– interventricularis
– – anterior A12.3.01.004 **91**
– – posterior A12.3.01.009 **91**
– intervertebralis A12.3.07.016 **96**
– intrarenales A08.1.04.001 **63, 97**
– jejunales A12.3.12.019 **98**
– jugularis
– – anterior A12.3.05.047 **93**
– – externa A12.3.05.045 **93**
– – interna A12.3.05.001 **93**
– labialis/es
– – anteriores ♀ A12.3.11.009 **98**
– – inferiores ♀ A12.3.05.026 **93**
– – posteriores ♀ A12.3.10.022 **97**
– – superior A12.3.05.025 **93**
– labyrinthi A12.3.05.114 **94, 153**
– lacrimalis A12.3.06.105 **95**
– laryngea
– – inferior A12.3.04.004 **92**
– – superior A12.3.05.017 **93**
– lateralis ventriculi lateralis A12.3.06.034 **94**
– lienalis A12.3.12.028 **99**
– lingualis A12.3.05.009 **93**
– lingularis A12.3.02.308 **92**
– lobi medii pulmonis dextri A12.3.02.111 **91**
– lumbales A12.3.07.012 **96**, A12.3.09.003 **96**
– lumbalis ascendens A12.3.07.011 **96**, A12.3.09.004 **97**
– magna cerebri A12.3.06.027 **94**
– marginalis
– – dextra A12.3.01.011 **91**
– – lateralis A12.3.11.020 **98**
– – – pedis A12.3.11.020 **98**
– – medialis A12.3.11.021 **98**
– – – pedis A12.3.11.021 **98**
– – sinistra A12.3.01.005 **91**
– maxillares A12.3.05.035 **93**
– media
– – profunda cerebri A12.3.06.020 **94**
– – superficialis cerebri A12.3.06.009 **94**
– medialis ventriculi lateralis A12.3.06.033 **94**
– mediana
– – antebrachii A12.3.08.020 **96**
– – cubiti A12.3.08.019 **96**
– mediastinales A12.3.04.008 **92**, A12.3.07.009 **95**
– medullae
– – oblongatae A12.3.06.048 **95**
– – spinalis A12.3.07.023 **96**
– medullaris/es
– – anterolateralis A12.3.06.050 **95**
– – dorsales A12.3.06.052 **95**
– – anteromediana A12.3.06.049 **95**
– – posteromediana A12.3.06.053 **95**
– – transversae A12.3.06.051 **95**
– membri
– – inferioris A12.3.11.001 **98**
– – superioris A12.3.08.001 **96**
– meningeae A12.3.05.008 **93**
– – mediae A12.3.05.037 **93**
– mesencephalica lateralis A12.3.06.042 **95**
– mesenterica
– – inferior A12.3.12.032 **99**
– – superior A12.3.12.018 **98**
– metacarpales
– – dorsales A12.3.08.025 **96**
– – palmares A12.3.08.035 **96**
– metatarsales
– – dorsales A12.3.11.013 **98**
– – plantares A12.3.11.017 **98**
– modioli communis A15.3.03.137 **153**
– musculophrenicae A12.3.04.021 **92**
– nasales externae A12.3.05.023 **93**
– nasofrontalis A12.3.06.103 **95**
– nuclei caudati A12.3.06.035 **95**
– nutricia/ens A12.0.00.034 **75**
– obliqua atrii sinistri A12.3.01.007 **91**
– obturatoriae A12.3.10.007 **97**
– occipitalis/es A12.3.04.013 **92**, A12.3.06.008 **94**
– oesophageales A12.3.04.011 **92**, A12.3.07.006 **95**
– ophthalmica
– – inferior A12.3.06.117 **95**
– – superior A12.3.06.102 **95**
– orbitae A12.3.06.015 **94**, A12.3.06.101 **95**
– ovarica
– – dextra ♀ A12.3.09.014 **97**
– – sinistra ♀ A12.3.09.012 **97**
– palatina externa A12.3.05.029 **93**
– palpebrales A12.3.06.115 **95**
– – inferiores A12.3.05.024 **93**
– – superiores A12.3.05.022 **93**
– pancreaticae A12.3.12.022 **99**, A12.3.12.029 **99**
– pancreaticoduodenalis/es A12.3.12.023 **99**
– – superior posterior A12.3.12.014 **98**
– paraumbilicales A12.3.12.013 **98**
– parietales A12.3.06.006 **94**
– parotideae A12.3.05.028 **93**, A12.3.05.041 **93**
– pectorales A12.3.08.003 **96**
– pedunculares A12.3.06.026 **94**
– perforantes A12.3.11.027 **98**
– pericardiacae A12.3.04.006 **92**, A12.3.07.008 **95**
– pericardiacophrenicae A12.3.04.007 **92**
– peroneae A12.3.11.033 **98**
– petrosa A12.3.06.062 **95**
– pharyngeae A12.3.05.007 **93**
– phrenicae
– – inferiores A12.3.09.002 **96**
– – superiores A12.3.07.010 **96**
– pontis A12.3.06.043 **95**
– – anterolateralis A12.3.06.045 **95**
– – anteromediana A12.3.06.044 **95**
– – lateralis A12.3.06.047 **95**
– – transversae A12.3.06.046 **95**
– pontomesencephalica A12.3.06.039 **95**
– poplitea A12.3.11.028 **98**
– portae hepatis A12.3.12.001 **98**
– portales hypophysiales A12.3.05.309 **94**
– posterior
– – corporis callosi A12.3.06.037 **95**
– – lobi superioris pulmonis dextri A12.3.02.108 **91**
– – septi pellucidi A12.3.06.032 **94**
– precentralis cerebelli A12.3.06.061 **95**
– prefrontales A12.3.06.004 **94**
– prepylorica A12.3.12.017 **98**
– profunda/e A12.0.00.035 **75**
– – cerebri A12.3.06.017 **94**
– – clitoridis ♀ A12.3.10.020 **97**
– – faciei A12.3.05.027 **93**
– – femoris A12.3.11.024 **98**
– – linguae A12.3.05.013 **93**
– – membri
– – – inferioris A12.3.11.022 **98**
– – – superioris A12.3.08.028 **96**
– – penis ♂ A12.3.10.020 **97**
– pubica A12.3.10.026 **97**
– pudenda/e
– – externae A12.3.11.004 **98**
– – interna A12.3.10.019 **97**
– pulmonalis/es A12.3.02.001 **91**
– – dextra
– – – inferior A12.3.02.201 **92**
– – – superior A12.3.02.101 **91**
– – sinistra
– – – inferior A12.3.02.401 **92**
– – – superior A12.3.02.301 **92**
– radiales A12.3.08.031 **96**

- recessus lateralis ventriculi quarti A12.3.06.054 **95**
- rectalis/es
- - inferiores A12.3.10.021 **97**
- - mediae A12.3.10.018 **97**
- - superior A12.3.12.035 **99**
- renales A12.3.09.009 **97**
- retromandibularis A12.3.05.031 **93**
- sacralis/es
- - laterales A12.3.10.008 **97**
- - mediana A12.3.10.002 **97**
- saphena
- - accessoria A12.3.11.007 **98**
- - magna A12.3.11.003 **98**
- - parva A12.3.11.010 **98**
- scalae
- - tympani A15.3.03.139 **153**
- - vestibuli A15.3.03.138 **153**
- scapularis dorsalis A12.3.08.004 **96**
- sclerales A12.3.06.110 **95**
- scrotales
- - anteriores ♂ A12.3.11.009 **98**
- - posteriores ♂ A12.3.10.022 **97**
- sigmoideae A12.3.12.034 **99**
- spinalis/es A12.3.07.017 **96**
- - anteriores A12.3.07.024 **96**
- - posteriores A12.3.07.025 **96**
- splenica A12.3.12.028 **99**
- stellatae renis A08.1.04.006 **63**
- sternocleidomastoidea A12.3.05.016 **93**
- stylomastoidea A12.3.05.044 **93**
- subclavia A12.3.08.002 **96**
- subcostalis A12.3.07.013 **96**
- subcutaneae abdominis A12.3.04.020 **92**
- sublingualis A12.3.05.012 **93**
- submentalis A12.3.05.030 **93**
- subscapularis A12.3.08.006 **96**
- superficialis/es A12.0.00.036 **75**
- - cerebri A12.3.06.002 **94**
- - membri
- - - inferioris A12.3.11.002 **98**
- - - superioris A12.3.08.014 **96**
- superior
- - cerebelli A12.3.06.059 **95**
- - cerebri A12.3.06.003 **94**
- - lobi inferioris pulmonis
- - - dextri A12.3.02.202 **92**
- - - sinistri A12.3.02.402 **92**
- - vermis A12.3.06.057 **95**
- supraorbitalis A12.3.05.021 **93**
- suprarenalis
- - dextra A12.3.09.013 **97**
- - sinistra A12.3.09.011 **97**
- suprascapularis A12.3.05.049 **93**
- supratrochleares A12.3.05.020 **93**
- surales A12.3.11.029 **98**
- temporalis/es
- - media A12.3.05.033 **93**
- - profundae A12.3.05.038 **93**
- - superficiales A12.3.05.032 **93**
- - v. inferioris cerebri A12.3.06.016 **94**
- - v. superioris cerebri A12.3.06.007 **94**
- terminalis A12.3.06.030 **94**
- testicularis
- - dextra ♂ A12.3.09.014 **97**
- - sinistra ♂ A12.3.09.012 **97**
- thalamostriata/e
- - inferiores A12.3.06.022 **94**
- - superior A12.3.06.030 **94**
- thoracica/e
- - internae A12.3.04.018 **92**
- - lateralis A12.3.08.011 **96**
- thoracoacromialis A12.3.08.016 **96**
- thoracodorsalis A12.3.08.008 **96**
- thoracoepigastricae A12.3.08.012 **96**
- thymicae A12.3.04.005 **92**
- thyroidea/e
- - inferior A12.3.04.002 **92**
- - mediae A12.3.05.015 **93**
- - superior A12.3.05.014 **93**
- tibiales
- - anteriores A12.3.11.031 **98**
- - posteriores A12.3.11.032 **98**
- tracheales A12.3.04.010 **92**
- transversa/e
- - cervicis A12.3.05.050 **93**
- - colli A12.3.05.050 **93**
- - faciei A12.3.05.034 **93**
- trunci encephali A12.3.06.038 **95**
- tympanicae A12.3.05.043 **93**
- ulnares A12.3.08.030 **96**
- umbilicalis A12.3.12.010 **98**
- uncalis A12.3.06.014 **94**
- uterinae ♀ A12.3.10.015 **97**
- ventriculi/aris/es
- - dextri/ae A12.3.01.015 **91**
- - - anteriores A12.3.01.012 **91**
- - inferior A12.3.06.024 **94**
- - sinistri/ae A12.3.01.017 **91**
- - - posteriores A12.3.01.006 **91**
- vertebralis A12.3.04.012 **92**
- - accessoria A12.3.04.015 **92**
- - anterior A12.3.04.014 **92**
- vesicales A12.3.10.011 **97**
- vestibularis
- - anterior A15.3.03.141 **153**
- - posterior A15.3.03.142 **153**
- vestibulocochlearis A15.3.03.140 **153**
- vorticosae A12.3.06.106 **95**

Venter A04.0.00.002 **33**
- anterior m. digastrici A04.2.03.003 **35**
- frontalis m. occipitofrontalis A04.1.03.004 **34**
- inferior m. omohyordeus A04.2.04.005 **35**
- occipitalis m. occipitofrontalis A04.1.03.005 **34**
- posterior m. digastrici A04.2.03.004 **35**
- superficialis m. omohyoidei inferior A04.2.04.005 **35**
- superior m. omohyoidei A04.2.04.004 **35**

Ventralis A01.0.00.013 **1**

Ventriculus
- cordis dexter/sinister A12.1.00.012 **76**
- dexter A12.1.02.001 **76**
- laryngis A06.2.09.010 **59**
- lateralis A14.1.09.272 **127**
- quartus A14.1.05.701 **115**
- sinister A12.1.04.001 **77**
- terminalis A14.1.02.006 **105**
- tertius A14.1.08.410 **120**

Venula/e A12.0.00.037 **75**
- macularis
- - inferior A15.2.04.049 **146**
- - media A15.2.04.050 **146**
- - superior A15.2.04.048 **146**
- nasalis retinae
- - inferior A15.2.04.047 **146**
- - superior A15.2.04.046 **146**
- rectae renis A08.1.04.005 **63**
- temporalis retinae
- - inferior A15.2.04.045 **146**
- - superior A15.2.04.044 **146**

Vermis cerebelli [I–X] A14.1.07.006 **118**

Vertebra/e A02.2.01.001 **16**
- cervicales [C I – C VII] A02.2.02.001 **16**
- lumbales [L I – L V] A02.2.04.001 **17**
- prominens [C VII] A02.2.02.301 **17**
- thoracicae [T I – T XII] A02.2.03.001 **17, 18**

Vertex A02.1.00.033 **8**
- corneae A15.2.02.015 **144**

Verticalis A01.0.00.001 **1**

Vesica
- biliaris/fellea A05.8.02.001 **56**
- urinaria A08.3.01.001 **64**

Vesicula seminalis A09.3.06.001 **68**

Vestibulocerebellum A14.1.07.007 **118**

Vestibulum
- aortae A12.1.04.009 **77**
- bursae omentalis A10.1.02.404 **72**
- labyrinthi A15.3.03.004 **151**
- laryngis A06.2.09.007 **59**
- nasi A06.1.02.009 **57**
- oris A05.1.01.003 **47**
- vaginae A09.2.01.012 **66**

Vestigium processus vaginalis A09.3.04.006 **68**

Vibrissae A16.0.00.020 **154**

Villi
- intestinales intestini tenuis A05.6.01.011 **52**
- synoviales A03.0.00.030 **25**

Vinculum/a
- breve digitorum manus A04.8.04.021 **45**
- longum digitorum manus A04.8.04.020 **45**
- tendinum digitorum
- - manus A04.8.04.019 **45**
- - pedis A04.8.06.018 **46**

Viscerocranium A02.1.00.008 **8**

Vola/aris A01.0.00.043 **1**, A01.1.00.028 **2**, A01.2.07.022 **5**

Vomer A02.1.11.001 **14**
Vortex/ices
- cordis A12.1.00.021 **76**
- pilorum A16.0.00.026 **154**
Vulva A09.2.01.001 **66**

Z

Zona/e
- externa medullae renalis A08.1.01.021 **63**
- glandularum periurethralium prostatae A09.3.08.004 **68**
- hypothalamicae A14.1.08.941 **124**
- incerta A14.1.08.707 **123**
- interna medullae renalis A08.1.01.026 **63**
- lateralis hypothalamicae A14.1.08.944 **124**
- medialis hypothalamicae A14.1.08.943 **124**
- orbicularis articulationis coxae A03.6.07.002 **30**
- periventricularis hypothalamicae A14.1.08.942 **124**
- transitionalis analis A05.7.05.007 **54**

Index of English Terms

Cecum *see* Caecum
Cecal *see* Caecal
Celiac *see* Coeliac
Esophageal *see* Oesophageal
Esophagus *see* Oesophagus
Gray *see* Grey

A

A1 segment of anterior cerebral artery A12.2.07.023 **82**
A2 segment of anterior cerebral artery A12.2.07.033 **83**
Abdomen A01.1.00.016 **2**
Abdominal
- aorta A12.2.12.001 **87**
- aortic nerve plexus A14.3.03.019 **143**
- cavity A01.1.00.051 **2**, A10.1.00.001 **72**
- extraperitoneal
- - fascia A04.5.02.004 **38**
- - ligament A04.5.02.005 **38**
- fascia A04.5.02.001 **38**
- lymph nodes A13.3.03.001 **102**
- ostium of uterine tube A09.1.02.002 **65**
- part
- - of oesophagus A05.4.01.006 **51**
- - of pectoralis major A04.4.01.005 **37**
- - of peripheral autonomic plexuses and ganglia A14.3.03.018 **143**
- - of thoracic duct A12.4.01.011 **99**
- - of ureter A08.2.01.002 **64**
- regions A01.2.04.001 **4**
Abdominopelvic cavity A01.1.00.050 **2**, A10.1.00.000 **72**
Abducens/t nerve [VI] A14.2.01.098 **135**
Abduction A03.0.00.053 **25**
Abductor
- digiti minimi
- - of hand A04.6.02.062 **41**
- - of foot A04.7.02.063 **43**
- hallucis A04.7.02.056 **43**
- muscle A04.0.00.020 **33**
- of fifth metatarsal A04.7.02.064 **43**
- pollicis
- - brevis A04.6.02.054 **41**
- - longus A04.6.02.049 **41**
Aberrant ductules of epididymis A09.3.02.007 **68**
Accessory
- branch of middle meningeal artery A12.2.05.062 **80**
- breast A16.0.02.003 **154**
- cephalic vein A12.3.08.017 **96**
- cuneate nucleus A14.1.04.209 **110**
- cusp of tooth A05.1.03.012 **48**
- hemi-azygos vein A12.3.07.005 **95**
- lacrimal glands A15.2.07.061 **148**
- lymph nodes A13.3.00.037 **101**
- medullary lamina of corpus striatum A14.1.09.513 **130**
- nasal cartilages A06.1.01.012 **57**
- nerve [XI] A14.2.01.184 **137**
- nuclei
- - of oculomotor nerve A14.1.06.303 **117**
- - of optic tract A14.1.06.314 **117**
- obturator
- - artery A12.2.16.006 **90**
- - nerve A14.2.07.019 **140**
- pancreas A05.9.01.018 **56**
- pancreatic duct A05.9.01.017 **56**
- parathyroid glands A11.4.00.004 **74**
- parotid gland A05.1.02.006 **47**
- phrenic nerves A14.2.02.031 **137**
- process of lumbar vertebra A02.2.04.002 **17**
- root of tooth A05.1.03.070 **49**
- saphenous vein A12.3.11.007 **98**
- spleen A13.2.01.022 **100**
- suprarenal glands A11.5.00.011 **74**
- thymic lobules A13.1.02.006 **100**
- thyroid glands A11.3.00.005 **74**
- vertebral vein A12.3.04.015 **92**
- visual structures A15.2.07.001 **147**
Acetabular
- branch
- - of medial circumflex femoral artery A12.2.16.024 **90**
- - of obturator artery A12.2.15.010 **89**
- fossa A02.5.01.004 **21**
- labrum A03.6.07.008 **30**
- margin A02.5.01.003 **21**
- notch A02.5.01.005 **21**
Acetabulum A02.5.01.002 **21**
Acoustic
- radiation A14.1.08.662 **122**, A14.1.09.545 **131**
- teeth A15.3.03.107 **153**
Acromial
- anastomosis of thoraco-acromial artery A12.2.09.007 **85**
- angle A02.4.01.011 **18**
- branch A12.2.08.052 **85**, A12.2.09.006 **85**
- - of suprascapular artery A12.2.08.052 **85**
- - of thoraco-acromial artery A12.2.09.006 **85**
- end of clavicle A02.4.02.007 **19**
- facet of clavicle A02.4.02.008 **19**
- part of deltoid A04.6.02.004 **40**
Acromioclavicular
- joint A03.5.03.001 **28**
- ligament A03.5.03.002 **28**
Acromion A02.4.01.009 **18**
Adduction A03.0.00.054 **25**
Adductor
- brevis A04.7.02.027 **42**
- canal A04.7.03.006 **43**
- compartment of thigh A04.7.01.004 **42**
- hallucis A04.7.02.060 **43**
- hiatus A04.7.03.008 **43**
- longus A04.7.02.026 **42**
- magnus A04.7.02.028 **42**
- minimus A04.7.02.029 **42**
- muscle A04.0.00.021 **33**
- pollicis A04.6.02.059 **41**
- tubercle of femur A02.5.04.023 **22**
Adenohypophysis A11.1.00.002 **74**
Aditus to mastoid antrum A15.3.02.021 **149**
Adrenal gland A11.5.00.001 **74**
Adrenergic cells in area postrema and anterior reticular nucleus A14.1.09.628 **132**
Adventitia
- of ductus deferens A09.3.05.008 **68**
- of oesophagus A05.4.01.009 **51**
- of renal pelvis A08.1.05.009 **64**
- of seminal gland A09.3.06.002 **68**
- of ureter A08.2.01.005 **64**
Afferent
- glomerular arteriole of kidney A08.1.03.005 **63**
- nerve fibres A14.2.00.017 **132**
Agger nasi A06.1.02.021 **57**
Aggregated lymphoid nodules
- of small intestine A05.6.01.014 **52, 101**
- of vermiform appendix A05.7.02.009 **53, 101**
Ala
- of crista galli A02.1.07.005 **13**
- of ilium A02.5.01.104 **21**
- of nose A06.1.01.005 **57**
- of sacrum A02.2.05.004 **17**
- of vomer A02.1.11.002 **14**
Alar
- folds of infrapatellar synovial fold A03.6.08.010 **30**
- ligaments A03.2.04.002 **27**
- part of nasalis A04.1.03.011 **34**
Alimentary system A05.0.00.000 **47**
Allocortex A14.1.09.305 **128**

Alveolar
– arch
– – of mandible A02.1.15.017 **15**
– – of maxilla A02.1.12.036 **14**
– canals of maxilla A02.1.12.015 **14**
– foramina of maxilla A02.1.12.014 **14**
– part of mandible A02.1.15.016 **15**
– process of maxilla A02.1.12.035 **14**
– yokes
– – of mandible A02.1.15.021 **15**
– – of maxilla A02.1.12.040 **14**
Alveus of hippocampus A14.1.09.333 **128**
Ambient cistern A14.1.01.213 **105**
Amiculum of olive A14.1.04.116 **109**
Aminergic cells A14.1.09.602 **131**
– in compact part of substantia nigra [A9] A14.1.09.610 **131**
– in reticular formation A14.1.09.607 **131**
– in ventral tegmental area [A10] A14.1.09.613 **131**
Ammon's horn A14.1.09.327 **128**
Amphiarthrosis A03.0.00.052 **25**
Ampulla
– of ductus deferens A09.3.05.006 **68**
– of duodenum A05.6.02.003 **52**
– of lacrimal canaliculus A15.2.07.067 **148**
– of uterine tube A09.1.02.006 **65**
Ampullary
– bony limbs A15.3.03.021 **151**
– crest A15.3.03.088 **152**
– cupula A15.3.03.090 **152**
– groove A15.3.03.089 **152**
– membranous limbs A15.3.03.072 **152**
– type of renal pelvis A08.1.05.008 **64**
Amygdaloclaustral area A14.1.09.403 **129**
Amygdalohippocampal area A14.1.09.404 **129**
Amygdaloid
– body A14.1.09.402 **129**
– complex A14.1.09.402 **129**
Amygdalopiriform transition area A14.1.09.405 **129**
Anal
– canal A05.7.05.001 **54**
– columns A05.7.05.004 **54**
– intersphincteric groove A05.7.05.012 **54**
– pecten A05.7.05.010 **54**
– sinuses A05.7.05.006 **54**
– transition zone A05.7.05.007 **54**
– triangle A01.2.06.002 **4**
– valves A05.7.05.005 **54**
Anastomotic
– branch
– – of lacrimal artery with middle meningeal artery A12.2.06.028 **82**
– – of middle meningeal artery with lacrimal artery A12.2.05.068 **81**
– vessel A12.0.00.024 **75**
Anatomical
– conjugate A02.5.02.013 **22**
– internal os A09.1.03.009 **65**
– neck of humerus A02.4.04.003 **19**
Anconeus A04.6.02.023 **40**
Angle
– of mandible A02.1.15.025 **15**
– of mouth A05.1.01.013 **47**
– of rib A02.3.02.010 **18**
Angular
– artery A12.2.05.029 **80**
– gyrus A14.1.09.124 **125**
– incisure of stomach A05.5.01.006 **51**
– vein A12.3.05.019 **93**
Ankle A01.1.00.041 **2**
– joint A03.6.10.002 **31**
– region A01.2.08.033 **6**
Anococcygeal
– body A04.5.04.016 **40, 71**
– ligament A04.5.04.016 **40, 71**
– nerve A14.2.07.045 **140**
Anocutaneous line A05.7.05.008 **54**
Anomalous tubercle of tooth A05.1.03.071 **49**
Anoperinealis A05.7.04.014 **54**
Anorectal
– flexure A05.7.05.002 **54**
– junction A05.7.05.003 **54**
Anorectoperineal muscles A05.7.04.012 **54**
Ansa
– cervicalis A14.2.02.013 **137**
– lenticularis
– – in corpus striatum A14.1.09.520 **130**
– – in thalamus A14.1.08.663 **122**
– peduncularis A14.1.08.665 **122, 129**
– subclavia A14.3.01.021 **141**
Anserine bursa A04.8.05.022 **45**
Ansiform lobule of cerebellum [H VII A] A14.1.07.207 **119**
Ansoparamedian fissure A14.1.07.211 **119**
Antebrachial
– fascia A04.6.03.008 **41**
– region A01.2.07.012 **4**
Anterior A01.0.00.011 **1**
– abdominal cutaneous branch of intercostal nerve A14.2.04.015 **139**
– acoustic stria A14.1.05.319 **113**
– ampullary nerve A14.2.01.128 **135**
– amygdaloid area A14.1.09.406 **129**
– and lateral thoracic regions A01.2.03.001 **4**
– ankle region A01.2.08.018 **5**
– arch of atlas A02.2.02.105 **16**
– articular facet of dens A02.2.02.204 **17**
– atlanto-occipital
– – ligament A03.1.08.003 **27**
– – membrane A03.1.08.002 **27**
– auricular
– – branches of superficial temporal artery A12.2.05.048 **80**
– – nerves A14.2.01.079 **134**
– – veins A12.3.05.040 **93**
– axillary
– – line A01.2.00.017 **3**
– – lymph nodes A13.3.01.006 **101**
– basal
– – branch of superior basal vein of lower lobe
– – – of left lung A12.3.02.407 **92**
– – – of right lung A12.3.02.207 **92**
– – segment
– – – of left lung [S VIII] A06.5.02.023 **61**
– – – of right lung [S VIII] A06.5.02.012 **61**
– – segmental
– – – artery A12.2.01.116 **78**, A12.2.01.217 **79**
– – – – of left lung A12.2.01.217 **79**
– – – – of right lung A12.2.01.116 **78**
– – – bronchus of left lung [B VIII] A06.4.02.023 **60**
– – – bronchus of right lung [B VIII] A06.4.02.012 **60**
– – vein
– – – of left lung A12.3.02.407 **92**
– – – of right lung A12.3.02.207 **92**
– belly of digastric A04.2.03.003 **35**
– bony ampulla A15.3.03.017 **151**
– border
– – of body of pancreas A05.9.01.011 **56**
– – of fibula A02.5.07.011 **23**
– – of lung A06.5.01.012 **60**
– – of radius A02.4.05.013 **20**
– – of testis A09.3.01.006 **67**
– – of tibia A02.5.06.017 **23**
– – of ulna A02.4.06.012 **20**
– branch/es
– – of great auricular nerve A14.2.02.020 **137**
– – of inferior
– – – pancreaticoduodenal artery A12.2.12.055 **88**
– – – suprarenal artery A12.2.12.078 **88**
– – of left superior pulmonary vein A12.3.02.305 **92**
– – of medial cutaneous nerve of forearm A14.2.03.029 **138**
– – of obturator
– – – artery A12.2.15.011 **89**
– – – nerve A14.2.07.013 **140**
– – of posteromedial central arteries A12.2.07.070 **83**
– – of right
– – – branch of portal vein A12.3.12.003 **98**
– – – hepatic duct A05.8.01.063 **56**
– – – superior pulmonary vein A12.3.02.105 **91**

– – of ulnar recurrent artery A12.2.09.043 **86**
– caecal artery A12.2.12.060 **88**
– cardiac veins A12.3.01.012 **91**
– cerebral
– – artery A12.2.07.022 **82, 83**
– – veins A12.3.06.019 **94**
– cervical
– – intertransversarii A04.3.01.012 **36**
– – lymph nodes A13.3.00.017 **101**
– – region A01.2.02.002 **3**
– chamber of eyeball A15.2.06.003 **146**
– choroidal artery A12.2.06.019 **81, 82**
– ciliary
– – arteries A12.2.06.034 **82**
– – veins A12.3.06.108 **95**
– circumflex humeral
– – artery A12.2.09.016 **86**
– – vein A12.3.08.010 **96**
– clinoid process A02.1.05.022 **11**
– cochlear nucleus A14.1.04.249 **111**
– column A14.1.02.102 **106**
– commissure of diencephalon A14.1.08.421 **121, 127, 131**
– – of labia majora A09.2.01.004 **66**
– communicating artery A12.2.07.029 **82, 84**
– compartment
– – of arm A04.6.01.002 **40**
– – of forearm A04.6.01.004 **40**
– – of leg A04.7.01.005 **42**
– – of thigh A04.7.01.002 **42**
– conjunctival arteries A12.2.06.035 **82**
– corneal epithelium A15.2.02.018 **144**
– corticospinal tract A14.1.02.205 **107**
– cranial fossa A02.1.00.048 **8**
– cruciate ligament A03.6.08.007 **30**
– cusp
– – of mitral valve A12.1.04.004 **77**
– – of tricuspid valve A12.1.02.004 **76**
– cutaneous
– – branch/es A14.2.07.005 **139**
– – – of femoral nerve A14.2.07.022 **140**
– – – of iliohypogastric nerve A14.2.07.005 **139**
– deep temporal artery A12.2.05.071 **81**
– divisions of brachial plexus A14.2.03.007 **138**
– ethmoidal
– – artery A12.2.06.039 **82**
– – cells A02.1.07.008 **13**, A06.1.03.006 **57**
– – foramen A02.1.00.079 **9**
– – nerve A14.2.01.030 **134**
– external
– – arcuate fibres of medulla A14.1.04.009 **108, 109**
– – vertebral venous plexus A12.3.07.019 **96**
– extremity of spleen A13.2.01.013 **100**
– facet on talus for calcaneus A02.5.10.006 **23**
– fascicle of palatopharyngeus A05.2.01.106 **50, 51**
– fasciculus proprius of spinal cord A14.1.02.203 **107**
– fold of malleus A15.3.02.065 **150**
– fontanelle A02.1.00.028 **8**
– fornix of vagina A09.1.04.003 **66**
– funiculus of spinal cord A14.1.02.202 **107**
– gastric branches of anterior vagal trunk A14.2.01.175 **136**
– gigantocellular reticular nucleus A14.1.04.304 **111**
– glandular branch of superior thyroid artery A12.2.05.007 **80**
– gluteal line A02.5.01.117 **21**
– grey
– – column of spinal cord A14.1.02.102 **106**
– – commissure of spinal cord A14.1.02.303 **108**
– horn
– – of lateral ventricle A14.1.09.273 **127**
– – of spinal cord A14.1.02.021 **106**, A14.1.02.103 **106**
– hypothalamic
– – area A14.1.08.902 **123**
– – nucleus A14.1.08.903 **123**
– – region A14.1.08.902 **123**
– inferior
– – cerebellar artery A12.2.08.019 **84**
– – fissure of cerebellum A14.1.07.218 **119**
– – iliac spine A02.5.01.112 **21**
– – segment of kidney A08.1.02.004 **63**
– – segmental artery of kidney A12.2.12.081 **88**
– intercavernous sinus A12.3.05.117 **94**
– intercondylar area A02.5.06.006 **23**
– intercostal
– – branches of internal thoracic artery A12.2.08.039 **85**
– – veins A12.3.04.022 **92**
– intermuscular septum of leg A04.7.03.022 **43**
– internal vertebral venous plexus A12.3.07.021 **96**
– interosseous
– – artery A12.2.09.048 **86**
– – nerve A14.2.03.034 **138**
– – veins A12.3.08.032 **96**
– interpositus nucleus A14.1.07.409 **120**
– interventricular
– – branch of left coronary artery A12.2.03.202 **79**
– – sulcus A12.1.00.009 **76**
– – vein A12.3.01.004 **91**
– intra-occipital synchondrosis A03.1.05.007 **27**
– jugular
– – lymph nodes A13.3.00.018 **101**
– – vein A12.3.05.047 **93**
– jugulo-omohyoid lymph nodes A13.3.00.035 **101**
– jugulodigastric lymph node A13.3.00.031 **101**
– labial
– – branches of deep external pudendal artery ♀ A12.2.16.015 **90**
– – nerves ♀ A14.2.07.007 **139**
– – veins ♀ A12.3.11.009 **98**
– lacrimal crest of maxilla A02.1.12.025 **14**
– lateral
– – malleolar artery A12.2.16.045 **90**
– – nasal branches of anterior ethmoidal artery A12.2.06.042 **82**
– – segment of liver A05.8.01.050 **55**
– layer
– – of rectus sheath A04.5.01.004 **38**
– – of thoracolumbar fascia A04.3.02.504 **37**
– ligament
– – of auricle A15.3.01.033 **148**
– – of fibular head A03.6.09.002 **31**
– – of malleus A15.3.02.054 **150**
– limb
– – of internal capsule A14.1.09.526 **130**
– – of stapes A15.3.02.035 **150**
– limiting lamina of cornea A15.2.02.019 **144**
– lip of external os A09.1.03.016 **66**
– lobe
– – of cerebellum A14.1.07.102 **118**
– – of pituitary gland A11.1.00.002 **74**
– longitudinal ligament A03.2.01.007 **27**
– malleolar fold A15.3.01.055 **149**
– medial
– – malleolar artery A12.2.16.046 **90**
– – nucleus A14.1.02.141 **106**, A14.1.06.305 **117**
– – segment of liver A05.8.01.047 **55**
– – visceral nucleus A14.1.06.305 **117**
– median
– – fissure
– – – of medulla A14.1.04.001 **108**
– – – of spinal cord A14.1.02.007 **105**
– – line A01.2.00.012 **3**
– mediastinum A07.1.02.104 **62**
– membranous ampulla A15.3.03.068 **152**

– meningeal branch
– – of anterior ethmoidal artery A12.2.06.040 **82**
– – of posterior ethmoidal nerve A14.2.01.029 **134**
– meniscofemoral ligament A03.6.08.003 **30**
– nasal spine of maxilla A02.1.12.011 **14**
– nerve of lesser curvature A14.2.01.176 **136**
– notch of auricle A15.3.01.018 **148**
– nuclei of thalamus A14.1.08.603 **121**
– nucleus
– – of lateral lemniscus A14.1.05.434 **114**
– – of pons A14.1.05.203 **112**
– – of spinal cord A14.1.02.106 **106**
– – of trapezoid body A14.1.05.422 **114**
– obturator tubercle A02.5.01.311 **22**
– olfactory nucleus A14.1.09.416 **129**
– palpebral margin A15.2.07.035 **147**
– papillary muscle
– – of left ventricle A12.1.04.007 **77**
– – of right ventricle A12.1.02.017 **77**
– paracentral gyrus A14.1.09.210 **126**
– paraventricular nucleus of thalamus A14.1.08.630 **122**
– parietal artery A12.2.07.067 **83**
– part
– – of anterior
– – – cochlear nucleus A14.1.04.250 **111**
– – – commissure A14.1.09.253 **127, 131**
– – – quadrangular lobule of cerebellum A14.1.07.117 **119**
– – of central lobule of cerebellum A14.1.07.106 **119**
– – of culmen A14.1.07.113 **119**
– – of diaphragmatic surface of liver A05.8.01.005 **54**
– – of lateral parabrachial nucleus A14.1.05.445 **114**
– – of tongue A05.1.04.005 **49**
– – of vagina A09.1.04.003 **66**
– pectoral cutaneous branch of intercostal nerve A14.2.04.013 **139**
– perforated substance A14.1.09.437 **129**
– perforating arteries A12.2.07.027 **82**
– periventricular nucleus A14.1.08.904 **123**
– pillar of fauces A05.2.01.005 **50**
– pole
– – of eyeball A15.2.01.002 **144**
– – of lens A15.2.05.008 **146**
– pontoreticulospinal tract A14.1.05.322 **113**
– pretectal nucleus A14.1.08.507 **121**
– process of malleus A15.3.02.048 **150**
– pulvinar nucleus A14.1.08.611 **121**
– quadrangular lobule of cerebellum [H IV et V] A14.1.07.116 **119**
– radiation of thalamus A14.1.08.666 **122**
– radicular artery A12.2.11.015 **87**
– ramus/i A14.2.02.011 **137**
– – of lateral cerebral sulcus A14.1.09.107 **125**
– – of lumbar nerves A14.2.05.008 **139**
– – of sacral nerves and coccygeal nerve A14.2.06.007 **139**
– – of spinal nerve A14.2.00.034 **133**
– – of thoracic nerves A14.2.04.006 **139**
– raphespinal tract A14.1.02.212 **107**, A14.1.04.123 **109**
– recess of tympanic membrane A15.3.02.068 **150**
– region
– – of arm A01.2.07.004 **4**
– – of elbow A01.2.07.009 **4**
– – of forearm A01.2.07.013 **4**
– – of knee A01.2.08.011 **5**
– – of leg A01.2.08.015 **5**
– – of thigh A01.2.08.007 **5**
– – of wrist A01.2.07.019 **5**
– reticulospinal tract A14.1.04.124 **109**
– root of spinal nerve A14.2.00.029 **133**
– sacral foramina A02.2.05.012 **17**
– sacro-iliac ligament A03.6.03.002 **30**
– sacrococcygeal ligament A03.2.08.004 **28**
– scalene A04.2.01.004 **35**
– scrotal
– – branches of deep external pudendal artery ♂ A12.2.16.015 **90**
– – nerves ♂ A14.2.07.007 **139**
– – veins ♂ A12.3.11.009 **98**
– segment
– – of eyeball A15.2.01.009 **144**
– – of left lung [S III] A06.5.02.017 **61**
– – of right lung [S III] A06.5.02.005 **61**
– segmental
– – artery
– – – of left lung A12.2.01.205 **78**
– – – of right branch of hepatic artery A12.2.12.033 **87**
– – – of right lung A12.2.01.104 **78**
– – bronchus of left lung [B III] A06.4.02.017 **60**
– – bronchus of right lung [B III] A06.4.02.005 **60**
– semicircular
– – canal A15.3.03.016 **151**
– – duct A15.3.03.067 **152**
– semilunar cusp of pulmonary valve A12.1.02.013 **77**
– septal branches of anterior ethmoidal artery A12.2.06.041 **82**
– solitary nucleus A14.1.04.240 **111**
– spinal
– – artery A12.2.08.016 **84**
– – veins A12.3.07.024 **96**
– spinocerebellar tract A14.1.02.226 **107**, A14.1.04.125 **109**, A14.1.05.323 **113**
– spinothalamic tract A14.1.02.214 **107**
– sternoclavicular ligament A03.5.04.003 **29**
– subnucleus of lateral parabrachial nucleus A14.1.05.445 **114**
– superior
– – alveolar
– – – arteries A12.2.05.079 **81**
– – – nerves A14.2.01.052 **134**
– – iliac spine A02.5.01.111 **21**
– – pancreaticoduodenal artery A12.2.12.025 **87**
– – segment of kidney A08.1.02.003 **63**
– – segmental artery of kidney A12.2.12.080 **88**
– surface
– – of cornea A15.2.02.016 **144**
– – of eyelid A15.2.07.027 **147**
– – of heart A12.1.00.003 **75**
– – of iris A15.2.03.023 **145**
– – of kidney A08.1.01.006 **63**
– – of lens A15.2.05.010 **146**
– – of maxilla A02.1.12.007 **14**
– – of patella A02.5.05.005 **23**
– – of petrous part of temporal bone A02.1.06.021 **12**
– – of prostate A09.3.08.007 **69**
– – of radius A02.4.05.008 **20**
– – of suprarenal gland A11.5.00.002 **74**
– – of ulna A02.4.06.008 **20**
– – of uterus A09.1.03.008 **65**
– talar articular surface of calcaneum A02.5.11.010 **24**
– talocrural region A01.2.08.018 **5**
– talofibular ligament A03.6.10.009 **31**
– tarsal tendinous sheaths A04.8.06.002 **45**
– tegmental
– – decussation A14.1.06.222 **117**
– – nuclei of midbrain A14.1.06.330 **117**
– – nucleus of pons A14.1.05.435 **114**
– temporal
– – artery A12.2.07.052 **83**
– – branch of middle cerebral artery A12.2.07.056 **83**

– – branches of lateral occipital artery A12.2.07.095 **84**
– – diploic vein A12.3.05.203 **94**
– thalamic
– – radiation A14.1.09.527 **130**
– – tubercle A14.1.08.102 **120**
– tibial
– – artery A12.2.16.042 **90**
– – lymph node A13.3.05.014 **103**
– – recurrent artery A12.2.16.043 **90**
– – veins A12.3.11.031 **98**
– tibiofibular ligament A03.6.05.003 **30**
– tibiotalar part of medial ligament of ankle joint A03.6.10.006 **31**
– transverse temporal gyrus A14.1.09.141 **125**
– triangle A01.2.02.002 **3**
– trigeminothalamic tract A14.1.05.311 **113**
– tubercle
– – of atlas A02.2.02.107 **16**
– – of calcaneum A02.5.11.005 **24**
– – of cervical vertebra A02.2.02.004 **16**
– tympanic artery A12.2.05.055 **80**
– vagal trunk A14.2.01.174 **136**
– vaginal column A09.1.04.014 **66**
– vein
– – of septum pellucidum A12.3.06.031 **94**
– – of upper lobe
– – – of left lung A12.3.02.305 **92**
– – – of right lung A12.3.02.105 **91**
– vein(s) of right ventricle A12.3.01.012 **91**
– ventrolateral nucleus of thalamus A14.1.08.650 **122**
– vertebral vein A12.3.04.014 **92**
– vestibular
– – artery A15.3.03.127 **153**
– – vein A15.3.03.141 **153**
– wall
– – of stomach A05.5.01.002 **51**
– – of vagina A09.1.04.006 **66**
– white commissure of spinal cord A14.1.02.305 **108**
Antero-inferior surface of body of pancreas A05.9.01.009 **56**
Anterodorsal nucleus of thalamus A14.1.08.604 **121**
Anterolateral
– central arteries A12.2.07.048 **83**
– medullary vein A12.3.06.050 **95**
– nucleus
– – of principal sensory nucleus of trigeminal nerve A14.1.05.408 **114**
– – of spinal cord A14.1.02.105 **106**
– pontine vein A12.3.06.045 **95**
– solitary nucleus A14.1.04.241 **111**
– sulcus
– – of medulla A14.1.04.005 **108**
– – of spinal cord A14.1.02.010 **105**
– surface
– – of arytenoid A06.2.04.004 **58**
– – of humerus A02.4.04.012 **19**
– system A14.1.04.137 **110, 113**, A14.1.06.215 **116**
– tracts A14.1.04.137 **110, 113**, A14.1.06.215 **116**
Anteromedial
– central arteries of anterior
– – cerebral artery A12.2.07.024 **82**
– – communicating artery A12.2.07.024 **82**
– frontal branch of callosomarginal artery A12.2.07.038 **83**
– intermuscular septum A04.7.03.007 **43**
– lobule of prostate A09.3.08.014 **69**
– nucleus
– – of spinal cord A14.1.02.107 **106**
– – of thalamus A14.1.08.605 **121**
– surface of humerus A02.4.04.011 **19**
Anteromedian
– medullary vein A12.3.06.049 **95**
– pontine vein A12.3.06.044 **95**
Anterosuperior surface of body of pancreas A05.9.01.007 **56**
Anteroventral nucleus of thalamus A14.1.08.606 **121**
Antihelical fossa A15.3.01.028 **148**
Antihelix A15.3.01.009 **148**
Antitragicus A15.3.01.042 **149**
Antitragus A15.3.01.016 **148**
Anular
– epiphysis A02.2.01.004 **16**
– ligament/s
– – of radius A03.5.09.007 **29**
– – of stapes A15.3.02.060 **150**
– – of trachea A06.3.01.006 **59**
– part of fibrous sheaths
– – of digits of hand A04.8.04.016 **45**
– – of toes A04.8.06.015 **46**
Anulo-olivary fibres A14.1.05.327 **113**
Anulus fibrosus A03.2.02.004 **27**
Anus A05.7.05.013 **54**
Aorta A12.2.02.001 **79**
Aortic
– arch A12.2.04.001 **79**
– bifurcation A12.2.13.001 **89**
– bulb A12.2.03.004 **79**
– glomera A12.2.04.003 **79**
– hiatus A04.4.02.010 **38**
– isthmus A12.2.04.002 **79**
– orifice A12.1.04.010 **77**
– sinus A12.2.03.002 **79**
– valve A12.1.04.012 **77**
– vestibule A12.1.04.009 **77**
Aorticorenal ganglia A14.3.03.028 **143**
Apex
– of arytenoid cartilage A06.2.04.012 **58**
– of auricle A15.3.01.021 **148**
– of bladder A08.3.01.002 **64**
– of cusp of tooth A05.1.03.011 **48**
– of dens A02.2.02.203 **17**
– of head of fibula A02.5.07.004 **23**
– of heart A12.1.00.007 **76**
– of lung A06.5.01.005 **60**
– of nose A06.1.01.004 **57**
– of patella A02.5.05.003 **23**
– of petrous part of temporal bone A02.1.06.012 **12**
– of posterior horn of spinal cord A14.1.02.116 **106**
– of prostate A09.3.08.006 **69**
– of sacrum A02.2.05.021 **17**
– of tongue A05.1.04.010 **49**
Apical A01.0.00.022 **1**
– branch of right superior pulmonary vein A12.3.02.102 **91**
– foramen A05.1.03.050 **48**
– ligament of dens A03.2.04.003 **27**
– segment of right lung [S I] A06.5.02.003 **61**
– segmental
– – artery
– – – of left lung A12.2.01.204 **78**
– – – of right lung A12.2.01.103 **78**
– – bronchus of right lung [B I] A06.4.02.003 **60**
– vein of upper lobe of right lung A12.3.02.102 **91**
Apical axillary lymph nodes A13.3.01.003 **101**
Apicoposterior
– branch of left superior pulmonary vein A12.3.02.302 **92**
– segment of left lung [S I + II] A06.5.02.016 **61**
– segmental bronchus of left lung [B I+II] A06.4.02.016 **60**
– vein of upper lobe of left lung A12.3.02.302 **92**
Aponeurosis A04.0.00.047 **34**
Apophysis A02.0.00.023 **7**
Appendicular
– artery A12.2.12.062 **88**
– lymph nodes A13.3.03.039 **102**
– nodes A13.3.03.039 **102**
– skeleton A02.0.00.010 **7**
– vein A12.3.12.025 **99**
Appendix A05.7.02.007 **53**
– of epididymis A09.3.02.011 **68**
– of testis A09.3.02.010 **68**
Approximal surface of tooth A05.1.03.042 **48**
Aqueduct of midbrain A14.1.06.501 **118**
Aqueous humor A15.2.06.002 **146**
Arachnoid
– granulations A14.1.01.205 **105**
– mater A14.1.01.201 **104**
– – and pia mater A14.1.01.003 **104**
– trabeculae A14.1.01.206 **105**
Arbor vitae A14.1.07.401 **119**
Arch
– of aorta A12.2.04.001 **79**
– of azygos vein A12.3.07.002 **95**
– of cricoid cartilage A06.2.03.002 **58**
– of thoracic duct A12.4.01.008 **99**

Archicerebellum A14.1.07.010 **118**
Archicortex A14.1.09.302 **128**
Arcuate
– arteries of kidney A08.1.03.003 **63**
– artery of foot A12.2.16.051 **90**
– crest of arytenoid A06.2.04.006 **58**
– eminence A02.1.06.023 **12**
– fasciculus A14.1.09.557 **131**
– fibres of telencephalon A14.1.09.554 **131**
– line
– – of ilium A02.5.01.105 **21**
– – of rectus sheath A04.5.01.006 **38**
– nucleus A14.1.04.256 **111**, A14.1.08.923 **123**
– popliteal ligament A03.6.08.014 **31**
– veins of kidney A08.1.04.003 **63**
Area postrema A14.1.04.258 **111**, **115**
Areola A16.0.02.012 **154**
Areolar
– glands A16.0.02.013 **155**
– tubercles A16.0.02.014 **155**
– venous plexus A12.3.08.013 **96**
Arm A01.1.00.022 **2**
Arrector muscle of hair A16.0.00.024 **154**
Arteriae lumbales imae A12.2.12.009 **87**
Arterial
– circle A12.0.00.006 **75**
– grooves A02.1.00.042 **8**
– plexus A12.0.00.012 **75**
Arteries A12.2.00.001 **78**
– of brain A12.2.07.001 **82**
– of lower limb A12.2.16.001 **90**
– of upper limb A12.2.09.001 **85**
Arteriole A12.0.00.005 **75**
Arteriolovenular anastomosis A12.0.00.002 **75**
Arteriovenous anastomosis A12.0.00.002 **75**
Artery A12.0.00.003 **75**
– of bulb
– – of penis ♂ A12.2.15.043 **89**
– – of vestibule ♀ A12.2.15.043 **89**
– of caudate lobe A12.2.12.032 **87**, A12.2.12.036 **87**
– of central sulcus A12.2.07.065 **83**
– of postcentral sulcus A12.2.07.066 **83**
– of precentral sulcus A12.2.07.064 **83**
– of pterygoid canal
– – internal carotid artery A12.2.06.006 **81**
– – maxillary artery A12.2.05.082 **81**
– of round ligament of uterus ♀ A12.2.16.007 **90**
– of tuber cinereum A12.2.07.073 **83**
– to ductus deferens A12.2.15.022 **89**
– to sciatic nerve A12.2.15.019 **89**
– to tail of pancreas A12.2.12.046 **88**
– to vas deferens ♂ A12.2.15.022 **89**
Articular
– branch/es A14.2.00.025 **133**
– – of descending genicular artery A12.2.16.019 **90**
– – of posterior branch of obturator nerve A14.2.07.018 **140**
– capsule A03.0.00.026 **25**
– cavity A03.0.00.022 **25**
– circumference
– – of head of radius A02.4.05.004 **20**
– – of ulna A02.4.06.016 **20**
– disc A03.0.00.032 **25**
– – of acromioclavicular joint A03.5.03.003 **28**
– – of distal radio-ulnar joint A03.5.10.002 **29**
– – of sternoclavicular joint A03.5.04.002 **29**
– – of temporomandibular joint A03.1.07.002 **27**
– facet
– – of head
– – – of fibula A02.5.07.003 **23**
– – – of radius A02.4.05.003 **19**
– – – of rib A02.3.02.003 **18**
– – of lateral malleolus A02.5.07.015 **23**
– – of tubercle of rib A02.3.02.009 **18**
– – on tibia for medial malleolus A02.5.06.022 **23**
– fossa A03.0.00.023 **25**
– head A03.0.00.024 **25**
– muscle of knee A04.7.02.024 **42**
– recess A03.0.00.038 **25**
– surface A02.0.00.036 **7**, A03.0.00.021 **25**
– – for cuboid on calcaneum A02.5.11.015 **24**
– – of arytenoid A06.2.04.002 **58**
– – of mandibular fossa of temporal bone A02.1.06.072 **13**
– – of patella A02.5.05.004 **23**
– system A03.0.00.000 **25**
– tubercle of temporal bone A02.1.06.073 **13**
– vascular plexus A12.0.00.014 **75**
– veins A12.3.05.042 **93**
Articularis
– cubiti A04.6.02.024 **40**
– genus A04.7.02.024 **42**
Articulations of auditory ossicles A15.3.02.049 **150**
Ary-epiglottic
– fold A06.2.09.003 **59**
– part of oblique arytenoid A06.2.08.011 **59**
Arytenoid
– articular surface on cricoid A06.2.03.004 **58**
– cartilage A06.2.04.001 **58**
Ascending
– aorta A12.2.03.001 **79**
– artery A12.2.12.070 **88**
– branch
– – of anterior segmental artery
– – – of left lung A12.2.01.206 **78**
– – – of right lung A12.2.01.105 **78**
– – of inferior epigastric artery A12.2.16.009 **90**
– – of lateral circumflex femoral artery A12.2.16.028 **90**
– – of medial circumflex femoral artery A12.2.16.025 **90**
– – of posterior segmental artery
– – – of left lung A12.2.01.209 **78**
– – – of right lung A12.2.01.108 **78**
– – of superior cervical artery A12.2.08.055 **85**
– cervical artery A12.2.08.049 **85**
– colon A05.7.03.002 **53**
– lumbar vein
– – azygos vein A12.3.07.011 **96**
– – inferior vena cava A12.3.09.004 **97**
– mesocolon A10.1.02.011 **72**
– palatine artery A12.2.05.021 **80**
– part
– – of duodenum A05.6.02.008 **52**
– – of trapezius A04.3.01.004 **36**
– pharyngeal artery A12.2.05.010 **80**
– ramus of lateral cerebral sulcus A14.1.09.106 **124**
Association
– fibre A14.1.00.016 **104**
– fibres of telencephalon A14.1.09.553 **131**
Asterion A02.1.00.020 **8**
Atlantic part of vertebral artery A12.2.08.009 **84**
Atlanto-occipital joint A03.1.08.001 **27**
Atlas [C I] A02.2.02.101 **16**
Atrial
– anastomotic branch of left coronary artery A12.2.03.207 **79**
– branches
– – of left coronary artery A12.2.03.214 **79**
– – of right coronary artery A12.2.03.105 **79**
Atrioventricular
– branches
– – of left coronary artery A12.2.03.208 **79**
– – of right coronary artery A12.2.03.102 **79**
– bundle A12.1.06.005 **77**
– nodal branch
– – of left coronary artery A12.2.03.213 **79**
– – of right coronary artery A12.2.03.110 **79**
– node A12.1.06.004 **77**
– septum A12.1.00.016 **76**
Atrium
– of lateral ventricle A14.1.09.281 **127**
– of middle meatus A06.1.02.025 **57**
Attachment A04.0.00.003 **33**

– of superficial external anal sphincter A04.5.04.019 **40**
Auditory
– commissure of pons A14.1.05.324 **113**
– ossicles A02.1.17.001 **16, 149**
– tube A15.3.02.073 **150**
Auricle A15.3.01.002 **148**
– of atrium A12.1.00.018 **76**
Auricular
– branch
– – of occipital artery A12.2.05.032 **80**
– – of posterior auricular
– – – artery A12.2.05.042 **80**
– – – nerve A14.2.01.104 **135**
– – of vagus A14.2.01.156 **136**
– cartilage A15.3.01.004 **148**
– muscles A15.3.01.036 **148**
– region A01.2.01.006 **3**
– surface
– – of ilium A02.5.01.121 **21**
– – of sacrum A02.2.05.007 **17**
– tubercle A15.3.01.020 **148**
Auricularis
– anterior A04.1.03.020 **34**
– posterior A04.1.03.022 **34**
– superior A04.1.03.021 **34**
Auriculotemporal nerve A14.2.01.074 **134**
Auscultatory triangle A01.2.05.006 **4**
Autonomic
– branch A14.2.00.040 **133**
– division A14.3.00.001 **141**
– ganglion A14.2.00.008 **132**
– nerve A14.2.00.039 **133**
– – fibres A14.2.00.020 **132**
– nuclei A14.1.06.304 **117**
– part of peripheral nervous system A14.3.00.001 **141**
– plexus A14.2.00.041 **133**
Axial A01.0.00.029 **1**
– skeleton A02.0.00.009 **7**
Axilla A01.1.00.021 **2**
Axillary
– artery A12.2.09.002 **85**
– fascia A04.6.03.002 **41**
– fossa A01.2.03.010 **4**
– hairs A16.0.00.021 **154**
– lymph nodes A13.3.01.002 **101**
– lymphatic plexus A12.4.01.004 **99**
– nerve A14.2.03.059 **139**
– process A16.0.02.007 **154**
– region A01.2.03.009 **4**
– tail A16.0.02.007 **154**
– vein A12.3.08.005 **96**
Axis
– [C II] A02.2.02.201 **17**
– of lens A15.2.05.012 **146**
– of pelvis A02.5.02.010 **22**
Azygos
– artery of vagina ♀ A12.2.15.032 **89**
– vein A12.3.07.001 **95**

B

Back A01.1.00.018 **2**
Ball and socket joint A03.0.00.050 **25**
Bare area of diaphragmatic surface of liver A05.8.01.008 **54**
Basal A01.0.00.023 **1**
– crest of cochlear duct A15.3.03.101 **152**
– forebrain A14.1.09.401 **129**
– group of inferior lobar arteries
– – of left lung A12.2.01.216 **79**
– – of right lung A12.2.01.115 **78**
– lamina
– – of choroid A15.2.03.007 **144**
– – of ciliary body A15.2.03.019 **145**
– – of spiral membrane A15.3.03.102 **152**
– nuclei and related structures A14.1.09.501 **130**
– nucleus of telencephalon A14.1.09.418 **129**
– part
– – of left inferior lobular artery A12.2.01.216 **79**
– – of right inferior lobular artery A12.2.01.115 **78**
– substance of telencephalon A14.1.09.417 **129**
– vein A12.3.06.018 **94**
– ventral medial nucleus of thalamus A14.1.08.645 **122**
Base
– of arytenoid cartilage A06.2.04.003 **58**
– of cochlea A15.3.03.027 **151**
– of heart A12.1.00.002 **75**
– of lung A06.5.01.004 **60**
– of mandible A02.1.15.003 **15**
– of metacarpal A02.4.09.002 **20**
– of metatarsal A02.5.17.002 **24**
– of modiolus cochleae A15.3.03.039 **151**
– of patella A02.5.05.002 **23**
– of peduncle A14.1.06.101 **116**
– of phalanx
– – of foot A02.5.18.006 **24**
– – of hand A02.4.10.006 **21**
– of posterior horn of spinal cord A14.1.02.123 **106**
– of prostate A09.3.08.002 **68**
– of sacrum A02.2.05.002 **17**
– of stapes A15.3.02.037 **150**
Basicranium A02.1.00.044 **8**
Basilar A01.0.00.024 **1**
– artery A12.2.07.081 **84**
– membrane of cochlear duct A15.3.03.102 **152**
– part
– – of occipital bone A02.1.04.005 **10**
– – of pons A14.1.05.101 **112**
– plexus A12.3.05.106 **93**
– sulcus A14.1.05.002 **112**
– venous plexus A12.3.05.106 **93**
Basilic vein A12.3.08.018 **96**
– of forearm A12.3.08.022 **96**
Basion A02.1.04.003 **10**
Basivertebral veins A12.3.07.022 **96**
Basolateral amygdaloid nucleus A14.1.09.407 **129**
Basomedial amygdaloid nucleus A14.1.09.408 **129**
Beard A16.0.00.018 **154**
Bed nucleus of stria terminalis A14.1.09.419 **129**
Belly A04.0.00.002 **33**
Biceps
– brachii A04.6.02.013 **40**
– femoris A04.7.02.032 **42**
Bicipital
– aponeurosis A04.6.02.016 **40**
– groove A02.4.04.007 **19**
Bicipitoradial bursa A04.8.03.014 **44**
Bicondylar joint A03.0.00.047 **25**
Bifurcate ligament A03.6.10.511 **31**
Bifurcation of pulmonary trunk A12.2.01.004 **78**
Bile duct A05.8.02.013 **56**
Biliaropancreatic ampulla A05.8.02.017 **56**
Bipennate muscle A04.0.00.016 **33**
Biventral lobule [H VIII] A14.1.07.216 **119**
Bladder A08.3.01.001 **64**
– mucosa A08.3.01.024 **64**
– neck part of detrusor A08.3.01.016 **64**
– serosa A08.3.01.008 **64**
– subserosa A08.3.01.009 **64**
Blood A12.0.00.009 **75**
– vessel A12.0.00.001 **75**
Body
– of bladder A08.3.01.003 **64**
– of breast A16.0.02.005 **154**
– of caudate nucleus A14.1.09.504 **130**
– of cerebellum A14.1.07.101 **118**
– of clavicle A02.4.02.005 **19**
– of clitoris A09.2.02.003 **67**
– of corpus callosum A14.1.09.244 **127**
– of epididymis A09.3.02.004 **68**
– of femur A02.5.04.012 **22**
– of fibula A02.5.07.006 **23**
– of fornix A14.1.09.258 **127**
– of gallbladder A05.8.02.004 **56**
– of humerus A02.4.04.010 **19**
– of hyoid bone A02.1.16.002 **16**
– of ilium A02.5.01.102 **21**
– of incus A15.3.02.039 **150**
– of ischium A02.5.01.202 **21**
– of lateral ventricle A14.1.09.274 **127**
– of mandible A02.1.15.002 **15**
– of maxilla A02.1.12.002 **14**
– of metacarpal A02.4.09.003 **20**
– of metatarsal A02.5.17.003 **24**
– of nail A16.0.01.004 **154**
– of pancreas A05.9.01.006 **56**
– of penis A09.4.01.003 **69**

– of phalanx A02.4.10.007 **21**, A02.5.18.007 **24**
– – of foot A02.5.18.007 **24**
– – of hand A02.4.10.007 **21**
– of pubis A02.5.01.302 **21**
– of radius A02.4.05.006 **20**
– of rib A02.3.02.007 **18**
– of sphenoid A02.1.05.002 **11**
– of sternum A02.3.03.006 **18**
– of stomach A05.5.01.012 **52**
– of talus A02.5.10.010 **24**
– of tibia A02.5.06.011 **23**
– of tongue A05.1.04.002 **49**
– of ulna A02.4.06.007 **20**
– of uterus A09.1.03.003 **65**
Bone marrow A13.1.01.001 **100**
Bones A02.0.00.000 **7**
– of cranium A02.1.01.001 **9**
– of foot A02.5.08.001 **23**
– of hand A02.4.07.001 **20**
– of lower limb A02.5.00.001 **21**
– of upper limb A02.4.00.001 **18**
Bony
– joints A03.0.00.002 **25**
– labyrinth A15.3.03.003 **151**
– nasal
– – cavity A02.1.00.086 **9**
– – septum A02.1.00.087 **9**
– palate A02.1.00.056 **9**
– part A02.0.00.001 **7**
– – of nasal septum A06.1.02.007 **57**
– – of pharyngotympanic tube A15.3.02.075 **150**
– union A03.0.00.019 **25**
Border
– of oval fossa A12.1.01.006 **76**
– of uterus A09.1.03.005 **65**
Brachial
– artery A12.2.09.018 **86**
– autonomic plexus A14.3.03.009 **143**
– fascia A04.6.03.005 **41**
– lymph nodes A13.3.01.010 **101**
– plexus A14.2.03.001 **137**
– region A01.2.07.003 **4**
– veins A12.3.08.029 **96**
Brachialis A04.6.02.018 **40**
Brachiocephalic
– lymph nodes A13.3.02.007 **102**
– trunk A12.2.04.004 **79**
– vein A12.3.04.001 **92**
Brachioradialis A04.6.02.039 **41**
Brachium
– of inferior colliculus A14.1.06.012 **115, 118, 122**
– of superior colliculus A14.1.06.013 **115, 118, 122**
Brain A14.1.03.001 **108**
– box A02.1.00.007 **8**
Brainstem A14.1.03.009 **108**
Branch/es
– of anterior choroidal artery to
– – amygdaloid body A12.2.07.015 **82**
– – anterior perforated substance A12.2.07.004 **82**
– – crus cerebri A12.2.07.021 **82**
– – globus pallidus A12.2.07.011 **82**
– – hippocampus A12.2.07.013 **82**
– – hypothalamic nuclei A12.2.07.017 **82**
– – internal capsule,
– – – genu A12.2.07.008 **82**
– – – posterior limb A12.2.07.009 **82**
– – – retrolentiform limb A12.2.07.010 **82**
– – lateral geniculate body A12.2.07.007 **82**
– – optic
– – – chiasma A12.2.07.005 **82**
– – – tract A12.2.07.006 **82**
– – red nucleus A12.2.07.020 **82**
– – substantia nigra A12.2.07.019 **82**
– – tail of caudate nucleus A12.2.07.012 **82**
– – thalamic nuclei A12.2.07.018 **82**
– – tuber cinereum A12.2.07.016 **82**
– – uncus A12.2.07.014 **82**
– of auriculotemporal nerve to tympanic membrane A14.2.01.076 **134**
– of cavernous part of internal carotid artery to
– – nerves A12.2.06.014 **81**
– – trigeminal ganglion A12.2.06.013 **81**
– of lingual nerve to isthmus of fauces A14.2.01.082 **135**
– of middle cerebral artery to angular gyrus A12.2.07.060 **83**
– of oculomotor nerve to ciliary ganglion A14.2.01.010 **133, 142**
– of posterior communicating artery to oculomotor nerve A12.2.07.079 **83**
– to amygdaloid body A12.2.07.015 **82**
– to angular gyrus A12.2.07.060 **83**
– to anterior perforated substance A12.2.07.004 **82**
– to ciliary ganglion A14.2.01.010 **133, 142**
– to crus cerebri A12.2.07.021 **82**
– to globus pallidus A12.2.07.011 **82**
– to hippocampus A12.2.07.013 **82**
– to hypothalamic nuclei A12.2.07.017 **82**
– to internal capsule,
– – genu A12.2.07.008 **82**
– – posterior limb A12.2.07.009 **82**
– – retrolentiform limb A12.2.07.010 **82**
– to isthmus of fauces A14.2.01.082 **135**
– to lateral geniculate body A12.2.07.007 **82**
– to nerves A12.2.06.014 **81**
– to oculomotor nerve A12.2.07.079 **83**
– to optic
– – chiasm(a) A12.2.07.005 **82**
– – tract A12.2.07.006 **82**
– to otic ganglion A14.2.01.067 **134, 142**
– to red nucleus A12.2.07.020 **82**
– to substantia nigra A12.2.07.019 **82**
– to tail of caudate nucleus A12.2.07.012 **82**
– to thalamic nuclei A12.2.07.018 **82**
– to trigeminal ganglion A12.2.06.013 **81**
– to tuber cinereum A12.2.07.016 **82**
– to tympanic membrane A14.2.01.076 **134**
– to uncus A12.2.07.014 **82**
Branching type of renal pelvis A08.1.05.002 **64**
Breast A16.0.02.001 **154**
Bregma A02.1.00.016 **8**
Broad ligament of uterus ♀ A10.1.02.505 **73**
Bronchi A06.4.01.001 **59**
Bronchial
– branches
– – of internal thoracic artery A12.2.08.032 **85**
– – of thoracic aorta A12.2.11.002 **86**
– – of vagus A14.2.01.171 **136**
– glands A06.4.02.030 **60**
– mucosa A06.4.02.029 **60**
– tree A06.4.01.002 **59**
– veins A12.3.04.009 **92**, A12.3.07.007 **95**
Bronchioles A06.5.02.026 **61**
Broncho-aortic constriction of oesophagus A05.4.01.004 **51**
Broncho-oesophageus A05.4.01.012 **51**
Bronchomediastinal
– lymphatic trunk A12.4.01.005 **99**
– trunk A12.4.01.005 **99**
Bronchopericardial membrane A12.1.08.004 **78**
Bronchopulmonary
– lymph nodes A13.3.02.015 **102**
– segments A06.5.02.001 **60**
Buccal
– artery A12.2.05.074 **81**
– branches of facial nerve A14.2.01.111 **135**
– cusp A05.1.03.019 **48**
– fat pad A05.1.01.015 **47**
– glands A05.1.02.015 **47**
– nerve A14.2.01.073 **134**
– region A01.2.01.013 **3**
– root A05.1.03.064 **49**
– surface of tooth A05.1.03.036 **48**
Buccinator A04.1.03.036 **35**
– lymph node A13.3.00.010 **101**
Buccopharyngeal
– fascia A04.1.04.010 **35**, A05.3.01.116 **51**

– part of superior constrictor A05.3.01.105 **51**
Bulb A14.1.03.003 **108**
– of occipital horn of lateral ventricle A14.1.09.284 **127**
– of penis A09.4.01.016 **69**
– of vestibule A09.2.01.013 **67**
Bulbar
– conjunctiva A15.2.07.050 **147**
– corticonuclear fibres A14.1.04.104 **109**
Bulbo-urethral gland A09.3.09.001 **69**
Bulboreticulospinal tract A14.1.02.221 **107**
Bulbospongiosus A09.5.02.005 **71**
Bursa
– of calcaneal tendon A04.8.05.032 **45**
– of piriformis A04.8.05.006 **45**
– of tendo calcaneus A04.8.05.032 **45**
– of tensor veli palatini A04.8.02.002 **44**
Bursae
– of lower limb A04.8.05.001 **45**
– of neck A04.8.02.001 **44**
– of upper limb A04.8.03.001 **44**
Buttocks A01.1.00.033 **2**

C

Caecal folds A10.1.02.423 **73**
Caecum A05.7.02.001 **53**
Caerulean nucleus A14.1.05.436 **114**
Caeruleospinal tract A14.1.02.232 **107**
Calcaneal
– anastomosis A12.2.16.076 **91**
– branches
– – of lateral malleolar branch of fibular artery A12.2.16.075 **91**
– – of posterior tibial artery A12.2.16.059 **91**
– process of cuboid A02.5.16.004 **24**
– sulcus A02.5.11.008 **24**
– tendon A04.7.02.048 **43**
– tubercle A02.5.11.005 **24**
– tuberosity A02.5.11.002 **24**
Calcaneocuboid
– joint A03.6.10.204 **31**
– ligament A03.6.10.513 **31**
Calcaneofibular ligament A03.6.10.011 **31**
Calcaneonavicular ligament A03.6.10.512 **31**
Calcaneus A02.5.11.001 **24**
Calcarine
– branch of medial occipital artery A12.2.07.102 **84**
– spur A14.1.09.285 **128**
– sulcus A14.1.09.225 **126**
Calf A01.1.00.039 **2**
Callosomarginal artery A12.2.07.037 **83**
Calvaria A02.1.00.032 **8**
Canal for
– auditory tube A02.1.06.019 **12**
– tensor tympani A02.1.06.018 **12**
– vertebral artery A02.2.02.110 **17**
Canaliculus for chorda tympani A02.1.06.011 **12**
Canine
– fossa A02.1.12.009 **14**, A05.1.03.061 **49**
– groove A05.1.03.060 **49**
– tooth A05.1.03.005 **48**
Capillary A12.0.00.025 **75**
– lamina of choroid A15.2.03.006 **144**
Capitate A02.4.08.011 **20**
Capitulum of humerus A02.4.04.022 **19**
Capsular
– branches
– – of intrarenal arteries A08.1.03.009 **63**
– – of renal artery A12.2.12.076 **88**
– ligaments A03.0.00.036 **25**
– veins A12.3.09.010 **97**
Capsule
– of crico-arytenoid joint A06.2.04.015 **58**
– of cricothyroid joint A06.2.03.007 **58**
– of ganglion A14.2.00.003 **132**
– of lens A15.2.05.007 **146**
– of lymph node A13.2.03.002 **100, 137**
– of prostate A09.3.08.017 **69**
Cardia A05.5.01.007 **51**
Cardiac
– branches of thoracic ganglia A14.3.01.025 **141**
– ganglia A14.3.03.014 **143**
– impression
– – on diaphragmatic surface of liver A05.8.01.004 **54**
– – on lung A06.5.01.009 **60**
– nerve plexus A14.3.03.012 **143**
– notch of left lung A06.5.01.013 **60**
– plexus A14.3.03.013 **143**
Cardial
– notch A05.5.01.011 **52**
– orifice A05.5.01.008 **51**
– part of stomach A05.5.01.007 **51**
Cardinal ligament A09.1.03.031 **66**
Cardiovascular system A12.0.00.000 **75**
Carina of trachea A06.3.01.009 **59**
Caroticotympanic
– arteries A12.2.06.005 **81**
– canaliculi A02.1.06.016 **12**
– nerves A14.2.01.142 **136, 142**
Carotid
– bifurcation A12.2.04.009 **79**
– body A12.2.04.007 **79**
– branch of glossopharyngeal nerve A14.2.01.146 **136**
– canal A02.1.06.013 **12**
– sheath A04.2.05.007 **36**
– sinus A12.2.04.008 **79**, A12.2.06.003 **81**
– sulcus A02.1.05.012 **11**
– syphon A12.2.06.023 **81**
– triangle A01.2.02.004 **3**
– tubercle A02.2.02.005 **16**
– wall of tympanic cavity A15.3.02.031 **149**
Carpal
– articular surface of radius A02.4.05.020 **20**
– bones A02.4.08.001 **20**
– groove A02.4.08.014 **20**
– joints A03.5.11.101 **29**
– region A01.2.07.018 **5**
– tendinous sheaths A04.8.04.003 **44**
– tunnel A03.5.11.201 **29**
Carpometacarpal
– joint of thumb A03.5.11.304 **29**
– joints A03.5.11.301 **29**
Cartilage
– of acoustic meatus A15.3.01.049 **149**
– of pharyngotympanic tube A15.3.02.079 **150**
– of tube A15.3.02.079 **150**
Cartilaginous
– external acoustic meatus A15.3.01.048 **149**
– joint A03.0.00.015 **25**
– part A02.0.00.005 **7**
– – of nasal septum A06.1.02.006 **57**
– – of pharyngotympanic tube A06.1.02.006 **57**
Carunculae hymenales A09.1.04.009 **66**
Cauda equina A14.2.00.036 **133**
Caudal A01.0.00.020 **1**
– fibres A14.1.09.565 **131**
– part of spinal nucleus of trigeminal nerve A14.1.04.212 **110**
– pontine reticular nucleus A14.1.05.502 **114**
– vertical occipital fibres A14.1.09.565 **131**
Caudate
– branches of left branch of portal vein A12.3.12.007 **98**
– lobe of liver A05.8.01.030 **55**, A05.8.01.043 **55**, A05.8.01.044 **55**
– nucleus A14.1.09.502 **130**
– process of caudate lobe of liver A05.8.01.032 **55**
Caudolenticular grey bridges A14.1.09.525 **130**
Caval opening A04.4.02.014 **38**
Cave of septum pellucidum A14.1.09.263 **127**
Cavernous
– branch of cavernous part of internal carotid artery A12.2.06.011 **81**
– nerve plexus A14.3.03.005 **142**
– nerves
– – of clitoris ♀ A14.3.03.056 **143**
– – of penis ♂ A14.3.03.056 **143**
– part of internal carotid artery A12.2.06.007 **81**
– plexus A14.3.03.006 **143**

– – of conchae A06.1.02.016 **57**
– sinus A12.3.05.116 **94**
– spaces
– – of corpora cavernosa A09.4.01.022 **69**
– – of corpus spongiosum A09.4.01.023 **69**
– veins of penis A09.4.01.025 **69**
Cavity/ies A01.1.00.047 **2**
– of concha A15.3.01.015 **148**
– of pharynx A05.3.01.002 **50**
Cell
– group
– – F A14.1.04.244 **111**
– – I A14.1.05.428 **114**
– – L A14.1.05.428 **114**
– – X A14.1.04.210 **110**
– – Y A14.1.04.246 **111**
– – Z A14.1.04.205 **110**
– nest region A14.1.04.203 **110**, A14.1.04.207 **110**
– – of cuneate nucleus A14.1.04.207 **110**
– – of gracile nucleus A14.1.04.203 **110**
Cellulae pneumaticae tubae auditivae A15.3.02.077 **150**
Cement/um A03.1.03.007 **26**, A05.1.03.057 **48**
Central A01.0.00.037 **1**
– amygdaloid nucleus A14.1.09.409 **129**
– axillary lymph nodes A13.3.01.007 **101**
– canal of spinal cord A14.1.02.019 **106, 108**
– cerebral sulcus A14.1.09.103 **124, 126**
– cord structures A14.1.02.301 **108**
– gelatinous substance of spinal cord A14.1.02.025 **106**
– grey substance A14.1.06.321 **117**
– intermediate
– – grey matter of spinal cord A14.1.02.134 **106**
– – substance A14.1.02.134 **106**
– lateral nucleus of thalamus A14.1.08.616 **121**
– lobule of cerebellum [II and III] A14.1.07.105 **119**
– medial nucleus of thalamus A14.1.08.617 **121**
– nervous system A14.1.00.001 **104**
– nucleus
– – of inferior colliculus A14.1.06.603 **118**
– – of spinal cord A14.1.02.111 **106**
– part
– – of cuneate nucleus A14.1.04.207 **110**
– – of gracile nucleus A14.1.04.203 **110**
– – of lateral ventricle A14.1.09.274 **127**
– precommissural nucleus A14.1.06.308 **117**
– reticular nucleus A14.1.04.314 **112**
– retinal
– – artery A12.2.06.024 **81**
– – vein A12.3.06.111 **95**
– sulcus A14.1.09.103 **124, 126**
– – of insula A14.1.09.153 **125**
– superior mesenteric lymph nodes A13.3.03.035 **102**
– tegmental tract A14.1.05.325 **113, 116**
– tendon of diaphragm A04.4.02.013 **38**
– thalamic radiation A14.1.08.667 **122**, A14.1.09.532 **130**
– vein/s
– – of liver A05.8.01.059 **55**
– – of suprarenal gland A11.5.00.010 **74**
Centromedian nucleus of thalamus A14.1.08.618 **121**
Cephalic vein A12.3.08.015 **96**
– of forearm A12.3.08.021 **96**
Ceratocricoid A06.2.08.005 **59**
– ligament A06.2.03.008 **58**
Ceratoglossus A05.1.04.104 **49**
Ceratopharyngeal part of middle constrictor A05.3.01.110 **51**
Cerebellar
– commissure A14.1.07.419 **120**
– cortex A14.1.07.402 **119**
– falx A14.1.01.106 **104**
– fissures A14.1.07.002 **118**
– fossa A02.1.04.037 **11**
– nuclei A14.1.07.406 **120**
– peduncles A14.1.07.412 **120**
– tentorium A14.1.01.104 **104**
– tonsillar branch A12.2.08.014 **84**
– veins A12.3.06.056 **95**
Cerebello-olivary fibres A14.1.05.328 **113, 116**
Cerebellopontine angle A14.1.05.004 **112**
Cerebellum A14.1.07.001 **118**
Cerebral
– aqueduct A14.1.06.501 **118**
– arterial circle A12.2.07.080 **83**
– cortex A14.1.09.003 **124**, A14.1.09.301 **128**
– crus A14.1.06.005 **115–116**
– falx A14.1.01.103 **104**
– fossa A02.1.04.036 **11**
– gyri A14.1.09.004 **124**
– hemisphere A14.1.09.002 **124**
– lobes A14.1.09.005 **124**
– part of internal carotid artery A12.2.06.015 **81**
– peduncle A14.1.06.004 **115–116**
– sulci A14.1.09.006 **124**
– surface
– – of sphenoid A02.1.05.025 **11**
– – of temporal bone A02.1.06.078 **13**
– veins A12.3.06.001 **94**
Cerebrospinal fluid A14.1.01.203 **105**
Cerebrum A14.1.09.001 **124**
Cervical
– branch of facial nerve A14.2.01.114 **135**
– canal A09.1.03.018 **66**
– enlargement A14.1.02.002 **105**
– fascia A04.2.05.001 **35**
– glands A09.1.03.020 **66**
– lordosis A02.2.00.006 **16**
– nerve plexus A14.2.02.012 **137**
– nerves [C1–C8] A14.2.02.002 **137**
– part
– – of internal carotid artery A12.2.06.002 **81**
– – of oesophagus A05.4.01.002 **51**
– – of spinal cord A14.1.02.014 **105**
– – of thoracic duct A12.4.01.009 **99**
– – of trachea A06.3.01.002 **59**
– – of vertebral artery A12.2.08.004 **84**
– pleura A07.1.02.006 **62**
– plexus A14.2.02.012 **137**
– rib A02.3.02.013 **18**
– segments [1–8] A14.1.02.014 **105**
– vertebrae [C I – C VII] A02.2.02.001 **16**
Cervicothoracic ganglion A14.3.01.020 **141**
Cervix
– of tooth A05.1.03.030 **48**
– of uterus A09.1.03.010 **65**
Chambers of eyeball A15.2.06.001 **146**
Check ligament of lateral rectus muscle A15.2.07.014 **147**
Cheek A01.1.00.008 **2**, A05.1.01.014 **47**
Chemically-defined cell groups A14.1.09.601 **131**
Chiasmatic
– branch of posterior communicating artery A12.2.07.072 **83**
– cistern A14.1.01.211 **105**
Chin A01.1.00.011 **2**
Choana/e A02.1.00.096 **9**, A06.1.02.003 **57**
Cholinergic cells A14.1.09.629 **132**
– of dorsal tegmental area [Ch5, Ch6, Ch8] A14.1.09.634 **132**
– of epithalamus [Ch7] A14.1.09.635 **132**
– of globus pallidus, accumbens nucleus and diagonal
– – band [Ch3] A14.1.09.632 **132**
– – gyrus [Ch2] A14.1.09.631 **132**
– of medial septal nuclei [Ch1] A14.1.09.630 **132**
– of substantia innominata, basal nucleus, amygdaloid body and olfactory tubercle [Ch4] A14.1.09.633 **132**
Chondrocranium A02.1.00.009 **8**
Chondroglossus A05.1.04.103 **49**
Chondropharyngeal part of middle constrictor A05.3.01.109 **51**
Chorda tympani A14.2.01.084 **135**, A14.2.01.118 **135, 142**, A14.3.02.012 **142**
Chordae tendineae of heart A12.1.00.023 **76**
Choroid A15.2.03.002 **144**

– blood vessels A15.2.03.008 **144**
– enlargement of lateral ventricle A14.1.09.283 **127**
– line of lateral ventricle A14.1.09.277 **127**
– membrane
– – of fourth ventricle A14.1.05.716 **115**
– – of third ventricle A14.1.01.305 **105, 121**
– plexus
– – of fourth ventricle A14.1.01.304 **105**, A14.1.05.715 **115**
– – of lateral ventricle A14.1.01.307 **105**, A14.1.09.279 **127**
– – of third ventricle A14.1.01.306 **105, 121**
Choroidal
– branch/es of anterior choroidal artery to
– – lateral ventricle A12.2.07.002 **82**
– – third ventricle A12.2.07.003 **82**
– of posterior inferior cerebellar artery to fourth ventricle A12.2.08.015 **84**
– enlargement A14.1.01.308 **105**
– fissure of lateral ventricle A14.1.09.278 **127**
Chyle cistern A12.4.01.012 **99**
Ciliary
– body A15.2.03.009 **144**
– bundle of palpebral part of orbicularis oculi A04.1.03.015 **34**
– ganglion A14.3.02.003 **142**
– glands A15.2.07.043 **147**
– margin of iris A15.2.03.022 **145**
– muscle A15.2.03.014 **144**
– part of retina A15.2.04.004 **145**
– plicae A15.2.03.012 **144**
– processes A15.2.03.011 **144**
– veins A12.3.06.107 **95**
– zonule A15.2.05.015 **146**
Cingular branch of callosomarginal artery A12.2.07.041 **83**
Cingulate
– gyrus A14.1.09.231 **126**
– sulcus A14.1.09.203 **126**
Cingulum of tooth A05.1.03.044 **48**
Circular
– fibres of ciliary muscle A15.2.03.018 **145**
– folds of small intestine A05.6.01.007 **52**
– muscle layer
– – of colon A05.7.03.017 **53**
– – of detrusor A08.3.01.018 **64**
– – of prostatic urethra A09.4.02.012 **70**
– – of rectum A05.7.04.015 **54**
– – of small intestine A05.6.01.006 **52**
– – of stomach A05.5.01.023 **52**
– – of urethra A09.2.03.008 **67**
– sulcus of insula A14.1.09.154 **125**
Circumduction A03.0.00.057 **26**
Circumferential pontine branches of pontine arteries A12.2.08.023 **84**
Circumflex
– branch of left coronary artery A12.2.03.206 **79**
– fibular branch of posterior tibial artery A12.2.16.056 **90**
– peroneal branch of posterior tibial artery A12.2.16.056 **90**
– scapular
– – artery A12.2.09.015 **86**
– – vein A12.3.08.007 **96**
Cistern/a A12.0.00.008 **75**
– ambiens A14.1.01.213 **105**
– chyli A12.4.01.012 **99**
– magna A14.1.01.208 **105**
– of great cerebral vein A14.1.01.217 **105**
– of lamina terminalis A14.1.01.216 **105**
– of lateral cerebral fossa A14.1.01.210 **105**
Claustrum A14.1.09.421 **129**
Clavicle A02.4.02.001 **19**
Clavicular
– branch of thoraco-acromial artery A12.2.09.008 **85**
– facet of scapula A02.4.01.010 **18**
– head of pectoralis major A04.4.01.003 **37**
– notch A02.3.03.003 **18**
– part of deltoid A04.6.02.003 **40**
Clavipectoral
– fascia A04.4.01.018 **37**
– triangle A01.2.03.004 **4**
Cleavage lines A16.0.00.008 **154**
Clinical
– crown of tooth A05.1.03.029 **48**
– root of tooth A05.1.03.033 **48**
Clitoris A09.2.02.001 **67**
Clivus A02.1.00.051 **8**, A02.1.04.006 **10**
– branches of cerebral part of internal carotid artery A12.2.06.021 **81**
Coccygeal
– body A12.2.12.011 **87**
– cornu A02.2.06.002 **17**
– foveola A01.2.05.004 **4**
– ligament A14.1.01.402 **105**
– nerve A14.2.07.043 **140**
– part of spinal cord A14.1.02.018 **105**
– plexus A14.2.07.044 **140**
– segments [1–3] A14.1.02.018 **105**
Coccygeus A04.5.04.011 **40**
Coccyx [coccygeal vertebrae I–IV] A02.2.06.001 **17**
Cochlea A15.3.03.025 **151**
Cochlear
– aqueduct A15.3.03.058 **152**
– area A15.3.03.053 **152**
– branch of vestibulocochlear artery A15.3.03.131 **153**
– canaliculus A02.1.06.042 **12**
– communicating branch of vestibular ganglion A14.2.01.124 **135**
– cupula A15.3.03.026 **151**
– duct A15.3.03.093 **152**
– ganglion A14.2.01.134 **136**
– labyrinth A15.3.03.091 **152**
– nerve A14.2.01.133 **136**
– nuclei
– – in medulla oblongata and pontile tegmentum A14.1.04.247 **111**
– – in pontile tegmentum A14.1.05.430 **114**
– recess A15.3.03.010 **151**
– septum A15.3.03.037 **151**
Coeliac
– branches of posterior vagal trunk A14.2.01.182 **137**
– ganglia A14.3.03.027 **143**
– lymph nodes A13.3.03.015 **102**
– nerve plexus A14.3.03.020 **143**
– plexus A14.3.03.021 **143**
– trunk A12.2.12.012 **87**
Coeliacoduodenal part of suspensory muscle of duodenum A05.6.02.013 **52**
Colic
– branch of ileocolic artery A12.2.12.064 **88**
– impression
– – on liver A05.8.01.021 **55**
– – on spleen A13.2.01.011 **100**
Collateral
– branch
– – of intercostal nerve A14.2.04.008 **139**
– – of posterior intercostal artery A12.2.11.017 **87**
– eminence of lateral ventricle A14.1.09.282 **127**
– ligaments
– – of interphalangeal joints
– – – of foot A03.6.10.902 **32**
– – – of hand A03.5.11.602 **30**
– – of metacarpophalangeal joints A03.5.11.502 **30**
– – of metatarsophalangeal joints A03.6.10.802 **32**
– sulcus A14.1.09.206 **126, 127**
– trigone A14.1.09.280 **127**
– vessel A12.0.00.026 **75**
Collicular artery A12.2.07.087 **84**
Colliculus of arytenoid A06.2.04.007 **58**
Colon A05.7.03.001 **53**
Column A14.1.00.007 **104**
– of fornix A14.1.08.420 **121, 127**
Commissural
– cusps of mitral valve A12.1.04.006 **77**
– fibre A14.1.00.017 **104**
– fibres of telencephalon A14.1.09.569 **131**
– nucleus
– – of solitary nuclei A14.1.04.232 **111**
– – of vagus nerve A14.1.04.252 **111**
Commissure/es A14.1.00.013 **104**

- of bulbs of vestibule
A09.2.01.014 **67**
- of fornix A14.1.09.260 **127**
- of inferior colliculus
A14.1.06.613 **118**
- of prostate A09.3.08.016 **69**
- of semilunar cusps
A12.1.02.016 **77**, A12.1.04.018 **77**
- - of aortic valve A12.1.04.018 **77**
- - of pulmonary valve
A12.1.02.016 **77**
- of superior colliculus
A14.1.06.614 **118**
Common
- anular tendon A15.2.07.015 **147**
- basal vein of lower lobe
- - of left lung A12.3.02.405 **92**
- - of right lung A12.3.02.205 **92**
- bony limb of semicircular canal
A15.3.03.020 **151**
- carotid
- - artery A12.2.04.006 **79**
- - nerve plexus A14.3.03.003 **142**
- cochlear artery A15.3.03.128 **153**
- fibular nerve A14.2.07.047 **140**
- flexor sheath of hand
A04.8.04.007 **44**
- hepatic
- - artery A12.2.12.015 **87**
- - duct A05.8.01.061 **56**
- iliac
- - artery A12.2.14.001 **89**
- - lymph nodes A13.3.04.003 **103**
- - vein A12.3.10.001 **97**
- interosseous artery
A12.2.09.047 **86**
- membranous limb of semicircular ducts A15.3.03.071 **152**
- modiolar vein A15.3.03.137 **153**
- nasal meatus A02.1.00.093 **9**, A06.1.02.031 **57**
- palmar digital
- - arteries A12.2.09.057 **86**
- - nerves
- - - of median nerve
A14.2.03.038 **138**
- - - of ulnar nerve
A14.2.03.046 **138**
- peroneal nerve A14.2.07.047 **140**
- plantar digital
- - arteries A12.2.16.068 **91**
- - nerves
- - - of medial plantar nerve
A14.2.07.067 **141**
- - - of lateral plantar nerve
A14.2.07.071 **141**
- tendinous
- - ring of extra-ocular muscles
A15.2.07.015 **147**
- - sheath
- - - of fibulares A04.8.06.011 **46**
- - - of peronei A04.8.06.011 **46**
Communicating
- branch/es A12.2.16.073 **91**
- - of anterior interosseous nerve with ulnar nerve
A14.2.03.037 **138**
- - of auriculotemporal nerve with facial nerve A14.2.01.078 **134**
- - of facial nerve with glossopharyngeal nerve
A14.2.01.107 **135**
- - of fibular artery
A12.2.16.073 **91**
- - of glossopharyngeal nerve with
- - - auriculotemporal nerve
A14.2.01.151 **136**
- - - chorda tympani
A14.2.01.152 **136**
- - - meningeal branch of vagus
A14.2.01.150 **136**
- - of internal laryngeal branch with recurrent laryngeal nerve A14.2.01.163 **136**
- - of lacrimal nerve with zygomatic nerve A14.2.01.019 **133**
- - of lingual nerve with hypoglossal nerve A14.2.01.083 **135**
- - of n. intermedius with tympanic plexus A14.2.01.119 **135**
- - of nasociliary nerve with cilary ganglion A14.2.01.026 **134**, **142**
- - of nervus intermedius with vagus nerve A14.2.01.120 **135**
- - of radial nerve with ulnar nerve
A14.2.03.057 **139**
- - of tympanic plexus with auricular branch of vagus nerve
A14.2.01.143 **136**
- - of vagus with glossopharyngeal nerve A14.2.01.143 **136**
- - with auricular branch of vagus nerve A14.2.01.143 **136**
- - with auriculotemporal nerve
A14.2.01.151 **136**
- - with chorda tympani
A14.2.01.152 **136**
- - with ciliary ganglion
A14.2.01.026 **134, 142**
- - with facial nerve
A14.2.01.078 **134**
- - with glossopharyngeal nerve
A14.2.01.107 **135**, A14.2.01.143 **136**
- - with hypoglossal nerve
A14.2.01.083 **135**
- - with meningeal branch
A14.2.01.150 **136**
- - with recurrent laryngeal nerve
A14.2.01.163 **136**
- - with tympanic plexus
A14.2.01.119 **135**
- - with ulnar nerve
A14.2.03.037 **138**, A14.2.03.057 **139**
- - with vagus nerve
A14.2.01.120 **135**
- - with zygomatic nerve
A14.2.01.019 **133**
Compact
- bone A02.0.00.003 **7**
- part
- - of pedunculopontine tegmental nucleus A14.1.06.337 **117, 118**
- - of substantia nigra
A14.1.06.112 **116**
- subnucleus of pedunculopontine tegmental nucleus
A14.1.06.337 **117, 118**
Compartment/s A04.0.00.030 **33**, A04.6.01.001 **40**, A04.7.01.001 **42**
Complex joint A03.0.00.042 **25**
Compressor urethrae ♀
A09.5.03.005 **71**
Concha of auricle
A15.3.01.013 **148**
Conchal crest
- of maxilla A02.1.12.019 **14**
- of palatine A02.1.13.009 **15**
Conducting system of heart
A12.1.06.002 **77**
Condylar
- canal A02.1.04.015 **10**
- emissary vein A12.3.05.304 **94**
- fossa A02.1.04.017 **10**
- joint A03.0.00.049 **25**
- process of mandible
A02.1.15.035 **16**
Condyle A02.0.00.029 **7**
- of humerus A02.4.04.021 **19**
Confluence of sinuses
A12.3.05.103 **93**
Conical lobules of epidiymis
A09.3.02.003 **68**
Conjoint tendon A04.5.01.020 **38**
Conjunctiva A15.2.07.047 **147**
Conjunctival
- glands A15.2.07.055 **147**
- ring A15.2.02.013 **144**
- sac A15.2.07.054 **147**
- veins A12.3.06.116 **95**
Conoid
- ligament A03.5.03.006 **28**
- tubercle A02.4.02.010 **19**
Contact zone of tooth
A05.1.03.043 **48**
Conus
- arteriosus A12.1.02.008 **76**
- branch
- - of left coronary artery
A12.2.03.203 **79**
- - of right coronary artery
A12.2.03.103 **79**
- elasticus A06.2.09.024 **59**
- medullaris A14.1.02.004 **105**
Convoluted seminiferous tubules
A09.3.01.022 **68**
Coraco-acromial ligament
A03.5.01.002 **28**
Coracobrachial bursa
A04.8.03.006 **44**
Coracobrachialis A04.6.02.017 **40**
Coracoclavicular ligament
A03.5.03.004 **28**
Coracohumeral ligament
A03.5.08.004 **29**
Coracoid process A02.4.01.023 **19**
Cord of umbilical artery
A12.2.15.026 **89**
Cords of brachial plexus
A14.2.03.009 **138**
Core region of nucleus accumbens
A14.1.09.441 **129**
Corium A16.0.00.010 **154**
Cornea A15.2.02.012 **144**

Corneal
– epithelium A15.2.02.018 **144**
– limbus A15.2.02.014 **144**
– vertex A15.2.02.015 **144**
Corneoscleral
– junction A15.2.02.014 **144**
– part of sclera A15.2.02.005 **144**
Corniculate
– cartilage A06.2.05.001 **58**
– tubercle A06.2.05.002 **58**, A06.2.09.004 **59**
Corona
– ciliaris A15.2.03.010 **144**
– of glans A09.4.01.008 **69**
– radiata A14.1.09.550 **131**
Coronal A01.0.00.004 **1**
– planes A01.2.00.001 **3**
– suture A03.1.02.002 **26**
Coronary
– ligament of liver A10.1.02.302 **72**
– sinus A12.3.01.002 **91**
– sulcus A12.1.00.011 **76**
Coronoid
– fossa A02.4.04.025 **19**
– process
– – of mandible A02.1.15.032 **15**
– – of ulna A02.4.06.003 **20**
Corpus
– albicans A09.1.01.016 **65**
– callosum A14.1.09.241 **127**
– – fibres A14.1.09.570 **131**
– cavernosum
– – of clitoris A09.2.02.005 **67**
– – penis A09.4.01.014 **69**
– luteum A09.1.01.015 **65**
– rubrum A09.1.01.014 **65**
– spongiosum penis A09.4.01.015 **69**
– striatum A14.1.09.515 **130**
Corrugator supercilii A04.1.03.018 **34**
Cortex
– corticis of kidney A08.1.01.017 **63**
– of lens A15.2.05.003 **146**
– of lymph node A13.2.03.005 **100**
– of suprarenal gland A11.5.00.007 **74**
– of thymus A13.1.02.004 **100**
Cortical
– amygdaloid nucleus A14.1.09.410 **129**
– bone A02.0.00.002 **7**
– labyrinth A08.1.01.016 **63**
– radiate
– – arteries of kidney A08.1.03.004 **63**
– – veins of kidney A08.1.04.004 **63**
Corticomesencephalic fibres A14.1.06.223 **117**
Corticonuclear fibres A14.1.06.104 **116**, A14.1.09.530 **130**
Corticopontine fibres A14.1.05.107 **112**, A14.1.06.105 **116**
Corticoreticular fibres A14.1.04.105 **109**, A14.1.05.106 **112**, A14.1.06.110 **116**, A14.1.09.533 **130**
Corticorubral fibres A14.1.09.534 **130**
Corticospinal fibres A14.1.04.103 **109**, A14.1.05.104 **112**, A14.1.06.103 **116**, A14.1.09.535 **130**
Corticotectal fibres A14.1.09.546 **131**
Corticothalamic fibres A14.1.09.536 **130**, A14.1.09.549 **131**
Costal
– arch A02.3.04.006 **18**
– cartilage A02.3.01.005 **17**
– groove A02.3.02.011 **18**
– margin A02.3.04.006 **18**
– notches A02.3.03.008 **18**
– part
– – of diaphragm A04.4.02.008 **38**
– – of parietal pleura A07.1.02.007 **62**
– process of lumbar vertebra A02.2.04.003 **17**
– surface
– – of lung A06.5.01.006 **60**
– – of scapula A02.4.01.002 **18**
Costocervical trunk A12.2.08.059 **85**
Costochondral joints A03.3.06.001 **28**
Costoclavicular ligament A03.5.04.005 **29**
Costodiaphragmatic recess A07.1.02.013 **62**
Costomediastinal recess A07.1.02.014 **62**
Costosternal joint A03.3.02.002 **28**
Costotransverse
– foramen A03.3.04.010 **28**
– joint A03.3.04.005 **28**
– ligament A03.3.04.006 **28**
Costovertebral joints A03.3.04.001 **28**
Costoxiphoid ligaments A03.3.05.005 **28**
Cotyloid joint A03.0.00.051 **25**
Coxal bone A02.5.01.001 **21**
Cranial A01.0.00.019 **1**
– arachnoid mater A14.1.01.204 **105**
– base A02.1.00.044 **8**
– cartilaginous joints A03.1.04.001 **27**
– cavity A01.1.00.048 **2**, A02.1.00.012 **8**
– dura mater A14.1.01.102 **104**
– fibrous joints A03.1.00.002 **26**
– nerve/s A14.2.00.038 **133**, A14.2.01.001 **133**
– part of parasympathetic part of autonomic division of nervous system A14.3.02.002 **142**
– pia mater A14.1.01.302 **105**
– root of accessory nerve A14.2.01.185 **137**
– sensory ganglion A14.2.00.007 **132**
– sutures A03.1.02.001 **26**
– synchondroses A03.1.05.001 **27**
– syndesmoses A03.1.01.001 **26**
– synovial joints A03.1.06.001 **27**
Craniocervical part of peripheral autonomic plexuses and ganglia A14.3.03.002 **142**
Craniospinal sensory ganglion A14.2.00.005 **132**
Cranium A02.1.00.001 **8**
Cremaster ♂ A04.5.01.018 **38**, A09.3.04.003 **68**
Cremasteric
– artery ♂ A12.2.16.007 **90**
– fascia ♂ A09.3.04.004 **68**
Crest A02.0.00.031 **7**
– of body of rib A02.3.02.012 **18**
– of greater tubercle A02.4.04.008 **19**
– of head of rib A02.3.02.004 **18**
– of lesser tubercle A02.4.04.009 **19**
– of neck of rib A02.3.02.006 **18**
– of round window A15.3.02.017 **149**
Cribriform
– area of renal papilla A08.1.01.030 **63**
– fascia A04.7.03.020 **43**
– foramina A02.1.07.003 **13**
– plate A02.1.07.002 **13**
Crico-arytenoid
– joint A06.2.04.014 **58**
– ligament A06.2.04.016 **58**
Crico-oesophageal tendon A05.4.01.011 **51**
Cricoid cartilage A06.2.03.001 **58**
Cricopharyngeal
– ligament A06.2.04.017 **58**
– part of inferior constrictor A05.3.01.113 **51**
Cricopharyngeus A05.3.01.113 **51**
Cricothyroid A06.2.08.001 **59**
– branch of superior thyroid artery A12.2.05.006 **80**
– joint A06.2.03.006 **58**
Cricotracheal ligament A06.2.03.010 **58**
Cricovocal membrane A06.2.09.024 **59**
Crista
– galli A02.1.07.004 **13**
– terminalis of right atrium A12.1.01.003 **76**
Crown of tooth A05.1.03.009 **48**
– pulp A05.1.03.052 **48**
Cruciate ligament of atlas A03.2.04.004 **27**
Cruciform
– eminence A02.1.04.028 **11**
– part of fibrous
– – sheath of digits of hand A04.8.04.017 **45**
– – sheaths of toes A04.8.06.016 **46**
Crura of antihelix A15.3.01.011 **148**
Crural interosseous nerve A14.2.07.060 **141**
Crus
– of clitoris A09.2.02.002 **67**

- of fornix A14.1.09.259 **127**
- of helix A15.3.01.006 **148**
- of penis A09.4.01.004 **69**
Cubital
- anastomosis A12.2.09.045 **86**
- fossa A01.2.07.010 **4**
- lymph nodes A13.3.01.011 **101**
- region A01.2.07.008 **4**
Cuboid A02.5.16.001 **24**
Culmen [IV and V] A14.1.07.112 **119**
Cuneate
- fasciculus A14.1.02.244 **107**, A14.1.04.016 **109**, A14.1.04.108 **109**
- nucleus A14.1.04.206 **110**
- transverse occipital fibres A14.1.09.567 **131**
- tubercle A14.1.04.017 **109**
Cuneiform
- cartilage A06.2.06.001 **58**
- nucleus A14.1.06.334 **117, 118**
- part of vomer A02.1.11.005 **14**
- tubercle A06.2.06.002 **58**, A06.2.09.005 **59**
Cuneocerebellar fibres A14.1.04.133 **110**
Cuneocuboid interosseous ligament A03.6.10.504 **31**
Cuneometatarsal interosseous ligaments A03.6.10.604 **32**
Cuneonavicular joint A03.6.10.301 **31**
Cuneospinal fibres A14.1.02.245 **108**
Cuneus A14.1.09.224 **126**
- fibres A14.1.09.567 **131**
Cupular
- caecum A15.3.03.120 **153**
- part of epitympanic recess A15.3.02.005 **149**
Cusp A12.0.00.021 **75**, A12.0.00.022 **75**
- of tooth A05.1.03.010 **48**
Cuspid A05.1.03.010 **48**
Cutaneous
- branch
- - of anterior branch of obturator nerve A14.2.07.014 **140**
- - of mixed nerve A14.2.00.024 **133**
- muscle A04.0.00.019 **33**
- vein A12.0.00.032 **75**
Cylindrical joint A03.0.00.044 **25**
Cymba conchae A15.3.01.014 **148**
Cystic
- artery A12.2.12.031 **87**
- duct A05.8.02.011 **56**
- lymph node A13.3.03.031 **102**
- vein A12.3.12.012 **98**
Cystohepatic triangle A10.1.02.428 **73**

D

Dartos
- fascia A09.4.03.003 **70**
- muscle A09.4.03.005 **70**
Deciduous teeth A05.1.03.076 **49**
Declive [VI] A14.1.07.203 **119**
Decussation A14.1.00.019 **104**
- of medial lemniscus A14.1.04.110 **109**
- of pyramids A14.1.04.004 **108**, A14.1.04.106 **109**
- of superior cerebellar peduncles A14.1.06.217 **116**
- of trochlear nerve fibres A14.1.06.615 **118**
Deep A01.0.00.034 **1**
- anterior cervical lymph nodes A13.3.00.019 **101**
- artery
- - of arm A12.2.09.020 **86**
- - of clitoris ♀ A12.2.15.045 **89**
- - of penis ♂ A12.2.15.045 **89**
- - of thigh A12.2.16.020 **90**
- auricular artery A12.2.05.054 **80**
- branch
- - of lateral plantar nerve A14.2.07.073 **141**
- - of medial
- - - circumflex femoral artery A12.2.16.023 **90**
- - - plantar artery A12.2.16.062 **91**
- - of radial nerve A14.2.03.054 **138**
- - of superior gluteal artery A12.2.15.015 **89**
- - of transverse cervical artery A12.2.08.057 **85**
- - of ulnar nerve A14.2.03.048 **138**
- cerebral veins A12.3.06.017 **94**
- cervical
- - artery A12.2.08.060 **85**
- - vein A12.3.04.017 **92**
- circumflex iliac
- - artery A12.2.16.008 **90**
- - vein A12.3.10.027 **97**
- dorsal vein
- - of clitoris ♀ A12.3.10.014 **97**
- - of penis ♂ A12.3.10.014 **97**
- external pudendal artery A12.2.16.014 **90**
- facial vein A12.3.05.027 **93**
- fascia of leg A04.7.03.021 **43**
- fibular nerve A14.2.07.055 **140**
- grey layer of superior colliculus A14.1.06.611 **118**
- head
- - of flexor pollicis brevis A04.6.02.057 **41**
- - of triceps brachii A04.6.02.022 **40**
- infrapatellar bursa A04.8.05.019 **45**
- inguinal
- - lymph nodes A13.3.05.007 **103**
- - ring A04.5.01.021 **38**
- investing fascia of abdomen A04.5.02.016 **39**
- layer
- - of levator palpebrae superioris A15.2.07.022 **147**
- - of temporal fascia A04.1.04.015 **35**
- lingual
- - artery A12.2.05.019 **80**
- - vein A12.3.05.013 **93**
- lymph
- - nodes of upper limb A13.3.01.014 **102**
- - vessel A12.0.00.040 **75**
- membranous layer of subcutaneous tissue A16.0.03.005 **155**
- middle cerebral vein A12.3.06.020 **94**
- palmar
- - arch A12.2.09.038 **86**
- - branch of ulnar artery A12.2.09.055 **86**
- parotid lymph nodes A13.3.00.005 **101**
- part
- - of anterior compartment of forearm A04.6.01.006 **40**
- - of external anal sphincter A04.5.04.015 **40, 54**
- - of masseter A04.1.04.004 **35**
- - of palpebral part of orbicularis oculi A04.1.03.016 **34**
- - of parotid gland A05.1.02.005 **47**
- - of posterior compartment of leg A04.7.01.008 **42**
- perineal
- - fascia A09.5.02.002 **71**
- - pouch A09.5.03.001 **71**
- - space A09.5.03.001 **71**
- peroneal nerve A14.2.07.055 **140**
- petrosal nerve A14.3.02.008 **142**
- plantar
- - arch A12.2.16.065 **91**
- - artery A12.2.16.054 **90**
- popliteal lymph nodes A13.3.05.013 **103**
- posterior sacrococcygeal ligament A03.2.08.003 **28**
- temporal
- - nerves A14.2.01.071 **134**
- - veins A12.3.05.038 **93**
- transverse
- - metacarpal ligament A03.5.11.504 **30**
- - metatarsal ligament A03.6.10.804 **32**
- - perineal muscle ♂ A09.5.03.004 **71**
- trigone A08.3.01.013 **64**
- vein/s A12.0.00.035 **75**
- - of clitoris ♀ A12.3.10.020 **97**
- - of lower limb A12.3.11.022 **98**
- - of penis ♂ A12.3.10.020 **97**
- - of thigh A12.3.11.024 **98**
- - of upper limb A12.3.08.028 **96**
- venous palmar arch A12.3.08.034 **96**
- white layer of superior colliculus A14.1.06.612 **118**
Deepest layer of subcutaneous tissue A16.0.03.006 **155**
Deferential
- nerve plexus A14.3.03.054 **143**
Deltoid A04.6.02.002 **40**
- branch

– – of profunda brachii artery A12.2.09.022 **86**
– – of thoraco-acromial artery A12.2.09.009 **85**
– fascia A04.6.03.004 **41**
– ligament A03.6.10.003 **31**
– region A01.2.07.002 **4**
– tubercle A02.4.01.006 **18**
– tuberosity A02.4.04.020 **19**
Deltopectoral
– lymph nodes A13.3.01.009 **101**
– triangle A01.2.03.004 **4**
Dens axis A02.2.02.202 **17**
Dental
– alveoli A03.1.03.008 **26**
– – of mandible A02.1.15.018 **15**
– – of maxilla A02.1.12.037 **14**
– branches
– – of inferior alveolar artery A12.2.05.057 **80**
– – of infra-orbital artery A12.2.05.080 **81**
– – of posterior superior alveolar artery A12.2.05.076 **81**
– papilla A05.1.03.054 **48**
– pulp A05.1.03.051 **48**
Dentate
– gyrus A14.1.09.237 **127**, A14.1.09.339 **128**
– nucleus A14.1.07.407 **120**
Denticulate
– ligament A14.1.01.310 **105**
– suture A03.0.00.013 **25**
Dentine A05.1.03.055 **48**
Dento-alveolar syndesmosis A03.1.03.001 **26**
Depression of optic disc A15.2.04.020 **145**
Depressor
– anguli oris A04.1.03.026 **34**
– labii inferioris A04.1.03.033 **34**
– septi nasi A04.1.03.012 **34**
– supercilii A04.1.03.019 **34**
Dermal ridges A16.0.00.004 **154**
Dermis A16.0.00.010 **154**
Descending
– aorta A12.2.10.001 **86**
– branch
– – of anterior segmental artery
– – – of left lung A12.2.01.207 **78**
– – – of right lung A12.2.01.106 **78**
– – of lateral circumflex femoral artery A12.2.16.029 **90**
– – of medial circumflex femoral artery A12.2.16.026 **90**
– – of occipital artery A12.2.05.036 **80**
– – of posterior segmental artery
– – – of left lung A12.2.01.210 **78**
– – – of right lung A12.2.01.109 **78**
– – of superior cervical artery A12.2.08.056 **85**
– colon A05.7.03.006 **53**
– genicular artery A12.2.16.017 **90**
– mesocolon A10.1.02.012 **72**
– palatine artery A12.2.05.084 **81**
– part
– – of duodenum A05.6.02.005 **52**
– – of iliofemoral ligament A03.6.07.005 **30**
– – of trapezius A04.3.01.002 **36**
Desmocranium A02.1.00.010 **8**
Desmodentium A03.1.03.006 **26**
Detrusor A08.3.01.014 **64**
Diagonal
– band A14.1.09.422 **129**
– conjugate A02.5.02.015 **22**
Diaphragm A04.4.02.001 **38**
Diaphragma sellae A14.1.01.107 **104**
Diaphragmatic
– constriction of oesophagus A05.4.01.005 **51**
– fascia A04.4.02.017 **38**
– part of parietal pleura A07.1.02.008 **62**
– surface
– – of heart A12.1.00.004 **75**
– – of liver A05.8.01.002 **54**
– – of lung A06.5.01.010 **60**
– – of spleen A13.2.01.007 **100**
Diaphysis A02.0.00.017 **7**
Diarthrosis A03.0.00.020 **25**
Diastema A05.1.03.078 **49**
Diencephalon A14.1.03.007 **108**, A14.1.08.001 **120**
Digastric A04.2.03.002 **35**
– branch of facial nerve A14.2.01.105 **135**
– fossa A02.1.15.009 **15**
Digits
– of foot A01.2.08.035 **6**
– of hand A01.2.07.026 **5**
Dilator
– muscle A04.0.00.029 **33**
– pupillae A15.2.03.030 **145**
Diploe A02.1.00.035 **8**
Diploic
– branch A12.2.06.038 **82**
– – of supra-orbital artery A12.2.06.038 **82**
– canals A02.1.00.036 **8**
– veins A12.3.05.201 **94**
Dissipated
– part of pedunculopontine tegmental nucleus A14.1.06.338 **117**
– subnucleus of pedunculopontine tegmental nucleus A14.1.06.338 **117**
Distal A01.0.00.036 **1**
– cusp A05.1.03.028 **48**
– deep inguinal lymph node A13.3.05.010 **103**
– fovea A05.1.03.063 **49**
– lateral striate branches of antero-lateral central arteries A12.2.07.050 **83**
– medial striate artery A12.2.07.034 **83**
– part
– – of prostate A09.3.08.005 **68**
– – of prostatic urethra A09.4.02.006 **70**
– phalanx
– – of foot A02.5.18.004 **24**
– – of hand A02.4.10.004 **21**
– radio-ulnar joint A03.5.10.001 **29**
– root A05.1.03.067 **49**
– surface of tooth A05.1.03.041 **48**
– transverse arch of foot A01.2.08.032 **5**
Distobuccal cusp A05.1.03.025 **48**
Distolingual cusp A05.1.03.027 **48**
Distopalatal cusp A05.1.03.026 **48**
Diverticula of ampulla of ductus deferens A09.3.05.007 **68**
Dome of pleura A07.1.02.006 **62**
Dopaminergic cells
– in arcuate nucleus [A12] A14.1.09.617 **132**
– in compact part of substantia nigra [A9] A14.1.09.611 **131**
– in medial zone and anterior area of hypothalamus [A14] A14.1.09.619 **132**
– in olfactory bulb [A15] A14.1.09.620 **132**
– in posterior hypothalamus [A11] A14.1.09.616 **132**
– in reticular formation [A8] A14.1.09.608 **131**
– in ventral tegmental area [A10] A14.1.09.614 **131**
– in zona incerta [A13] A14.1.09.618 **132**
Dorsal A01.0.00.014 **1**
– accessory
– – nucleus of optic tract A14.1.06.315 **117**
– – olivary nucleus A14.1.04.225 **110**
– acoustic stria A14.1.05.321 **113**
– artery
– – of clitoris ♀ A12.2.15.044 **89**
– – of foot A12.2.16.048 **90**
– – of penis ♂ A12.2.15.044 **89**
– branch/es
– – of lumbar artery A12.2.12.005 **87**
– – of medial occipital artery to corpus callosum A12.2.07.099 **84**
– – of posterior intercostal
– – – artery A12.2.11.008 **86**
– – – vein A12.3.07.015 **96**
– – of second posterior intercostal artery A12.2.08.064 **85**
– – of subcostal artery A12.2.11.021 **87**
– – of ulnar nerve A14.2.03.042 **138**
– – to corpus callosum A12.2.07.099 **84**
– calcaneocuboid ligament A03.6.10.515 **31**
– carpal
– – arch A12.2.09.033 **86**
– – branch
– – – of radial artery A12.2.09.032 **86**
– – – of ulnar atery A12.2.09.053 **86**
– – tendinous sheaths A04.8.04.008 **44**

- carpometacarpal ligaments A03.5.11.302 **29**
- cochlear nucleus A14.1.04.248 **111**
- column of spinal cord A14.1.02.239 **107**
- cuboideonavicular ligament A03.6.10.510 **31**
- cuneocuboid ligament A03.6.10.509 **31**
- cuneonavicular ligament A03.6.10.514 **31**
- digital
- - arteries
- - - of hand A12.2.09.035 **86**
- - - of foot A12.2.16.053 **90**
- - branches of radial nerve A14.2.03.058 **139**
- - nerves
- - - of deep fibular nerve A14.2.07.057 **140**
- - - of superficial fibular nerve A14.2.07.054 **140**
- - - of ulnar nerve A14.2.03.043 **138**
- - veins of foot A12.3.11.014 **98**
- external arcuate fibres A14.1.04.121 **109**
- fascia
- - of foot A04.7.03.030 **44**
- - of hand A04.6.03.009 **41**
- fasciculus proprius A14.1.02.240 **107**
- funiculus of spinal cord A14.1.02.239 **107**
- grey
- - column A14.1.02.114 **106**
- - commissure A14.1.02.304 **108**
- horn
- - of spinal cord A14.1.02.023 **106**, A14.1.02.115 **106**
- hypothalamic
- - area A14.1.08.916 **123**
- - region A14.1.08.916 **123**
- intercarpal ligaments A03.5.11.104 **29**
- intercuneiform ligament A03.6.10.508 **31**
- intermediate sulcus of spinal cord A14.1.02.012 **105**
- interossei
- - of foot A04.7.02.070 **43**
- - of hand A04.6.02.066 **41**
- lamella of principal olivary nucleus A14.1.04.221 **110**
- lateral geniculate nucleus A14.1.08.802 **123**
- lingual
- - branches of lingual artery A12.2.05.017 **80**
- - veins A12.3.05.010 **93**
- longitudinal fasciculus A14.1.04.114 **109**, A14.1.05.305 **112**, A14.1.06.211 **116**, A14.1.08.946 **124**
- median
- - septum of spinal cord A14.1.02.009 **105**
- - sulcus
- - - of medulla A14.1.04.020 **109**
- - - of spinal cord A14.1.02.008 **105**
- medullary veins A12.3.06.052 **95**
- metacarpal
- - arteries A12.2.09.034 **86**
- - ligaments A03.5.11.402 **29**
- - veins A12.3.08.025 **96**
- metatarsal
- - arteries A12.2.16.052 **90**
- - ligaments A03.6.10.703 **32**
- - veins A12.3.11.013 **98**
- nasal artery A12.2.06.049 **82**
- nerve
- - of clitoris ♀ A14.2.07.042 **140**
- - of penis ♂ A14.2.07.042 **140**
- nucleus/i A14.1.06.306 **117**, A14.1.06.315 **117**
- - of hypothalamus A14.1.08.921 **123**
- - of lateral lemniscus A14.1.05.432 **114**
- - of medial geniculate body A14.1.08.810 **123**
- - of pons A14.1.05.208 **112**
- - of thalamus A14.1.08.607 **121**
- - of vagus nerve A14.1.04.229 **110**
- pallidum A14.1.09.519 **130**
- pancreatic artery A12.2.12.042 **88**
- paraflocculаris [H VIII B] A14.1.07.219 **119**
- paragigantocellular reticular nucleus A14.1.04.313 **112**
- paramedian nucleus A14.1.04.228 **110**
- part/s
- - of anterior quadrangular lobule of cerebellum [H V] A14.1.07.118 **119**
- - of central
- - - lobule of cerebellum [III] A14.1.07.107 **119**
- - - reticular nucleus A14.1.04.315 **112**
- - of culmen [V] A14.1.07.115 **119**
- - of intertransversarii laterales lumborum A04.3.01.015 **36**
- - of lateral parabrachial nucleus A14.1.05.444 **114**
- - of wing of central lobule of cerebellum [H III] A14.1.07.110 **119**
- premammillary nucleus A14.1.08.934 **124**
- radiocarpal ligament A03.5.11.003 **29**
- rami
- - of cervical nerves A14.2.02.003 **137**
- - of lumbar nerves A14.2.05.002 **139**
- - of sacral nerves and coccygeal nerve A14.2.06.002 **139**
- - of thoracic nerves A14.2.04.002 **139**
- raphe nucleus A14.1.05.604 **115**, **117**
- region of foot A01.2.08.024 **5**
- root A14.2.00.030 **133**
- - ganglion A14.2.00.006 **132**
- scapular
- - artery A12.2.08.057 **85**, A12.2.08.058 **85**
- - nerve A14.2.03.011 **138**
- - vein A12.3.08.004 **96**
- septal nucleus A14.1.09.267 **127**, A14.1.09.444 **129**
- solitary nucleus A14.1.04.238 **111**
- spinocerebellar tract A14.1.02.227 **107**, A14.1.04.132 **110**
- striatum A14.1.09.517 **130**
- subdivision of nucleus of posterior commissure A14.1.06.312 **117**
- subnucleus of lateral parabrachial nucleus A14.1.05.444 **114**
- supra-optic commissure A14.1.08.947 **124**
- surface/s
- - of fingers A01.2.07.033 **5**
- - of sacrum A02.2.05.013 **17**
- - of toes A01.2.08.042 **6**
- tarsal ligaments A03.6.10.506 **31**
- tarsometatarsal ligaments A03.6.10.602 **31**
- tegmental
- - decussation A14.1.06.221 **117**
- - nucleus A14.1.05.449 **114**
- thalamus A14.1.08.101 **120**
- thoracic nucleus A14.1.02.135 **106**
- trigeminothalamic tract A14.1.05.312 **113**
- tubercle A02.4.05.017 **20**
- ulnocarpal ligament A03.5.11.005 **29**
- vein
- - of corpus callosum A12.3.06.037 **95**
- - of posterior intercostal vein A12.3.07.015 **96**
- venous
- - arch of foot A12.3.11.012 **98**
- - network
- - - of foot A12.3.11.011 **98**
- - - of hand A12.3.08.023 **96**
- visceral nucleus A14.1.06.306 **117**
- white
- - column A14.1.02.239 **107**
- - commissure A14.1.02.306 **108**

Dorsalis pedis artery A12.2.16.048 **90**

Dorsolateral
- nucleus
- - of pons A14.1.05.209 **112**
- - of spinal cord A14.1.02.108 **106**
- part of supra-optic nucleus A14.1.08.913 **123**

– solitary nucleus
A14.1.04.239 **111**
– sulcus
– – of medulla A14.1.04.012 **108**
– – of spinal cord A14.1.02.011 **105**
– tract A14.1.02.228 **107**
Dorsomedial
– nucleus
– – of dorsal hypothalamus
A14.1.08.917 **123**
– – of intermediate hypothalamus
A14.1.08.922 **123**
– – of pons A14.1.05.210 **112**
– – of principal sensory nucleus of trigeminal nerve
A14.1.05.407 **114**
– – of spinal cord A14.1.02.110 **106**
– – of thalamus A14.1.08.622 **122**
– part
– – of red nucleus
A14.1.06.326 **117**
– – of supra-optic nucleus
A14.1.08.914 **123**
Dorsum
– of foot A01.1.00.045 **2**, A01.2.08.024 **5**
– of hand A01.1.00.029 **2**, A01.2.07.021 **5**
– of nose A06.1.01.003 **57**
– of penis A09.4.01.005 **69**
– of tongue A05.1.04.004 **49**
– sellae A02.1.05.010 **11**
Downy hair A16.0.00.015 **154**
Duct
– of bulbo-urethral gland
A09.3.09.002 **69**
– of epididymis A09.3.02.006 **68**
Ductus
– deferens A09.3.05.001 **68**
– reuniens A15.3.03.081 **152**
Duodenal
– branches
– – of anterior superior pancreaticoduodenal artery
A12.2.12.027 **87**
– – of posterior superior pancreaticoduodenal artery
A12.2.12.020 **87**
– cap A05.6.02.003 **52**
– glands A05.6.02.017 **53**
– impression on liver
A05.8.01.020 **55**
Duodenojejunal
– flexure A05.6.02.009 **52**
– fold A10.1.02.410 **72**
Duodenomesocolic fold
A10.1.02.412 **73**
Duodenum A05.6.02.001 **52**
Dura mater A14.1.01.002 **104**, A14.1.01.101 **104**
Dural
– part of filum terminale
A14.1.01.402 **105**
– venous sinuses A12.3.05.101 **93**

E

Ear A01.1.00.005 **2**, A15.3.00.001 **148**
Efferent
– ductules A09.3.01.025 **68**
– glomerular arteriole of kidney
A08.1.03.006 **63**
– nerve fibres A14.2.00.018 **132**
Ejaculatory duct A09.3.07.001 **68**
Elbow A01.1.00.023 **2**
– joint A03.5.09.001 **29**
Ellipsoid joint A03.0.00.049 **25**
Elliptical recess A15.3.03.005 **151**
Emboliform nucleus
A14.1.07.409 **120**
Eminence A02.0.00.027 **7**
Eminentia
– conchae A15.3.01.029 **148**
– fossae triangularis
A15.3.01.031 **148**
– scaphae A15.3.01.030 **148**
Emissary
– vein/s A12.0.00.033 **75**, A12.3.05.301 **94**
Emptying internal urethral orifice
A09.4.02.002 **70**
Enamel A05.1.03.056 **48**
Endo-abdominal fascia
A04.5.02.006 **38**
Endocardium A12.1.05.001 **77**
Endocrine glands A11.0.00.000 **74**
Endolemniscal nucleus
A14.1.04.259 **111**
Endolymph A15.3.03.061 **152**
Endolymphatic
– duct A15.3.03.079 **152**
– sac A15.3.03.080 **152**
– space A15.3.03.060 **152**
Endometrium A09.1.03.027 **66**
Endomysium A04.0.00.043 **34**
Endoneurium A14.2.00.014 **132**
Endopeduncular nucleus
A14.1.08.918 **123**
Endopelvic fascia A04.5.03.007 **39**
Endosteum A02.0.00.038 **7**
Endothelium of anterior chamber of eyeball A15.2.02.022 **144**
Endothoracic fascia
A04.4.01.020 **37, 62**
Enteric
– nerve plexus A14.3.03.039 **143**
Ependyma A14.1.00.022 **104**
Epicardium A12.1.08.007 **78**
Epicondyle A02.0.00.030 **7**
Epicranial aponeurosis
A04.1.03.007 **34**
Epicranius A04.1.03.002 **34**
Epidermis A16.0.00.009 **154**
Epididymal branches of testicular artery ♂ A12.2.12.088 **88**
Epididymis A09.3.02.001 **68**
Epidural space A14.1.01.110 **104**, A14.1.01.112 **104**
Epigastric
– fold A10.1.02.434 **73**
– fossa A01.2.04.003 **4**
– region A01.2.04.003 **4**
Epiglottic
– cartilage A06.2.07.002 **58**
– tubercle A06.2.07.004 **58**
– vallecula A05.3.01.020 **50**
Epiglottis A06.2.07.001 **58**
Epimysium A04.0.00.041 **34**
Epinephric cells in area postrema and anterior reticular nucleus [C1, C2] A14.1.09.628 **132**
Epineurium A14.2.00.016 **132**
Epiphysial
– cartilage A02.0.00.019 **7**, A03.0.00.018 **25**
– line A02.0.00.021 **7**
– plate A02.0.00.020 **7**
Epiphysis A02.0.00.018 **7**
Epiploic foramen A10.1.02.403 **72**
Episcleral
– arteries A12.2.06.036 **82**
– layer A15.2.02.008 **144**
– space A15.2.07.006 **147**
– veins A12.3.06.114 **95**
Epithalamus A14.1.08.002 **120**, A14.1.08.501 **121**
Epitympanic recess
A15.3.02.004 **149**
Eponychium A16.0.01.010 **154**
Epoophoron A09.1.05.001 **66**
Equator
– of eyeball A15.2.01.004 **144**
– of lens A15.2.05.013 **146**
Erector spinae A04.3.02.002 **36**
– aponeurosis A04.3.02.003 **36**
Ethmoid A02.1.07.001 **13**
Ethmoidal
– bone A02.1.07.001 **13**
– bulla A02.1.07.015 **13**, A06.1.02.026 **57**
– cells A06.1.03.005 **57**
– crest
– – of maxilla A02.1.12.027 **14**
– – of palatine A02.1.13.010 **15**
– groove A02.1.10.002 **14**
– infundibulum A02.1.07.017 **13**, A06.1.02.027 **57**
– labyrinth A02.1.07.007 **13**
– notch A02.1.03.028 **10**
– process of inferior concha
A02.1.08.004 **13**
– veins A12.3.06.104 **95**
Ethmoidolacrimal suture
A03.1.02.020 **26**
Ethmoidomaxillary suture
A03.1.02.019 **26**
Excretory duct/s
– of lacrimal gland
A15.2.07.060 **148**
– of seminal gland
A09.3.06.005 **68**
Extension A03.0.00.059 **26**
Extensor A01.0.00.046 **1**
– carpi
– – radialis
– – – brevis A04.6.02.041 **41**
– – – longus A04.6.02.040 **41**
– – ulnaris A04.6.02.045 **41**
– compartment
– – of arm A04.6.01.003 **40**
– – of forearm A04.6.01.007 **40**
– – of leg A04.7.01.005 **42**
– – of thigh A04.7.01.002 **42**
– digiti minimi A04.6.02.044 **41**
– digitorum A04.6.02.042 **41**
– – brevis A04.7.02.055 **43**

– – longus A04.7.02.038 **42**
– hallucis
– – brevis A04.7.02.054 **43**
– – longus A04.7.02.040 **42**
– indicis A04.6.02.052 **41**
– muscle A04.0.00.024 **33**
– pollicis
– – brevis A04.6.02.050 **41**
– – longus A04.6.02.051 **41**
– retinaculum of hand A04.6.03.010 **41**
External A01.0.00.030 **1**
– acoustic
– – aperture A15.3.01.046 **149**
– – meatus A02.1.06.055 **13**, A15.3.01.045 **149**
– – opening A02.1.06.054 **13**
– – pore A15.3.01.046 **149**
– anal sphincter A04.5.04.012 **40, 54, 71**
– axis of eyeball A15.2.01.006 **144**
– branch
– – of accessory nerve A14.2.01.189 **137**
– – of superior laryngeal nerve A14.2.01.161 **136**
– capsule A14.1.09.551 **131**
– carotid
– – artery A12.2.05.001 **79**
– – nerve plexus A14.3.03.007 **143**
– – nerves A14.3.01.013 **141**
– conjugate A02.5.02.018 **22**
– ear A15.3.01.001 **148**
– granular layer of isocortex [Layer II] A14.1.09.310 **128**
– iliac
– – artery A12.2.16.002 **90**
– – lymph nodes A13.3.04.009 **103**
– – vein A12.3.10.024 **97**
– intercostal
– – membrane A03.3.01.002 **28, 37**
– – muscle A04.4.01.012 **37**
– jugular vein A12.3.05.045 **93**
– longitudinal layer of detrusor A08.3.01.017 **64**
– medullary lamina
– – of corpus striatum A14.1.09.508 **130**
– – of thalamus A14.1.08.660 **122**
– nasal
– – artery A12.2.06.049 **82**
– – branches of infra-orbital nerve A14.2.01.061 **134**
– – nerve A14.2.01.034 **134**
– – veins A12.3.05.023 **93**
– nucleus of inferior colliculus A14.1.06.604 **118**
– oblique A04.5.01.008 **38**
– occipital
– – crest A02.1.04.023 **11**
– – protuberance A02.1.04.022 **11**
– opening of carotid canal A02.1.06.014 **12**
– os of uterus A09.1.03.015 **66**
– palatine vein A12.3.05.029 **93**
– pudendal veins A12.3.11.004 **98**
– pyramidal layer of isocortex [Layer III] A14.1.09.311 **128**
– rotation A03.0.00.055 **25**
– spermatic fascia A09.3.04.002 **68**
– surface
– – of cochlear duct A15.3.03.095 **152**
– – of cranial base A02.1.00.053 **8**
– – of frontal bone A02.1.03.003 **10**
– – of parietal bone A02.1.02.007 **9**
– table of calvaria A02.1.00.034 **8**
– urethral
– – orifice A09.2.03.005 **67**, A09.4.02.030 **70**
– – sphincter ♀ A09.2.03.006 **67, 71**
– – sphincter ♂ A09.4.02.016 **70, 71**
– urinary meatus A09.4.02.030 **70**
Extra-ocular muscles A04.1.01.001 **34, 147**
Extracapsular ligaments A03.0.00.037 **25**
Extradural space A14.1.01.110 **104**
Extra-ocular part of central retinal
– artery A12.2.06.025 **81**
– vein A12.3.06.112 **95**
Extraperitoneal
– fascia A04.5.02.004 **38**, A04.5.03.005 **39**
– ligament A04.5.02.005 **38**, A04.5.03.006 **39**
– space A10.1.01.001 **72**
Extraserosal fascia A04.0.00.035 **33**
Extreme capsule A14.1.09.552 **131**
Extrinsic muscles of eyeball A04.1.01.001 **34, 147**
Eye A01.1.00.007 **2**, A15.2.00.001 **144**
Eyeball A15.2.01.001 **144**
Eyebrow/s A15.2.07.023 **147**, A16.0.00.017 **154**
Eyelash/es A15.2.07.037 **147**, A15.2.07.038 **147, 154**
Eyelids A15.2.07.024 **147**

F

Face A01.1.00.006 **2**
Facet
– for calcaneonavicular part of bifurcate ligament A02.5.10.005 **23**
– for dens A02.2.02.106 **16**
– for plantar calcaneonavicular ligament A02.5.10.004 **23**
– on atlas for dens A02.2.02.106 **16**
– on talus for
– – calcaneonavicular part of bifurcate ligament A02.5.10.005 **23**
– – plantar calcaneonavicular ligament A02.5.10.004 **23**
Facial
– area of internal acoustic meatus A15.3.03.048 **151**
– artery A12.2.05.020 **80**
– aspect A02.1.00.002 **8**
– canal A02.1.06.009 **12**
– colliculus A14.1.05.705 **115**
– lymph nodes A13.3.00.009 **101**
– muscles A04.1.03.001 **34**
– nerve [VII] A14.2.01.099 **135**
– region A01.2.01.008 **3**
– skeleton A02.1.00.008 **8**
– vein A12.3.05.018 **93**
Falciform
– ligament of liver A10.1.02.303 **72**
– margin of saphenous opening A04.7.03.017 **43**
– process of sacrotuberous ligament A03.6.03.006 **30**
False
– chordae tendineae of heart A12.1.00.024 **76**
– pelvis A02.5.02.005 **22**
– ribs [VIII–XII] A02.3.01.003 **17**
Falx
– cerebelli A14.1.01.106 **104**
– cerebri A14.1.01.103 **104**
Fascia A04.0.00.031 **33**
– iliaca A04.5.02.007 **39**
– lata A04.7.03.002 **43**
– of clitoris A09.2.02.007 **67**
– of head and neck A04.0.00.032 **33**
– of individual
– – abdominal organ A04.5.02.003 **38**
– – extraperitoneal
– – – abdominal organ A04.5.03.003 **39**
– – – pelvic organ A04.5.03.008 **39**
– – muscle A04.0.00.040 **34**
– – pelvic organ A04.5.03.003 **39**
– of limbs A04.0.00.037 **34**
– of lower limb A04.7.03.001 **43**
– of muscles A04.0.00.038 **34**
– of penis A09.4.01.026 **69**
– of trunk A04.0.00.033 **33**
– of upper limb A04.6.03.001 **41**
Fascial sheath of eyeball A15.2.07.004 **147**
Fascicle A14.1.00.012 **104**
Fasciculus A14.1.00.012 **104**
– peduncularis A14.1.09.427 **129**
– retroflexus A14.1.08.502 **121**
Fasciolar gyrus A14.1.09.233 **126**
Fastigial nucleus A14.1.07.411 **120**
Fastigiospinal tract A14.1.02.217 **107**
Fastigium A14.1.05.714 **115**
Fat body of ischio-anal fossa A09.5.04.002 **71**
Fatty
– appendices of colon A05.7.03.010 **53**
– layer of subcutaneous tissue A16.0.03.002 **155**
– – of abdomen A04.5.02.024 **39**
Fauces A05.2.01.001 **50**
Female
– external genitalia A09.2.00.001 **66, 71**
– genital system A09.0.00.001 **65**

– internal genitalia
A09.1.00.001 **65**
– urethra A08.4.01.001 **64, 67**
Femoral
– artery A12.2.16.010 **90**
– branch A14.2.07.010 **140**
– canal A04.7.03.012 **43**
– nerve A14.2.07.020 **140**
– – plexus A14.3.03.044 **143**
– nutrient arteries
A12.2.16.032 **90**
– region A01.2.08.006 **5**
– ring A04.7.03.014 **43**
– septum A04.7.03.015 **43**
– triangle A01.2.08.008 **5**,
A04.7.03.013 **43**
– vein A12.3.11.023 **98**
Femur A02.5.04.001 **22**
Fibre/Fiber A14.1.00.015 **104**
Fibres of stria terminalis
A14.1.08.948 **124**
Fibro-elastic membrane of larynx
A06.2.09.021 **59**
Fibrocartilaginous ring of tympanic
membrane A15.3.01.060 **149**
Fibromusculocartilaginous layer of
bronchus A06.4.02.027 **60**
Fibrous
– appendix of liver
A05.8.01.028 **55**
– capsule
– – of kidney A08.1.01.013 **63**
– – of liver A05.8.01.054 **55**
– – of spleen A13.2.01.002 **100**
– – of thyroid gland
A11.3.00.006 **74**
– joint A03.0.00.004 **25**
– layer
– – in or on deep aspect of fatty
layer of subcutaneous tissue
A16.0.03.004 **155**
– – of articular capsule
A03.0.00.027 **25**
– – of eyeball A15.2.02.001 **144**
– membrane A03.0.00.027 **25**
– pericardium A12.1.08.002 **78**
– sheath/s A04.8.01.006 **44**
– – of digits of hand
A04.8.04.015 **45**
– – of toes A04.8.06.014 **46**
Fibula A02.5.07.001 **23**
Fibular A01.0.00.041 **1**
– artery A12.2.16.071 **91**
– articular facet on tibia
A02.5.06.005 **23**
– border of foot A01.2.08.026 **5**
– collateral ligament
A03.6.08.011 **30**
– compartment of leg
A04.7.01.009 **42**
– lymph node A13.3.05.016 **103**
– notch A02.5.06.023 **23**
– nutrient artery A12.2.16.077 **91**
– tarsal tendinous sheaths
A04.8.06.010 **46**
– trochlea A02.5.11.014 **24**
– veins A12.3.11.033 **98**
Fibularis
– brevis A04.7.02.042 **42**
– longus A04.7.02.041 **42**
– tertius A04.7.02.039 **42**
Fifth toe [V] A01.2.08.040 **6**
Filiform papillae A05.1.04.014 **49**
Filling internal urethral orifice
A09.2.03.001 **67**, A09.4.02.001 **70**
Filum
– terminale A14.1.01.401 **105**
– – externum A14.1.01.402 **105**
– – internum A14.1.01.403 **105**
– terminale, spinal part
A14.1.02.005 **105**
Fimbria/e A14.1.09.332 **128**
– of hippocampus
A14.1.09.239 **127**,
A14.1.09.332 **128**
– of uterine tube A09.1.02.004 **65**
Fimbriated fold of tongue
A05.1.04.008 **49**
Fimbriodentate sulcus
A14.1.09.238 **127**
Fingers including thumb
A01.1.00.030 **2**, A01.2.07.026 **5**
First
– crus of ansiform lobule of cere-
bellum [H VII A]
A14.1.07.208 **119**
– posterior intercostal artery
A12.2.08.062 **85**
– rib [I] A02.3.02.014 **18**
Fissura antitragohelicina
A15.3.01.026 **148**
Fissure for
– ligamentum
– – teres A05.8.01.014 **54**
– – venosum A05.8.01.010 **54**
– round ligament A05.8.01.014 **54**
Fixed end A04.0.00.004 **33**
Flank A01.2.04.004 **4**
Flat
– bone A02.0.00.013 **7**
– muscle A04.0.00.007 **33**
Flexion A03.0.00.058 **26**
Flexor A01.0.00.045 **1**
– accessorius A04.7.02.068 **43**
– carpi
– – radialis A04.6.02.028 **41**
– – ulnaris A04.6.02.030 **41**
– compartment
– – of arm A04.6.01.002 **40**
– – of forearm A04.6.01.004 **40**
– – of leg A04.7.01.006 **42**
– – of thigh A04.7.01.003 **42**
– digiti minimi brevis
– – of hand A04.6.02.063 **41**
– – of foot A04.7.02.066 **43**
– digitorum
– – brevis A04.7.02.067 **43**
– – longus A04.7.02.052 **43**
– – profundus A04.6.02.036 **41**
– – superficialis A04.6.02.033 **41**
– hallucis
– – brevis A04.7.02.057 **43**
– – longus A04.7.02.053 **43**
– muscle A04.0.00.023 **33**
– pollicis
– – brevis A04.6.02.055 **41**
– – longus A04.6.02.037 **41**
– retinaculum
– – of foot A04.7.03.026 **43**
– – of hand A04.6.03.013 **41**
Floating ribs [XI–XII]
A02.3.01.004 **17**
Flocculonodular lobe
A14.1.07.301 **119**
Flocculus [H X] A14.1.07.304 **119**
Floor
– of fourth ventricle
A14.1.05.702 **115**
– of orbit A02.1.00.076 **9**
– of tympanic cavity
A15.3.02.006 **149**
Fold/s
– of chorda tympani
A15.3.02.066 **150**
– of incus A15.3.02.071 **150**
– of iris A15.2.03.027 **145**
– of left vena cava A12.1.08.010 **78**
– of stapedius A15.3.02.072 **150**
– of superior laryngeal nerve
A05.3.01.025 **50**
– of uterine tube A09.1.02.014 **65**
Foliate papillae A05.1.04.017 **49**
Folium/ia
– of cerebellum A14.1.07.003 **118**
– of vermis [VII A]
A14.1.07.206 **119**
Fontanelles A02.1.00.027 **8**
Foot A01.1.00.040 **2**
– region A01.2.08.022 **5**
Footplate A15.3.02.037 **150**
Foramen
– caecum
– – of frontal bone A02.1.03.018 **10**
– – of medulla oblongata
A14.1.04.002 **108**
– – of tongue A05.1.04.020 **49**
– lacerum A02.1.00.055 **8**
– magnum A02.1.04.002 **10**
– ovale A02.1.05.036 **11**,
A12.1.01.007 **76**
– petrosum A02.1.05.039 **11**
– rotundum A02.1.05.035 **11**
– singulare A15.3.03.052 **152**
– spinosum A02.1.05.038 **11**
– transversarium of cervical
vertebra A02.2.02.003 **16**
Foramina nervosa
A15.3.03.033 **151**
Forearm A01.1.00.024 **2**
Forebrain A14.1.03.006 **108**
Forehead A01.1.00.002 **2**,
A02.1.00.013 **8**
Foreskin A09.4.01.011 **69**
Fornix
– cerebrae A14.1.08.949 **124**,
A14.1.09.255 **127**
– of lacrimal sac A15.2.07.069 **148**
– of stomach A05.5.01.010 **51**
– of vagina A09.1.04.002 **??**
Fossa A02.0.00.034 **7**
– antihelica A15.3.01.028 **148**
– for gallbladder A05.8.01.013 **54**
– for lacrimal
– – – gland A02.1.03.026 **10**
– – – sac A02.1.00.082 **9**
– of incus A15.3.02.025 **149**

– of oval window
A15.3.02.010 **149**
– of round window
A15.3.02.016 **149**
– ovalis A12.1.01.005 **76**
Four-headed muscle
A04.0.00.014 **33**
Fourchette A09.2.01.008 **66**
Fourth
– toe [IV] A01.2.08.039 **6**
– ventricle A14.1.05.701 **115**
Fovea
– centralis A15.2.04.022 **145**
– for ligament of head
A02.5.04.003 **22**
Foveola A15.2.04.023 **145**
Free
– border
– – of nail A16.0.01.008 **154**
– – of ovary A09.1.01.005 **65**
– part
– – of lower limb A02.5.03.001 **22**
– – of upper limb A02.4.03.001 **19**
– taenia A05.7.03.016 **53**
Frenulum
– of clitoris A09.2.01.010 **66**
– of ileal orifice A05.7.02.004 **53**
– of labia minora A09.2.01.008 **66**
– of lower lip A05.1.01.011 **47**
– of prepuce A09.4.01.012 **69**
– of superior medullary vellum
A14.1.05.720 **115**,
A14.1.06.010 **115**
– of tongue A05.1.04.012 **49**
– of upper lip A05.1.01.010 **47**
– veli A14.1.05.005 **112**
Front of chest A01.1.00.015 **2**
Frontal A01.0.00.015 **1**
– angle of parietal bone
A02.1.02.015 **10**
– aspect A02.1.00.002 **8**
– belly of occipitofrontalis
A04.1.03.004 **34**
– bone A02.1.03.001 **10**
– border of parietal bone
A02.1.02.014 **10**
– branch
– – of middle meningeal artery
A12.2.05.063 **81**
– – of superficial temporal artery
A12.2.05.051 **80**
– crest A02.1.03.016 **10**
– diploic vein A12.3.05.202 **94**
– eminence A02.1.03.004 **10**
– forceps A14.1.09.250 **127**
– horn of lateral ventricle
A14.1.09.273 **127**
– lobe A14.1.09.110 **125–126**
– margin of sphenoid
A02.1.05.032 **11**
– nerve A14.2.01.020 **133**
– notch/foramen A02.1.03.010 **10**
– operculum A14.1.09.112 **125**
– planes A01.2.00.001 **3**
– pole A14.1.09.111 **125**
– process
– – of maxilla A02.1.12.024 **14**
– – of zygomatic A02.1.14.006 **15**
– region A01.2.01.002 **3**
– sinus A02.1.03.029 **10**,
A06.1.03.004 **57**
– suture A02.1.03.007 **10, 26**
– tuber A02.1.03.004 **10**
– veins A12.3.06.005 **94**
Fronto-ethmoidal suture
A03.1.02.014 **26**
Frontolacrimal suture
A03.1.02.016 **26**
Frontomaxillary suture
A03.1.02.015 **26**
Frontonasal suture
A03.1.02.013 **26**
Frontopontine fibres
A14.1.06.106 **116**, A14.1.09.528 **130**
Frontozygomatic suture
A03.1.02.017 **26**
Fundiform ligament
– of clitoris ♀ A04.5.02.023 **39, 67, 70**
– of penis ♂ A04.5.02.023 **39, 67, 70**
Fundus
– of bladder A08.3.01.004 **64**
– of gallbladder A05.8.02.002 **56**
– of internal acoustic meatus
A15.3.03.046 **151**
– of stomach A05.5.01.009 **51**
– of uterus A09.1.03.002 **65**
Fungiform papillae
A05.1.04.015 **49**
Funicular part of ductus deferens
A09.3.05.003 **68**
Funiculi of spinal cord
A14.1.02.013 **105**
Funiculus A14.1.00.010 **104**
– separans A14.1.05.711 **115**
Fusiform muscle A04.0.00.006 **33**

G

Gallbladder A05.8.02.001 **56**
– mucosa A05.8.02.009 **56**
Ganglion A14.2.00.002 **132**
– impar A14.3.01.037 **142**
– of sympathetic trunk
A14.3.01.003 **141**
Ganglionic
– branches
– – of lingual nerve to
– – – sublingual ganglion
A14.2.01.088 **135, 142**
– – – submandibular ganglion
A14.2.01.087 **135**
– – of mandibular nerve to otic ganglion A14.2.01.067 **134, 142**
– – of maxillary nerve to pterygopalatine ganglion
A14.2.01.039 **134, 142**
– – to otic ganglion
A14.2.01.067 **134, 142**
– – to pterygopalatine ganglion
A14.2.01.039 **134, 142**
– – to sublingual ganglion
A14.2.01.088 **135, 142**
– – to submandibular ganglion
A14.2.01.087 **135**
– layer of retina A15.2.04.016 **145**
Gastric
– areas A05.5.01.030 **52**
– branches
– – of left gastro-omental artery
A12.2.12.048 **88**
– – of right gastro-omental artery
A12.2.12.023 **87**
– canal A05.5.01.013 **52**
– folds A05.5.01.028 **52**
– glands A05.5.01.033 **52**
– impression
– – on liver A05.8.01.019 **54**
– – on spleen A13.2.01.010 **100**
– mucosa A05.5.01.027 **52**
– nerve plexuses A14.3.03.024 **143**
– pits A05.5.01.032 **52**
– rugae A05.5.01.028 **52**
Gastrocnemius A04.7.02.044 **43**
Gastrocolic ligament
A10.1.02.205 **72**
Gastroduodenal artery
A12.2.12.016 **87**
Gastropancreatic fold
A10.1.02.408 **72**
Gastrophrenic ligament
A10.1.02.202 **72**
Gastrosplenic ligament
A10.1.02.203 **72**
Gelatinous
– solitary nucleus
A14.1.04.233 **111**
– subnucleus of spinal nucleus of trigeminal nerve
A14.1.04.214 **110**
– substance of posterior horn of spinal cord A14.1.02.119 **106**
Gemellus
– inferior A04.7.02.014 **42**
– superior A04.7.02.013 **42**
Genicular
– anastomosis A12.2.16.040 **90**
– veins A12.3.11.030 **98**
Geniculate ganglion
A14.2.01.116 **135**
Geniculocalcarine fibres
A14.1.09.542 **130**
Geniculotemporal fibres
A14.1.09.545 **131**
Geniculum of facial
– canal A02.1.06.010 **12**
– nerve A14.2.01.100 **135**
Genioglossus A05.1.04.101 **49**
Geniohyoid A04.2.03.007 **35**
Genital
– branch A14.2.07.009 **140**
– systems A09.0.00.000 **65**
Genitofemoral nerve
A14.2.07.008 **139**
Genu
– of corpus callosum
A14.1.09.243 **127**
– of facial nerve A14.1.05.314 **113**
– of internal capsule
A14.1.09.529 **130**
Gigantocellular reticular nucleus
A14.1.04.302 **111**
Gingiva A03.1.03.003 **26**,
A05.1.01.108 **47**
Gingival

– branches of mental nerve A14.2.01.097 **135**
– groove A05.1.01.111 **47**
– margin A05.1.01.109 **47**
– papilla A05.1.01.110 **47**
– sulcus A05.1.01.111 **47**
Glabella A02.1.03.006 **10**
Glands
– of bile duct A05.8.02.019 **56**
– of mouth A05.1.02.001 **47**
Glandular branches
– of facial artery A12.2.05.024 **80**
– of inferior thyroid artery A12.2.08.045 **85**
Glans
– of clitoris A09.2.02.004 **67**
– penis A09.4.01.007 **69**
Glenohumeral
– joint A03.5.08.001 **29**
– ligaments A03.5.08.003 **29**
Glenoid
– cavity of scapula A02.4.01.019 **19**
– labrum of scapula A03.5.08.002 **29**
Globose nucleus A14.1.07.410 **120**
Globus pallidus
– external segment A14.1.09.509 **130**
– internal segment A14.1.09.511 **130**
– lateral segment A14.1.09.509 **130**
– medial segment A14.1.09.511 **130**
Glossopharyngeal
– nerve [IX] A14.2.01.135 **136**
– part of superior constrictor A05.3.01.107 **51**
Glottis A06.2.09.012 **59**
Gluteal
– aponeurosis A04.7.02.009 **42**
– fold A01.2.08.004 **5**
– lymph nodes A13.3.04.019 **103**
– region A01.2.08.002 **5**
– surface of ilium A02.5.01.116 **21**
– tuberosity A02.5.04.017 **22**
Gluteus
– maximus A04.7.02.006 **42**
– medius A04.7.02.007 **42**
– minimus A04.7.02.008 **42**
Gomphosis A03.0.00.006 **25**, A03.1.03.001 **26**
Gonion A02.1.00.021 **8**
Gracile
– fasciculus A14.1.02.243 **107**, A14.1.04.018 **109**, A14.1.04.107 **109**
– lobule A14.1.07.213 **119**
– nucleus A14.1.04.202 **110**
– tubercle A14.1.04.019 **109**
Gracilespinal fibres A14.1.02.246 **108**
Gracilis A04.7.02.030 **42**
Granular
– foveolae A02.1.00.039 **8**
– layer A14.1.07.403 **119**, A14.1.09.342 **128**
– – of cerebellar cortex A14.1.07.403 **119**
– – of dentate gyrus A14.1.09.342 **128**
Great
– auricular nerve A14.2.02.018 **137**
– cardiac vein A12.3.01.003 **91**
– cerebral vein A12.3.06.027 **94**
– saphenous vein A12.3.11.003 **98**
– toe [I] A01.2.08.036 **6**
Greater
– curvature of stomach A05.5.01.004 **51**
– horn of hyoid A02.1.16.004 **16**
– occipital nerve A14.2.02.008 **137**
– omentum A10.1.02.201 **72**
– palatine
– – artery A12.2.05.085 **81**
– – canal A02.1.00.057 **9**
– – foramen A02.1.00.058 **9**
– – groove A02.1.12.022 **14**, A02.1.13.006 **15**
– – nerve A14.2.01.045 **134**
– pancreatic artery A12.2.12.045 **88**
– pelvis A02.5.02.005 **22**
– petrosal nerve A14.2.01.117 **135**, **142**
– sciatic
– – foramen A03.6.03.008 **30**
– – notch A02.5.01.009 **21**
– splanchnic nerve A14.3.01.028 **141**
– supraclavicular fossa A01.2.02.011 **3**
– trochanter A02.5.04.005 **22**
– tubercle A02.4.04.005 **19**
– tympanic spine A02.1.06.056 **13**
– vestibular gland A09.2.01.016 **67**
– wing of sphenoid A02.1.05.024 **11**
Grey
– columns of spinal cord A14.1.02.101 **106**
– line A14.1.05.712 **115**
– matter/substance A14.1.00.002 **104**
– – of basilar part of pons A14.1.05.201 **112**
– – of medulla A14.1.04.201 **110**
– – of midbrain tegmentum A14.1.06.301 **117**
– – of pontile tegmentum A14.1.05.401 **113**
– – of spinal cord A14.1.02.020 **106**
– – of thalamus A14.1.08.602 **121**
– ramus communicans A14.3.01.006 **141**
Groin A01.2.04.006 **4**
Groove/s A02.0.00.035 **7**
– for arteries A02.1.02.006 **9**
– for extensor muscle tendons A02.4.05.018 **20**
– for greater petrosal nerve A02.1.06.025 **12**
– for inferior petrosal sinus A02.1.00.052 **8**, A02.1.04.008 **10**, A02.1.06.038 **12**
– for lesser petrosal nerve A02.1.06.027 **12**
– for marginal sinus A02.1.04.034 **11**
– for middle
– – meningeal artery A02.1.02.005 **9**
– – temporal artery A02.1.06.066 **13**
– for occipital sinus A02.1.04.033 **11**
– for popliteus A02.5.04.026 **22**
– for radial nerve A02.4.04.014 **19**
– for sigmoid sinus A02.1.02.003 **9**, A02.1.04.032 **11**, A02.1.06.006 **12**
– for spinal nerve A02.2.02.007 **16**
– for subclavian
– – artery A02.3.02.016 **18**
– – vein A02.3.02.017 **18**
– for subclavius A02.4.02.006 **19**
– for superior
– – petrosal sinus A02.1.06.030 **12**
– – sagittal sinus A02.1.00.038 **8**, A02.1.02.004 **9**, A02.1.03.017 **10**
– for tendon
– – of fibularis longus A02.5.11.013 **24**, A02.5.16.002 **24**
– – of flexor hallucis longus A02.5.10.017 **24**, A02.5.11.007 **24**
– – of peroneus longus A02.5.11.013 **24**, A02.5.16.002 **24**
– for transverse sinus A02.1.04.031 **11**
– for ulnar nerve A02.4.04.028 **19**
– for vena cava A05.8.01.009 **54**
– for vertebral artery A02.2.02.109 **17**
– of crus of helix A15.3.01.027 **148**
– of promontory of tympanic cavity A15.3.02.012 **149**
– of pterygoid hamulus A02.1.05.052 **12**
Growth plate A02.0.00.020 **7**
Gum A03.1.03.004 **26**, A05.1.01.108 **47**
Gustatory organ A15.4.00.001 **153**

H

Habenula A14.1.08.003 **120**
Habenular
– commissure A14.1.08.414 **121**
– sulcus A14.1.08.004 **120**
– trigone A14.1.08.005 **120**
Habenulo-interpeduncular tract A14.1.08.502 **121**
Hair
– crosses A16.0.00.027 **154**
– follicle A16.0.00.023 **154**
– streams A16.0.00.025 **154**
– whorls A16.0.00.026 **154**
Hairs A16.0.00.014 **154**
– of head A16.0.00.016 **154**
– of tragus A16.0.00.019 **154**

– of vestibule of nose A16.0.00.020 **154**
Hamate A02.4.08.012 **20**
Hamulus of spiral lamina A15.3.03.034 **151**
Hand A01.1.00.025 **2**
– region A01.2.07.017 **5**
Handle of malleus A15.3.02.044 **150**
Hard palate A05.1.01.103 **47**
Haustra of colon A05.7.03.009 **53**
Head
– of caudate nucleus A14.1.09.503 **130**
– of epididymis A09.3.02.002 **68**
– of femur A02.5.04.002 **22**
– of fibula A02.5.07.002 **23**
– of humerus A02.4.04.002 **19**
– of malleus A15.3.02.045 **150**
– of mandible A02.1.15.036 **16**
– of metacarpal A02.4.09.004 **20**
– of metatarsal A02.5.17.004 **24**
– of pancreas A05.9.01.002 **56**
– of phalanx
– – of foot A02.5.18.008 **24**
– – of hand A02.4.10.008 **21**
– of posterior horn of spinal cord A14.1.02.118 **106**
– of radius A02.4.05.002 **19**
– of rib A02.3.02.002 **18**
– of stapes A15.3.02.034 **149**
– of talus A02.5.10.002 **23**
– of ulna A02.4.06.015 **20**
Heart A12.1.00.001 **75**
Heel A01.1.00.042 **2**
– region A01.2.08.023 **5**
Helicine
– arteries of penis A09.4.01.024 **69**
– branches of uterine artery ♀ A12.2.15.030 **89**
Helicis
– major A15.3.01.037 **148**
– minor A15.3.01.038 **148**
Helicotrema A15.3.03.044 **151**
Helix A15.3.01.005 **148**
Hemi-azygos vein A12.3.07.004 **95**
Hemisphere of cerebellum [H II – H X] A14.1.07.004 **118**
Hepatic
– artery proper A12.2.12.029 **87**
– branches of anterior vagal trunk A14.2.01.177 **136**
– flexure A05.7.03.003 **53**
– lymph nodes A13.3.03.030 **102**
– nerve plexus A14.3.03.022 **143**
– portal vein A12.3.12.001 **98**
– segmentation: lobes, parts, divisions and segments A05.8.01.033 **55**
– veins A12.3.09.005 **97**
Hepato-oesophageal ligament A10.1.02.103 **72**
Hepatocolic ligament A10.1.02.106 **72**
Hepatoduodenal ligament A10.1.02.105 **72**
Hepatogastric ligament A10.1.02.104 **72**
Hepatopancreatic
– ampulla A05.8.02.017 **56**
– fold A10.1.02.409 **72**
Hepatophrenic ligament A10.1.02.102 **72**
Hepatorenal
– ligament A10.1.02.306 **72**
– recess of subhepatic space A10.1.02.427 **73**
Hiatus
– for greater petrosal nerve A02.1.06.024 **12**
– for lesser petrosal nerve A02.1.06.026 **12**
– semilunaris A02.1.07.018 **13**
Hidden
– border of nail A16.0.01.006 **154**
– part of duodenum A05.6.02.010 **52**
Highest
– nasal concha A06.1.02.012 **57**
– nuchal line A02.1.04.024 **11**
Hilum
– of dentate nucleus A14.1.07.408 **120**
– of inferior olivary nucleus A14.1.04.224 **110**
– of kidney A08.1.01.004 **63**
– of lung A06.5.01.015 **60**
– of lymph node A13.2.03.004 **100**
– of ovary A09.1.01.002 **65**
– of suprarenal gland A11.5.00.009 **74**
Hindbrain A14.1.03.002 **108**
Hinge joint A03.0.00.046 **25**
Hip A01.1.00.034 **2**
– bone A02.5.01.001 **21**
– joint A03.6.07.001 **30**
– region A01.2.08.005 **5**
Hippocampal
– commissure A14.1.09.571 **131**
– digitations A14.1.09.324 **128**
– sulcus A14.1.09.236 **126**
Hippocampus A14.1.09.321 **128**
– proper A14.1.09.327 **128**
Histological internal os A09.1.03.013 **65**
Hook of hamate A02.4.08.013 **20**
Horizontal A01.0.00.002 **1**
– fissure
– – of cerebellum A14.1.07.209 **119**
– – of right lung A06.5.01.022 **60**
– limb of diagonal band A14.1.09.423 **129**
– part
– – of duodenum A05.6.02.007 **52**
– – of middle cerebral artery A12.2.07.047 **83**
– planes A01.2.00.002 **3**
– plate of palatine A02.1.13.013 **15**
Humeral
– head
– – of extensor carpi ulnaris A04.6.02.046 **41**
– – of flexor carpi ulnaris A04.6.02.031 **41**
– – of pronator teres A04.6.02.026 **40**
– lymph nodes A13.3.01.004 **101**
– nutrient arteries A12.2.09.021 **86**
Humero-ulnar
– head of flexor digitorum superficialis A04.6.02.034 **41**
– joint A03.5.09.002 **29**
Humeroradial joint A03.5.09.003 **29**
Humerus A02.4.04.001 **19**
Hyaloid
– artery A15.2.06.009 **146**
– canal A15.2.06.010 **146**
– fossa A15.2.06.011 **146**
Hymen A09.1.04.008 **66**
Hymenal caruncles A09.1.04.009 **66**
Hyo-epiglottic ligament A06.2.07.006 **59**
Hyoglossus A05.1.04.102 **49**
Hyoid bone A02.1.16.001 **16**
Hypochondrium A01.2.04.002 **4**
Hypoconulid A05.1.03.028 **48**
Hypogastric nerve A14.3.03.047 **143**
Hypoglossal
– canal A02.1.04.016 **10**
– nerve [XII] A14.2.01.191 **137**
– trigone A14.1.05.708 **115**
Hyponychium A16.0.01.011 **154**
Hypopharynx A05.3.01.023 **50**
Hypophysial fossa A02.1.05.009 **11**
Hypothalamic
– branch of posterior communicating artery A12.2.07.077 **83**
– sulcus A14.1.08.427 **121**
Hypothalamohypophysial tract A14.1.08.950 **124**
Hypothalamospinal
– fibres A14.1.02.233 **107**, A14.1.04.126 **109**, A14.1.06.203 **116**
– tract A14.1.05.329 **113**
Hypothalamus A14.1.08.401 **120**, A14.1.08.901 **123**
Hypothenar eminence A01.2.07.024 **5**

I

Ileal
– arteries A12.2.12.058 **88**
– branch of ileocolic artery A12.2.12.063 **88**
– diverticulum A05.6.04.003 **53**
– orifice A05.7.02.003 **53**
– papilla A05.7.02.002 **53**
– veins A12.3.12.020 **99**
Ileocaecal
– fold A10.1.02.421 **73**
– lip A05.7.02.006 **53**
Ileocolic
– artery A12.2.12.059 **88**
– lip A05.7.02.005 **53**
– lymph nodes A13.3.03.036 **102**
– vein A12.3.12.024 **99**
Ileum A05.6.04.001 **53**
Iliac
– crest A02.5.01.106 **21**

– fascia A04.5.02.009 **39**, A04.7.03.009 **43**
– fossa A02.5.01.115 **21**
– nerve plexus A14.3.03.043 **143**
– tuberosity A02.5.01.122 **21**
Iliacus A04.7.02.003 **42**
– branch of iliolumbar artery A12.2.15.005 **89**
Ilio-inguinal nerve A14.2.07.006 **139**
Iliococcygeal raphe A04.5.04.018 **40**
Iliococcygeus A04.5.04.008 **40**
Iliocostalis A04.3.02.005 **36**
– cervicis A04.3.02.009 **36**
– lumborum A04.3.02.006 **36**
Iliofemoral ligament A03.6.07.003 **30**
Iliohypogastric nerve A14.2.07.003 **139**
Iliolumbar
– artery A12.2.15.002 **89**
– ligament A03.2.07.002 **27**
– vein A12.3.10.003 **97**
Iliopectineal
– arch A04.5.02.010 **39, 43**
– bursa A04.8.05.011 **45**
Iliopsoas A04.7.02.002 **42**
– fascia A04.5.02.007 **39**
Iliopubic
– eminence A02.5.01.307 **21**
– nerve A14.2.07.003 **139**
– ramus A02.5.01.307 **21**
– tract A04.5.02.013 **39**
Iliotibial tract A04.7.03.003 **43**
Ilium A02.5.01.101 **21**
Impression for costoclavicular ligament A02.4.02.004 **19**
Impressions of cerebral gyri A02.1.00.040 **8**
Incisal margin of tooth A05.1.03.046 **48**
Incisive
– bone A02.1.12.031 **14**
– canal/s A02.1.00.061 **9, 14**
– duct A06.1.02.033 **57**
– foramina A02.1.00.062 **9, 14**
– fossa A02.1.00.060 **9**
– papilla A05.1.01.107 **47**
– suture A02.1.12.032 **14**
Incisor tooth A05.1.03.004 **48**
Incisura of tentorium A14.1.01.105 **104**
Incudomallear joint A15.3.02.050 **150**
Incudostapedial joint A15.3.02.051 **150**
Incus A15.3.02.038 **150**
Index finger A01.2.07.028 **5**
Indusium griseum A14.1.09.246 **127**
Inferior A01.0.00.018 **1**
– aberrant ductule of epididymis A09.3.02.009 **68**
– alveolar
– – artery A12.2.05.056 **80**
– – nerve A14.2.01.089 **135**
– anal nerves A14.2.07.038 **140**
– anastomotic vein A12.3.06.010 **94**
– angle of scapula A02.4.01.016 **19**
– articular
– – facet of vertebra A02.2.01.017 **16**
– – process of vertebra A02.2.01.016 **16**
– – surface
– – – of atlas A02.2.02.104 **16**
– – – of tibia A02.5.06.024 **23**
– aspect A02.1.00.006 **8**
– basal vein of lower lobe
– – of left lung A12.3.02.410 **92**
– – of right lung A12.3.02.210 **92**
– belly of omohyoid A04.2.04.005 **35**
– border
– – of body of pancreas A05.9.01.012 **56**
– – of liver A05.8.01.024 **55**
– – of lung A06.5.01.014 **60**
– – of spleen A13.2.01.015 **100**
– branch/es
– – of oculomotor nerve A14.2.01.009 **133**
– – of superior gluteal artery A12.2.15.017 **89**
– – of transverse cervical nerve A14.2.02.023 **137**
– bulb of jugular vein A12.3.05.005 **93**
– calyx of kidney A08.1.05.006 **64**
– cerebellar peduncle A14.1.04.013 **109**, A14.1.07.413 **120**
– cerebral veins A12.3.06.013 **94**
– cervical
– – cardiac
– – – branches of vagus A14.2.01.165 **136**
– – – nerve A14.3.01.022 **141**
– – ganglion A14.3.01.019 **141**
– choroid vein A12.3.06.025 **94**
– clunial nerves A14.2.07.034 **140**
– colliculus A14.1.06.014 **115, 118**
– conjunctival fornix A15.2.07.053 **147**
– constrictor A05.3.01.111 **51**
– cortical branches of middle cerebral artery A12.2.07.055 **83**
– costal facet A02.2.03.003 **17**
– deep
– – branch of superior gluteal artery A12.2.15.017 **89**
– – lateral cervical lymph nodes A13.3.00.032 **101**
– dental
– – branches A14.2.01.092 **135**
– – nerve plexus A14.2.01.091 **135**
– – nerves A14.2.01.092 **135**
– diaphragmatic lymph nodes A13.3.03.012 **102**
– duodenal
– – flexure A05.6.02.006 **52**
– – fold A10.1.02.412 **73**
– – fossa A10.1.02.413 **73**
– epigastric
– – artery A12.2.16.003 **90**
– – lymph nodes A13.3.03.013 **102**
– – vein A12.3.10.025 **97**
– extensor retinaculum of foot A04.7.03.027 **43**
– extremity of kidney A08.1.01.009 **63**
– eyelid A15.2.07.026 **147**
– fascia of pelvic diaphragm A04.5.03.020 **39**
– fibular retinaculum A04.7.03.029 **44**
– fovea of sulcus limitans A14.1.05.726 **115**
– frontal
– – gyrus A14.1.09.113 **125**
– – sulcus A14.1.09.117 **125**
– ganglion
– – of glossopharyngeal nerve A14.2.01.137 **136**
– – of vagus A14.2.01.157 **136**
– gemellus A04.7.02.014 **42**
– genial spine A02.1.15.011 **15**
– gingival
– – branches A14.2.01.093 **135**
– – nerves A14.2.01.093 **135**
– gluteal
– – artery A12.2.15.018 **89**
– – line A02.5.01.119 **21**
– – lymph nodes A13.3.04.021 **103**
– – nerve A14.2.07.032 **140**
– – veins A12.3.10.006 **97**
– head of lateral pterygoid A04.1.04.008 **35**
– hemi-azygos vein A12.3.07.004 **95**
– horn
– – of falciform margin of saphenous opening A04.7.03.019 **43**
– – of lateral ventricle A14.1.09.287 **128**
– – of thyroid cartilage A06.2.02.011 **58**
– hypogastric nerve plexus A14.3.03.048 **143**
– hypophysial artery A12.2.06.012 **81**
– ileocaecal recess A10.1.02.420 **73**
– labial
– – branch of facial artery A12.2.05.025 **80**
– – veins A12.3.05.026 **93**
– laryngeal
– – artery A12.2.08.044 **85**
– – vein A12.3.04.004 **92**
– lateral
– – brachial cutaneous nerve A14.2.03.051 **138**
– – cutaneous nerve of arm A14.2.03.051 **138**
– – flexure of rectum A05.7.04.006 **54**
– – genicular artery A12.2.16.038 **90**
– ligament of epididymis A09.3.01.012 **67**
– limb of ansa cervicalis A14.2.02.015 **137**

– linear nucleus A14.1.06.402 **117**
– lingular
– – artery A12.2.01.212 **79**
– – bronchus [B V] A06.4.02.019 **60**
– – segment of left lung [S V] A06.5.02.019 **61**
– lip A05.7.02.006 **53**
– lobar arteries
– – of left lung A12.2.01.214 **79**
– – of right lung A12.2.01.113 **78**
– lobe A06.5.01.020 **60**
– – of left lung A06.5.02.020 **61**
– – of right lung A06.5.02.009 **61**
– longitudinal
– – fasciculus A14.1.09.556 **131**
– – muscle of tongue A05.1.04.107 **49**
– lumbar triangle A01.2.05.009 **4**
– lymph nodes A13.3.03.025 **102**
– macular
– – arteriole A15.2.04.042 **146**
– – venule A15.2.04.049 **146**
– medial genicular artery A12.2.16.039 **90**
– mediastinum A07.1.02.103 **62**
– medullary velum A14.1.05.721 **115**
– mental spine A02.1.15.011 **15**
– mesenteric
– – artery A12.2.12.069 **88**
– – ganglion A14.3.03.037 **143**
– – lymph nodes A13.3.03.043 **103**
– – nerve plexus A14.3.03.036 **143**
– – vein A12.3.12.032 **99**
– nasal
– – concha A02.1.08.001 **13**, A06.1.02.015 **57**
– – meatus A02.1.00.091 **9**, A06.1.02.029 **57**
– – retinal
– – – arteriole A15.2.04.040 **146**
– – – venule A15.2.04.047 **146**
– nodes A13.3.03.025 **102**
– nuchal line A02.1.04.026 **11**
– oblique A15.2.07.019 **147**
– occipitofrontal fasciculus A14.1.09.561 **131**
– olivary complex A14.1.04.219 **110**
– olive A14.1.04.008 **108**
– ophthalmic vein A12.3.06.117 **95**
– orbital fissure A02.1.00.084 **9**
– palpebral
– – arch A12.2.06.046 **82**
– – branches of infra-orbital nerve A14.2.01.060 **134**
– – veins A12.3.05.024 **93**
– pancreatic
– – artery A12.2.12.043 **88**
– – lymph nodes A13.3.03.026 **102**
– pancreaticoduodenal
– – artery A12.2.12.054 **88**
– – lymph nodes A13.3.03.029 **102**
– parathyroid gland A11.4.00.003 **74**
– parietal lobule A14.1.09.125 **125**
– part
– – of duodenum A05.6.02.007 **52**
– – of lingular vein A12.3.02.310 **92**
– – of trapezius A04.3.01.004 **36**
– – of vestibular ganglion A14.2.01.130 **136**
– – of wing of central lobule of cerebellum A14.1.07.109 **119**
– peroneal retinaculum A04.7.03.029 **44**
– petrosal sinus A12.3.05.113 **94**
– phrenic
– – artery A12.2.12.002 **87**
– – veins A12.3.09.002 **96**
– pole
– – of kidney A08.1.01.009 **63**
– – of testis A09.3.01.003 **67**
– pubic
– – ligament A03.6.02.004 **30**
– – ramus A02.5.01.313 **22**
– pulvinar nucleus A14.1.08.612 **121**
– recess of omental bursa A10.1.02.406 **72**
– rectal
– – artery A12.2.15.039 **89**
– – nerve plexus A14.3.03.050 **143**
– – nerves A14.2.07.038 **140**
– – veins A12.3.10.021 **97**
– rectus A15.2.07.011 **147**
– root of ansa cervicalis A14.2.02.015 **137**
– sagittal sinus A12.3.05.111 **94**
– salivatory nucleus A14.1.04.255 **111**
– segment of kidney A08.1.02.005 **63**
– segmental artery A12.2.12.082 **88**
– semilunar lobule of cerebellum A14.1.07.210 **119**
– sphincter A05.8.02.016 **56**
– subtendinous bursa of biceps femoris A04.8.05.023 **45**
– superficial inguinal lymph nodes A13.3.05.006 **103**
– suprarenal artery A12.2.12.077 **88**
– surface
– – of heart A12.1.00.004 **75**
– – of petrous part of temporal bone A02.1.06.040 **12**
– – of tongue A05.1.04.007 **49**
– synovial membrane of temporo-mandibular joint A03.1.07.006 **27**
– tarsal muscle A15.2.07.046 **147**
– tarsus A15.2.07.039 **147**
– temporal
– – gyrus A14.1.09.148 **125, 126**
– – line of parietal bone A02.1.02.009 **9**
– – retinal
– – – arteriole A15.2.04.038 **146**
– – – venule A15.2.04.045 **146**
– – sulcus A14.1.09.147 **125, 126**
– terminal branches of middle cerebral artery A12.2.07.055 **83**
– thalamic radiation A14.1.08.668 **122**
– thalamostriate veins A12.3.06.022 **94**
– thoracic aperture A02.3.04.004 **18**
– thyroid
– – artery A12.2.08.043 **85**
– – notch A06.2.02.006 **58**
– – tubercle A06.2.02.008 **58**
– – vein A12.3.04.002 **92**
– tibiofibular joint A03.6.05.001 **30**
– tracheobronchial lymph nodes A13.3.02.014 **102**
– transverse scapular ligament A03.5.01.004 **28**
– trunk of brachial plexus A14.2.03.006 **138**
– tympanic artery A12.2.05.013 **80**
– ulnar collateral artery A12.2.09.026 **86**
– vein of vermis A12.3.06.058 **95**
– veins of cerebellar hemisphere A12.3.06.060 **95**
– vena cava A12.3.09.001 **96**
– ventricular vein A12.3.06.024 **94**
– vertebral notch A02.2.01.010 **16**
– vesical artery A12.2.15.027 **89**
– vestibular
– – area of internal acoustic meatus A15.3.03.051 **151**
– – nucleus A14.1.04.243 **111**
Inferior basal vein of lower lobe of left lung A12.3.02.410 **92**
Inferodextral lateral flexure of rectum A05.7.04.006 **54**
Inferolateral
– lobule of prostate A09.3.08.012 **69**
– margin of cerebral hemisphere A14.1.09.012 **124**
– surface of prostate A09.3.08.009 **69**
Inferomedial margin of cerebral hemisphere A14.1.09.011 **124**
Inferoposterior lobule of prostate A09.3.08.011 **69**
Infra-auricular lymph nodes A13.3.00.007 **101**
Infra-orbital
– artery A12.2.05.078 **81**
– canal A02.1.12.004 **14**
– foramen A02.1.12.008 **14**
– groove A02.1.12.005 **14**
– margin A02.1.00.072 **9**
– – of maxilla A02.1.12.006 **14**
– nerve A14.2.01.059 **134**
– region A01.2.01.012 **3**
Infraclavicular
– fossa A01.2.03.003 **4**
– lymph nodes A13.3.01.009 **101**
– part of brachial plexus A14.2.03.020 **138**
Infraglenoid tubercle A02.4.01.021 **19**
Infraglottic cavity A06.2.09.018 **59**
Infrahyoid
– branch of superior thyroid artery A12.2.05.003 **79**

– bursa A04.8.02.004 **44**, A06.2.02.016 **58**
– lymph nodes A13.3.00.020 **101**
– muscles A04.2.04.001 **35**
Infralobar part of posterior branch of right superior pulmonary vein A12.3.02.109 **91**
Inframammary region A01.2.03.008 **4**
Infrapalpebral sulcus A01.2.01.011 **3**
Infrapatellar
– branch of saphenous nerve A14.2.07.024 **140**
– fat pad A03.6.08.018 **31**
– synovial fold A03.6.08.009 **30**
Infrascapular region A01.2.05.007 **4**
Infraspinatus A04.6.02.008 **40**
Infraspinous
– fascia A04.6.02.009 **40**
– fossa A02.4.01.008 **18**
Infrasternal angle A02.3.04.008 **18**
Infratemporal
– crest of sphenoid A02.1.05.028 **11**
– fossa A02.1.00.024 **8**
– surface
– – of maxilla A02.1.12.013 **14**
– – of sphenoid A02.1.05.027 **11**
Infratrochlear nerve A14.2.01.035 **134**
Infundibular
– nucleus A14.1.08.923 **123**
– recess A14.1.08.422 **121**
Infundibulopelvic ligament ♀ A09.1.01.018 **65, 73**
Infundibulum
– of gallbladder A05.8.02.003 **56**
– of pituitary gland A11.1.00.007 **74, 120**
– of right ventricle A12.1.02.008 **76**
– of uterine tube A09.1.02.003 **65**
Inguinal
– branches of deep external pudendal artery A12.2.16.016 **90**
– canal A04.5.01.026 **38**
– falx A04.5.01.020 **38**
– ligament A04.5.01.009 **38**
– lymph nodes A13.3.05.002 **103**
– part of ductus deferens A09.3.05.004 **68**
– region A01.2.04.006 **4**
– triangle A10.1.02.433 **73**
Inion A02.1.00.018 **8**
Inner
– border of iris A15.2.03.026 **145**
– layer of eyeball A15.2.04.001 **145**
– limiting layer of retina A15.2.04.018 **145**
– lip of iliac crest A02.5.01.110 **21**
– nuclear layer of retina A15.2.04.014 **145**
– plexiform layer of retina A15.2.04.015 **145**
– sheath of optic nerve A15.2.04.033 **146**
– spiral sulcus A15.3.03.123 **153**
– stripe of renal medulla A08.1.01.023 **63**
– zone of renal medulla A08.1.01.026 **63**
Innermost intercostal muscle A04.4.01.014 **37**
Innominate substance A14.1.09.426 **129**
Inserting periodontium A03.1.03.005 **26**
Insula A14.1.09.149 **125**
Insular
– arteries A12.2.07.054 **83**
– gyri A14.1.09.150 **125**
– lobe A14.1.09.149 **125**
– part of middle cerebral artery A12.2.07.053 **83**
– threshold A14.1.09.155 **125**
– veins A12.3.06.021 **94**
Interalveolar septa
– of mandible A02.1.15.019 **15**
– of maxilla A02.1.12.038 **14**
Interarytenoid
– fold of rima glottidis A06.2.09.017 **59**
– notch A06.2.09.006 **59**
Interatrial septum A12.1.00.019 **76**
Interbundle region of renal medulla A08.1.01.025 **63**
Intercalated nucleus A14.1.04.264 **111**
Intercapitular veins
– of foot A12.3.11.019 **98**
– of hand A12.3.08.024 **96**
Intercarpal joints A03.5.11.101 **29**
Intercartilaginous part of rima glottidis A06.2.09.016 **59**
Interchondral joints A03.3.07.001 **28**
Interclavicular ligament A03.5.04.006 **29**
Intercollicular vein A12.3.06.041 **95**
Intercondylar
– eminence A02.5.06.008 **23**
– fossa A02.5.04.028 **22**
– line A02.5.04.029 **23**
Intercostal
– lymph nodes A13.3.02.004 **102**
– nerves A14.2.04.006 **139**
– nodes A13.3.02.004 **102**
– space A02.3.04.007 **18**
Intercostobrachial nerves A14.2.04.012 **139**
Intercristal
– diameter A02.5.02.020 **22**
– distance A02.5.02.020 **22**
Intercrural
– fibres of superficial inguinal ring A04.5.01.016 **38**
– fissure of cerebellum A14.1.07.209 **119**
Intercuneiform
– interosseous ligaments A03.6.10.505 **31**
– joints A03.6.10.401 **31**
Interdental papilla A05.1.01.110 **47**
Interfascicular
– fasciculus A14.1.02.242 **107**
– nucleus
– – of hypoglossal nerve A14.1.04.306 **111**
– – of tegmentum of midbrain A14.1.06.331 **117**
Interfoveolar ligament A04.5.02.012 **39**
Interganglionic branches of sympathetic trunk A14.3.01.004 **141**
Intergeniculate leaf A14.1.08.807 **123**
Intergluteal cleft A01.2.08.003 **5**
Interiliac lymph nodes A13.3.04.016 **103**
Interlobar
– arteries of kidney A08.1.03.002 **63**
– cerebral sulci A14.1.09.102 **124, 125**
– surface of lung A06.5.01.011 **60**
– veins of kidney A08.1.04.002 **63**
Interlobular
– arteries
– – of kidney A08.1.03.004 **63**
– – of liver A05.8.01.057 **55**
– bile ducts A05.8.01.060 **56**
– veins
– – of kidney A08.1.04.004 **63**
– – of liver A05.8.01.058 **55**
Intermammary cleft A16.0.02.002 **154**
Intermaxillary suture A03.1.02.029 **26**
Intermediate A01.0.00.008 **1**
– acoustic stria A14.1.05.320 **113**
– atrial branch
– – of left coronary artery A12.2.03.210 **79**
– – of right coronary artery A12.2.03.107 **79**
– branch of hepatic artery A12.2.12.039 **88**
– cervical septum A14.1.01.311 **105**
– common iliac lymph nodes A13.3.04.005 **103**
– cuneiform A02.5.14.001 **24**
– deep inguinal lymph node A13.3.05.009 **103**
– dorsal cutaneous nerve A14.2.07.053 **140**
– external iliac lymph nodes A13.3.04.011 **103**
– ganglia A14.3.01.008 **141**
– grey
– – column A14.1.02.130 **106**
– – layer of superior colliculus A14.1.06.609 **118**
– – zone A14.1.02.130 **106**
– hepatic vein A12.3.09.007 **97**
– hypothalamic
– – area A14.1.08.920 **123**
– – region A14.1.08.920 **123**
– investing fascia of abdomen A04.5.02.017 **39**
– lacunar external iliac lymph node A13.3.04.014 **103**
– lateral flexure of rectum A05.7.04.005 **54**

– linear nucleus A14.1.06.403 **118**
– lumbar lymph nodes A13.3.03.007 **102**
– lymph node of vascular lacuna A13.3.04.014 **103**
– nerve A14.2.01.115 **135**
– nucleus of lateral lemniscus A14.1.05.433 **114**
– part of urethra A09.4.02.017 **70, 71**
– reticular nucleus A14.1.04.307 **111**
– sacral crest A02.2.05.016 **17**
– solitary nucleus A14.1.04.234 **111**
– supraclavicular nerves A14.2.02.026 **137**
– temporal branches of lateral occipital artery A12.2.07.096 **84**
– tendon A04.0.00.045 **34**
– white layer of superior colliculus A14.1.06.610 **118**
– zone
– – of iliac crest A02.5.01.109 **21**
– – of spinal grey A14.1.02.130 **106**
Intermediolateral nucleus of spinal cord A14.1.02.133 **106**
Intermediomedial
– frontal branch of callosomarginal artery A12.2.07.039 **83**
– nucleus of spinal cord A14.1.02.137 **106**
Intermediosinistral lateral flexure of rectum A05.7.04.005 **54**
Intermembranous part of rima glottidis A06.2.09.015 **59**
Intermesenteric nerve plexus A14.3.03.031 **143**
Intermetacarpal joints A03.5.11.401 **29**
Intermetatarsal
– joints A03.6.10.701 **32**
– spaces A03.6.10.705 **32**
Intermuscular
– gluteal bursae A04.8.05.009 **45**
– septum A04.3.02.004 **36**
– – of erector spinae A04.3.02.004 **36**
Internal A01.0.00.031 **1**
– acoustic
– – meatus A02.1.06.033 **12, 151**
– – opening A02.1.06.032 **12, 151**
– anal sphincter A05.7.05.011 **54**
– arcuate fibres A14.1.04.109 **109**
– axis of eyeball A15.2.01.007 **144**
– basilar nucleus of spinal cord A14.1.02.126 **106**
– branch
– – of accessory nerve A14.2.01.188 **137**
– – of superior laryngeal nerve A14.2.01.162 **136**
– capsule A14.1.09.524 **130**
– carotid
– – artery A12.2.06.001 **81, 83**
– – nerve A14.3.01.011 **141**
– – – plexus A14.3.03.004 **142**
– – venous plexus A12.3.05.308 **94**
– cerebral veins A12.3.06.028 **94**
– ear A15.3.03.001 **151**
– granular layer of isocortex [Layer IV] A14.1.09.312 **128**
– iliac
– – artery A12.2.15.001 **89**
– – lymph nodes A13.3.04.018 **103**
– – nodes A13.3.04.018 **103**
– – vein A12.3.10.004 **97**
– intercostal
– – membrane A03.3.01.003 **28, 37**
– – muscle A04.4.01.013 **37**
– jugular vein A12.3.05.001 **93**
– longitudinal layer of detrusor A08.3.01.019 **64**
– medullary lamina
– – of corpus striatum A14.1.09.510 **130**
– – of thalamus A14.1.08.661 **122**
– nasal branches
– – of anterior ethmoidal nerve A14.2.01.031 **134**
– – of infra-orbital nerve A14.2.01.062 **134**
– oblique A04.5.01.017 **38**
– occipital
– – crest A02.1.04.030 **11**
– – protuberance A02.1.04.029 **11**
– opening
– – of carotid canal A02.1.06.015 **12**
– – of cochlear canaliculus A15.3.03.036 **151**
– – of vestibular canaliculus A15.3.03.006 **151**
– pudendal
– – artery A12.2.15.038 **89**
– – vein A12.3.10.019 **97**
– pyramidal layer of isocortex [Layer V] A14.1.09.313 **128**
– rotation A03.0.00.056 **26**
– spermatic fascia A09.3.04.005 **68**
– surface
– – of cranial base A02.1.00.045 **8**
– – of frontal bone A02.1.03.015 **10**
– – of parietal bone A02.1.02.002 **9**
– table of calvaria A02.1.00.037 **8**
– thoracic
– – artery A12.2.08.029 **85**
– – veins A12.3.04.018 **92**
– urethral
– – orifice A08.3.01.027 **64, 67, 70**
– – sphincter A09.2.03.009 **67**, A09.4.02.013 **70**
– urinary meatus A08.3.01.028 **64, 67, 70**
Internasal suture A03.1.02.025 **26**
Interosseous
– border
– – of fibula A02.5.07.012 **23**
– – of radius A02.4.05.012 **20**
– – of tibia A02.5.06.019 **23**
– – of ulna A02.4.06.011 **20**
– cubital bursa A04.8.03.015 **44**
– intercarpal ligaments A03.5.11.106 **29**
– membrane A03.0.00.007 **25**
– – of forearm A03.5.06.002 **29**
– – of leg A03.6.05.002 **30**
– metacarpal
– – ligaments A03.5.11.404 **29**
– – spaces A03.5.11.405 **30**
– nerve of leg A14.2.07.060 **141**
– sacro-iliac ligament A03.6.03.003 **30**
Interparietal bone A02.1.04.013 **10**
Interpectoral lymph nodes A13.3.01.008 **101**
Interpeduncular
– cistern A14.1.01.212 **105**
– fossa A14.1.06.001 **115**
– nucleus A14.1.06.313 **117**
– veins A12.3.06.040 **95**
Interphalangeal joints
– of foot A03.6.10.901 **32**
– of hand A03.5.11.601 **30**
Interpolar part of spinal nucleus of trigeminal nerve A14.1.04.216 **110**
Interpositospinal tract A14.1.02.218 **107**
Interproximal surface of tooth A05.1.03.042 **48**
Interpubic
– disc A03.6.02.002 **30**
– fibrocartilage A03.6.02.002 **30**
Interradicular septa
– of mandible A02.1.15.020 **15**
– of maxilla A02.1.12.039 **14**
Intersegmental part
– of anterior
– – basal vein of lower lobe
– – – of left lung A12.3.02.409 **92**
– – – of right lung A12.3.02.209 **92**
– – vein of upper lobe
– – – of left lung A12.3.02.307 **92**
– – – of right lung A12.3.02.107 **91**
– of apical vein of upper lobe of right lung A12.3.02.104 **91**
– of apicoposterior vein of upper lobe of left lung A12.3.02.304 **92**
– of superior vein of lower lobe
– – of left lung A12.3.02.404 **92**
– – of right lung A12.3.02.204 **92**
Intersigmoid recess A10.1.02.417 **73**
Intersphincteric groove A05.7.05.012 **54**
Interspinales A04.3.02.301 **37**
– cervicis A04.3.02.304 **37**
– lumborum A04.3.02.302 **37**
– thoracis A04.3.02.303 **37**
Interspinous
– diameter A02.5.02.019 **22**
– distance A02.5.02.019 **22**
– ligaments A03.2.01.002 **27**
– plane A01.2.00.011 **3**
Interstitial
– amygdaloid nucleus A14.1.09.411 **129**
– nuclei
– – of anterior hypothalamus A14.1.08.905 **123**

– – of medial longitudinal fasciculus A14.1.05.438 **114**
– nucleus A14.1.06.307 **117**
– solitary nucleus A14.1.04.235 **111**
– subdivision of nucleus of posterior commissure A14.1.06.311 **117**
Interstitiospinal tract A14.1.02.210 **107**, A14.1.04.127 **109**, A14.1.05.330 **113**
Intertendinous connections of extensor digitorum A04.6.02.043 **41**
Interthalamic adhesion A14.1.08.103 **120, 121**
Intertragic
– incisure A15.3.01.019 **148**
– notch A15.3.01.019 **148**
Intertransversarii A04.3.02.401 **37**
– laterales lumborum A04.3.01.014 **36**
Intertransverse ligaments A03.2.01.004 **27**
Intertrochanteric
– crest A02.5.04.010 **22**
– diameter A02.5.02.021 **22**
– distance A02.5.02.021 **22**
– line A02.5.04.009 **22**
Intertubercular
– plane A01.2.00.010 **3**
– sulcus A02.4.04.007 **19**
– tendon sheath A04.8.04.002 **44**
Interureteric crest A08.3.01.025 **64**
Intervenous tubercle A12.1.01.014 **76**
Interventricular
– foramen A14.1.08.411 **120, 127**
– septal branches
– – of left coronary artery A12.2.03.205 **79**
– – of right coronary artery A12.2.03.109 **79**
– septum A12.1.00.013 **76**
Intervertebral
– disc A03.2.02.003 **27**
– foramen A02.2.01.008 **16**
– foramina A02.2.05.011 **17**
– joint A03.2.02.002 **27**
– surface A02.2.01.003 **16**
– vein A12.3.07.016 **96**
Intestinal
– glands
– – of large intestine A05.7.01.008 **53**
– – of small intestine A05.6.01.012 **52**
– lymphatic trunks A12.4.01.014 **99**
– surface of uterus A09.1.03.006 **65**
– trunks A12.4.01.014 **99**
– villi A05.6.01.011 **52**
Intra-articular
– ligament of head of rib A03.3.04.004 **28**
– sternocostal ligament A03.3.05.002 **28**
Intra-ocular part of optic nerve A15.2.04.028 **145**
Intrabiventral fissure A14.1.07.218 **119**
Intracapsular ligaments A03.0.00.035 **25**
Intracranial part
– of optic nerve A15.2.04.025 **145**
– of vertebral artery A12.2.08.010 **84**
Intraculminate fissure A14.1.07.114 **119**
Intraglandular lymph nodes of parotid A13.3.00.008 **101**
Intrajugular process A02.1.04.021 **11**, A02.1.06.046 **13**
Intralaminar
– nuclei of thalamus A14.1.08.615 **121**
– part of optic nerve A15.2.04.030 **145**
Intralobar part of posterior branch of right superior pulmonary vein A12.3.02.110 **91**
Intramural part
– of ureter A08.2.01.004 **64**
– of urethra ♀ A09.2.03.003 **67**
– of urethra ♂ A09.4.02.003 **70**
– of uterine tube A09.1.02.008 **65**
Intraocular part of central retinal
– artery A12.2.06.026 **81, 146**
– vein A12.3.06.113 **95, 146**
Intraparietal sulcus A14.1.09.127 **125**
Intrapulmonary
– blood vessels A06.5.01.023 **60**
– lymph nodes A13.3.02.016 **102**
– nodes A13.3.02.016 **102**
Intrarenal
– arteries A08.1.03.001 **63, 88**
– veins A08.1.04.001 **63, 97**
Intrasegmental
– bronchi A06.4.02.026 **60**
– part
– – of anterior basal vein of lower lobe
– – – of left lung A12.3.02.408 **92**
– – – of right lung A12.3.02.208 **92**
– – of apical vein of upper lobe of right lung A12.3.02.103 **91**
– – of apicoposterior vein of upper lobe of left lung A12.3.02.303 **92**
– – of superior vein of lower lobe
– – – of left lung A12.3.02.403 **92**
– – – of right lung A12.3.02.203 **92**
– – of vein of upper lobe
– – – of left lung A12.3.02.306 **92**
– – – of right lung A12.3.02.106 **91**
Intratendinous olecranon bursa A04.8.03.012 **44**
Intrathalamic fibres A14.1.08.669 **122**
Intratonsillar cleft A05.2.01.013 **50**
Investing
– abdominal fascia A04.5.02.015 **39**
– layer A04.0.00.039 **34**
– – of cervical fascia A04.2.05.002 **35**
Iridial part of retina A15.2.04.005 **145**
Iridocorneal angle A15.2.06.004 **146**
Iris A15.2.03.020 **145**
Irregular bone A02.0.00.014 **7**
Ischial
– spine A02.5.01.205 **21**
– tuberosity A02.5.01.204 **21**
Ischio-anal fossa A09.5.04.001 **71**
Ischiocavernosus A09.5.02.004 **71**
Ischiococcygeus A04.5.04.011 **40**
Ischiofemoral ligament A03.6.07.006 **30**
Ischiopubic ramus A02.5.01.007 **21**
Ischiorectal fossa A09.5.04.001 **71**
Ischium A02.5.01.201 **21**
Isocortex A14.1.09.307 **128**
Isthmus
– of cartilaginous auricle A15.3.01.024 **148**
– of cingulate gyrus A14.1.09.232 **126**
– of fauces A05.2.01.002 **50**
– of pharyngotympanic tube A15.3.02.076 **150**
– of prostate A09.3.08.016 **69**
– of thyroid gland A11.3.00.003 **74**
– of uterine tube A09.1.02.007 **65**
– of uterus A09.1.03.012 **65**

J

Jejunal
– arteries A12.2.12.057 **88**
– veins A12.3.12.019 **98**
Jejunum A05.6.03.001 **53**
Joint A03.0.00.001 **25**
– capsule A03.0.00.026 **25**
– of head of rib A03.3.04.002 **28**
Joints A03.0.00.000 **25**
– of foot A03.6.10.001 **31**
– of free
– – lower limb A03.6.04.001 **30**
– – upper limb A03.5.05.001 **29**
– of hand A03.5.11.001 **29**
– of lower limb A03.6.00.001 **30**
– of pectoral girdle A03.5.00.002 **28**
– of pelvic girdle A03.4.00.001 **30**
– of skull A03.1.00.001 **26**
– of upper limb A03.5.00.001 **28**
Jugular
– body A12.3.05.003 **93**
– foramen A02.1.00.054 **8**
– fossa A02.1.06.041 **12**
– lymphatic trunk A12.4.01.002 **99**
– nerve A14.3.01.010 **141**
– notch
– – of occipital bone A02.1.04.019 **10**
– – of petrous temporal bone A02.1.06.039 **12**, A02.1.06.045 **13**

– – of sternum A02.3.03.004 **18**
– process A02.1.04.020 **11**
– trunk A12.4.01.002 **99**
– tubercle A02.1.04.018 **10**
– venous arch A12.3.05.048 **93**
– wall A15.3.02.006 **149**
– – of tympanic cavity A15.3.02.006 **149**
Jugulo-omohyoid lymph node A13.3.00.033 **101**
Jugulodigastric lymph node A13.3.00.029 **101**
Jugum sphenoidale A02.1.05.003 **11**
Juxta-intestinal mesenteric lymph nodes A13.3.03.034 **102**
Juxta-oesophageal lymph nodes A13.3.02.017 **102**
Juxta-oral organ A05.1.01.016 **47**
Juxtacolic artery A12.2.12.068 **88**
Juxtarestiform body A14.1.04.119 **109**, A14.1.07.415 **120**

K

Kidney A08.1.01.001 **63**
– lobes A08.1.01.014 **63**
Knee A01.1.00.036 **2**
– joint A03.6.08.001 **30**
– region A01.2.08.010 **5**
Koniocellular layer of dorsal nucleus of lateral geniculate body A14.1.08.803 **123**

L

Labial
– branches of mental nerve A14.2.01.096 **135**
– commissure of mouth A05.1.01.012 **47**
– glands A05.1.02.014 **47**
– part of orbicularis oris A04.1.03.025 **34**
– surface of tooth A05.1.03.037 **48**
Labium
– majus A09.2.01.003 **66**
– minus A09.2.01.007 **66**
Labrum A03.0.00.025 **25**
Labyrinthine
– arteries A12.2.08.020 **84, 153**
– veins A12.3.05.114 **94, 153**
– wall of tympanic cavity A15.3.02.008 **149**
Lacrimal
– apparatus A15.2.07.056 **147**
– artery A12.2.06.027 **81**
– bone A02.1.09.001 **13**
– canaliculus A15.2.07.066 **148**
– caruncle A15.2.07.049 **147**
– fold A15.2.07.071 **148**
– fossa A02.1.03.026 **10**
– gland A15.2.07.057 **148**
– groove A02.1.00.081 **9**
– – in lacrimal bone A02.1.09.003 **14**
– – in maxilla A02.1.12.018 **14**
– hamulus A02.1.09.004 **14**
– lake A15.2.07.063 **148**
– margin of maxilla A02.1.12.020 **14**
– nerve A14.2.01.018 **133**
– notch A02.1.12.026 **14**
– nucleus A14.1.05.414 **114**
– papilla A15.2.07.064 **148**
– pathway A15.2.07.062 **148**
– process of inferior concha A02.1.08.002 **13**
– punctum A15.2.07.065 **148**
– sac A15.2.07.068 **148**
– vein A12.3.06.105 **95**
Lacrimoconchal suture A03.1.02.028 **26**
Lacrimomaxillary suture A03.1.02.027 **26**
Lactiferous
– duct A16.0.02.010 **154**
– sinus A16.0.02.011 **154**
Lacunar inguinal ligament A04.5.01.010 **38**
Lacunar-molecular layer of hippocampus A14.1.09.335 **128**
Lacus lacrimalis A15.2.07.063 **148**
Lambda A02.1.00.017 **8**
Lambdoid
– border of occipital bone A02.1.04.012 **10**
– suture A03.1.02.004 **26**
Lamina A14.1.00.008 **104**
– affixa A14.1.09.276 **127**
– cribrosa of sclera A15.2.02.011 **144**
– of cricoid cartilage A06.2.03.003 **58**
– of modiolus A15.3.03.040 **151**
– – cochleae A15.3.03.040 **151**
– of septum pellucidum A14.1.09.264 **127**
– of vertebral arch A02.2.01.007 **16**
– terminalis A14.1.08.419 **127**, A14.1.08.424 **121**
Large intestine A05.7.01.001 **53**
Laryngeal
– cartilages and joints A06.2.02.001 **58**
– cavity A06.2.09.001 **59**
– glands A06.2.09.020 **59**
– inlet A06.2.09.002 **59**
– mucosa A06.2.09.019 **59**
– muscles A04.2.07.001 **36, 59**
– prominence A06.2.02.003 **58**
– saccule A06.2.09.011 **59**
– ventricle A06.2.09.010 **59**
– vestibule A06.2.09.007 **59**
Laryngopharyngeal branches of superior cervical ganglion A14.3.01.014 **141**
Laryngopharynx A05.3.01.023 **50**
Larynx A06.2.01.001 **58**
Lateral A01.0.00.010 **1**
– abdominal cutaneous branch A14.2.04.011 **139**
– – of intercostal nerve A14.2.04.011 **139**
– accessory nucleus of optic tract A14.1.06.316 **117**
– ampullary nerve A14.2.01.129 **136**
– amygdaloid nucleus A14.1.09.412 **129**
– angle
– – of eye A15.2.07.033 **147**
– – of scapula A02.4.01.017 **19**
– antebrachial cutaneous nerve A14.2.03.026 **138**
– aortic lymph nodes A13.3.03.004 **102**
– aperture A14.1.05.718 **115**
– arcuate ligament A04.4.02.007 **38**
– aspect A02.1.00.005 **8**
– atlanto-axial joint A03.2.05.001 **27**
– atlanto-occipital ligament A03.1.08.005 **27**
– axillary lymph nodes A13.3.01.004 **101**
– basal
– – segment
– – – of left lung [S IX] A06.5.02.024 **61**
– – – of right lung [S IX] A06.5.02.013 **61**
– – segmental
– – – artery
– – – – of left lung A12.2.01.218 **79**
– – – – of right lung A12.2.01.117 **78**
– – – bronchus [B IX]
– – – – of left lung A06.4.02.024 **60**
– – – – of right lung A06.4.02.013 **60**
– bicipital groove A01.2.07.005 **4**
– bony ampulla A15.3.03.023 **151**
– border
– – of foot A01.2.08.026 **5**
– – of forearm A01.2.07.015 **5**
– – of humerous A02.4.04.018 **19**
– – of kidney A08.1.01.002 **63**
– – of nail A16.0.01.007 **154**
– – of scapula A02.4.01.013 **19**
– branch/es
– – of artery of tuber cinereum A12.2.07.075 **83**
– – of left
– – – coronary artery A12.2.03.204 **79**
– – – hepatic duct A05.8.01.066 **56**
– – of pontine arteries A12.2.08.023 **84**
– – of posterior ramus
– – – of cervical nerve A14.2.02.005 **137**
– – – of lumbar nerve A14.2.05.004 **139**
– – – of thoracic nerve A14.2.04.004 **139**
– – of sacral or coccygeal nerve A14.2.06.004 **139**
– – of superior cerebellar artery A12.2.08.028 **85**
– – of supra-orbital nerve A14.2.01.022 **133**

– – of umbilical part of left branch of portal vein A12.3.12.009 **98**
– bulboreticulospinal tract A14.1.04.129 **109**
– calcaneal branches of sural nerve A14.2.07.064 **141**
– caval lymph nodes A13.3.03.009 **102**
– cerebellomedullary cistern A14.1.01.209 **105**
– cerebral
– – fossa A14.1.09.009 **124**
– – sulcus A14.1.09.104 **124**
– cervical
– – lymph nodes A13.3.00.026 **101**
– – nucleus A14.1.02.127 **106**
– – region A01.2.02.009 **3**
– circumflex femoral
– – artery A12.2.16.027 **90**
– – veins A12.3.11.026 **98**
– common iliac lymph nodes A13.3.04.006 **103**
– compartment of leg A04.7.01.009 **42**
– condyle
– – of femur A02.5.04.024 **22**
– – of tibia A02.5.06.004 **23**
– cord of brachial plexus A14.2.03.021 **138**
– corticospinal tract A14.1.02.219 **107**
– costal branch of internal thoracic artery A12.2.08.038 **85**
– costotransverse ligament A03.3.04.008 **28**
– crico-arytenoid A06.2.08.006 **59**
– crus
– – of major alar cartilage of nose A06.1.01.010 **57**
– – of superficial inguinal ring A04.5.01.015 **38**
– cuneiform A02.5.15.001 **24**
– cutaneous
– – branch
– – – of dorsal branch of posterior intercostal artery A12.2.11.010 **86**
– – – of iliohypogastric nerve A14.2.07.004 **139**
– – – of posterior intercostal artery A12.2.11.018 **87**
– – nerve
– – – of forearm A14.2.03.026 **138**
– – – of thigh A14.2.07.011 **140**
– direct veins of lateral ventricle A12.3.06.036 **95**
– division of lumbar erector spinae A04.3.02.007 **36**
– dorsal
– – cutaneous nerve A14.2.07.063 **141**
– – nucleus of thalamus A14.1.08.608 **121**
– epicondyle
– – of femur A02.5.04.025 **22**
– – of humerus A02.4.04.029 **19**
– external iliac lymph nodes A13.3.04.012 **103**
– fasciculus proprius A14.1.02.216 **107**
– femoral
– – cutaneous nerve A14.2.07.011 **140**
– – intermuscular septum A04.7.03.004 **43**
– fibres of vertical occipital fasciculi A14.1.09.564 **131**
– flexures of rectum A05.7.04.003 **53**
– fornix of vagina A09.1.04.005 **66**
– frontobasal artery A12.2.07.062 **83**
– funiculus
– – of medulla A14.1.04.007 **108**
– – of spinal cord A14.1.02.215 **107**
– geniculate body A14.1.08.302 **120**
– glandular branch of superior thyroid artery A12.2.05.009 **80**
– glosso-epiglottic fold A05.3.01.022 **50**
– groove of midbrain A14.1.06.006 **115**
– habenular nucleus A14.1.08.503 **121**
– head
– – of flexor hallucis brevis A04.7.02.059 **43**
– – of gastrocnemius A04.7.02.045 **43**
– – of triceps brachii A04.6.02.021 **40**
– horn
– – of spinal cord A14.1.02.022 **106**, A14.1.02.132 **106**
– hypothalamic area A14.1.08.929 **124**
– inguinal fossa A10.1.02.435 **73**
– intercondylar tubercle A02.5.06.010 **23**
– intermediate
– – grey matter of spinal cord A14.1.02.136 **106**
– – substance A14.1.02.136 **106**
– intermuscular septum of arm A04.6.03.007 **41**
– internal nasal branches of anterior ethmoidal nerve A14.2.01.032 **134**
– jugulo-omohyoid lymph node A13.3.00.034 **101**
– jugulodigastric lymph node A13.3.00.030 **101**
– lacunae of superior sagittal sinus A12.3.05.110 **94**
– lacunar external iliac lymph node A13.3.04.015 **103**
– lamella of principal olivary nucleus A14.1.04.223 **110**
– lamina of cartilage of pharyngotympanic tube A15.3.02.081 **150**
– lemniscus A14.1.05.317 **113**, A14.1.06.204 **116**, A14.1.08.670 **122**
– ligament
– – of ankle joint A03.6.10.008 **31**
– – of bladder A04.5.03.016 **39**
– – of malleus A15.3.02.056 **150**
– – of rectum A05.7.04.016 **54**
– – of temporomandibular joint A03.1.07.003 **27**
– lip
– – of bicipital groove A02.4.04.008 **19**
– – of linea aspera A02.5.04.014 **22**
– longitudinal stria A14.1.09.247 **127**
– lymph node of vascular lacuna A13.3.04.015 **103**
– malleolar
– – arterial network A12.2.16.047 **90**
– – branches of fibular artery A12.2.16.074 **91**
– – facet of talus A02.5.10.013 **24**
– malleolus A02.5.07.014 **23**
– mammary branches
– – of intercostal nerve A14.2.04.010 **139**
– – of lateral
– – – cutaneous branch of posterior intercostal artery A12.2.11.019 **87**
– – – thoracic artery A12.2.09.012 **85**
– margin
– – of humerus A02.4.04.018 **19**
– – of orbit A02.1.00.073 **9**
– marginal vein of foot A12.3.11.020 **98**
– mass of atlas A02.2.02.102 **16**
– medullary
– – branches of vertebral artery A12.2.08.018 **84**
– – lamina of corpus striatum A14.1.09.508 **130**
– membranous ampulla A15.3.03.074 **152**
– meniscus A03.6.08.002 **30**
– mesencephalic vein A12.3.06.042 **95**
– nasal branch/es
– – of facial artery A12.2.05.028 **80**
– – of anterior ethmoidal nerve A14.2.01.032 **134**
– nucleus/i
– – of mammillary body A14.1.08.935 **124**
– – of medial dorsal nucleus of thalamus A14.1.08.623 **122**
– – of pons A14.1.05.204 **112**
– – of trapezoid body A14.1.05.423 **114**
– occipital artery A12.2.07.094 **84**
– occipitotemporal gyrus A14.1.09.227 **126**
– olfactory
– – gyrus A14.1.09.220 **126**
– – stria A14.1.09.436 **129**
– orbitofrontal artery A12.2.07.062 **83**
– palpebral

– – arteries A12.2.06.029 **82**
– – commissure A15.2.07.031 **147**
– – ligament A15.2.07.040 **147**
– parabrachial nucleus A14.1.05.441 **114**
– paragigantocellular reticular nucleus A14.1.04.305 **111**
– part
– – of biventral lobule A14.1.07.217 **119**
– – of globus pallidus A14.1.09.512 **130**
– – of lateral parabrachial nucleus A14.1.05.442 **114**
– – of longitudinal arch of foot A01.2.08.029 **5**
– – of medial parabrachial nucleus A14.1.05.448 **114**
– – of middle lobe vein of right lung A12.3.02.112 **91**
– – of nucleus accumbens A14.1.09.441 **129**
– – of occipital bone A02.1.04.009 **10**
– – of posterior compartment of forearm A04.6.01.008 **40**
– – of sacrum A02.2.05.006 **17**
– – of substantia nigra A14.1.06.113 **116**
– – of vagina A09.1.04.005 **66**
– patellar retinaculum A03.6.08.017 **31**
– pectoral
– – cutaneous branch of intercostal nerve A14.2.04.009 **139**
– – nerve A14.2.03.018 **138**
– – region A01.2.03.006 **4**
– pericardial lymph nodes A13.3.02.010 **102**
– pericuneate nucleus A14.1.04.261 **111**
– periolivary nuclei A14.1.05.420 **114**
– pharyngeal space A05.3.01.119 **51**
– plantar
– – artery A12.2.16.064 **91**
– – nerve A14.2.07.069 **141**
– plate of sphenoid A02.1.05.043 **12**
– pontine vein A12.3.06.047 **95**
– posterior
– – cervical intertransversarii A04.3.01.013 **36**
– – nucleus of thalamus A14.1.08.609 **121**
– preoptic nucleus A14.1.08.906 **123**
– process
– – of calcaneal tuberosity A02.5.11.004 **24**
– – of malleus A15.3.02.047 **150**
– – of septal nasal cartilage A06.1.01.014 **57**
– – of talus A02.5.10.014 **24**
– pterygoid A04.1.04.006 **35**
– puboprostatic ligament ♂ A04.5.03.015 **39**
– pubovesical ligament ♀ A04.5.03.015 **39**
– pulvinar nucleus A14.1.08.613 **121**
– raphespinal tract A14.1.02.234 **107**, A14.1.04.128 **109**
– recess of fourth ventricle A14.1.05.717 **115**
– rectus A15.2.07.013 **147**
– region of abdomen A01.2.04.004 **4**
– reticular nucleus A14.1.04.308 **111**
– reticulospinal tract A14.1.02.221 **107**
– retromalleolar region A01.2.08.020 **5**
– root
– – of median nerve A14.2.03.033 **138**
– – of optic tract A14.1.08.405 **120**
– rotation A03.0.00.055 **25**
– sacral
– – arteries A12.2.15.006 **89**
– – branches of median sacral artery A12.2.12.010 **87**
– – crest A02.2.05.017 **17**
– – veins A12.3.10.008 **97**
– sacrococcygeal ligament A03.2.08.005 **28**
– segment of right lung [S IV] A06.5.02.007 **61**
– segmental
– – artery
– – – of hepatic artery A12.2.12.038 **87**
– – – of right lung A12.2.01.112 **78**
– – bronchus [B IV] A06.4.02.007 **60**
– semicircular
– – canal A15.3.03.022 **151**
– – duct A15.3.03.073 **152**
– septal nucleus A14.1.09.268 **127**, A14.1.09.445 **129**
– spinothalamic tract A14.1.02.225 **107**
– stria A14.1.09.436 **129**
– subnucleus
– – of lateral parabrachial nucleus A14.1.05.442 **114**
– – of medial parabrachial nucleus A14.1.05.448 **114**
– subtendinous bursa of gastrocnemius A04.8.05.025 **45**
– sulcus A14.1.09.104 **124**
– superior
– – cerebellar artery A12.2.08.028 **85**
– – olivary nucleus A14.1.05.416 **114**
– supraclavicular nerves A14.2.02.027 **137**
– supracondylar line A02.5.04.020 **22**
– sural cutaneous nerve A14.2.07.048 **140**
– surface
– – of fibula A02.5.07.007 **23**
– – of ovary A09.1.01.004 **65**
– – of radius A02.4.05.010 **20**
– – of testis A09.3.01.004 **67**
– – of tibia A02.5.06.016 **23**
– – of zygomatic A02.1.14.002 **15**
– talocalcaneal ligament A03.6.10.102 **31**
– tarsal artery A12.2.16.049 **90**
– tectobulbar tract A14.1.06.206 **116**
– thoracic
– – artery A12.2.09.011 **85**
– – vein A12.3.08.011 **96**
– thyrohyoid ligament A06.2.02.017 **58**
– tuberal nuclei A14.1.08.927 **123**, A14.1.08.930 **124**
– tubercle of talus A02.5.10.018 **24**
– umbilical fold A10.1.02.434 **73**
– vein of lateral ventricle A12.3.06.034 **94**
– ventricle A14.1.09.272 **127**
– vertical occipital fibres A14.1.09.564 **131**
– vesical lymph nodes A13.3.04.027 **103**
– vestibular nucleus A14.1.05.427 **114**
– vestibulospinal tract A14.1.02.206 **107**, A14.1.04.131 **110**
– wall
– – of orbit A02.1.00.077 **9**
– – of tympanic cavity A15.3.02.032 **149**
– – triangle of pelvis ♀ A10.1.02.509 **73**
– zone of hypothalamus A14.1.08.944 **124**
Laterodorsal tegmental nucleus A14.1.06.318 **117**
Lateroposterior tegmental nucleus A14.1.06.318 **117**
Latissimus dorsi A04.3.01.006 **36**
Layer/s
– I of superior colliculus A14.1.06.606 **118**
– II of superior colliculus A14.1.06.607 **118**
– III of superior colliculus A14.1.06.608 **118**
– IV of superior colliculus A14.1.06.609 **118**
– of ammon's horn A14.1.09.334 **128**
– of dentate gyrus A14.1.09.340 **128**
– of hippocampus A14.1.09.334 **128**
– of inner and outer segments of retina A15.2.04.010 **145**
– of isocortex A14.1.09.308 **128**
– of nerve fibres of retina A15.2.04.017 **145**
– V of superior colliculus A14.1.06.610 **118**
– VI of superior colliculus A14.1.06.611 **118**

– VII of superior colliculus A14.1.06.612 **118**
Least splanchnic nerve A14.3.01.032 **142**
Left A01.0.00.007 **1**
– anterior lateral segment of liver A05.8.01.040 **55**
– atrial veins A12.3.01.016 **91**
– atrioventricular
– – orifice A12.1.04.002 **77**
– – valve A12.1.04.003 **77**
– atrium A12.1.03.001 **77**
– auricle A12.1.03.002 **77**
– branch
– – of atrioventricular bundle A12.1.06.007 **77**
– – of hepatic artery A12.2.12.035 **87**
– – of portal vein A12.3.12.005 **98**
– bundle of atrioventricular bundle A12.1.06.007 **77**
– colic
– – artery A12.2.12.071 **88**
– – flexure A05.7.03.005 **53**
– – lymph nodes A13.3.03.042 **103**
– – vein A12.3.12.033 **99**
– coronary
– – artery A12.2.03.201 **79**
– – cusp of aortic valve A12.1.04.014 **77**
– crus of diaphragm A04.4.02.004 **38**
– duct of caudate lobe of liver A05.8.01.069 **56**
– fibrous trigone of heart A12.1.00.026 **76**
– gastric
– – artery A12.2.12.013 **87**
– – vein A12.3.12.015 **98**
– gastro-epiploic
– – artery A12.2.12.047 **88**
– – vein A12.3.12.031 **99**
– gastro-omental
– – artery A12.2.12.047 **88**
– – vein A12.3.12.031 **99**
– hepatic
– – duct A05.8.01.065 **56**
– – vein A12.3.09.008 **97**
– inferior
– – lobar bronchus A06.4.02.020 **60**
– – pulmonary vein A12.3.02.401 **92**
– lateral division of liver A05.8.01.038 **55**
– liver A05.8.01.037 **55**
– lobe
– – of liver A05.8.01.027 **55**
– – of prostate A09.3.08.010 **69**
– – of thyroid gland A11.3.00.001 **74**
– lumbar lymph nodes A13.3.03.003 **102**
– lung A06.5.01.002 **60**
– main bronchus A06.4.01.004 **59**
– marginal
– – artery of left coronary artery A12.2.03.209 **79**
– – vein of great cardiac vein A12.3.01.005 **91**
– medial
– – division of liver A05.8.01.041 **55**
– – segment of liver A05.8.01.042 **55**
– ovarian vein ♀ A12.3.09.012 **97**
– part of liver A05.8.01.037 **55**
– posterior lateral segment of liver A05.8.01.039 **55**
– pulmonary artery A12.2.01.201 **78**
– semilunar cusp
– – of aortic valve A12.1.04.014 **77**
– – of pulmonary valve A12.1.02.012 **77**
– superior
– – intercostal vein A12.3.04.024 **92**
– – lobar bronchus A06.4.02.015 **60**
– – pulmonary vein A12.3.02.301 **92**
– suprarenal vein A12.3.09.011 **97**
– testicular vein ♂ A12.3.09.012 **97**
– triangular ligament of liver A10.1.02.305 **72**
– ventricle A12.1.04.001 **77**
– ventricular veins A12.3.01.017 **91**
Leg A01.1.00.038 **2**
– region A01.2.08.014 **5**
Lemniscus A14.1.00.014 **104**
Lens A15.2.05.001 **146**
– epithelium A15.2.05.006 **146**
– fibres A15.2.05.005 **146**
– substance A15.2.05.002 **146**
Lenticular
– fasciculus [H2] A14.1.09.521 **130**, A14.1.08.664 **122**
– nucleus A14.1.09.506 **130**
– process of incus A15.3.02.041 **150**
Lenticulostriate arteries A12.2.07.048 **83**
Lentiform nucleus A14.1.09.506 **130**
Leptomeningeal space A14.1.01.202 **104**
– of optic nerve A15.2.04.034 **146**
Leptomeninx A14.1.01.003 **104**
Lesser
– curvature of stomach A05.5.01.005 **51**
– horn of hyoid A02.1.16.003 **16**
– occipital nerve A14.2.02.017 **137**
– omentum A10.1.02.101 **72**
– palatine
– – arteries A12.2.05.086 **81**
– – canals A02.1.13.008 **15**
– – foramina A02.1.00.059 **9**, A02.1.13.016 **15**
– – nerves A14.2.01.047 **134**
– pelvis A02.5.02.006 **22**
– petrosal nerve A14.2.01.149 **136**, **142**
– sac A10.1.02.402 **72**
– sciatic
– – foramen A03.6.03.009 **30**
– – notch A02.5.01.206 **21**
– splanchnic nerve A14.3.01.030 **141**
– supraclavicular fossa A01.2.02.008 **3**
– trochanter A02.5.04.007 **22**
– tubercle A02.4.04.006 **19**
– tympanic spine A02.1.06.057 **13**
– vestibular glands A09.2.01.017 **67**
– wing of sphenoid A02.1.05.020 **11**
Levator
– anguli oris A04.1.03.034 **34**
– ani A04.5.04.002 **39**
– glandulae thyroideae A04.2.04.008 **35**
– labii superioris A04.1.03.031 **34**
– – alaeque nasi A04.1.03.032 **34**
– palpebrae superioris A15.2.07.020 **147**
– prostatae ♂ A04.5.04.005 **39, 69**
– scapulae A04.3.01.009 **36**
– veli palatini A05.2.01.102 **50**
Levatores costarum A04.4.01.009 **37**
– breves A04.4.01.011 **37**
– longi A04.4.01.010 **37**
Lienorenal ligament A10.1.02.207 **72**
Ligament
– of head of femur A03.6.07.010 **30**
– of left vena cava A12.3.01.008 **91**
– of ovary A09.1.01.017 **65**
Ligamenta flava A03.2.01.003 **27**
Ligaments A03.0.00.034 **25**
– of auditory ossicles A15.3.02.053 **150**
– of auricle A15.3.01.032 **148**
Ligamentum
– arteriosum (Ductus arteriosus) A12.2.01.202 **78**
– nuchae A03.2.01.006 **27**
– venosum A05.8.01.011 **54, 98**
Limbic lobe A14.1.09.230 **126**
Limbous suture A03.0.00.011 **25**
Limbus
– fossae ovalis A12.1.01.006 **76**
– of osseous spiral lamina A15.3.03.104 **152**
– of sphenoid A02.1.05.004 **11**
Limen
– insulae A14.1.09.155 **125**
– nasi A06.1.02.010 **57**
Line A02.0.00.032 **7**
Linea
– alba A04.5.01.022 **38**
– aspera A02.5.04.013 **22**
– semilunaris A04.5.01.025 **38**
– terminalis of pelvis A02.5.02.007 **22**
Lingual
– aponeurosis A05.1.04.025 **49**
– artery A12.2.05.015 **80**
– branch/es

– – of accessory nerve A14.2.01.192 **137**
– – of facial nerve A14.2.01.112 **135**
– – of glossopharyngeal nerve A14.2.01.148 **136**
– – of lingual nerve A14.2.01.086 **135**
– cusp of tooth A05.1.03.021 **48**
– fibres of transverse occipital fasciculi A14.1.09.568 **131**
– glands A05.1.02.018 **47**
– gyrus A14.1.09.226 **126**
– lymph nodes A13.3.00.014 **101**
– nerve A14.2.01.081 **135**
– papillae A05.1.04.013 **49**
– septum A05.1.04.024 **49**
– surface of tooth A05.1.03.038 **48**
– tonsil A05.1.04.022 **49, 100**
– transverse occipital fibres A14.1.09.568 **131**
– vein A12.3.05.009 **93**
Lingula
– of cerebellum [I] A14.1.07.103 **118**
– of left lung A06.5.01.018 **60**
– of mandible A02.1.15.029 **15**
Lingular
– artery A12.2.01.211 **78**
– branch of left superior pulmonary vein A12.3.02.308 **92**
– vein A12.3.02.308 **92**
Linguofacial trunk A12.2.05.014 **80**
Lips A05.1.01.005 **47**
– of mouth A05.1.01.005 **47**
Little
– finger A01.2.07.031 **5**
– toe A01.2.08.040 **6**
Liver A05.8.01.001 **54**
Lobar and segmental bronchi A06.4.02.001 **60**
Lobe/s
– of ear A15.3.01.003 **148**
– of mammary gland A16.0.02.008 **154**
– of thyroid gland A11.3.00.002 **74**
– of thymus A13.1.02.002 **100**
Lobule/s
– of auricle A15.3.01.003 **148**
– of epididymis A09.3.02.003 **68**
– of liver A05.8.01.056 **55**
– of mammary gland A16.0.02.009 **154**
– of lung A06.5.02.027 **61**
– of testis A09.3.01.020 **67**
– of thymus A13.1.02.003 **100**
– of thyroid gland A11.3.00.009 **74**
Locus caeruleus A14.1.05.706 **115**
Long
– association fibres of telencephalon A14.1.09.558 **131**
– bone A02.0.00.011 **7**
– ciliary nerves A14.2.01.027 **134**
– gyrus of insula A14.1.09.151 **125**
– head
– – of biceps
– – – brachii A04.6.02.014 **40**
– – – femoris A04.7.02.033 **42**
– – of triceps brachii A04.6.02.020 **40**
– limb of incus A15.3.02.040 **150**
– pitch helicoidal muscle layer of small intestine A05.6.01.005 **52**
– plantar ligament A03.6.10.517 **31**
– posterior ciliary arteries A12.2.06.032 **82**
– saphenous vein A12.3.11.003 **98**
– thoracic nerve A14.2.03.012 **138**
Longissimus A04.3.02.010 **36**
– capitis A04.3.02.014 **36**
– cervicis A04.3.02.013 **36**
– thoracis A04.3.02.011 **36**
Longitudinal A01.0.00.028 **1**
– arch of foot A01.2.08.028 **5**
– bands A03.2.04.005 **27**
– canals of modiolus cochleae A15.3.03.042 **151**
– cerebral fissure A14.1.09.007 **124**
– duct of epoophoron A09.1.05.002 **66**
– fibres of ciliary muscle A15.2.03.016 **145**
– fold of duodenum A05.6.02.014 **53**
– muscle layer
– – of colon A05.7.03.012 **53**
– – of intermediate urethra A09.4.02.019 **70**
– – of prostatic urethra A09.4.02.014 **70**
– – of rectum A05.7.04.010 **54**
– – of small intestine A05.6.01.005 **52**
– – of spongy urethra A09.4.02.028 **70**
– – of stomach A05.5.01.022 **52**
– – of urethra A09.2.03.010 **67**
– pontine fibres A14.1.05.103 **112**
Longus
– capitis A04.2.01.003 **35**
– colli A04.2.01.002 **35**
Loose connective tissue A16.0.03.006 **155**
– of abdomen A04.5.02.020 **39**
Lower
– dental arcade A05.1.03.003 **48**
– eyelid A15.2.07.026 **147**
– head of lateral pterygoid A04.1.04.008 **35**
– limb A01.1.00.031 **2**
– lip A05.1.01.009 **47**
– lobe of lung A06.5.01.020 **60**
– pole of testis A09.3.01.003 **67**
– trunk of brachial plexus A14.2.03.006 **138**
Lowest splanchnic nerve A14.3.01.032 **142**
Lumbar
– arteries A12.2.12.004 **87**
– branch of iliolumbar artery A12.2.15.003 **89**
– cistern A14.1.01.219 **105**
– ganglia A14.3.01.033 **142**
– lordosis A02.2.00.007 **16**
– lymphatic trunk A12.4.01.013 **99**
– nerves [L1–L5] A14.2.05.001 **139**
– part
– – of diaphragm A04.4.02.002 **38**
– – of iliocostalis lumborum A04.3.02.007 **36**
– – of longissimus thoracis A04.3.02.012 **36**
– – of spinal cord A14.1.02.016 **105**
– plexus A14.2.07.002 **139**
– region A01.2.05.008 **4**
– rib A02.3.02.020 **18**
– segments [1–5] A14.1.02.016 **105**
– splanchnic nerves A14.3.01.034 **142**
– veins A12.3.07.012 **96**, A12.3.09.003 **96**
– vertebrae [L I – L V] A02.2.04.001 **17**
Lumbocostal
– ligament A03.3.04.009 **28**
– triangle A04.4.02.016 **38**
Lumbosacral
– enlargement A14.1.02.003 **105**
– joint A03.2.07.001 **27**
– plexus A14.2.07.001 **139**
– trunk A14.2.07.026 **140**
Lumbricals
– of foot A04.7.02.069 **43**
– of hand A04.6.02.065 **41**
Luminal A01.0.00.032 **1**
Lunate A02.4.08.005 **20**
– sulcus A14.1.09.134 **125**
– surface of acetabulum A02.5.01.006 **21**
Lungs A06.5.01.001 **60**
Lunogracile fissure A14.1.07.211 **119**
Lunule of nail A16.0.01.005 **154**
Lunules of semilunar cusps
– of aortic valve A12.1.04.017 **77**
– of pulmonary valve A12.1.02.015 **77**
Lymph A12.0.00.043 **75**
– node/s A13.2.03.001 **100**
– – around cardia A13.3.03.017 **102**
– – of abdomen A13.3.03.001 **102**
– – of anterior border of omental foramen A13.3.03.032 **101**
– – of arch of azygos vein A13.3.02.009 **102**
– – of head and neck A13.3.00.001 **101**
– – of ligamentum arteriosum A13.3.02.008 **102**
– – of lower limb A13.3.05.001 **103**
– – of pelvis A13.3.04.001 **103**
– – of thorax A13.3.02.001 **102**
– – of upper limb A13.3.01.001 **101**
– nodules of vermiform appendix A05.7.02.009 **53, 101**
Lymphatic
– capillary A12.0.00.044 **75**
– plexus A12.0.00.041 **75**
– rete A12.0.00.045 **75**

- trunks and ducts
 A12.4.01.001 **99**
- valvule A12.0.00.042 **75**
- vessel A12.0.00.038 **75**
Lymphoid
- nodules
- - of lingual tonsil
 A05.1.04.023 **49, 100**
- - of pharyngeal tonsil
 A05.3.01.009 **50, 100**
- system A13.0.00.000 **100**

M

M1 segment of middle cerebral
 artery A12.2.07.047 **83**
M2 segment of middle cerebral
 artery A12.2.07.053 **83**,
 A12.2.07.055 **83**, A12.2.07.061 **83**
Macula/e
- cribrosa/e A15.3.03.011 **151**
- - inferior A15.3.03.014 **151**
- - media A15.3.03.013 **151**
- - superior A15.3.03.012 **151**
- of retina A15.2.04.021 **145**
- of saccule A15.3.03.084 **152**
- of utricle A15.3.03.083 **152**
- utriculosacculares
 A15.3.03.082 **152**
Magnocellular
- division of ventral anterior nucleus of thalamus
 A14.1.08.653 **122**
- layers of dorsal nucleus of lateral geniculate body
 A14.1.08.804 **123**
- nucleus of medial dorsal nucleus of thalamus A14.1.08.624 **122**
- part
- - of inferior vestibular nucleus
 A14.1.04.244 **111**
- - of lateral reticular nucleus
 A14.1.04.309 **112**
- - of red nucleus
 A14.1.06.324 **117**
- subnucleus of spinal nucleus of trigeminal nerve
 A14.1.04.215 **110**
Magnus raphe nucleus
 A14.1.04.321 **112, 115**
Main portal fissure
 A05.8.01.035 **55**
Major
- alar cartilage of nose
 A06.1.01.007 **57**
- calices A08.1.05.003 **64**
- circulus arteriosus of iris
 A15.2.03.034 **145**
- duodenal papilla
 A05.6.02.015 **53**
- forceps A14.1.09.251 **127**
- renal calyces A08.1.05.003 **64**
- salivary glands A05.1.02.002 **47**
- sublingual duct A05.1.02.009 **47**
Malar lymph node
 A13.3.00.012 **101**
Male
- external genitalia
 A09.4.00.001 **69, 71**
- genital system A09.0.00.002 **65**
- internal genitalia
 A09.3.00.001 **67**
- urethra A08.5.01.001 **64, 70**
Malleolar
- fossa A02.5.07.016 **23**
- groove A02.5.06.021 **23**,
 A02.5.07.017 **23**
- prominence A15.3.01.057 **149**
- stria A15.3.01.058 **149**
Malleus A15.3.02.043 **150**
Mamillary process of lumbar vertebra A02.2.04.004 **17**
Mammary
- gland A16.0.02.006 **154**
- region A01.2.03.007 **4**
Mammelons A05.1.03.059 **49**
Mammillary
- arteries A12.2.07.078 **83**
- body A14.1.08.402 **120**
- line A01.2.00.016 **3**
- process A02.2.04.004 **17**
Mammillotegmental fasciculus
 A14.1.08.953 **124**
Mammillothalamic fasciculus
 A14.1.08.671 **122**, A14.1.08.954 **124**
Mandible A02.1.15.001 **15**
Mandibular
- canal A02.1.15.030 **15**
- dental arcade A05.1.03.003 **48**
- division [Vc; V3]
 A14.2.01.064 **134**
- foramen A02.1.15.028 **15**
- fossa A02.1.06.071 **13**
- lymph node A13.3.00.013 **101**
- nerve A14.2.01.064 **134**
- notch A02.1.15.034 **15**
- symphysis A02.1.15.004 **15**
- torus A02.1.15.013 **15**
Manubriosternal
- joint A03.3.02.006 **28**
- synchondrosis A03.3.02.007 **28**
Manubrium of sternum
 A02.3.03.002 **18**
Margin of tongue A05.1.04.009 **49**
Marginal
- arcade A12.2.12.068 **88**
- artery A12.2.12.068 **88**
- branch
- - of cingulate sulcus
 A14.1.09.204 **126**
- - of parieto-occipital sulcus
 A14.1.09.204 **126**
- mandibular branch of facial nerve
 A14.2.01.113 **135**
- nucleus
- - of restiform body
 A14.1.04.246 **111**
- - of spinal cord A14.1.02.117 **106**
- part of orbicularis oris
 A04.1.03.024 **34**
- ridge of tooth A05.1.03.045 **48**
- sinus A12.3.05.104 **93**
- sulcus A14.1.09.204 **126**
- tubercle A02.1.14.008 **15**
Marrow cavity A02.0.00.037 **7**
Massa intermedia
 A14.1.08.103 **120, 121**
Masseter A04.1.04.002 **35**
Masseteric
- artery A12.2.05.070 **81**
- fascia A04.1.04.011 **35**
- nerve A14.2.01.070 **134**
- tuberosity A02.1.15.026 **15**
Masticatory muscles
 A04.1.04.001 **35**
Mastoid
- angle of parietal bone
 A02.1.02.018 **10**
- antrum A15.3.02.028 **149**
- border of occipital bone
 A02.1.04.011 **10**
- branch
- - of occipital artery
 A12.2.05.031 **80**
- - of posterior tympanic artery
 A12.2.05.040 **80**
- canaliculus A02.1.06.044 **13**
- cells A15.3.02.029 **149**
- emissary vein A12.3.05.303 **94**
- fontanelle A02.1.00.031 **8**
- foramen A02.1.06.008 **12**
- lymph nodes A13.3.00.003 **101**
- notch A02.1.06.005 **12**
- process A02.1.06.004 **12**
- region A01.2.01.007 **3**
- wall of tympanic cavity
 A15.3.02.020 **149**
Maxilla A02.1.12.001 **14**
Maxillary
- artery A12.2.05.053 **80**
- dental arcade A05.1.03.002 **48**
- division [Vb; V3]
 A14.2.01.037 **134**
- hiatus A02.1.12.021 **14**
- nerve A14.2.01.037 **134**
- process of inferior concha
 A02.1.08.003 **13**
- sinus A02.1.12.023 **14**,
 A06.1.03.002 **57**
- surface
- - of palatine A02.1.13.004 **14**
- - of sphenoid A02.1.05.029 **11**
- tuberosity A02.1.12.016 **14**
- veins A12.3.05.035 **93**
Medial A01.0.00.009 **1**
- accessory
- - nucleus of optic tract
 A14.1.06.317 **117**
- - olivary nucleus
 A14.1.04.226 **110**
- amygdaloid nucleus
 A14.1.09.413 **129**
- and inferior surfaces of cerebral hemisphere A14.1.09.201 **125**
- angle of eye A15.2.07.034 **147**
- antebrachial cutaneous nerve
 A14.2.03.028 **138**
- arcuate ligament
 A04.4.02.006 **38**
- basal
- - segment
- - - of left lung [S VII]
 A06.5.02.022 **61**
- - - of right lung [S VII]
 A06.5.02.011 **61**
- - segmental
- - - artery

- - - - of left lung A12.2.01.219 **79**
- - - - of right lung A12.2.01.118 **78**
- - - bronchus
- - - - of left lung [B VII] A06.4.02.022 **60**
- - - - of right lung [B VII] A06.4.02.011 **60**
- bicipital groove A01.2.07.006 **4**
- border
- - of forearm A01.2.07.016 **5**
- - of foot A01.2.08.027 **5**
- - of humerus A02.4.04.015 **19**
- - of kidney A08.1.01.003 **63**
- - of scapula A02.4.01.012 **18**
- - of suprarenal gland A11.5.00.006 **74**
- - of tibia A02.5.06.018 **23**
- brachial cutaneous nerve A14.2.03.027 **138**
- branch/es
- - of artery of tuber cinereum A12.2.07.074 **83**
- - of left hepatic duct A05.8.01.067 **56**
- - of pontine arteries A12.2.08.022 **84**
- - of posterior ramus
- - - of cervical nerve A14.2.02.004 **137**
- - - of lumbar nerve A14.2.05.003 **139**
- - - of thoracic nerve A14.2.04.003 **139**
- - of sacral or coccygeal nerve A14.2.06.003 **139**
- - of superior cerebellar artery A12.2.08.026 **85**
- - of supra-orbital nerve A14.2.01.023 **133**
- - of umbilical part of left branch of portal vein A12.3.12.011 **98**
- calcaneal branches of tibial nerve A14.2.07.065 **141**
- canthic fold A15.2.07.028 **147**
- cervical nucleus A14.1.02.128 **106**
- circumflex femoral
- - artery A12.2.16.021 **90**
- - veins A12.3.11.025 **98**
- clunial nerves A14.2.06.006 **139**
- collateral artery A12.2.09.023 **86**
- common iliac lymph nodes A13.3.04.004 **103**
- compartment of thigh A04.7.01.004 **42**
- condyle
- - of femur A02.5.04.021 **22**
- - of tibia A02.5.06.003 **23**
- cord of brachial plexus A14.2.03.022 **138**
- crest of fibula A02.5.07.010 **23**
- crural cutaneous nerve A14.2.07.025 **140**
- crus
- - of major alar cartilage of nose A06.1.01.008 **57**
- - of superficial inguinal ring A04.5.01.014 **38**
- cuneiform A02.5.13.001 **24**
- cutaneous
- - branch of dorsal branch of posterior intercostal artery A12.2.11.009 **86**
- - nerve
- - - of arm A14.2.03.027 **138**
- - - of forearm A14.2.03.028 **138**
- - - of leg A14.2.07.025 **140**
- division of lumbar erector spinae A04.3.02.012 **36**
- dorsal
- - cutaneous nerve A14.2.07.052 **140**
- - nucleus of thalamus A14.1.08.622 **122**
- eminence of floor of fourth ventricle A14.1.05.704 **115**
- epicondyle
- - of femur A02.5.04.022 **22**
- - of humerus A02.4.04.027 **19**
- external iliac lymph nodes A13.3.04.010 **103**
- femoral intermuscular septum A04.7.03.005 **43**
- forebrain bundle A14.1.08.955 **124**
- frontal gyrus A14.1.09.207 **126**
- frontobasal artery A12.2.07.035 **83**
- geniculate
- - body A14.1.08.303 **120**
- - nuclei A14.1.08.808 **123**
- habenular nucleus A14.1.08.504 **121**
- head
- - of flexor hallucis brevis A04.7.02.058 **43**
- - of gastrocnemius A04.7.02.046 **43**
- - of triceps brachii A04.6.02.022 **40**
- inguinal fossa A10.1.02.432 **73**
- intercondylar tubercle A02.5.06.009 **23**
- intermuscular septum of arm A04.6.03.006 **41**
- internal nasal branches of anterior ethmoidal nerve A14.2.01.033 **134**
- lacunar external iliac lymph node A13.3.04.013 **103**
- lamina of cartilage of pharyngotympanic tube A15.3.02.080 **150**
- lemniscus A14.1.04.111 **109, 112**, A14.1.06.207 **116**, A14.1.08.672 **122**
- ligament
- - of ankle joint A03.6.10.003 **31**
- - of temporomandibular joint A03.1.07.004 **27**
- lip
- - of bicipital groove A02.4.04.009 **19**
- - of linea aspera A02.5.04.015 **22**
- longitudinal
- - fasciculus A14.1.04.113 **109**, A14.1.05.304 **112**, A14.1.06.209 **116**
- - stria A14.1.09.248 **127**
- lumbar intertransversarii A04.3.02.402 **37**
- lymph node of vascular lacuna A13.3.04.013 **103**
- magnocellular nucleus A14.1.08.811 **123**
- - of medial geniculate body A14.1.08.811 **123**
- malleolar
- - arterial network A12.2.16.058 **91**
- - branches of posterior tibial artery A12.2.16.057 **91**
- - facet of talus A02.5.10.015 **24**
- malleolus A02.5.06.020 **23**
- mammary branches
- - of intercostal nerve A14.2.04.014 **139**
- - of perforating branches of internal thoracic artery A12.2.08.037 **85**
- margin of orbit A02.1.00.074 **9**
- marginal vein of foot A12.3.11.021 **98**
- medullary
- - branches of vertebral artery A12.2.08.017 **84**
- - lamina of corpus striatum A14.1.09.510 **130**
- meniscus A03.6.08.005 **30**
- nasal branches A14.2.01.033 **134**
- nucleus/i
- - of mammillary body A14.1.08.936 **124**
- - of medial dorsal nucleus of thalamus A14.1.08.624 **122**
- - of thalamus A14.1.08.621 **121**
- - of trapezoid body A14.1.05.424 **114**
- occipital artery A12.2.07.098 **84**
- occipitotemporal gyrus A14.1.09.228 **126**
- olfactory
- - gyrus A14.1.09.221 **126**
- - stria A14.1.09.435 **129**
- orbitofrontal artery A12.2.07.035 **83**
- palpebral
- - arteries A12.2.06.044 **82**
- - commissure A15.2.07.032 **147**
- - ligament A15.2.07.041 **147**
- parabrachial nucleus A14.1.05.446 **114**
- part
- - of biventral lobule A14.1.07.219 **119**
- - of globus pallidus A14.1.09.514 **130**
- - of lateral parabrachial nucleus A14.1.05.443 **114**
- - of longitudinal arch of foot A01.2.08.030 **5**
- - of medial parabrachial nucleus A14.1.05.447 **114**

– – of middle lobe vein of right lung A12.3.02.113 **91**
– – of nucleus accumbens A14.1.09.442 **129**
– patellar retinaculum A03.6.08.016 **31**
– pectoral nerve A14.2.03.017 **138**
– pericuneate nucleus A14.1.04.260 **111**
– periolivary nuclei A14.1.05.419 **114**
– plantar
– – artery A12.2.16.061 **91**
– – nerve A14.2.07.066 **141**
– plate of sphenoid A02.1.05.044 **12**
– posterior cervical intertransversarii A04.3.02.404 **37**
– preoptic nucleus A14.1.08.907 **123**
– process of calcaneal tuberosity A02.5.11.003 **24**
– pterygoid A04.1.04.009 **35**
– puboprostatic ligament ♂ A04.5.03.013 **39**
– pubovesical ligament ♀ A04.5.03.013 **39**
– pulvinar nucleus A14.1.08.614 **121**
– rectus A15.2.07.012 **147**
– reticular nucleus A14.1.04.317 **112**
– reticulospinal tract A14.1.02.209 **107**
– retromalleolar region A01.2.08.021 **5**
– root
– – of median nerve A14.2.03.032 **138**
– – of optic tract A14.1.08.406 **120**
– rotation A03.0.00.056 **26**
– segment of right lung [S V] A06.5.02.008 **61**
– segmental
– – artery
– – – of hepatic artery A12.2.12.037 **87**
– – – of right lung A12.2.01.111 **78**
– – bronchus [B V] A06.4.02.008 **60**
– septal nucleus A14.1.09.269 **127**, A14.1.09.446 **129**
– solitary nucleus A14.1.04.236 **111**
– stria A14.1.09.435 **129**
– subnucleus
– – of lateral parabrachial nucleus A14.1.05.443 **114**
– – of medial parabrachial nucleus A14.1.05.447 **114**
– subtendinous bursa of gastrocnemius A04.8.05.026 **45**
– superior
– – cerebellar artery A12.2.08.026 **85**
– – olivary nucleus A14.1.05.417 **114**
– supraclavicular nerves A14.2.02.025 **137**
– supracondylar
– – line A02.5.04.019 **22**
– – ridge A02.4.04.016 **19**, A02.4.04.019 **19**
– supraepicondylar ridge A02.4.04.016 **19**, A02.4.04.019 **19**
– sural cutaneous nerve A14.2.07.061 **141**
– surface
– – of arytenoid A06.2.04.010 **58**
– – of fibula A02.5.07.008 **23**
– – of ovary A09.1.01.003 **65**
– – of testis A09.3.01.005 **67**
– – of tibia A02.5.06.013 **23**
– – of ulna A02.4.06.010 **20**
– talocalcaneal ligament A03.6.10.103 **31**
– tarsal arteries A12.2.16.050 **90**
– tubercle of talus A02.5.10.019 **24**
– umbilical fold A10.1.02.431 **73**
– vein of lateral ventricle A12.3.06.033 **94**
– ventral nucleus of thalamus A14.1.08.626 **122**
– vestibular nucleus/i
– – in medulla oblongata A14.1.04.245 **111**
– – in pontile tegmentum A14.1.05.426 **114**
– vestibulospinal tract A14.1.02.207 **107**
– wall
– – of orbit A02.1.00.078 **9**
– – of tympanic cavity A15.3.02.008 **149**
– zone of hypothalamus A14.1.08.943 **124**
Median A01.0.00.003 **1**
– antebrachial vein A12.3.08.020 **96**
– aperture A14.1.05.722 **115**
– arcuate ligament A04.4.02.005 **38**
– artery A12.2.09.049 **86**
– atlanto-axial joint A03.2.04.001 **27**
– callosal artery A12.2.07.032 **83**
– commissural artery A12.2.07.031 **82**
– conjugate A02.5.02.017 **22**
– cricothyroid ligament A06.2.03.009 **58**
– cubital vein A12.3.08.019 **96**
– eminence of hypothalamus A14.1.08.409 **120**
– glosso-epiglottic fold A05.3.01.021 **50**
– nerve A14.2.03.031 **138**
– nucleus/i A14.1.05.205 **112**
– – of pons A14.1.05.205 **112**
– – of thalamus A14.1.08.627 **122**
– palatine suture A03.1.02.032 **26**
– plane A01.2.00.004 **3**
– preoptic nucleus A14.1.08.908 **123**
– raphe nucleus A14.1.05.603 **115**
– sacral
– – artery A12.2.12.008 **87**
– – crest A02.2.05.014 **17**
– – vein A12.3.10.002 **97**
– sagittal plane A01.2.00.004 **3**
– sulcus
– – of fourth ventricle A14.1.05.703 **115**
– – of tongue A05.1.04.018 **49**
– thyrohyoid ligament A06.2.02.014 **58**
– umbilical
– – fold A10.1.02.429 **73**
– – ligament A08.3.01.007 **64**
– vein of forearm A12.3.08.020 **96**
Mediastinal
– branches
– – of internal thoracic artery A12.2.08.030 **85**
– – of thoracic aorta A12.2.11.005 **86**
– part of parietal pleura A07.1.02.009 **62**
– surface of lung A06.5.01.008 **60**
– veins A12.3.04.008 **92**, A12.3.07.009 **95**
Mediastinum A07.1.02.101 **62**
– of testis A09.3.01.018 **67**
Medulla A11.5.00.008 **74**, A13.2.03.006 **101**
– oblongata A14.1.03.003 **108**
– of lymph node A13.2.03.006 **101**
– of suprarenal gland A11.5.00.008 **74**
– of thymus A13.1.02.005 **100**
Medullary
– cavity A02.0.00.037 **7**
– cone A14.1.02.004 **105**
– rays of kidney A08.1.01.018 **63**
– reticulospinal
– – fibres A14.1.04.130 **110**
– – tract A14.1.02.221 **107**
– stria/e of fourth ventricle A14.1.05.318 **113**, A14.1.05.707 **115**
Medullopontine sulcus A14.1.05.001 **112**
Membranous
– labyrinth A15.3.03.059 **152**
– lamina of pharyngotympanic tube A15.3.02.082 **150**
– layer of subcutaneous tissue A16.0.03.005 **155**
– – of abdomen A04.5.02.022 **39**
– – of perineum A09.5.00.007 **71**
– part A02.0.00.006 **7**
– – of interventricular septum A12.1.00.015 **76**
– – of nasal septum A06.1.02.005 **57**
– urethra A09.4.02.017 **70, 71**
– wall
– – of tympanic cavity A15.3.02.032 **149**
– – of trachea A06.3.01.007 **59**
Meningeal
– branch/es

– – of cavernous part of internal carotid artery A12.2.06.010 **81**
– – of cerebral part of internal carotid artery A12.2.06.022 **81**
– – of mandibular nerve A14.2.01.065 **134**
– – of maxillary nerve A14.2.01.038 **134**
– – of occipital artery A12.2.05.035 **80**
– – of spinal nerve A14.2.00.032 **133**
– – of vagus A14.2.01.155 **136**
– – of vertebral artery A12.2.08.011 **84**
– veins A12.3.05.008 **93**, A12.3.05.037 **93**
Meninges A14.1.01.001 **104**
Meniscus A03.0.00.033 **25**
Mental
– branch of inferior alveolar artery A12.2.05.059 **80**
– branches of mental nerve A14.2.01.095 **135**
– foramen A02.1.15.007 **15**
– nerve A14.2.01.094 **135**
– protuberance A02.1.15.005 **15**
– region A01.2.01.020 **3**
– tubercle A02.1.15.006 **15**
Mentalis A04.1.03.037 **35**
Mentolabial sulcus A01.2.01.019 **3**
Meridians A15.2.01.005 **144**
Meridional fibres of ciliary muscle A15.2.03.015 **144**
Mesencephalic
– arteries A12.2.08.024 **84**
– corticonuclear fibres A14.1.06.202 **116**
– nucleus of trigeminal nerve A14.1.05.409 **114, 117**
– tract of trigeminal nerve A14.1.05.313 **113**, A14.1.06.210 **116**
Mesencephalon A14.1.03.005 **108, 115**
Mesentery A10.1.02.007 **72**
Mesial
– fovea A05.1.03.062 **49**
– root A05.1.03.066 **49**
– surface A05.1.03.040 **48**
– – of tooth A05.1.03.040 **48**
Mesiobuccal
– cusp A05.1.03.022 **48**
– root A05.1.03.068 **49**
Mesiolingual
– cusp A05.1.03.024 **48**
– root A05.1.03.069 **49**
Mesiopalatal cusp A05.1.03.023 **48**
Meso-appendix A10.1.02.014 **72**
Mesocolic
– lymph nodes A13.3.03.040 **103**
– taenia A05.7.03.014 **53**
Mesocolon A10.1.02.009 **72**
Mesocortex A14.1.09.306 **128**
Mesometrium ♀ A10.1.02.506 **73**
Mesosalpinx ♀ A10.1.02.507 **73**
Mesotendon A04.8.01.008 **44**
Mesovarian border of ovary A09.1.01.006 **65**
Mesovarium ♀ A10.1.02.508 **73**
Metacarpal region A01.2.07.025 **5**
Metacarpals [I–V] A02.4.09.001 **20**
Metacarpophalangeal joints A03.5.11.501 **30**
Metacarpus A01.1.00.027 **2**
Metaphysis A02.0.00.022 **7**
Metatarsal
– interosseous ligaments A03.6.10.702 **32**
– region A01.2.08.034 **6**
Metatarsals [I–V] A02.5.17.001 **24**
Metatarsophalangeal joints A03.6.10.801 **32**
Metatarsus A01.1.00.043 **2**
Metathalamus A14.1.08.301 **120**, A14.1.08.801 **123**
Metencephalon A14.1.03.004 **108**
Metopic suture A02.1.03.007 **10, 26**
Midaxillary line A01.2.00.018 **3**
Midbrain A14.1.03.005 **108, 115**
Midcarpal joint A03.5.11.102 **29**
Midclavicular line A01.2.00.015 **3**
Middle A01.0.00.025 **1**
– calyx of kidney A08.1.05.005 **64**
– cardiac vein A12.3.01.009 **91**
– cerebellar peduncle A14.1.05.003 **112**, A14.1.07.416 **120**
– cerebral artery A12.2.07.046 **83, 84**
– cervical
– – cardiac nerve A14.3.01.018 **141**
– – ganglion A14.3.01.016 **141**
– clinoid process A02.1.05.008 **11**
– colic
– – artery A12.2.12.067 **88**
– – lymph nodes A13.3.03.042 **103**
– – vein A12.3.12.027 **99**
– constrictor A05.3.01.108 **51**
– cranial fossa A02.1.00.049 **8**
– cuneiform A02.5.14.001 **24**
– ear A15.3.02.001 **149**
– ethmoidal cells A02.1.07.009 **13**, A06.1.03.007 **58**
– facet on talus for calcaneus A02.5.10.008 **24**
– finger A01.2.07.029 **5**
– frontal gyrus A14.1.09.118 **125**
– genicular artery A12.2.16.036 **90**
– layer of thoracolumbar fascia A04.3.02.503 **37**
– lobar
– – artery of right lung A12.2.01.110 **78**
– – bronchus A06.4.02.006 **60**
– lobe A09.3.08.015 **69**
– – branch of right superior pulmonary vein A12.3.02.111 **91**
– – of prostate A09.3.08.015 **69**
– – of right lung A06.5.01.019 **60**, A06.5.02.006 **61**
– – vein of right lung A12.3.02.111 **91**
– macular
– – arteriole A15.2.04.043 **146**
– – venule A15.2.04.050 **146**
– mediastinum A07.1.02.105 **62**
– meningeal
– – artery A12.2.05.061 **80**
– – veins A12.3.05.037 **93**
– nasal
– – concha A02.1.07.014 **13**, A06.1.02.014 **57**
– – meatus A02.1.00.090 **9**, A06.1.02.024 **57**
– part of trapezius A04.3.01.003 **36**
– phalanx
– – of foot A02.5.18.003 **24**
– – of hand A02.4.10.003 **20**
– rectal
– – artery A12.2.15.036 **89**
– – nerve plexus A14.3.03.049 **143**
– – veins A12.3.10.018 **97**
– scalene A04.2.01.005 **35**
– superior alveolar
– – branch A14.2.01.051 **134**
– – nerve A14.2.01.051 **134**
– suprarenal artery A12.2.12.074 **88**
– talar articular surface of calcaneum A02.5.11.011 **24**
– temporal
– – artery A12.2.05.050 **80**
– – branch/es A12.2.07.057 **83**
– – – of lateral occipital artery A12.2.07.096 **84**
– – – of middle cerebral artery A12.2.07.057 **83**
– – gyrus A14.1.09.146 **125**
– – vein A12.3.05.033 **93**
– thyroid veins A12.3.05.015 **93**
– trunk of brachial plexus A14.2.03.005 **137**
Midline groove of tongue A05.1.04.018 **49**
Minor
– alar cartilages of nose A06.1.01.011 **57**
– calices A08.1.05.007 **64**
– circulus arteriosus of iris A15.2.03.035 **145**
– duodenal papilla A05.6.02.016 **53**
– forceps A14.1.09.250 **127**
– renal calyces A08.1.05.007 **64**
– salivary glands A05.1.02.013 **47**
– sublingual ducts A05.1.02.010 **47**
Mitral valve A12.1.04.003 **77**
Mixed nerve A14.2.00.023 **133**
Mobile
– end A04.0.00.005 **33**
– part of nasal septum A06.1.01.009 **57**
Moderator band A12.1.02.020 **77**
Modiolus
– anguli oris A04.1.03.035 **34**
– cochleae A15.3.03.038 **151**
Molar
– glands A05.1.02.016 **47**
– tooth A05.1.03.007 **48**
– tubercle A05.1.03.073 **49**

Molecular layer
- of cerebellar cortex A14.1.07.405 **119**
- of dentate gyrus A14.1.09.341 **128**
- of isocortex [Layer I] A14.1.09.309 **128**
Mons pubis A09.2.01.002 **66**
Motor
- decussation A14.1.04.004 **108**, A14.1.04.106 **109**
- nerve A14.2.00.021 **133**
- nucleus
- - of facial nerve A14.1.05.412 **114**
- - of trigeminal nerve A14.1.05.410 **114**
- root
- - of spinal nerve A14.2.00.029 **133**
- - of trigeminal nerve A14.2.01.015 **133**
Mouth A01.1.00.010 **2**, A05.1.00.001 **47**
Mucosal folds of gallbladder A05.8.02.010 **56**
Mucous membrane
- of bladder A08.3.01.023 **64**
- of bronchus A06.4.02.029 **60**
- of ductus deferens A09.3.05.010 **68**
- of gallbladder A05.8.02.009 **56**
- of intermediate urethra A09.4.02.020 **70**
- of large intestine A05.7.01.006 **53**
- of larynx A06.2.09.019 **59**
- of mouth A05.1.01.002 **47**
- of nose A06.1.02.017 **57**
- of oesophagus A05.4.01.015 **51**
- of pharyngotympanic tube A15.3.02.083 **151**
- of pharynx A05.3.01.029 **51**
- of prostatic urethra A09.4.02.015 **70**
- of renal pelvis A08.1.05.011 **64**
- of seminal gland A09.3.06.004 **68**
- of small intestine A05.6.01.009 **52**
- of spongy urethra A09.4.02.029 **70**
- of stomach A05.5.01.027 **52**
- of tongue A05.1.04.011 **49**
- of trachea A06.3.01.010 **59**
- of tympanic cavity A15.3.02.063 **150**
- of ureter A08.2.01.007 **64**
- of urethra A09.2.03.012 **67**
- of uterine tube A09.1.02.013 **65**
- of vagina A09.1.04.011 **66**
Multifidus A04.3.02.202 **37**
- cervicis A04.3.02.205 **37**
- lumborum A04.3.02.203 **37**
- thoracis A04.3.02.204 **37**
Multiform layer
- of dentate gyrus A14.1.09.343 **128**
- of isocortex [Layer VI] A14.1.09.314 **128**
Multipennate muscle A04.0.00.017 **33**
Muscle/s A04.0.00.000 **33**
- layer A16.0.03.003 **155**
- - in fatty layer of subcutaneous tissue A16.0.03.003 **155**
- - of pharynx A04.2.06.001 **36, 51**
- of abdomen A04.5.00.001 **38**
- of anal triangle A09.5.00.003 **71**
- of auditory ossicles A04.1.02.001 **34, 150**
- of back A04.3.00.001 **36**
- - proper A04.3.02.001 **36**
- of head A04.1.00.001 **34**
- of lower limb A04.7.00.001 **42**
- of neck A04.2.00.001 **35**
- of soft palate and fauces A04.1.06.001 **35, 50**
- of terminal notch of auricle A15.3.01.040 **148**
- of thorax A04.4.00.001 **37**
- of tongue A04.1.05.001 **35, 49**
- of upper limb A04.6.00.001 **40**
- of urogenital triangle A09.5.00.004 **71**
- sheath A04.0.00.040 **34**
Muscular
- arteries A12.2.06.033 **82**
- branch/es
- - of accessory nerve A14.2.01.190 **137**
- - of anterior
- - - branch of obturator nerve A14.2.07.015 **140**
- - - interosseous nerve A14.2.03.035 **138**
- - of axillary nerve A14.2.03.060 **139**
- - of deep fibular nerve A14.2.07.056 **140**
- - of femoral nerve A14.2.07.021 **140**
- - of intercostal nerves A14.2.04.007 **139**
- - of musculocutaneous nerve A14.2.03.025 **138**
- - of perineal nerves A14.2.07.041 **140**
- - of posterior branch of obturator nerve A14.2.07.017 **140**
- - of radial nerve A14.2.03.053 **138**
- - of spinal nerve A14.2.00.026 **133**
- - of superficial fibular nerve A14.2.07.051 **140**
- - of supraclavicular part of brachial plexus A14.2.03.019 **138**
- - of tibial nerve A14.2.07.059 **141**
- - of ulnar nerve A14.2.03.041 **138**
- - of vertebral artery A12.2.08.008 **84**
- fascia of eyeball A15.2.07.008 **147**
- layer
- - of bladder A08.3.01.010 **64**
- - of colon A05.7.03.011 **53**
- - of ductus deferens A09.3.05.009 **68**
- - of gallbladder A05.8.02.008 **56**
- - of intermediate urethra A09.4.02.018 **70**
- - of large intestine A05.7.01.004 **53**
- - of oesophagus A05.4.01.010 **51**
- - of prostatic urethra A09.4.02.011 **70**
- - of rectum A05.7.04.009 **54**
- - of renal pelvis A08.1.05.010 **64**
- - of seminal gland A09.3.06.003 **68**
- - of small intestine A05.6.01.004 **52**
- - of spongy urethra A09.4.02.027 **70**
- - of stomach A05.5.01.021 **52**
- - of ureter A08.2.01.006 **64**
- - of urethra A09.2.03.007 **67**
- - of uterine tube A09.1.02.012 **65**
- - of vagina A09.1.04.010 **66**
- part of interventricular septum A12.1.00.014 **76**
- process of arytenoid A06.2.04.013 **58**
- space A04.7.03.010 **43**
- system A04.0.00.000 **33**
- tissue of prostate A09.3.08.020 **69**
- triangle A01.2.02.005 **3**
- trochlea A04.0.00.049 **34**
Muscularis mucosae
- of large intestine A05.7.01.007 **53**
- of oesophagus A05.4.01.016 **51**
- of small intestine A05.6.01.010 **52**
- of stomach A05.5.01.029 **52**
Musculi pectinati
- of left atrium A12.1.03.003 **77**
- of right atrium A12.1.01.008 **76**
Musculocutaneous nerve A14.2.03.024 **138**
Musculophrenic
- artery A12.2.08.040 **85**
- veins A12.3.04.021 **92**
Musculotubal canal A02.1.06.017 **12**
Musculus uvulae A05.2.01.104 **50**
Myelencephalon A14.1.03.003 **108**
Myenteric nerve plexus A14.3.03.041 **143**
Mylohyoid A04.2.03.006 **35**
- branch of inferior alveolar artery A12.2.05.060 **80**
- groove A02.1.15.031 **15**
- line A02.1.15.012 **15**
Mylopharyngeal part of superior constrictor A05.3.01.106 **51**
Myocardium A12.1.06.001 **77**
Myometrium A09.1.03.025 **66**

N

Nail A16.0.01.001 **154**
– matrix A16.0.01.002 **154**
– wall A16.0.01.003 **154**
Nares A06.1.02.002 **57**
Nasal
– bone A02.1.10.001 **14**
– cartilages A06.1.01.006 **57**
– cavity A06.1.02.001 **57**
– crest
– – of maxilla A02.1.12.030 **14**
– – of palatine A02.1.13.018 **15**
– foramina A02.1.10.003 **14**
– glands A06.1.02.020 **57**
– margin of frontal bone A02.1.03.021 **10**
– mucosa A06.1.02.017 **57**
– notch A02.1.12.010 **14**
– part of frontal bone A02.1.03.019 **10**
– region A01.2.01.016 **3**
– septal branch of superior labial branch of facial artery A12.2.05.027 **80**
– septum A06.1.02.004 **57**
– spine of frontal bone A02.1.03.020 **10**
– surface
– – of maxilla A02.1.12.017 **14**
– – of palatine A02.1.13.003 **14**, A02.1.13.014 **15**
– vestibule A06.1.02.009 **57**
Nasalis A04.1.03.009 **34**
Nasion A02.1.00.015 **8**
Nasociliary
– nerve A14.2.01.025 **133**
– root of ciliary ganglion A14.2.01.026 **134, 142**
Nasofrontal vein A12.3.06.103 **95**
Nasolabial
– lymph node A13.3.00.011 **101**
– sulcus A01.2.01.017 **3**
Nasolacrimal
– canal A02.1.00.085 **9**
– duct A15.2.07.070 **148**
Nasomaxillary suture A03.1.02.026 **26**
Nasopalatine nerve A14.2.01.043 **134**
Nasopharyngeal meatus A02.1.00.095 **9**, A06.1.02.032 **57**
Nasopharynx A05.3.01.003 **50**
Natal cleft A01.2.08.003 **5**
Navicular A02.5.12.001 **24**
– articular surface of talus A02.5.10.003 **23**
– fossa A09.4.02.022 **70**
Neck A01.1.00.012 **2**
– of bladder A08.3.01.005 **64**
– of femur A02.5.04.004 **22**
– of fibula A02.5.07.005 **23**
– of gallbladder A05.8.02.005 **56**
– of glans A09.4.01.010 **69**
– of malleus A15.3.02.046 **150**
– of mandible A02.1.15.037 **16**
– of pancreas A05.9.01.005 **56**
– of posterior horn of spinal cord A14.1.02.120 **106**
– of radius A02.4.05.005 **20**
– of rib A02.3.02.005 **18**
– of scapula A02.4.01.022 **19**
– of talus A02.5.10.007 **24**
– of tooth A05.1.03.030 **48**
Neocerebellum A14.1.07.012 **118**
Neocortex A14.1.09.304 **128**
Neostriatum A14.1.09.516 **130**
Nerve A14.2.00.013 **132**
– fibre A13.0.00.001 **104**
– of pterygoid canal A14.3.02.007 **142**
– plexus of ductus deferens ♂ A14.3.03.053 **143**
– terminals A16.0.00.031 **154**
– to external acoustic meatus A14.2.01.075 **134**
– to lateral pterygoid A14.2.01.072 **134**
– to medial pterygoid A14.2.01.066 **134**
– to mylohyoid A14.2.01.090 **135**
– to obturator internus A14.2.07.028 **140**
– to piriformis A14.2.07.029 **140**
– to quadratus femoris A14.2.07.030 **140**
– to stapedius A14.2.01.101 **135**
– to tensor
– – tympani A14.2.01.069 **134**
– – veli palatini A14.2.01.068 **134**
Nervous system A14.0.00.000 **104**
Nervus spinosus A14.2.01.065 **134**
Neural
– layer of retina A15.2.04.009 **145**
– lobe of pituitary gland A11.1.00.008 **74, 120**
Neurocranium A02.1.00.007 **8**
Neuroglia A14.0.00.005 **104**
Neurohypophysis A11.1.00.006 **74, 120, 124**
Neuron A14.0.00.002 **104**
Nipple A16.0.02.004 **154**
– line A01.2.00.016 **3**
Nodule of vermis [X] A14.1.07.302 **119**
Nodules of semilunar cusps
– of aortic valve A12.1.04.016 **77**
– of pulmonary valve A12.1.02.014 **77**
Noncoronary cusp of aortic valve A12.1.04.015 **77**
Nonvisual retina A15.2.04.003 **145**
Noradrenergic/Norepinephric cells
– in caudolateral pons [A5] A14.1.09.606 **131**
– in compact part of substantia nigra [A9] A14.1.09.612 **131**
– in locus caeruleus [A6] A14.1.09.605 **131**
– in medulla [A1, A2] A14.1.09.603 **131**
– in nucleus of lateral lemniscus [A7] A14.1.09.604 **131**
– in reticular formation [A8] A14.1.09.609 **131**
– in ventral tegmental area [A10] A14.1.09.615 **131**
Nose A01.1.00.009 **2**, A06.1.01.001 **57**
Nostrils A06.1.02.002 **57**
Notch A02.0.00.033 **7**
– for ligamentum teres A05.8.01.025 **55**
– in cartilage of acoustic meatus A15.3.01.050 **149**
– of cardiac apex A12.1.00.008 **76**
Nuchal
– fascia A04.3.01.017 **36**
– ligament A03.2.01.006 **27**
Nuclei
– of inferior colliculus A14.1.06.602 **118**
– of lateral lemniscus A14.1.05.431 **114**
– of perizonal fields of subthalamus [H, H1, H2] A14.1.08.703 **123**
– of solitary tract A14.1.04.230 **111**
– of trapezoid body A14.1.05.421 **114**
Nucleus A14.1.00.003 **104**
– accumbens A14.1.09.440 **129**
– ambiguus A14.1.04.253 **111**
– lateralis cerebelli A14.1.07.407 **120**
– limitans A14.1.08.635 **122**
– medialis cerebelli A14.1.07.411 **120**
– of abducens nerve A14.1.05.411 **114**
– of accessory nerve A14.1.02.112 **106**
– of ansa lenticularis A14.1.08.919 **123**
– of cranial nerve A14.1.00.004 **104**
– of diagonal band A14.1.09.425 **129**
– of dorsal field of subthalamus [H1] A14.1.08.705 **123**
– of hypoglossal nerve A14.1.04.227 **110**
– of lateral olfactory tract A14.1.09.414 **129**
– of lens A15.2.05.004 **146**
– of medial field of subthalamus [H] A14.1.08.704 **123**
– of oculomotor nerve A14.1.06.302 **117**
– of optic tract A14.1.08.508 **121**
– of origin A14.1.00.005 **104**
– of phrenic nerve A14.1.02.113 **106**
– of posterior commissure A14.1.06.309 **117**
– of pudendal nerve A14.1.02.139 **106**
– of trochlear nerve A14.1.06.319 **117**
– of ventral field of subthalamus [H2] A14.1.08.706 **123**
– proprius of spinal cord A14.1.02.121 **106**
– pulposus A03.2.02.005 **27**
– reuniens A14.1.08.632 **122**
Nutrient
– artery A12.0.00.004 **75**

– – of radius A12.2.09.029 **86**
– – of ulna A12.2.09.046 **86**
– canal A02.0.00.042 **7**
– foramen A02.0.00.041 **7**
– vein A12.0.00.034 **75**

O

Obex A14.1.04.021 **109**, A14.1.05.723 **115**
Oblique
– arytenoid A06.2.08.010 **59**
– cord of interosseous membrane of forearm A03.5.06.003 **29**
– diameter of pelvis A02.5.02.012 **22**
– fibres of pyloric sphincter A05.5.01.025 **52**
– fissure of lung A06.5.01.021 **60**
– head of adductor
– – hallucis A04.7.02.061 **43**
– – pollicis A04.6.02.060 **41**
– line
– – of mandible A02.1.15.008 **15**
– – of thyroid cartilage A06.2.02.009 **58**
– muscle of auricle A15.3.01.044 **149**
– part of cricothyroid A06.2.08.003 **59**
– pericardial sinus A12.1.07.002 **78**
– popliteal ligament A03.6.08.013 **31**
– ridge of tooth A05.1.03.016 **48**
– vein of left atrium A12.3.01.007 **91**
Obliquus capitis
– inferior A04.2.02.007 **35**
– superior A04.2.02.006 **35**
Oblong fovea of arytenoid A06.2.04.008 **58**
Obscurus raphe nucleus A14.1.04.319 **112**
Obturator
– artery A12.2.15.008 **89**
– branch of pubic branch of inferior epigastric artery A12.2.16.005 **90**
– canal A03.6.01.003 **30**
– crest A02.5.01.309 **21**
– externus A04.7.02.031 **42**
– fascia A04.5.03.009 **39**
– foramen A02.5.01.008 **21**
– groove A02.5.01.310 **22**
– internus A04.7.02.012 **42**
– lymph nodes A13.3.04.017 **103**
– membrane A03.6.01.002 **30**
– nerve A14.2.07.012 **140**
– veins A12.3.10.007 **97**
Occipital A01.0.00.016 **1**
– angle of parietal bone A02.1.02.016 **10**
– artery A12.2.05.030 **80**
– aspect A02.1.00.004 **8**
– belly of occipitofrontalis A04.1.03.005 **34**
– bone A02.1.04.001 **10**
– border of parietal bone A02.1.02.011 **9**
– branch
– – of occipital artery A12.2.05.034 **80**
– – of posterior auricular
– – – artery A12.2.05.043 **80**
– – – nerve A14.2.01.103 **135**
– condyle A02.1.04.014 **10**
– diploic vein A12.3.05.205 **94**
– emissary vein A12.3.05.305 **94**
– forceps A14.1.09.251 **127**
– groove A02.1.06.007 **12**
– horn of lateral ventricle A14.1.09.286 **128**
– line A14.1.09.318 **128**
– – of internal granular layer of isocortex A14.1.09.318 **128**
– lobe A14.1.09.132 **125, 126**
– lymph nodes A13.3.00.002 **101**
– margin of temporal bone A02.1.06.003 **12**
– plane A02.1.04.027 **11**
– pole A14.1.09.133 **125**
– region A01.2.01.004 **3**
– sinus A12.3.05.105 **93**
– stripe of internal granular layer of isocortex A14.1.09.318 **128**
– vein/s A12.3.04.013 **92**, A12.3.06.008 **94**
Occipitofrontalis A04.1.03.003 **34**
Occipitomastoid suture A03.1.02.005 **26**
Occipitopontine fibres A14.1.06.107 **116**, A14.1.09.540 **130**
Occipitotectal fibres A14.1.09.541 **130**
Occipitotemporal
– branch of medial occipital artery A12.2.07.103 **84**
– sulcus A14.1.09.229 **126**
Occiput A01.1.00.003 **2**, A02.1.00.014 **8**
Occluded part of umbilical artery A12.2.15.025 **89**
Occlusal
– curves A05.1.03.075 **49**
– fissure A05.1.03.017 **48**
– fossa A05.1.03.018 **48**
– surface of tooth A05.1.03.034 **48**
Oculomotor
– nerve [III] A14.2.01.007 **133**
– root of ciliary ganglion A14.2.01.010 **133, 142**
– sulcus A14.1.06.003 **115**
Oesophageal
– branches A12.2.08.047 **85**
– – of inferior thyroid artery A12.2.08.047 **85**
– – of left gastric artery A12.2.12.014 **87**
– – of recurrent laryngeal nerve A14.2.01.168 **136**
– – of thoracic
– – – aorta A12.2.11.003 **86**
– – – ganglia A14.3.01.027 **141**
– glands A05.4.01.017 **51**
– hiatus A04.4.02.011 **38**
– impression on liver A05.8.01.018 **54**
– mucosa A05.4.01.015 **51**
– nerve plexus A14.2.01.173 **136**, A14.3.03.015 **143**
– veins A12.3.04.011 **92**, A12.3.07.006 **95**
Oesophagus A05.4.01.001 **51**
Olecranon A02.4.06.002 **20**
– fossa A02.4.04.024 **19**
Olfactory
– area A15.1.00.002 **144**
– bulb A14.1.09.429 **129**
– glands A15.1.00.003 **144**
– groove A06.1.02.011 **57**
– islets A14.1.09.428 **129**
– nerve [I] A14.2.01.004 **133**
– nerves A14.2.01.005 **133**
– organ A15.1.00.001 **144**
– part of nasal mucosa A15.1.00.002 **144**
– peduncle A14.1.09.430 **129**
– region of nasal mucosa A06.1.02.019 **57**
– striae A14.1.09.434 **129**
– sulcus A14.1.09.219 **126**
– tract A14.1.09.431 **129**
– trigone A14.1.09.432 **129**
– tubercle A14.1.09.433 **129**
Olivary pretectal nucleus A14.1.08.509 **121**
Olivocerebellar tract A14.1.04.118 **109**
Olivocochlear tract A14.1.05.316 **113**
Olivospinal fibres A14.1.02.213 **107**, A14.1.02.223 **107**
Omental
– appendices A05.7.03.010 **53**
– branches
– – of left gastro-omental artery A12.2.12.049 **88**
– – of right gastro-omental artery A12.2.12.024 **87**
– bursa A10.1.02.402 **72**
– eminence of pancreas A05.9.01.013 **56**
– foramen A10.1.02.403 **72**
– taenia A05.7.03.015 **53**
– tuberosity of liver A05.8.01.017 **54**
Omoclavicular triangle A01.2.02.010 **3**
Omohyoid A04.2.04.003 **35**
Omotracheal triangle A01.2.02.005 **3**
Opening/s
– of aqueduct of midbrain A14.1.06.502 **118, 121**
– of cerebral aqueduct A14.1.06.502 **118, 121**
– of cochlear canaliculus A02.1.06.043 **12**
– of coronary sinus A12.1.01.009 **76**
– of frontal sinus A02.1.03.030 **10**
– of inferior vena cava A12.1.01.010 **76**
– of nasolacrimal

– – canal A02.1.00.092 **9**
– – duct A06.1.02.030 **57**
– of papillary ducts A08.1.01.031 **63**
– of pulmonary
– – trunk A12.1.02.009 **76**
– – veins A12.1.03.004 **77**
– of renal papillary ducts A08.1.01.031 **63**
– of smallest cardiac veins A12.1.01.004 **76**
– of sphenoidal sinus A02.1.05.018 **11**
– of superior vena cava A12.1.01.011 **76**
– of vestibular canaliculus A02.1.06.036 **12**
Opercular part of inferior frontal gyrus A14.1.09.116 **125**
Ophthalmic
– artery A12.2.06.016 **81**
– division [Va; V3] A14.2.01.016 **133**
– nerve A14.2.01.016 **133**
Opisthion A02.1.04.004 **10**
Opponens
– digiti minimi
– – of hand A04.6.02.064 **41**
– – of foot A04.7.02.065 **43**
– muscle A04.0.00.027 **33**
– pollicis A04.6.02.058 **41**
Opposition A03.0.00.062 **26**
Optic
– axis A15.2.01.008 **144**
– canal A02.1.05.021 **11**
– chiasm A14.1.08.403 **120**
– chiasma A14.1.08.403 **120**
– disc A15.2.04.019 **145**
– layer of superior colliculus A14.1.06.608 **118**
– nerve [II] A14.2.01.006 **133**, A15.2.04.024 **145**
– part of retina A15.2.04.007 **145**
– radiation A14.1.08.673 **122**, A14.1.09.542 **130**, A14.1.09.547 **131**
– tract A14.1.08.404 **120**
Ora serrat retinae A15.2.04.006 **145**
Oral
– cavity A05.1.01.001 **47**
– – proper A05.1.01.101 **47**
– fissure A05.1.01.004 **47**
– opening A05.1.01.004 **47**
– pontine reticular nucleus A14.1.05.503 **114**
– region A01.2.01.018 **3**
– subnucleus of spinal nucleus of trigeminal nerve A14.1.05.405 **113**
– vestibule A05.1.01.003 **47**
Orbicular muscle A04.0.00.018 **33**
Orbicularis
– oculi A04.1.03.013 **34**
– oris A04.1.03.023 **34**
Orbiculus ciliaris A15.2.03.013 **144**
Orbit A02.1.00.067 **9**
Orbital
– branch/es
– – of middle meningeal artery A12.2.05.064 **81**
– – of maxillary nerve A14.2.01.040 **134**
– cavity A02.1.00.068 **9**
– fat body A15.2.07.007 **147**
– gyri A14.1.09.216 **126**
– margin A02.1.00.070 **9**
– muscle A15.2.07.009 **147**
– opening A02.1.00.069 **9**
– part
– – of frontal bone A02.1.03.022 **10**
– – of inferior frontal gyrus A14.1.09.114 **125**
– – of lacrimal gland A15.2.07.058 **148**
– – of optic nerve A15.2.04.027 **145**
– – of orbicularis oculi A04.1.03.017 **34**
– plate of ethmoid A02.1.07.011 **13**
– process of palatine A02.1.13.011 **15**
– region A01.2.01.010 **3**
– septum A15.2.07.003 **147**
– sulci A14.1.09.217 **126**
– surface
– – of frontal bone A02.1.03.023 **10**
– – of maxilla A02.1.12.003 **14**
– – of sphenoid A02.1.05.030 **11**
– – of zygomatic A02.1.14.004 **15**
– tubercle A02.1.14.007 **15**
– veins A12.3.06.015 **94**, A12.3.06.101 **95**
Orbitalis A15.2.07.009 **147**
Oriens layer of hippocampus A14.1.09.336 **128**
Orifice
– of ileal papilla A05.7.02.003 **53**
– of vermiform appendix A05.7.02.008 **53**
Oropharyngeal isthmus A05.2.01.002 **50**
Oropharynx A05.3.01.019 **50**
Os
– centrale A02.4.08.002 **20**
– trigonum A02.5.10.021 **24**
Osseous spiral lamina A15.3.03.029 **151**
Ossification centre A02.0.00.043 **7**
Otic ganglion A14.3.02.014 **142**
Otolith A15.3.03.086 **152**
Otolithic membrane A15.3.03.085 **152**
Outer
– border of iris A15.2.03.025 **145**
– limiting layer of retina A15.2.04.011 **145**
– lip of iliac crest A02.5.01.107 **21**
– nuclear layer of retina A15.2.04.012 **145**
– plexiform layer of retina A15.2.04.013 **145**
– sheath of optic nerve A15.2.04.032 **145**
– spiral sulcus A15.3.03.124 **153**
– stripe of renal medulla A08.1.01.022 **63**
– zone of renal medulla A08.1.01.021 **63**
Oval
– fossa A12.1.01.005 **76**
– window A15.3.02.009 **149**
Ovarian
– artery ♀ A12.2.12.086 **88**
– branches of uterine artery ♀ A12.2.15.033 **89**
– cortex A09.1.01.011 **65**
– fimbria A09.1.02.005 **65**
– fossa ♀ A10.1.02.510 **73**
– medulla A09.1.01.012 **65**
– nerve plexus ♀ A14.3.03.035 **143**
– stroma A09.1.01.010 **65**
Ovary A09.1.01.001 **65**

P

P1 segment of posterior cerebral artery A12.2.07.083 **84**
P2 segment of posterior cerebral artery A12.2.07.088 **84**
P3 segment of posterior cerebral artery A12.2.07.094 **84**
P4 segment of posterior cerebral artery A12.2.07.098 **84**
Pachymeninx A14.1.01.002 **104**
Palatal
– cusp A05.1.03.020 **48**
– root A05.1.03.065 **49**
– surface
– – of palatine A02.1.13.015 **15**
– – of tooth A05.1.03.039 **48**
Palate A05.1.01.102 **47**
Palatine
– aponeurosis A05.2.01.101 **50**
– bone A02.1.13.001 **14**
– crest of palatine A02.1.13.019 **15**
– glands A05.1.02.017 **47**
– grooves A02.1.12.034 **14**
– process of maxilla A02.1.12.029 **14**
– raphe A05.1.01.105 **47**
– rugae A05.1.01.106 **47**
– spines A02.1.12.033 **14**
– surface A02.1.13.015 **15**
– tonsil A05.2.01.011 **50, 100**
– torus A02.1.00.063 **9**
Palato-ethmoidal suture A03.1.02.031 **26**
Palatoglossal arch A05.2.01.005 **50**
Palatoglossus A05.1.04.110 **49, 50**
Palatomaxillary suture A03.1.02.030 **26**
Palatopharyngeal
– arch A05.2.01.007 **50**
– ridge A05.3.01.018 **50**
– sphincter A05.2.01.107 **50**
Palatopharyngeus A05.2.01.105 **50, 51**
Palatovaginal
– canal A02.1.00.064 **9**
– groove A02.1.05.049 **12**
Paleocerebellum A14.1.07.011 **118**

Paleocortex A14.1.09.303 **128**
Paleostriatum A14.1.09.518 **130**
Pallidal raphe nucleus
A14.1.04.320 **112**
Pallidum A14.1.09.518 **130**
Palm A01.1.00.028 **2**,
A01.2.07.022 **5**
Palmar A01.0.00.043 **1**
– aponeurosis A04.6.03.012 **41**
– branch
– – of anterior interosseous nerve
A14.2.03.036 **138**
– – of ulnar nerve
A14.2.03.044 **138**
– carpal
– – branch
– – – of radial artery
A12.2.09.030 **86**
– – – of ulnar atery
A12.2.09.054 **86**
– – tendinous sheaths
A04.8.04.004 **44**
– carpometacarpal ligaments
A03.5.11.303 **29**
– digital veins A12.3.08.027 **96**
– intercarpal ligaments
A03.5.11.105 **29**
– interossei A04.6.02.067 **41**
– ligaments
– – of interphalangeal joints of
hand A03.5.11.603 **30**
– – of metacarpophalangeal joints
A03.5.11.503 **30**
– metacarpal
– – arteries A12.2.09.039 **86**
– – ligaments A03.5.11.403 **29**
– – veins A12.3.08.035 **96**
– radiocarpal ligament
A03.5.11.004 **29**
– region A01.2.07.022 **5**
– surfaces of fingers
A01.2.07.032 **5**
– ulnocarpal ligament
A03.5.11.006 **29**
Palmaris
– brevis A04.6.02.053 **41**
– longus A04.6.02.029 **41**
Palmate folds of cervical canal
A09.1.03.019 **66**
Palpebral
– branches of infratrochlear nerve
A14.2.01.036 **134**
– conjunctiva A15.2.07.051 **147**
– fissure A15.2.07.030 **147**
– part
– – of lacrimal gland
A15.2.07.059 **148**
– – of orbicularis oculi
A04.1.03.014 **34**
– veins A12.3.06.115 **95**
Palpebronasal fold
A15.2.07.028 **147**
Pampiniform venous plexus
A12.3.09.015 **97**
Pancreas A05.9.01.001 **56**
Pancreatic
– branches
– – of anterior superior pancreaticoduodenal artery
A12.2.12.026 **87**
– – of posterior superior pancreaticoduodenal artery
A12.2.12.019 **87**
– – of splenic atery
A12.2.12.041 **88**
– duct A05.9.01.015 **56**
– impression on spleen
A13.2.01.012 **100**
– islets A05.9.01.019 **56, 74**
– lymph nodes A13.3.03.023 **102**
– nerve plexus A14.3.03.025 **143**
– notch A05.9.01.004 **56**
– veins A12.3.12.022 **99**,
A12.3.12.029 **99**
Pancreaticocolic ligament
A10.1.02.209 **72**
Pancreaticoduodenal
– lymph nodes A13.3.03.027 **102**
– veins A12.3.12.023 **99**
Pancreaticosplenic ligament
A10.1.02.208 **72**
Papilla of parotid duct
A05.1.01.017 **47**
Papillae
– of dermis A16.0.00.012 **154**
– of tongue A05.1.04.013 **49**
Papillary
– layer of dermis A16.0.00.011 **154**
– muscles of heart
A12.1.00.022 **76**
– process of caudate lobe of liver
A05.8.01.031 **55**
– ridges A16.0.00.004 **154**
Para-aortic bodies
A12.2.04.003 **79**
Para-umbilical veins
A12.3.12.013 **98**
Para-urethral ducts
A09.2.03.015 **67**, A09.4.02.026 **70**
Para-uterine lymph nodes ♀
A13.3.04.028 **103**
Parabigeminal nucleus
A14.1.06.320 **117**
Parabrachial
– nuclei A14.1.05.439 **114**
– pigmented nucleus
A14.1.06.332 **117**
Paracentral
– branches A12.2.07.042 **83**
– lobule A14.1.09.209 **126**
– nucleus of thalamus
A14.1.08.619 **121**
– sulcus A14.1.09.208 **126**
Paracervix A09.1.03.022 **66**
Paracolic
– gutters A10.1.02.424 **73**
– lymph nodes A13.3.03.041 **103**
Paracommissural solitary nucleus
A14.1.04.237 **111**
Paradidymis A09.3.03.001 **68**
Paraduodenal
– fold A10.1.02.414 **73**
– recess A10.1.02.415 **73**
Parafascicular nucleus of thalamus
A14.1.08.620 **121**
Parahippocampal gyrus
A14.1.09.234 **126**
Paralaminar part of medial dorsal nucleus of thalamus
A14.1.08.625 **122**
Paralemniscal nucleus
A14.1.05.504 **114**
Paramammary lymph nodes
A13.3.02.002 **102**
Paramastoid process
A02.1.04.035 **11**
Paramedian
– arteries A12.2.07.084 **84**
– lobule [H VII B] A14.1.07.213 **119**
– nucleus of pons
A14.1.05.206 **112**
– planes A01.2.00.005 **3**
– pontine branches of pontine arteries A12.2.08.022 **84**
– reticular nucleus
A14.1.05.505 **115**
Parametrium A09.1.03.021 **66**
Paramolar
– cusp A05.1.03.072 **49**
– tubercle A05.1.03.072 **49**
Paranasal sinuses A06.1.03.001 **57**
Paranephric fat A08.1.01.011 **63**
Paranigral nucleus
A14.1.06.333 **117, 118**
Paraolfactory
– area A14.1.09.213 **126**
– gyri A14.1.09.214 **126**
– sulci A14.1.09.215 **126**
Parapeduncular nucleus
A14.1.06.702 **118**
Parapharyngeal space
A05.3.01.119 **51**
Pararectal
– fossa A10.1.02.514 **73**
– lymph nodes A13.3.04.030 **103**
Pararenal fat body A08.1.01.011 **63**
Parasolitary nucleus
A14.1.04.231 **111**
Parasternal
– line A01.2.00.014 **3**
– lymph nodes A13.3.02.003 **102**
Parasubiculum A14.1.09.322 **128**
Parasympathetic
– ganglion A14.2.00.012 **132**
– part of autonomic division of nervous system A14.3.02.001 **142**
– root
– – of ciliary ganglion
A14.2.01.010 **133, 142**
– – of otic ganglion
A14.2.01.149 **136, 142**
– – of pelvic ganglia
A14.3.02.018 **142**
– – of pterygopalatine ganglion
A14.2.01.117 **135, 142**
– – of sublingual ganglion
A14.3.02.012 **142**
– – of submandibular ganglion
A14.2.01.118 **135, 142**
Parataenial nucleus
A14.1.08.628 **122**
Paraterminal gyrus
A14.1.09.212 **126**
Parathyroid gland A11.4.00.001 **74**

Paratracheal lymph nodes A13.3.00.024 **101**, A13.3.02.011 **102**
Paravaginal lymph nodes ♀ A13.3.04.029 **103**
Paraventricular
– fibres A14.1.08.951 **124**
– nuclei of thalamus A14.1.08.629 **122**
– nucleus of hypothalamus A14.1.08.909 **123**
Paraventriculohypophysial tract A14.1.08.956 **124**
Paravertebral line A01.2.00.021 **3**
Paravesical
– fossa A10.1.02.502 **73**
– lymph nodes A13.3.04.024 **103**
Parenchyma
– of prostate A09.3.08.018 **69**
– of testis A09.3.01.021 **68**
– of thyroid gland A11.3.00.008 **74**
Parietal
– abdominal
– – fascia A04.5.02.006 **38**
– – lymph nodes A13.3.03.002 **102**
– bone A02.1.02.001 **9**
– border of temporal bone A02.1.06.062 **13**
– branch
– – of medial occipital artery A12.2.07.100 **84**
– – of middle meningeal artery A12.2.05.065 **81**
– – of superficial temporal artery A12.2.05.052 **80**
– eminence A02.1.02.010 **9**
– emissary vein A12.3.05.302 **94**
– fascia A04.0.00.034 **33**
– – of abdomen A04.5.02.006 **39**
– – of thorax A04.4.01.020 **37, 62**
– – of pelvis A04.5.03.007 **39**
– foramen A02.1.02.019 **10**
– layer
– – of serous pericardium A12.1.08.006 **78**
– – of tunica vaginalis testis A09.3.01.009 **67**
– lobe A14.1.09.123 **125, 126**
– lymph nodes A13.3.03.002 **102**
– margin
– – of frontal bone A02.1.03.012 **10**
– – of sphenoid A02.1.05.033 **11**
– notch A02.1.06.063 **13**
– operculum A14.1.09.126 **125**
– pelvic
– – fascia A04.5.03.007 **39**
– – lymph nodes A13.3.04.002 **103**
– peritoneum A10.1.02.005 **72**
– pleura A07.1.02.005 **62**
– region A01.2.01.003 **3**
– serosa A07.1.02.010 **62**
– subserosa A07.1.02.011 **62**
– tuber A02.1.02.010 **9**
– veins A12.3.06.006 **94**
Parieto-occipital
– branch/es
– – of medial occipital artery A12.2.07.101 **84**
– – of pericallosal artery A12.2.07.045 **83**
– sulcus A14.1.09.108 **125, 126**
Parietomastoid suture A03.1.02.011 **26**
Parietopontine fibres A14.1.06.108 **116**, A14.1.09.537 **130**
Paroophoron A09.1.06.001 **66**
Parotid
– branch/es
– – of auriculotemporal nerve A14.2.01.077 **134**
– – of deep facial vein A12.3.05.028 **93**
– – of posterior auricular artery A12.2.05.044 **80**
– – of superficial temporal artery A12.2.05.046 **80**
– duct A05.1.02.007 **47**
– fascia A04.1.04.012 **35**
– gland A05.1.02.003 **47**
– lymph nodes A13.3.00.004 **101**, A13.3.00.005 **101**
– nerve plexus A14.2.01.108 **135**
– region A01.2.01.014 **3**
– veins A12.3.05.028 **93**, A12.3.05.041 **93**
Pars
– alpha of gigantocellular reticular nucleus A14.1.04.303 **111**
– anterior of pituitary gland A11.1.00.005 **74**
– copularis [H VIII A] A14.1.07.217 **119**
– distalis of pituitary gland A11.1.00.005 **74**
– flaccida of tympanic membrane A15.3.01.053 **149**
– intermedia
– – of pituitary gland A11.1.00.004 **74**
– – urethrae A09.4.02.017 **70, 71**
– laminaris A14.1.08.625 **122**
– membranacea urethrae A09.4.02.017 **70, 71**
– nervosa of pituitary gland A11.1.00.008 **74, 120**
– paralaminaris of medial dorsal nucleus of thalamus A14.1.08.625 **122**
– tensa of tympanic membrane A15.3.01.054 **149**
– tuberalis of pituitary gland A11.1.00.003 **74**
Part of optic nerve in canal A15.2.04.026 **145**
Parvocellular
– layers of dorsal nucleus of lateral geniculate body A14.1.08.805 **123**
– nucleus of medial dorsal nucleus of thalamus A14.1.08.623 **122**
– part
– – of lateral
– – – reticular nucleus A14.1.04.310 **112**
– – – vestibular nucleus A14.1.05.428 **114**
– – of red nucleus A14.1.06.325 **117**
– of ventral posteromedial nucleus of thalamus A14.1.08.643 **122**
– reticular nucleus A14.1.04.312 **112**
Patella A02.5.05.001 **23**
Patellar
– anastomosis A12.2.16.041 **90**
– ligament A03.6.08.015 **31**
– surface of femur A02.5.04.027 **22**
Patent part of umbilical artery A12.2.15.021 **89**
Pecten pubis A02.5.01.308 **21**
Pectinate
– line of anal canal A05.7.05.009 **54**
– muscles
– – of left atrium A12.1.03.003 **77**
– – of right atrium A12.1.01.008 **76**
Pectineal
– inguinal ligament A04.5.01.011 **38**
– line
– – of femur A02.5.04.016 **22**
– – of pubis A02.5.01.308 **21**
Pectineus A04.7.02.025 **42**
Pectoral
– branches of thoraco-acromial artery A12.2.09.010 **85**
– fascia A04.4.01.017 **37**
– girdle A01.1.00.020 **2**, A02.4.00.002 **18**
– lymph nodes A13.3.01.006 **101**
– region A01.2.03.005 **4**
– veins A12.3.08.003 **96**
Pectoralis
– major A04.4.01.002 **37**
– minor A04.4.01.006 **37**
Pedicle of vertebral arch A02.2.01.006 **16**
Peduncle of flocculus A14.1.07.303 **119**
Peduncular
– branches of posterior cerebral artery A12.2.07.093 **84**
– loop A14.1.08.665 **122, 129**
– nucleus of pons A14.1.05.207 **112**
– veins A12.3.06.026 **94**
Pedunculopontine tegmental nucleus A14.1.06.336 **117, 118**
Pelvic
– bone A02.5.01.001 **21**
– cavity A01.1.00.052 **2**, A02.5.02.002 **22**, A10.1.00.002 **72**
– diaphragm A04.5.04.001 **39**
– fascia A04.5.03.001 **39**
– floor A04.5.04.001 **39**
– ganglia A14.3.02.017 **142**
– girdle A01.1.00.032 **2**, A02.5.00.002 **21**
– inclination A02.5.02.022 **22**
– inlet A02.5.02.008 **22**
– lateral wall triangle ♀ A10.1.02.509 **73**
– lymph nodes A13.3.04.001 **103**

– nerve plexus A14.3.03.048 **143**
– outlet A02.5.02.009 **22**
– part
– – of ductus deferens A09.3.05.005 **68**
– – of parasympathetic part of autonomic division of nervous system A14.3.02.016 **142**, A14.3.03.045 **143**
– – of ureter A08.2.01.003 **64**
– splanchnic nerves A14.3.02.018 **142**
– surface of sacrum A02.2.05.009 **17**
Pelvis A01.1.00.017 **2**, A02.5.02.001 **22**
– of kidney A08.1.05.001 **64**
Penicilli A13.2.01.020 **100**
Penis A09.4.01.001 **69**
Pennate muscle A04.0.00.016 **33**
Perforating
– arteries
– of deep femoral artery A12.2.16.031 **90**
– – of penis ♂ A12.2.15.046 **89**
– branch/es
– – of deep palmar arch A12.2.09.040 **86**
– – of fibular artery A12.2.16.072 **91**
– – of internal thoracic artery A12.2.08.036 **85**
– – of plantar metatarsal artery A12.2.16.067 **91**
– – of posterior interosseous artery A12.2.09.051 **86**
– cutaneous nerve A14.2.07.036 **140**
– radiate arteries of kidney A08.1.03.007 **63**
– veins A12.3.11.027 **98**
Peri-olivary nuclei A14.1.05.418 **114**
Peri-urethral gland zone of prostate A09.3.08.004 **68**
Periamygdaloid cortex A14.1.09.415 **129**
Periaqueductal grey substance A14.1.06.321 **117**
Periarterial nerve plexus A14.2.00.044 **133**
Pericallosal
– artery A12.2.07.043 **83**
– cistern A14.1.01.214 **105**
Pericardiacophrenic
– artery A12.2.08.034 **85**
– veins A12.3.04.007 **92**
Pericardial
– branch/es
– – of phrenic nerve A14.2.02.029 **137**
– – of thoracic aorta A12.2.11.004 **86**
– cavity A06.6.03.001 **77**, A07.1.03.001 **62**
– serosa A12.1.08.008 **78**
– subserosa A12.1.08.009 **78**
– veins A12.3.04.006 **92**, A12.3.07.008 **95**
Pericardium A12.1.08.001 **78**
Pericentral nucleus of inferior colliculus A14.1.06.605 **118**
Perichondrium A02.0.00.008 **7**
Perichoroidal space A15.2.03.004 **144**
Pericranium A02.1.00.011 **8**
Peridental branches
– of inferior alveolar artery A12.2.05.058 **80**
– of infra-orbital artery A12.2.05.081 **81**
– of posterior superior alveolar artery A12.2.05.077 **81**
Perifornical nucleus A14.1.08.931 **124**
Perihypoglossal nuclei A14.1.04.262 **111**
Perikaryon A14.0.00.003 **104**
Perilymph A15.3.03.056 **152**
Perilymphatic space A15.3.03.055 **152**
Perimetrium A09.1.03.023 **66**
Perimysium A04.0.00.042 **34**
Perineal
– artery A12.2.15.040 **89**
– body A09.5.00.005 **71**
– branches of posterior cutaneous nerve of thigh A14.2.07.035 **140**
– fascia A09.5.02.002 **71**
– flexure A05.7.05.002 **54**
– membrane A09.5.03.002 **71**
– muscles A04.5.05.001 **40, 71**
– nerves A14.2.07.039 **140**
– raphe A09.5.00.002 **71**
– region A01.2.06.001 **4**
Perinephric fat A08.1.01.012 **63**
Perineum A09.5.00.001 **71**
Perineurium A14.2.00.015 **132**
Periodontal
– fibre A03.1.03.006 **26**
– membrane A03.1.03.002 **26**
Periodontium A03.1.03.002 **26**, A05.1.03.058 **49**
Perionyx A16.0.01.009 **154**
Periorbita A15.2.07.002 **147**
Periosteum A02.0.00.007 **7**
Peripeduncular nucleus
– of mesencephalon A14.1.06.322 **117**
– of pons A14.1.05.207 **112**
Peripharyngeal space A05.3.01.117 **51**
Peripheral A01.0.00.038 **1**
– autonomic plexuses and ganglia A14.3.03.001 **142**
– nervous system A14.2.00.001 **132**
Perirenal fat capsule A08.1.01.012 **63**
Peritoneal
– attachments of liver A10.1.02.301 **72**
– cavity A10.1.02.001 **72**
– serosa A10.1.02.003 **72**
– subserosa A10.1.02.004 **72**
Peritoneum A10.1.02.002 **72**
Peritrigeminal nucleus A14.1.04.266 **111**
Perivascular fibrous capsule of liver A05.8.01.055 **55**
Periventricular
– fibres A14.1.08.674 **122**, A14.1.08.957 **124**
– nucleus A14.1.08.924 **123**
– preoptic nucleus A14.1.08.910 **123**
– zone of hypothalamus A14.1.08.942 **124**
Permanent teeth A05.1.03.077 **49**
Peroneal A01.0.00.041 **1**
– artery A12.2.16.071 **91**
– border of foot A01.2.08.026 **5**
– compartment of leg A04.7.01.009 **42**
– lymph node A13.3.05.016 **103**
– trochlea A02.5.11.014 **24**
– tubercle A02.5.11.014 **24**
– veins A12.3.11.033 **98**
Peroneus
– brevis A04.7.02.042 **42**
– longus A04.7.02.041 **42**
– tertius A04.7.02.039 **42**
Perpendicular plate
– of ethmoid A02.1.07.006 **13**
– of palatine A02.1.13.002 **14**
Pes hippocampi A14.1.09.323 **128**
Petro-occipital
– fissure A02.1.00.047 **8**
– synchondrosis A03.1.05.004 **27**
Petrosal
– branch of middle meningeal artery A12.2.05.066 **81**
– fossula A02.1.06.050 **13**
– vein A12.3.06.062 **95**
Petrosphenoidal fissure A02.1.00.046 **8**
Petrosquamous
– fissure A02.1.06.075 **13**
– sinus A12.3.05.107 **93**
Petrotympanic fissure A02.1.06.074 **13**
Petrous part
– of internal carotid artery A12.2.06.004 **81**
– of temporal bone A02.1.06.002 **12**
Phalanx/Phalanges
– of hand A02.4.10.001 **20**
– of foot A02.5.18.001 **24**
Pharyngeal
– branch/es
– – of artery of pterygoid canal A12.2.05.083 **81**
– – of ascending pharyngeal artery A12.2.05.012 **80**
– – of descending palatine artery A12.2.05.087 **81**
– – of glossopharyngeal nerve A14.2.01.144 **136**
– – of inferior thyroid artery A12.2.08.046 **85**
– – of recurrent laryngeal nerve A14.2.01.169 **136**
– – of vagus A14.2.01.158 **136**
– bursa A05.3.01.010 **50**

– glands A05.3.01.030 **51**
– hypophysis A05.3.01.005 **50**
– lymphoid
– – nodules A05.3.01.009 **50, 100**
– – ring A13.2.02.001 **100**
– mucosa A05.3.01.029 **51**
– muscles A04.2.06.001 **36, 51**
– nerve A14.2.01.044 **134**
– – plexus A14.2.01.159 **136**
– opening A15.3.02.085 **151**
– – of auditory tube A05.3.01.011 **50**
– – of pharyngotympanic tube A15.3.02.085 **151**
– raphe A05.3.01.101 **51**
– recess A05.3.01.017 **50**
– tonsil A05.3.01.006 **50, 100**
– tubercle A02.1.04.007 **10**
– veins A12.3.05.007 **93**
– venous plexus A12.3.05.006 **93**
Pharyngo-oesophageal constriction A05.3.01.026 **50**
Pharyngobasilar fascia A05.3.01.027 **50**
Pharyngotympanic tube A15.3.02.073 **150**
Pharynx A05.3.01.001 **50**
Philtrum A05.1.01.007 **47**
Phrenic
– ganglia A14.3.03.020 **143**
– nerve A14.2.02.028 **137**
– nucleus A14.1.02.113 **106**
Phrenico-abdominal branches of phrenic nerve A14.2.02.030 **137**
Phrenico-oesophageal ligament A04.4.02.012 **38**
Phrenicocoeliac part of suspensory muscle of duodenum A05.6.02.012 **52**
Phrenicocolic ligament A10.1.02.211 **72**
Phrenicomediastinal recess A07.1.02.015 **62**
Phrenicopleural fascia A07.1.02.019 **62**
Phrenicosplenic ligament A10.1.02.206 **72**
Physiological cup A15.2.04.020 **145**
Pia mater A14.1.01.301 **105**
Pial
– filament A14.1.01.403 **105**
– part of filum terminale A14.1.01.403 **105**
Pigmented
– epithelium of iris A15.2.03.032 **145**
– layer of retina A15.2.04.008 **145**
Pineal
– body A11.2.00.001 **74, 120**
– gland A11.2.00.001 **74, 120**
– nerve A14.3.01.012 **141**
– recess A14.1.08.415 **121**
Pinna A15.3.01.002 **148**
Piriform
– aperture A02.1.00.088 **9**
– fossa A05.3.01.024 **50**
– recess A05.3.01.024 **50**
Piriformis A04.7.02.011 **42**
– fascia A04.5.03.011 **39**
Pisiform A02.4.08.007 **20**
– joint A03.5.11.107 **29**
Pisohamate ligament A03.5.11.108 **29**
Pisometacarpal ligament A03.5.11.109 **29**
Pituitary gland A11.1.00.001 **74**
Pivot joint A03.0.00.045 **25**
Plane
– joint A03.0.00.043 **25**
– suture A03.0.00.009 **25**
Planes, lines and regions A01.2.00.000 **3**
Plantar A01.0.00.044 **1**
– aponeurosis A04.7.03.031 **44**
– calcaneocuboid ligament A03.6.10.518 **31**
– calcaneonavicular ligament A03.6.10.203 **31**
– cuboideonavicular ligament A03.6.10.520 **31**
– cuneocuboid ligament A03.6.10.522 **31**
– cuneonavicular ligaments A03.6.10.519 **31**
– digital
– – arteries proper A12.2.16.069 **91**
– – veins A12.3.11.018 **98**
– intercuneiform ligaments A03.6.10.521 **31**
– interossei A04.7.02.071 **43**
– ligaments
– – of interphalangeal joints of foot A03.6.10.903 **32**
– – of metatarsophalangeal joints A03.6.10.803 **32**
– metatarsal
– – arteries A12.2.16.066 **91**
– – ligaments A03.6.10.704 **32**
– – veins A12.3.11.017 **98**
– region A01.2.08.025 **5**
– surfaces of toes A01.2.08.041 **6**
– tarsal ligaments A03.6.10.516 **31**
– tarsometatarsal ligaments A03.6.10.603 **32**
– tendinous sheath
– – of fibularis longus A04.8.06.012 **46**
– – of peroneus longus A04.8.06.012 **46**
– venous
– – arch A12.3.11.016 **98**
– – network A12.3.11.015 **98**
Plantaris A04.7.02.049 **43**
Platysma A04.2.01.001 **35**
Pleura A07.1.02.001 **62**
Pleural
– cavity A07.1.01.001 **62**
– cupula A07.1.02.006 **62**
– recesses A07.1.02.012 **62**
Pleuro-oesophageus A05.4.01.013 **51**
Plexus of ductus deferens ♂ A14.3.03.054 **143**
Plica semilunaris conjunctivae A15.2.07.048 **147**
Pneumatized bone A02.0.00.015 **7**
Polar
– frontal artery A12.2.07.036 **83**
– temporal artery A12.2.07.051 **83**
Pons A14.1.03.010 **108, 112**
Pontine
– arteries A12.2.08.021 **84**
– corticonuclear fibres A14.1.05.105 **112**
– nuclei A14.1.05.202 **112**
– raphe nucleus A14.1.05.602 **115**
– veins A12.3.06.043 **95**
Pontobulbar nucleus A14.1.04.267 **111**
Pontocerebellar
– cistern A14.1.01.215 **105**
– fibres A14.1.05.110 **112**
Pontocerebellum A14.1.07.009 **118**
Pontomesencephalic vein A12.3.06.039 **95**
Pontoreticulospinal tract A14.1.02.209 **107**
Popliteal
– artery A12.2.16.033 **90**
– fossa A01.2.08.013 **5**
– lymph nodes A13.3.05.011 **103**
– surface of femur A02.5.04.018 **22**
– vein A12.3.11.028 **98**
Popliteus A04.7.02.050 **43**
Porta hepatis A05.8.01.016 **54**
Portal veins of hypophysis A12.3.05.309 **94**
Postaortic lymph nodes A13.3.03.006 **102**
Postcaval lymph nodes A13.3.03.011 **102**
Postcentral
– branch of spinal branch of dorsal branch of posterior intercostal artery A12.2.11.012 **87**
– fissure of cerebellum A14.1.07.111 **119**
– gyrus A14.1.09.128 **125**
– sulcus A14.1.09.129 **125**
Postclival fissure A14.1.07.205 **119**
Postcommissural fibres of column of fornix A14.1.09.257 **127**
Postcommunicating part
– of anterior cerebral artery A12.2.07.033 **83**
– of posterior cerebral artery A12.2.07.088 **84**
Posterior A01.0.00.012 **1**
– accessory
– – nucleus of optic tract A14.1.06.315 **117**
– – olivary nucleus A14.1.04.225 **110**
– acoustic stria A14.1.05.321 **113**
– ampullary nerve A14.2.01.131 **136**
– ankle region A01.2.08.019 **5**
– antebrachial cutaneous nerve A14.2.03.052 **138**
– arch of atlas A02.2.02.108 **17**
– articular facet of dens A02.2.02.205 **17**
– atlanto-occipital membrane A03.1.08.004 **27**

– attachment of linea alba A04.5.01.024 **38**
– auricular
– – artery A12.2.05.037 **80**
– – groove A15.3.01.022 **148**
– – nerve A14.2.01.102 **135**
– – vein A12.3.05.046 **93**
– axillary
– – line A01.2.00.019 **3**
– – lymph nodes A13.3.01.005 **101**
– basal
– – segment
– – – of left lung [S X] A06.5.02.025 **61**
– – – of right lung [S X] A06.5.02.014 **61**
– – segmental
– – – artery
– – – – of left lung A12.2.01.220 **79**
– – – – of right lung A12.2.01.119 **78**
– – – bronchus
– – – – of left lung [B X] A06.4.02.025 **60**
– – – – of right lung [B X] A06.4.02.014 **60**
– belly of digastric A04.2.03.004 **35**
– bony ampulla A15.3.03.019 **151**
– border
– – of fibula A02.5.07.013 **23**
– – of petrous part of temporal bone A02.1.06.037 **12**
– – of radius A02.4.05.014 **20**
– – of testis A09.3.01.007 **67**
– – of ulna A02.4.06.013 **20**
– brachial cutaneous nerve A14.2.03.050 **138**
– branch/es
– – of great auricular nerve A14.2.02.019 **137**
– – of inferior
– – – pancreaticoduodenal artery A12.2.12.056 **88**
– – – suprarenal artery A12.2.12.083 **88**
– – of medial cutaneous nerve of forearm A14.2.03.030 **138**
– – of obturator
– – – artery A12.2.15.012 **89**
– – – nerve A14.2.07.016 **140**
– – of posteromedial central arteries A12.2.07.071 **83**
– – of right
– – – branch of portal vein A12.3.12.004 **98**
– – – hepatic duct A05.8.01.064 **56**
– – – superior pulmonary vein A12.3.02.108 **91**
– – of ulnar recurrent artery A12.2.09.044 **86**
– caecal artery A12.2.12.061 **88**
– calcaneal articular facet A02.5.10.020 **24**
– cerebellomedullary cistern A14.1.01.208 **105**
– cerebral artery A12.2.07.082 **84, 85**
– cervical
– – nerve plexus A14.2.02.010 **137**
– – region A01.2.02.012 **4**
– chamber A15.2.06.005 **146**
– – of eyeball A15.2.06.005 **146**
– circumflex humeral
– – artery A12.2.09.017 **86**
– – vein A12.3.08.009 **96**
– clinoid process A02.1.05.011 **11**
– cochlear nucleus A14.1.04.248 **111**
– column of spinal cord
– – grey A14.1.02.114 **106**
– – white A14.1.02.239 **107**
– commissure
– – of diencephalon A14.1.08.416 **121**
– – of labia majora A09.2.01.005 **66**
– communicating artery A12.2.06.018 **81, 83, 84**
– compartment
– – of arm A04.6.01.003 **40**
– – of forearm A04.6.01.007 **40**
– – of leg A04.7.01.006 **42**
– – of thigh A04.7.01.003 **42**
– conjunctival arteries A12.2.06.045 **82**
– cord of brachial plexus A14.2.03.023 **138**
– cranial fossa A02.1.00.050 **8**
– crico-arytenoid A06.2.08.004 **59**
– cruciate ligament A03.6.08.008 **30**
– cusp
– – of mitral valve A12.1.04.005 **77**
– – of tricuspid valve A12.1.02.005 **76**
– cutaneous
– – branch/nerve
– – – of posterior ramus
– – – – of cervical nerve A14.2.02.006 **137**
– – – – of lumbar nerve A14.2.05.005 **139**
– – – – of thoracic nerve A14.2.04.005 **139**
– – – of sacral or coccygeal nerve A14.2.06.005 **139**
– – nerve
– – – of arm A14.2.03.050 **138**
– – – of forearm A14.2.03.052 **138**
– – – of thigh A14.2.07.033 **140**
– deep temporal artery A12.2.05.072 **81**
– divisions of brachial plexus A14.2.03.008 **138**
– ethmoidal
– – artery A12.2.06.043 **82**
– – cells A02.1.07.010 **13**, A06.1.03.008 **58**
– – foramen A02.1.00.080 **9**
– – nerve A14.2.01.028 **134**
– external
– – arcuate fibres A14.1.04.121 **109**
– – vertebral venous plexus A12.3.07.020 **96**
– extremity of spleen A13.2.01.014 **100**
– facet on talus for calcaneus A02.5.10.020 **24**
– fascicle of palatopharyngeus A05.2.01.107 **50**
– fasciculus proprius A14.1.02.240 **107**
– femoral cutaneous nerve A14.2.07.033 **140**
– fold of malleus A15.3.02.064 **150**
– fontanelle A02.1.00.029 **8**
– fornix of vagina A09.1.04.004 **66**
– funiculus of spinal cord A14.1.02.239 **107**
– gastric
– – artery A12.2.12.052 **88**
– – branches of posterior vagal trunk A14.2.01.180 **137**
– glandular branch of superior thyroid artery A12.2.05.008 **80**
– gluteal line A02.5.01.118 **21**
– grey
– – column of spinal cord A14.1.02.114 **106**
– – commissure of spinal cord A14.1.02.304 **108**
– horn
– – of lateral ventricle A14.1.09.286 **128**
– – of spinal cord A14.1.02.023 **106**, A14.1.02.115 **106**
– hypothalamic
– – area A14.1.08.933 **124**
– – region A14.1.08.933 **124**
– inferior
– – cerebellar artery A12.2.08.012 **84**
– – iliac spine A02.5.01.114 **21**
– – nasal nerves A14.2.01.046 **134**
– intercavernous sinus A12.3.05.118 **94**
– intercondylar area A02.5.06.007 **23**
– intercostal
– – arteries A12.2.11.007 **86**
– – veins A12.3.07.014 **96**
– intermediate sulcus of spinal cord A14.1.02.012 **105**
– intermuscular septum of leg A04.7.03.023 **43**
– internal vertebral venous plexus A12.3.07.026 **96**
– interosseous
– – artery A12.2.09.050 **86**
– – nerve A14.2.03.055 **138**
– – veins A12.3.08.033 **96**
– interpositus nucleus A14.1.07.410 **120**
– interventricular
– – branch of right coronary artery A12.2.03.108 **79**
– – sulcus A12.1.00.010 **76**
– – vein A12.3.01.009 **91**
– intra-occipital synchondrosis A03.1.05.006 **27**
– labial
– – branches of perineal artery ♀ A12.2.15.041 **89**
– – nerves ♀ A14.2.07.040 **140**

– – veins ♀ A12.3.10.022 **97**
– lacrimal crest A02.1.09.002 **14**
– lateral
– – choroidal branches of posterior cerebral artery A12.2.07.092 **84**
– – nasal arteries A12.2.05.089 **81**
– – segment of liver A05.8.01.051 **55**
– layer
– – of rectus sheath A04.5.01.005 **38**
– – of thoracolumbar fascia A04.3.02.502 **37**
– left ventricular branch of left coronary artery A12.2.03.211 **79**
– ligament
– – of auricle A15.3.01.035 **148**
– – of fibular head A03.6.09.003 **31**
– – of incus A15.3.02.058 **150**
– limb
– – of internal capsule A14.1.09.531 **130**
– – of stapes A15.3.02.036 **150**
– limiting lamina of cornea A15.2.02.021 **144**
– lip of external os A09.1.03.017 **66**
– liver A05.8.01.043 **55**
– lobe
– – of cerebellum A14.1.07.201 **119**
– – of pituitary gland A11.1.00.006 **74, 120, 124**
– longitudinal
– – fasciculus A14.1.04.114 **109**, A14.1.05.305 **112**, A14.1.06.211 **116**, A14.1.08.946 **124**
– – ligament A03.2.01.008 **27**
– lumbar nerve plexus A14.2.05.007 **139**
– malleolar fold A15.3.01.056 **149**
– medial
– – choroidal branches of posterior cerebral artery A12.2.07.091 **84**
– – segment of liver A05.8.01.048 **55**
– median
– – line A01.2.00.022 **3**
– – septum of spinal cord A14.1.02.009 **105**
– – sulcus
– – – of medulla A14.1.04.020 **109**
– – – of spinal cord A14.1.02.008 **105**
– mediastinum A07.1.02.106 **62**
– membranous ampulla A15.3.03.070 **152**
– meningeal artery A12.2.05.011 **80**
– meniscofemoral ligament A03.6.08.004 **30**
– nasal
– – aperture/s A02.1.00.096 **9**, A06.1.02.003 **57**
– – spine of palatine A02.1.13.017 **15**
– nerve of lesser curvature A14.2.01.181 **137**
– nuclear complex of thalamus A14.1.08.634 **122**
– nucleus
– – of accessory
– – – oculomotor nuclei A14.1.06.306 **117**
– – – nuclei of optic tract A14.1.06.315 **117**
– – of hypothalamus A14.1.08.939 **124**
– – of lateral
– – – funiculus of spinal cord A14.1.02.129 **106**
– – – lemniscus A14.1.05.432 **114**
– – of pons A14.1.05.208 **112**
– – of thalamus A14.1.08.636 **122**
– – of vagus nerve A14.1.04.229 **110**
– obturator tubercle A02.5.01.312 **22**
– palpebral margin A15.2.07.036 **147**
– papillary muscle
– – of left ventricle A12.1.04.008 **77**
– – of right ventricle A12.1.02.018 **77**
– paracentral gyrus A14.1.09.222 **126**
– paragigantocellular reticular nucleus A14.1.04.313 **112**
– paramedian nucleus of medulla A14.1.04.228 **110**
– paraventricular nucleus of thalamus A14.1.08.631 **122**
– parietal artery A12.2.07.068 **83**
– part
– – of anterior
– – – cochlear nucleus A14.1.04.251 **111**
– – – commissure A14.1.09.254 **127, 131**
– – – quadrangular lobule of cerebellum A14.1.07.118 **119**
– – of central lobule of cerebellum A14.1.07.107 **119**
– – of culmen A14.1.07.115 **119**
– – of diaphragmatic surface of liver A05.8.01.007 **54**
– – of knee A01.1.00.037 **2**
– – of lateral
– – – funiculus of spinal cord A14.1.02.229 **107**
– – – parabrachial nucleus A14.1.05.444 **114**
– – of liver A05.8.01.043 **55**
– – of tongue A05.1.04.006 **49**
– – of vagina A09.1.04.004 **66**
– perforated substance A14.1.06.002 **115**
– periventricular nucleus A14.1.08.925 **123**
– pillar of fauces A05.2.01.007 **50**
– plexus of lumbar nerves A14.2.05.007 **139**
– pole
– – of eyeball A15.2.01.003 **144**
– – of lens A15.2.05.009 **146**
– pretectal nucleus A14.1.08.510 **121**
– process
– – of septal nasal cartilage A06.1.01.015 **57**
– – of talus A02.5.10.016 **24**
– quadrangular lobule of cerebellum [H VI] A14.1.07.204 **119**
– radicular artery A12.2.11.014 **87**
– rami
– – of cervical nerves A14.2.02.003 **137**
– – of lumbar nerves A14.2.05.002 **139**
– – of sacral nerves and coccygeal nerve A14.2.06.002 **139**
– – of thoracic nerves A14.2.04.002 **139**
– ramus
– – of lateral cerebral sulcus A14.1.09.105 **124**
– – of spinal nerve A14.2.00.035 **133**
– raphe nucleus A14.1.05.604 **115, 117**
– recess of tympanic membrane A15.3.02.070 **150**
– region
– – of arm A01.2.07.007 **4**
– – of elbow A01.2.07.011 **4**
– – of forearm A01.2.07.014 **5**
– – of knee A01.2.08.012 **5**
– – of leg A01.2.08.016 **5**
– – of thigh A01.2.08.009 **5**
– – of wrist A01.2.07.020 **5**
– root of spinal nerve A14.2.00.030 **133**
– sacral foramina A02.2.05.015 **17**
– sacro-iliac ligament A03.6.03.004 **30**
– scalene A04.2.01.006 **35**
– scrotal
– – branches of perineal artery ♂ A12.2.15.041 **89**
– – nerves ♂ A14.2.07.040 **140**
– – veins ♂ A12.3.10.022 **97**
– segment
– – of eyeball A15.2.01.010 **144**
– – of kidney A08.1.02.006 **63**
– – of liver A05.8.01.044 **55**
– – of right lung [S II] A06.5.02.004 **61**
– segmental
– – artery
– – – of kidney A12.2.12.084 **88**
– – – of left lung A12.2.01.208 **78**
– – – of liver A12.2.12.034 **87**
– – – of right lung A12.2.01.107 **78**
– – bronchus [B II] A06.4.02.004 **60**
– semicircular
– – canal A15.3.03.018 **151**
– – duct A15.3.03.069 **152**
– semilunar cusp of aortic valve A12.1.04.015 **77**
– septal branches of sphenopalatine artery A12.2.05.090 **81**

- sinus of tympanic cavity A15.3.02.026 **149**
- solitary nucleus A14.1.04.238 **111**
- spinal
- – artery A12.2.08.013 **84**
- – veins A12.3.07.025 **96**
- spinocerebellar tract A14.1.02.227 **107**, A14.1.04.132 **110**
- sternoclavicular ligament A03.5.04.004 **29**
- subnucleus of lateral parabrachial nucleus A14.1.05.444 **114**
- superior
- – alveolar
- – – artery A12.2.05.075 **81**
- – – branches A14.2.01.050 **134**
- – – nerves A14.2.01.050 **134**
- – fissure of cerebellum A14.1.07.205 **119**
- – iliac spine A02.5.01.113 **21**
- – lateral nasal branches of maxillary nerve A14.2.01.041 **134**
- – medial nasal branches of maxillary nerve A14.2.01.042 **134**
- – pancreaticoduodenal artery A12.2.12.018 **87**
- surface
- – of arytenoid A06.2.04.011 **58**
- – of body of pancreas A05.9.01.008 **56**
- – of cornea A15.2.02.017 **144**
- – of eyelid A15.2.07.029 **147**
- – of fibula A02.5.07.009 **23**
- – of humerus A02.4.04.013 **19**
- – of iris A15.2.03.024 **145**
- – of kidney A08.1.01.007 **63**
- – of lens A15.2.05.011 **146**
- – of petrous part of temporal bone A02.1.06.031 **12**
- – of prostate A09.3.08.008 **69**
- – of radius A02.4.05.009 **20**
- – of scapula A02.4.01.004 **18**
- – of suprarenal gland A11.5.00.003 **74**
- – of tibia A02.5.06.014 **23**
- – of ulna A02.4.06.009 **20**
- – of uterus A09.1.03.006 **65**
- talar articular surface of calcaneum A02.5.11.012 **24**
- talocalcaneal ligament A03.6.10.104 **31**
- talocrural region A01.2.08.019 **5**
- talofibular ligament A03.6.10.010 **31**
- tegmental
- – decussation A14.1.06.221 **117**
- – nucleus A14.1.05.449 **114**
- temporal
- – branch/es
- – – of middle cerebral artery A12.2.07.058 **83**
- – – of lateral occipital artery A12.2.07.097 **84**
- – diploic vein A12.3.05.204 **94**
- thalamic radiation A14.1.08.675 **122**, A14.1.09.543 **131**
- thoracic nucleus A14.1.02.135 **106**
- tibial
- – artery A12.2.16.055 **90**
- – lymph node A13.3.05.015 **103**
- – recurrent artery A12.2.16.044 **90**
- – veins A12.3.11.032 **98**
- tibiofibular ligament A03.6.05.004 **30**
- tibiotalar part of medial ligament of ankle joint A03.6.10.007 **31**
- transverse temporal gyrus A14.1.09.142 **125**
- triangle A01.2.02.009 **3**
- trigeminothalamic tract A14.1.05.312 **113**
- tubercle
- – of atlas A02.2.02.111 **17**
- – of cervical vertebra A02.2.02.006 **16**
- tympanic artery A12.2.05.039 **80**
- vagal trunk A14.2.01.179 **137**
- vaginal column A09.1.04.015 **66**
- vein
- – of corpus callosum A12.3.06.037 **95**
- – of septum pellucidum A12.3.06.032 **94**
- – of upper lobe of right lung A12.3.02.108 **91**
- vein(s) of left ventricle A12.3.01.006 **91**
- ventrolateral nucleus of thalamus A14.1.08.651 **122**
- vestibular
- – branch of vestibulocochlear artery A15.3.03.131 **153**
- – vein A15.3.03.142 **153**
- visceral nucleus A14.1.06.306 **117**
- wall
- – of stomach A05.5.01.003 **51**
- – of tympanic cavity A15.3.02.020 **149**
- – of vagina A09.1.04.007 **66**
- white
- – column of spinal cord A14.1.02.239 **107**
- – commissure of spinal cord A14.1.02.306 **108**

Posterolateral
- central arteries A12.2.07.089 **84**
- fissure of cerebellum A14.1.07.223 **119**
- nucleus
- – of pons A14.1.05.209 **112**
- – of spinal cord A14.1.02.108 **106**
- solitary nucleus A14.1.04.239 **111**
- sulcus
- – of medulla A14.1.04.012 **108**
- – of spinal cord A14.1.02.011 **105**
- tract A14.1.02.228 **107**

Posteromedial
- central arteries
- – from posterior
- – – cerebral artery A12.2.07.084 **84**
- – – communicating artery A12.2.07.069 **83**
- frontal branch of callosomarginal artery A12.2.07.040 **83**
- nucleus
- – of pons A14.1.05.210 **112**
- – of principal sensory nucleus of trigeminal nerve A14.1.05.407 **114**
- – of spinal cord A14.1.02.110 **106**
- part of red nucleus A14.1.06.326 **117**

Posteromedian medullary vein A12.3.06.053 **95**

Postganglionic nerve fibres A14.2.00.010 **132**

Postlaminar part of optic nerve A15.2.04.029 **145**

Postlingual fissure A14.1.07.104 **119**

Postpyramidal fissure of cerebellum A14.1.07.220 **119**

Postremal chamber of eyeball A15.2.06.006 **146**

Postsulcal part of tongue A05.1.04.006 **49**

Postvesical lymph nodes A13.3.04.026 **103**

Pre-accessory cuneate nucleus A14.1.04.210 **110**

Pre-aortic lymph nodes A13.3.03.005 **102**

Pre-auricular lymph nodes A13.3.00.006 **101**

Pre-epiglottic fat body A06.2.07.007 **59**

Pre-occipital notch A14.1.09.109 **125**

Pre-olivary groove A14.1.04.006 **108**

Pre-optic
- area A14.1.08.407 **120, 124**
- arteries A12.2.07.028 **82**

Prebiventral fissure A14.1.07.214 **119**

Precaecal lymph nodes A13.3.03.037 **102**

Precaecocolic fascia A05.7.02.010 **53**

Precaval lymph nodes A13.3.03.010 **102**

Precentral
- cerebellar vein A12.3.06.061 **95**
- fissure of cerebellum A14.1.07.104 **119**
- gyrus A14.1.09.119 **125**
- sulcus A14.1.09.120 **125**

Prechiasmatic sulcus A02.1.05.005 **11**

Preclival fissure A14.1.07.119 **119**

Precommissural
- fibres of column of fornix A14.1.09.256 **127**
- septal nucleus A14.1.09.265 **127**

Precommunicating part
- of anterior cerebral artery A12.2.07.023 **82**

– of posterior cerebral artery A12.2.07.083 **84**
Preculminate fissure A14.1.07.111 **119**
Precuneal branches of pericallosal artery A12.2.07.044 **83**
Precuneus A14.1.09.223 **126**
Prefrontal
– artery A12.2.07.063 **83**
– veins A12.3.06.004 **94**
Preganglionic nerve fibres A14.2.00.009 **132**
Pregeniculate nucleus A14.1.08.806 **123**
Prelaminar
– branch of spinal branch of dorsal branch of posterior intercostal artery A12.2.11.013 **87**
– part of optic nerve A15.2.04.031 **145**
Prelaryngeal lymph nodes A13.3.00.021 **101**
Premammillary artery A12.2.07.076 **83**
Premaxilla A02.1.12.031 **14**
Premolar tooth A05.1.03.006 **48**
Prepancreatic artery A12.2.12.044 **88**
Prepericardial lymph nodes A13.3.02.006 **102**
Prepositus nucleus A14.1.04.265 **111**
Preprostatic
– part of urethra A09.4.02.003 **70**
– sphincter A09.4.02.013 **70**
Prepuce
– of clitoris A09.2.01.009 **66**
– of penis A09.4.01.011 **69**
Preputial glands A09.4.01.028 **70**
Prepyloric vein A12.3.12.017 **98**
Prepyramidal fissure of cerebellum A14.1.07.214 **119**
Presacral
– fascia A04.5.03.018 **39**
– nerve A14.3.03.046 **143**
Presplenic fold A10.1.02.204 **72**
Presternal region A01.2.03.002 **4**
Presubiculum A14.1.09.325 **128**
Presulcal part of tongue A05.1.04.005 **49**
Pretectal
– area A14.1.08.505 **121**
– nuclei A14.1.08.506 **121**
Pretecto-olivary fibres A14.1.05.306 **113, 117**
Pretracheal
– layer of cervical fascia A04.2.05.004 **35**
– lymph nodes A13.3.00.023 **101**
Prevertebral
– layer of cervical fascia A04.2.05.006 **36**
– lymph nodes A13.3.02.018 **102**
– part of vertebral artery A12.2.08.003 **84**
Prevesical lymph nodes A13.3.04.025 **103**
Primary A02.0.00.044 **7**
– cartilaginous joint A03.0.00.018 **25**
– curvature A02.2.00.002 **16**
– fissure of cerebellum A14.1.07.119 **119**
– hair A16.0.00.015 **154**
– lymphoid organs A13.1.00.001 **100**
Princeps pollicis artery A12.2.09.036 **86**
Principal
– division of ventral anterior nucleus of thalamus A14.1.08.654 **122**
– olivary nucleus A14.1.04.220 **110**
– sensory nucleus of trigeminal nerve A14.1.05.406 **113**
– ventral medial nucleus of thalamus A14.1.08.646 **122**
Procerus A04.1.03.008 **34**
Process/us A02.0.00.028 **7**
– cochleariformis A15.3.02.018 **149**
Profunda
– brachii artery A12.2.09.020 **86**
– femoris vein A12.3.11.024 **98**
Projection fibre A14.1.00.018 **104**
Prominence
– of facial canal A15.3.02.023 **149**
– of lateral semicircular canal A15.3.02.022 **149**
Promontorial lymph nodes A13.3.04.008 **103**
Promontory
– of sacrum A02.2.05.003 **17**
– of tympanic cavity A15.3.02.011 **149**
Pronation A03.0.00.060 **26**
Pronator
– muscle A04.0.00.025 **33**
– quadratus A04.6.02.038 **41**
– teres A04.6.02.025 **40**
– tuberosity A02.4.05.011 **20**
Proper
– cochlear artery A15.3.03.132 **153**
– palmar digital
– – arteries A12.2.09.058 **86**
– – nerves A14.2.03.039 **138**, A14.2.03.047 **138**
– plantar digital nerves A14.2.07.068 **141**, A14.2.07.072 **141**
Prosencephalon A14.1.03.006 **108**
Prostate A09.3.08.001 **68**
Prostatic
– branches
– – of inferior vesical artery ♂ A12.2.15.028 **89**
– – of middle rectal artery ♂ A12.2.15.037 **89**
– ducts A09.3.08.019 **69**
– nerve plexus ♂ A14.3.03.052 **143**
– sinus A09.4.02.010 **70**
– urethra A09.4.02.004 **70**
– utricle A09.4.02.009 **70**
– venous plexus ♂ A12.3.10.013 **97**
Proximal A01.0.00.035 **1**
– deep inguinal lymph node A13.3.05.008 **103**
– lateral striate branches of anterolateral central arteries A12.2.07.049 **83**
– medial striate arteries A12.2.07.025 **82**
– part
– – of prostate A09.3.08.003 **68**
– – of prostatic urethra A09.4.02.005 **70**
– phalanx
– – of foot A02.5.18.002 **24**
– – of hand A02.4.10.002 **20**
– radio-ulnar joint A03.5.09.004 **29**
– transverse arch of foot A01.2.08.031 **5**
Psoas
– fascia A04.5.02.008 **39**
– major A04.7.02.004 **42**
– minor A04.7.02.005 **42**
Pterion A02.1.00.019 **8**
Pterygoid
– branches of posterior deep temporal artery A12.2.05.073 **81**
– canal A02.1.05.053 **12**
– fossa A02.1.05.046 **12**
– fovea A02.1.15.038 **16**
– hamulus A02.1.05.051 **12**
– notch A02.1.05.045 **12**
– process of sphenoid A02.1.05.042 **12**
– tuberosity A02.1.15.027 **15**
– venous plexus A12.3.05.036 **93**
Pterygomandibular raphe A05.3.01.102 **51**
Pterygomaxillary fissure A02.1.00.026 **8**
Pterygomeningeal artery A12.2.05.069 **81**
Pterygopalatine
– fossa A02.1.00.025 **8**
– ganglion A14.3.02.006 **142**
Pterygopharyngeal part of superior constrictor A05.3.01.104 **51**
Pterygospinous
– ligament A03.1.01.002 **26**
– process A02.1.05.054 **12**
Pubic
– arch A02.5.02.003 **22**
– branch
– – of inferior epigastric
– – – artery A12.2.16.004 **90**
– – – vein A12.3.10.026 **97**
– – of obturator artery A12.2.15.009 **89**
– crest A02.5.01.305 **21**
– hairs A16.0.00.022 **154**
– region A01.2.04.007 **4**
– symphysis A03.6.02.001 **30**
– tubercle A02.5.01.303 **21**
– vein A12.3.10.026 **97**
Pubis A02.5.01.301 **21**
Pubo-analis A04.5.04.006 **39**
Pubocervical ligament A09.1.03.030 **66**
Pubococcygeal tendon A04.5.04.017 **40**

Pubococcygeus A04.5.04.003 **39**
Pubofemoral ligament A03.6.07.007 **30**
Puboperineales A04.5.04.004 **39**
Puboprostatic ligament A04.5.03.015 **39**
Puboprostaticus A04.5.04.005 **39, 69**
Puborectalis A04.5.04.007 **40**
Pubovaginalis ♀ A04.5.04.005 **39, 69**
Pubovesical ligament A04.5.03.013 **39**
Pubovesicalis A04.5.03.014 **39**, A08.3.01.020 **64**
Pudendal
- canal A09.5.04.003 **71**
- cleft A09.2.01.006 **66**
- nerve A14.2.07.037 **140**
Pudendum A09.2.01.001 **66**
Pulmonary
- branches
- - of pulmonary nerve plexus A14.3.03.016 **143**
- - of thoracic ganglia A14.3.01.026 **141**
- groove A02.3.04.005 **18**
- ligament A07.1.02.017 **62**
- lobule A06.5.02.027 **61**
- nerve plexus A14.2.01.172 **136**, A14.3.03.016 **143**
- pleura A07.1.02.002 **62**
- trunk A12.2.01.001 **78**
- valve A12.1.02.010 **76**
- veins A12.3.02.001 **91**
Pulp
- canal A05.1.03.049 **48**
- cavity A05.1.03.047 **48**
- - of crown A05.1.03.048 **48**
Pulvinar A14.1.08.104 **120**
- nuclei A14.1.08.610 **121**
Pupil A15.2.03.028 **145**
Pupillary
- margin of iris A15.2.03.021 **145**
- membrane A15.2.03.036 **145**
Purkinje cell layer of cerebellar cortex A14.1.07.404 **119**
Putamen A14.1.09.507 **130**
Pyloric
- antrum A05.5.01.015 **52**
- branch of anterior vagal trunk A14.2.01.178 **136**
- canal A05.5.01.016 **52**
- lymph nodes A13.3.03.019 **102**
- orifice A05.5.01.018 **52**
- part of stomach A05.5.01.014 **52**
- sphincter A05.5.01.024 **52**
Pylorus A05.5.01.017 **52**
Pyramid A14.1.04.003 **108**
- of medulla A14.1.04.003 **108**
- of vermis [VIII] A14.1.07.215 **119**
- of vestibule A15.3.03.008 **151**
Pyramidal
- eminence A15.3.02.024 **149**
- layer of hippocampus A14.1.09.337 **128**
- lobe of thyroid gland A11.3.00.004 **74**
- muscle of auricle A15.3.01.041 **148**
- process of palatine A02.1.13.007 **15**
- tract A14.1.04.102 **109**, A14.1.06.102 **116**
Pyramidalis A04.5.01.007 **38**
Pyramis [VIII] A14.1.07.215 **119**

Q

Quadrangular membrane A06.2.09.022 **59**
Quadrate
- ligament A03.5.09.008 **29**
- lobe of liver A05.8.01.029 **55**
- muscle A04.0.00.010 **33**
- tubercle A02.5.04.011 **22**
Quadratus
- femoris A04.7.02.015 **42**
- lumborum A04.5.01.027 **38**
- - fascia A04.3.02.504 **37**
- plantae A04.7.02.068 **43**
Quadriceps femoris A04.7.02.017 **42**
Quadrigeminal
- artery A12.2.07.087 **84**
- cistern A14.1.01.217 **105**
- plate A14.1.06.011 **115, 118**

R

Radial A01.0.00.039 **1**
- artery A12.2.09.027 **86**
- border of forearm A01.2.07.015 **5**
- collateral
- - artery A12.2.09.024 **86**
- - ligament
- - - of elbow joint A03.5.09.006 **29**
- - - of wrist joint A03.5.11.008 **29**
- fibres of ciliary muscle A15.2.03.017 **145**
- fossa A02.4.04.026 **19**
- groove A02.4.04.014 **19**
- head of flexor digitorum superficialis A04.6.02.035 **41**
- nerve A14.2.03.049 **138**
- notch A02.4.06.005 **20**
- part of posterior compartment of forearm A04.6.01.008 **40**
- recurrent artery A12.2.09.028 **86**
- styloid process A02.4.05.015 **20**
- tuberosity A02.4.05.007 **20**
- veins A12.3.08.031 **96**
Radialis indicis artery A12.2.09.037 **86**
Radiate
- carpal ligament A03.5.11.103 **29**
- layer of hippocampus A14.1.09.338 **128**
- ligament of head of rib A03.3.04.003 **28**
- sternocostal ligaments A03.3.05.003 **28**
Radiation of corpus callosum A14.1.09.249 **127**
Radicular branches of spinal branches of vertebral artery A12.2.08.006 **84**
Radii of lens A15.2.05.014 **146**
Radio-ulnar syndesmosis A03.5.06.001 **29**
Radius A02.4.05.001 **19**
Rami communicantes A14.3.01.005 **141**
Ramus A02.5.01.203 **21**
- communicans A14.2.00.033 **133**
- of ischium A02.5.01.203 **21**
- of mandible A02.1.15.024 **15**
- of pubis A02.5.01.306 **21**, A02.5.01.313 **22**
Raphe
- nuclei
- - of medulla oblongata A14.1.04.257 **111**, A14.1.04.318 **112**
- - of pontile tegmentum A14.1.05.402 **113**, A14.1.05.601 **115**
- - of tegmentum of midbrain A14.1.06.401 **117**
- of medulla oblongata A14.1.04.122 **109**
- of penis A09.4.01.013 **69**
- of pons A14.1.05.303 **112**
- of scrotum A09.4.03.002 **70**
Recesses of tympanic membrane A15.3.02.067 **150**
Recesses, fossae and folds A10.1.02.401 **72**
Rectal
- ampulla A05.7.04.008 **54**
- stalk A05.7.04.016 **54**
- venous plexus A12.3.10.010 **97**
Recto-urethral muscles A05.7.04.012 **54**
- inferior A05.7.04.014 **54**
- superior A05.7.04.013 **54**
Recto-uterine
- fold ♀ A10.1.02.511 **73**
- ligament A09.1.03.032 **66**
- pouch ♀ A10.1.02.512 **73**
Recto-uterinus A09.1.03.026 **66**
Recto-vesical pouch ♂ A10.1.02.513 **73**
Rectococcygeus A05.7.04.011 **54**
Rectoperinealis A05.7.04.013 **54**
Rectoprostatic fascia A04.5.03.004 **39**
Rectosacral fascia A04.5.03.019 **39**
Rectovaginal
- fascia A04.5.03.004 **39**
- septum ♀ A04.5.03.004 **39**
Rectovesical septum ♂ A04.5.03.004 **39**
Rectovesicalis A04.5.03.017 **39, 54, 64**
Rectum A05.7.04.001 **53**
Rectus
- abdominis A04.5.01.001 **38**
- capitis
- - anterior A04.2.02.002 **35**
- - lateralis A04.2.02.003 **35**
- - posterior
- - - major A04.2.02.004 **35**

– – – minor A04.2.02.005 **35**
– femoris A04.7.02.018 **42**
– sheath A04.5.01.003 **38**
Recurrent
– branch A14.2.00.032 **133**
– interosseous artery A12.2.09.052 **86**
– laryngeal nerve A14.2.01.166 **136**
– meningeal branch of ophthalmic artery A12.2.06.030 **82**
Red
– bone marrow A02.0.00.040 **7**
– nucleus A14.1.06.323 **117**
– pulp A13.2.01.005 **100**
Reflected
– head of rectus femoris A04.7.02.020 **42**
– inguinal ligament A04.5.01.012 **38**
Region
– I of hippocampus proper [CA1] A14.1.09.328 **128**
– II of hippocampus proper [CA2] A14.1.09.329 **128**
– III of hippocampus proper [CA3] A14.1.09.330 **128**
– IV of hippocampus proper [CA4] A14.1.09.331 **128**
Regional lymph nodes A12.4.02.001 **99, 101**
Regions
– of back A01.2.05.001 **4**
– of head A01.2.01.001 **3**
– of lower limb A01.2.08.001 **5**
– of neck A01.2.02.001 **3**
– of upper limb A01.2.07.001 **4**
Renal
– artery A12.2.12.075 **88**
– branch/es
– – of lesser splanchnic nerve A14.3.01.031 **141**
– – of vagus A14.2.01.183 **137**
– columns A08.1.01.019 **63**
– cortex A08.1.01.015 **63**
– – corticis A08.1.01.017 **63**
– cortical labyrinth A08.1.01.016 **63**
– crest A08.1.01.028 **63**
– fascia A08.1.01.010 **63**
– ganglia A14.3.03.033 **143**
– impression
– – on liver A05.8.01.022 **55**
– – on spleen A13.2.01.009 **100**
– medulla A08.1.01.020 **63**
– nerve plexus A14.3.03.032 **143**
– papilla A08.1.01.027 **63**
– pelvis A08.1.05.001 **64**
– pyramids A08.1.01.029 **63**
– segments A08.1.02.001 **63**
– sinus A08.1.01.005 **63**
– surface of suprarenal gland A11.5.00.004 **74**
– veins A12.3.09.009 **97**
Reposition A03.0.00.063 **26**
Respiratory
– region of nasal mucosa A06.1.02.018 **57**
– system A06.0.00.000 **57**
Restiform body A14.1.04.014 **109**, A14.1.07.414 **120**
Rete
– mirabile A12.0.00.013 **75**
– testis A09.3.01.024 **68**
Reticular
– formation A14.1.00.021 **104**, A14.1.05.403 **113**, A14.1.06.327 **117**
– layer of dermis A16.0.00.013 **154**
– membrane of spiral organ A15.3.03.122 **153**
– nucleus/i
– – of medulla oblongata A14.1.04.301 **111**
– – of mesencephalon A14.1.06.701 **118**
– – of pontile tegmentum A14.1.05.501 **114**
– – of thalamus A14.1.08.638 **122**
– part of substantia nigra A14.1.06.114 **116**
Reticulospinal fibres A14.1.02.208 **107**
Reticulotegmental nucleus of pons A14.1.05.211 **112**, A14.1.05.506 **115**
Retina A15.2.04.002 **145**
Retinaculum caudale A16.0.00.006 **154**
Retinal blood vessels A15.2.04.035 **146**
Retinohypothalamic tract A14.1.08.960 **124**
Retro-ambiguus nucleus A14.1.04.254 **111**
Retro-inguinal
– muscular space A04.7.03.010 **43**
– space A10.1.01.004 **72**
– vascular space A04.7.03.011 **43**
Retro-olivary
– area A14.1.04.011 **108**
– groove A14.1.04.010 **108**
Retrobulbar
– fat A15.2.07.007 **147**
– nucleus [A8] A14.1.09.607 **131**
Retrocaecal
– lymph nodes A13.3.03.038 **102**
– recess A10.1.02.422 **73**
Retrocalcaneal bursa A04.8.05.032 **45**
Retrochiasmatic
– area A14.1.08.926 **123**
– region A14.1.08.926 **123**
Retrodorsal lateral nucleus of spinal cord A14.1.02.109 **106**
Retroduodenal
– arteries A12.2.12.021 **87**
– recess A10.1.02.416 **73**
Retrofacial nucleus A14.1.04.218 **110**
Retrohyoid bursa A04.8.02.005 **44**, A06.2.02.015 **58**
Retrolenticular limb A14.1.09.539 **130**
Retrolentiform limb A14.1.09.539 **130**
Retromandibular vein A12.3.05.031 **93**
Retromolar
– fossa A02.1.15.023 **15**
– triangle A02.1.15.022 **15**
Retroperitoneal space A10.1.01.002 **72**
Retropharyngeal
– lymph nodes A13.3.00.025 **101**, A13.3.00.038 **101**
– space A05.3.01.118 **51**
Retroposterior lateral nucleus of spinal cord A14.1.02.109 **106**
Retropubic space A10.1.01.003 **72**
Retropyloric lymph nodes A13.3.03.022 **102**
Retrorubral part of substantia nigra A14.1.06.115 **116**
Retrotrigeminal nucleus A14.1.04.217 **110**
Retrozonular space A15.2.06.007 **146**
Rhinal sulcus A14.1.09.240 **127**
Rhombencephalon A14.1.03.002 **108**
Rhomboid
– fossa A14.1.05.702 **115**
– major A04.3.01.007 **36**
– minor A04.3.01.008 **36**
– nucleus A14.1.08.633 **122**
Ribs [I–XII] A02.3.01.001 **17**
Ridge A02.0.00.031 **7**
Right A01.0.00.006 **1**
– atrial veins A12.3.01.014 **91**
– atrioventricular
– – orifice A12.1.02.002 **76**
– – valve A12.1.02.003 **76**
– atrium A12.1.01.001 **76**
– auricle A12.1.01.002 **76**
– border of heart A12.1.00.006 **76**
– branch
– – of atrioventricular bundle A12.1.06.006 **77**
– – of hepatic artery A12.2.12.030 **87**
– – of portal vein A12.3.12.002 **98**
– bundle of atrioventricular bundle A12.1.06.006 **77**
– colic
– – artery A12.2.12.065 **88**
– – flexure A05.7.03.003 **53**
– – lymph nodes A13.3.03.042 **103**
– – vein A12.3.12.026 **99**
– coronary
– – artery A12.2.03.101 **79**
– – cusp of aortic valve A12.1.04.013 **77**
– crus of diaphragm A04.4.02.003 **38**
– duct of caudate lobe of liver A05.8.01.068 **56**
– fibrous trigone of heart A12.1.00.025 **76**
– flexural artery A12.2.12.066 **88**
– gastric
– – artery A12.2.12.028 **87**
– – vein A12.3.12.016 **98**
– gastro-epiploic
– – artery A12.2.12.022 **87**
– – vein A12.3.12.021 **99**
– gastro-omental
– – artery A12.2.12.022 **87**

– – vein A12.3.12.021 **99**
– hepatic
– – duct A05.8.01.062 **56**
– – vein A12.3.09.006 **97**
– inferior
– – lobar bronchus A06.4.02.009 **60**
– – pulmonary vein A12.3.02.201 **92**
– lateral division of liver A05.8.01.049 **55**
– liver A05.8.01.045 **55**
– lobe
– – of liver A05.8.01.026 **55**
– – of prostate A09.3.08.010 **69**
– – of thyroid gland A11.3.00.001 **74**
– lumbar lymph nodes A13.3.03.008 **102**
– lung A06.5.01.003 **60**
– – inferior lobe A06.5.02.009 **61**
– – middle lobe A06.5.02.006 **61**
– – superior lobe A06.5.02.002 **60**
– lymphatic duct A12.4.01.006 **99**
– main bronchus A06.4.01.003 **59**
– marginal
– – branch of right coronary artery A12.2.03.106 **79**
– – vein A12.3.01.011 **91**
– medial division of liver A05.8.01.046 **55**
– ovarian vein ♀ A12.3.09.014 **97**
– part
– – of diaphragmatic surface of liver A05.8.01.006 **54**
– – of liver A05.8.01.045 **55**
– portal fissure A05.8.01.036 **55**
– posterolateral branch of right coronary artery A12.2.03.111 **79**
– pulmonary artery A12.2.01.101 **78**
– semilunar cusp
– – of aortic valve A12.1.04.013 **77**
– – of pulmonary valve A12.1.02.011 **77**
– superior
– – intercostal vein A12.3.07.003 **95**
– – lobar bronchus A06.4.02.002 **60**
– – pulmonary vein A12.3.02.101 **91**
– suprarenal vein A12.3.09.013 **97**
– testicular vein ♂ A12.3.09.014 **97**
– thoracic duct A12.4.01.006 **99**
– triangular ligament of liver A10.1.02.304 **72**
– ventricle A12.1.02.001 **76**
– ventricular veins A12.3.01.015 **91**
Right/left
– atrium A12.1.00.017 **76**
– fibrous ring of heart A12.1.00.027 **76**
– gastric lymph nodes A13.3.03.016 **102**
– gastro-omental lymph nodes A13.3.03.018 **102**
– lamina of thyroid cartilage A06.2.02.004 **58**
– pulmonary surface of heart A12.1.00.005 **75**
– ventricle A12.1.00.012 **76**
Right/middle/left colic nodes A13.3.03.042 **103**
Rima
– glottidis A06.2.09.014 **59**
– vestibuli A06.2.09.009 **59**
Ring finger A01.2.07.030 **5**
Risorius A04.1.03.028 **34**
Roof A02.1.00.075 **9**
– of fourth ventricle A14.1.05.713 **115**
– of orbit A02.1.00.075 **9**
Root/s
– apex of tooth A05.1.03.032 **48**
– canal of tooth A05.1.03.049 **48**
– of brachial plexus A14.2.03.002 **??**
– of lung A06.5.01.016 **60**
– of mesentery A10.1.02.008 **72**
– of nose A06.1.01.002 **57**
– of penis A09.4.01.002 **69**
– of tongue A05.1.04.003 **49**
– of tooth A05.1.03.031 **48**
– pulp of tooth A05.1.03.053 **48**
Rootlets of spinal nerve A14.2.00.028 **133**
Rostral A01.0.00.021 **1**
– part
– – of cuneate nucleus A14.1.04.208 **110**
– – of gracile nucleus A14.1.04.204 **110**
Rostrodorsal subnucleus of gracile nucleus A14.1.04.205 **110**
Rostrum of corpus callosum A14.1.09.242 **127**
Rotator muscle A04.0.00.022 **33**
Rotatores A04.3.02.210 **37**
– cervicis A04.3.02.213 **37**
– lumborum A04.3.02.211 **37**
– thoracis A04.3.02.212 **37**
Round
– ligament
– – of liver A05.8.01.015 **54, 98**
– – of uterus A09.1.03.029 **66**
– window A15.3.02.015 **149**
Rubro-olivary
– fibres A14.1.05.326 **113, 116**
– tract A14.1.04.135 **110**, A14.1.06.214 **116**
Rubrobulbar tract A14.1.04.134 **110**
Rubronuclear tract A14.1.06.212 **116**
Rubropontine tract A14.1.05.331 **113**
Rubrospinal tract A14.1.02.220 **107**, A14.1.04.136 **110**, A14.1.05.332 **113**, A14.1.06.213 **116**
Rugae of gallbladder A05.8.02.010 **56**

S

Sacciform recess
– of distal radio-ulnar joint A03.5.10.003 **29**
– of elbow joint A03.5.09.009 **29**
Saccular
– duct A15.3.03.078 **152**
– nerve A14.2.01.132 **136**
– recess A15.3.03.009 **151**
Saccule A15.3.03.065 **152**
Sacral
– canal A02.2.05.019 **17**
– cornu A02.2.05.018 **17**
– flexure of rectum A05.7.04.002 **53**
– ganglia A14.3.01.035 **142**
– hiatus A02.2.05.020 **17**
– horn A02.2.05.018 **17**
– kyphosis A02.2.00.004 **16**
– lymph nodes A13.3.04.022 **103**
– nerves and coccygeal nerve [S1–S5, Co] A14.2.06.001 **139**
– parasympathetic nuclei A14.1.02.138 **106**
– part of spinal cord A14.1.02.017 **105**
– plexus A14.2.07.027 **140**
– region A01.2.05.003 **4**
– segments [1–5] A14.1.02.017 **105**
– splanchnic nerves A14.3.01.036 **142**
– tuberosity A02.2.05.008 **17**
– venous plexus A12.3.10.009 **97**
Sacro-iliac joint A03.6.03.001 **30**
Sacrococcygeal joint A03.2.08.001 **27**
Sacropelvic surface of ilium A02.5.01.120 **21**
Sacrospinous ligament A03.6.03.007 **30**
Sacrotuberous ligament A03.6.03.005 **30**
Sacrum [sacral vertebrae I–V] A02.2.05.001 **17, 21**
Saddle joint A03.0.00.048 **25**
Sagittal A01.0.00.005 **1**
– border of parietal bone A02.1.02.013 **10**
– planes A01.2.00.003 **3**
– suture A03.1.02.003 **26**
Sagulum nucleus A14.1.06.328 **117**
Salpingopalatine fold A05.3.01.014 **50**
Salpingopharyngeal fold A05.3.01.013 **50**
Salpingopharyngeus A05.3.01.115 **51**
Saphenous
– branch of descending genicular artery A12.2.16.018 **90**
– nerve A14.2.07.023 **140**
– opening A04.7.03.016 **43**
Sartorius A04.7.02.016 **42**
Scala
– media A15.3.03.092 **152**
– tympani A15.3.03.045 **151**
– vestibuli A15.3.03.043 **151**
Scalene tubercle A02.3.02.015 **18**
Scalenus
– anterior A04.2.01.004 **35**
– medius A04.2.01.005 **35**

- minimus A04.2.01.007 **35**
- posterior A04.2.01.006 **35**
Scapha A15.3.01.012 **148**
Scaphoid A02.4.08.003 **20**
- fossa A02.1.05.047 **12**
Scapula A02.4.01.001 **18**
Scapular
- line A01.2.00.020 **3**
- region A01.2.05.005 **4**
Schindylesis A03.0.00.014 **25**
Sciatic
- bursa
- - of gluteus maximus A04.8.05.010 **45**
- - of obturator internus A04.8.05.007 **45**
- nerve A14.2.07.046 **140**
Sclera A15.2.02.002 **144**
Scleral
- spur A15.2.02.007 **144**
- veins A12.3.06.110 **95**
- venous sinus A12.3.06.109 **95, 144**
Scoliosis A02.2.00.008 **16**
Scrotal part of ductus deferens A09.3.05.002 **68**
Scrotum A09.4.03.001 **70**
Sebaceous glands A15.2.07.044 **147**, A16.0.00.030 **154**
Second
- crus of ansiform lobule of cerebellum [H VII A] A14.1.07.210 **119**
- posterior intercostal artery A12.2.08.063 **85**
- rib [II] A02.3.02.018 **18**
- toe [II] A01.2.08.037 **6**
Secondary A02.0.00.045 **7**
- cartilaginous joint A03.0.00.017 **25**
- curvatures A02.2.00.005 **16**
- fissure of cerebellum A14.1.07.220 **119**
- lymphoid organs A13.2.00.001 **100**
- spiral lamina A15.3.03.035 **151**
- tympanic membrane A15.3.02.019 **149**
- visceral grey
- - matter/substance of spinal cord A14.1.02.125 **106**
Segmental medullary artery A12.2.08.007 **84**, A12.2.11.016 **87**, A12.2.12.007 **87**
Segmentation
- of bronchi A06.4.02.001 **60**
- of liver A05.8.01.033 **55**
- of lungs A06.5.02.001 **60**
- of kidneys A08.1.02.001 **63**
- of spinal cord A14.1.02.014 **105**
- of vertebral column A02.2.02.001 **16**, A02.2.03.001 **17, 18**, A02.2.04.001 **17**, A02.2.05.001 **17, 21**
Sella turcica A02.1.05.006 **11**
Sellar diaphragm A14.1.01.107 **104**
Semicircular
- canals A15.3.03.015 **151**
- ducts A15.3.03.066 **152**
Semilunar
- fold A05.2.01.008 **50**
- folds of colon A05.7.03.008 **53**
- hiatus A06.1.02.028 **57**
- lobules of cerebellum A14.1.07.207 **119**
Semimembranosus A04.7.02.036 **42**
- bursa A04.8.05.027 **45**
Seminal
- colliculus A09.4.02.008 **70**
- gland A09.3.06.001 **68**
- vesicle A09.3.06.001 **68**
Seminiferous tubules A09.3.01.022 **68**
Semipennate muscle A04.0.00.015 **33**
Semispinalis A04.3.02.206 **37**
- capitis A04.3.02.209 **37**
- cervicis A04.3.02.208 **37**
- thoracis A04.3.02.207 **37**
Semitendinosus A04.7.02.035 **42**
Sense organs A15.0.00.000 **144**
Sensory
- decussation A14.1.04.110 **109**
- nerve A14.2.00.022 **133**
- root
- - of ciliary ganglion A14.2.01.026 **134, 142**
- - of otic ganglion A14.2.01.067 **134, 142**
- - of pelvic ganglia A14.3.02.020 **142**
- - of pterygopalatine ganglion A14.2.01.039 **134, 142**
- - of sublingual ganglion A14.2.01.088 **135, 142**
- - of submandibular ganglion A14.2.01.087 **135**, A14.2.01.088 **135, 142**
- - of trigeminal nerve A14.2.01.013 **133**
Septa testis A09.3.01.019 **67**
Septal
- area A14.1.09.443 **129**
- cusp of tricuspid valve A12.1.02.006 **76**
- nasal cartilage A06.1.01.013 **57**
- nuclei and related structures A14.1.09.266 **127**
- papillary muscle of right ventricle A12.1.02.019 **77**
Septofimbrial nucleus A14.1.09.270 **127**, A14.1.09.447 **129**
Septomarginal
- fasciculus A14.1.02.241 **107**
- trabecula A12.1.02.020 **77**
Septum
- of corpora cavernosa A09.2.02.006 **67**
- of frontal sinuses A02.1.03.031 **10**
- of glans A09.4.01.009 **69**
- of musculotubal canal A02.1.06.020 **12**
- of scrotum A09.4.03.004 **70**
- of sphenoidal sinuses A02.1.05.017 **11**
- pellucidum A14.1.09.262 **127**
- penis A09.4.01.019 **69**
Serotoninergic cells
- adjacent to medial vestibular nucleus and prepositus nucleus [B4] A14.1.09.624 **132**
- in dorsal raphe nucleus [B7] A14.1.09.627 **132**
- in magnus raphe nucleus [B3] A14.1.09.623 **132**
- in median raphe nucleus [B6] A14.1.09.626 **132**
- in obscurus raphe nucleus [B2] A14.1.09.622 **132**
- in pallidal raphe nucleus [B1] A14.1.09.621 **132**
- in pontine raphe nucleus [B5] A14.1.09.625 **132**
Serous coat
- of bladder A08.3.01.008 **64**
- of gallbladder A05.8.02.006 **56**
- of large intestine A05.7.01.002 **53**
- of liver A05.8.01.052 **55**
- of oesophagus A05.4.01.007 **51**
- of parietal pleura A07.1.02.010 **62**
- of pericardium A12.1.08.008 **78**
- of peritoneum A10.1.02.003 **72**
- of small intestine A05.6.01.002 **52**
- of spleen A13.2.01.018 **100**
- of stomach A05.5.01.019 **52**
- of testis A09.3.01.014 **67**
- of uterine tube A09.1.02.010 **65**
- of uterus A09.1.03.023 **66**
- of visceral pleura A07.1.02.003 **62**
- pericardium A12.1.08.005 **78**
Serrate suture A03.0.00.012 **25**
Serratus
- anterior A04.4.01.008 **37**
- posterior
- - inferior A04.3.01.010 **36**
- - superior A04.3.01.011 **36**
Sesamoid
- bone A02.0.00.016 **7**
- bones
- - of foot A02.5.19.001 **24**
- - of hand A02.4.11.001 **21**
- cartilage of cricopharyngeal ligament A06.2.04.018 **58**
Shaft
- of clavicle A02.4.02.005 **19**
- of femur A02.5.04.012 **22**
- of fibula A02.5.07.006 **23**
- of humerus A02.4.04.010 **19**
- of metacarpal A02.4.09.003 **20**
- of metatarsal A02.5.17.003 **24**
- of phalanx
- - of foot A02.5.18.007 **24**
- - of hand A02.4.10.007 **21**
- of radius A02.4.05.006 **20**
- of rib A02.3.02.007 **18**
- of tibia A02.5.06.011 **23**
- of ulna A02.4.06.007 **20**

Sheath of styloid process
A02.1.06.060 **13**
Shell region
– of cuneate nucleus
A14.1.04.208 **110**
– of gracile nucleus
A14.1.04.204 **110**
– of nucleus accumbens
A14.1.09.442 **129**
Short
– association fibres of telencephalon
A14.1.09.559 **131**
– bone A02.0.00.012 **7**
– ciliary nerves A14.3.02.005 **142**
– circumferential arteries
A12.2.07.085 **84**
– gastric
– – arteries A12.2.12.050 **88**
– – veins A12.3.12.030 **99**
– gyri of insula A14.1.09.152 **125**
– head of biceps
– – brachii A04.6.02.015 **40**
– – femoris A04.7.02.034 **42**
– limb of incus A15.3.02.042 **150**
– pitch helicoidal muscle layer of small intestine
A05.6.01.006 **52**
– plantar ligament
A03.6.10.518 **31**
– posterior ciliary arteries
A12.2.06.031 **82**
– saphenous vein A12.3.11.010 **98**
Shoulder
– girdle A01.1.00.020 **2**, A02.4.00.002 **18**
– joint A03.5.08.001 **29**
Sigmoid
– arteries A12.2.12.072 **88**
– colon A05.7.03.007 **53**
– lymph nodes A13.3.03.044 **103**
– mesocolon A10.1.02.013 **72**
– sinus A12.3.05.108 **93**
– veins A12.3.12.034 **99**
Simple
– bony limb of semicircular canal
A15.3.03.024 **151**
– joint A03.0.00.041 **25**
– lobule of cerebellum [H VI and VI]
A14.1.07.202 **119**
– membranous limb of semicircular ducts A15.3.03.075 **152**
Sinu-atrial
– nodal branch
– – of left coronary artery
A12.2.03.212 **79**
– – of right coronary artery
A12.2.03.104 **79**
– node A12.1.06.003 **77**
Sinus
– of epididymis A09.3.01.013 **67**
– of pulmonary trunk
A12.2.01.002 **78**
– of venae cavae A12.1.01.012 **76**
– tympani A15.3.02.014 **149**
– venosus A12.0.00.016 **75**
Sinusoid A12.0.00.027 **75**
Skeletal system A02.0.00.000 **7**
Skin A16.0.00.002 **154**
– glands A16.0.00.028 **154**
– ligaments A16.0.00.005 **154**
– sulci A16.0.00.003 **154**
Small
– cardiac vein A12.3.01.010 **91**, A12.3.01.013 **91**
– intestine A05.6.01.001 **52**
– saphenous vein A12.3.11.010 **98**
Socket A03.0.00.006 **25**
Soft palate A05.1.01.104 **47**, A05.2.01.003 **50**
Sole A01.1.00.044 **2**, A01.2.08.025 **5**
Soleal line A02.5.06.015 **23**
Soleus A04.7.02.047 **43**
Solitariospinal tract
A14.1.02.235 **107**
Solitary
– lymphoid nodules of small intestine A05.6.01.013 **52, 101**
– nuclei A14.1.04.230 **111**
– tract A14.1.04.120 **109**
Somatic nerve fibres
A14.2.00.019 **132**
Spaces of iridocorneal angle
A15.2.03.033 **145**
Spermatic cord A09.3.04.001 **68**
Spheno-ethmoidal
– recess A02.1.00.094 **9**, A06.1.02.022 **57**
– suture A03.1.02.007 **26**
– synchondrosis A03.1.05.008 **27**
Spheno-occipital synchondrosis
A03.1.05.002 **27**
Sphenofrontal suture
A03.1.02.006 **26**
Sphenoid A02.1.05.001 **11**
– part of middle cerebral artery
A12.2.07.047 **83**
– process of septal nasal cartilage
A06.1.01.015 **57**
Sphenoidal
– angle A02.1.02.017 **10**
– – of parietal bone
A02.1.02.017 **10**
– bone A02.1.05.001 **11**
– concha A02.1.05.019 **11**
– crest A02.1.05.014 **11**
– emissary foramen
A02.1.05.037 **11**
– fontanelle A02.1.00.030 **8**
– lingula A02.1.05.013 **11**
– margin
– – of frontal bone
A02.1.03.027 **10**
– – of temporal bone
A02.1.06.064 **13**
– process of palatine
A02.1.13.012 **15**
– rostrum A02.1.05.015 **11**
– sinus A02.1.05.016 **11**, A06.1.03.003 **57**
– yoke A02.1.05.003 **11**
Sphenomandibular ligament
A03.1.07.007 **27**
Sphenomaxillary suture
A03.1.02.023 **26**
Sphenopalatine
– artery A12.2.05.088 **81**
– foramen A02.1.00.097 **9**
– notch A02.1.13.005 **14**
Sphenoparietal
– sinus A12.3.05.119 **94**
– suture A03.1.02.009 **26**
Sphenopetrosal
– fissure A02.1.00.046 **8**
– synchondrosis A03.1.05.003 **27**
Sphenosquamous suture
A03.1.02.008 **26**
Sphenovomerine suture
A03.1.02.021 **26**
Sphenozygomatic suture
A03.1.02.022 **26**
Spherical recess A15.3.03.009 **151**
Spheroidal joint A03.0.00.050 **25**
Sphincter
– muscle A04.0.00.028 **33**
– of ampulla A05.8.02.018 **56**
– of bile duct A05.8.02.014 **56**
– of hepatopancreatic ampulla
A05.8.02.018 **56**
– of pancreatic duct
A05.9.01.016 **56**
– pupillae A15.2.03.029 **145**
– urethrovaginalis ♀
A09.5.03.006 **71**
Spinal
– arachnoid mater
A14.1.01.218 **105**
– area X A14.1.02.302 **108**
– branch/es
– – of ascending cervical artery
A12.2.08.050 **85**
– – of dorsal branch of posterior intercostal
– – – artery A12.2.11.011 **87**
– – – vein A12.3.07.017 **96**
– – of iliolumbar artery
A12.2.15.004 **89**
– – of lateral sacral artery
A12.2.15.007 **89**
– – of lumbar artery
A12.2.12.006 **87**
– – of second posterior intercostal artery A12.2.08.065 **85**
– – of subcostal artery
A12.2.11.022 **87**
– – of vertebral artery
A12.2.08.005 **84**
– cord A14.1.02.001 **105**
– dura mater A14.1.01.111 **104**
– ganglion A14.2.00.006 **132**
– lamina/e
– – I A14.1.02.117 **106**
– – II A14.1.02.119 **106**
– – III and IV A14.1.02.121 **106**
– – V A14.1.02.122 **106**
– – VI A14.1.02.124 **106**
– – VII A14.1.02.131 **106**
– – VII–IX A14.1.02.104 **106**
– – X A14.1.02.302 **108**
– lemniscus A14.1.04.137 **110, 113**, A14.1.06.215 **116**, A14.1.08.676 **122**
– nerve/s A14.2.00.027 **133**, A14.2.02.001 **137**
– – plexus A14.2.00.037 **133**

– nucleus of trigeminal nerve A14.1.04.211 **110**, A14.1.05.404 **113**
– part
– – of accessory nerve A14.2.01.186 **137**
– – of deltoid A04.6.02.005 **40**
– – of filum terminale A14.1.02.005 **105**
– pia mater A14.1.01.309 **105**
– reticular formation A14.1.02.140 **106**
– root of accessory nerve A14.2.01.186 **137**
– tract of trigeminal nerve A14.1.04.115 **109**, A14.1.05.309 **113**
– vein A12.3.07.017 **96**
Spinalis A04.3.02.015 **36**
– capitis A04.3.02.018 **36**
– cervicis A04.3.02.017 **36**
– thoracis A04.3.02.016 **36**
Spine
– of helix A15.3.01.007 **148**
– of scapula A02.4.01.005 **18**
– of sphenoid bone A02.1.05.040 **11**
Spino-olivary
– fibres A14.1.04.145 **110, 113**
– tract A14.1.02.230 **107**, A14.1.04.117 **109**
Spinobulbar fibres A14.1.04.144 **110, 113**
Spinocerebellum A14.1.07.008 **118**
Spinocervical tract A14.1.02.236 **107**
Spinocuneate fibres A14.1.02.247 **108**
Spinogracile fibres A14.1.02.248 **108**
Spinohypothalamic fibres A14.1.04.143 **110, 113, 116**
Spinomesencephalic fibres A14.1.04.140 **110, 113, 116**
Spinoperiaqueductal fibres A14.1.04.142 **110, 113, 116**
Spinoreticular
– fibres A14.1.04.139 **110, 113, 116**
– tract A14.1.02.231 **107**
Spinotectal
– fibres A14.1.04.141 **110, 113, 116**
– tract A14.1.02.224 **107**
Spinothalamic fibres A14.1.04.138 **110, 113, 116**
Spinotransversales A04.3.02.101 **36**
Spinous process of vertebra A02.2.01.012 **16**
Spinovestibular tract A14.1.02.237 **107**, A14.1.04.146 **110**
Spiral
– canal
– – of cochlea A15.3.03.028 **151**
– – of modiolus cochleae A15.3.03.041 **151**
– crest of cochlear duct A15.3.03.101 **152**
– fold A05.8.02.012 **56**
– ganglion A14.2.01.134 **136**, A15.3.03.125 **153**
– ligament of cochlear duct A15.3.03.099 **152**
– limbus A15.3.03.104 **152**
– line of femur A02.5.04.016 **22**
– membrane A15.3.03.100 **152**
– modiolar artery A15.3.03.133 **153**
– organ A15.3.03.121 **153**
– prominence of cochlear duct A15.3.03.097 **152**
Spleen A13.2.01.001 **100**
Splenic
– artery A12.2.12.040 **88**
– branches of splenic artery A12.2.12.051 **88**
– flexure A05.7.03.005 **53**
– hilum A13.2.01.017 **100**
– lymph nodes A13.3.03.026 **102**
– lymphoid nodules A13.2.01.021 **100**
– nerve plexus A14.3.03.023 **143**
– pulp A13.2.01.004 **100**
– recess of omental bursa A10.1.02.407 **72**
– sinus A13.2.01.019 **100**
– trabeculae A13.2.01.003 **100**
– vein A12.3.12.028 **99**
Splenium of corpus callosum A14.1.09.245 **127**
Splenius A04.3.02.102 **36**
– capitis A04.3.02.103 **37**
– cervicis A04.3.02.104 **37**
Splenocolic ligament A10.1.02.210 **72**
Splenorenal ligament A10.1.02.207 **72**
Spongy
– bone A02.0.00.004 **7**
– layer
– – of urethra A09.2.03.011 **67**
– – of vagina A09.1.04.017 **66**
– urethra A09.4.02.021 **70**
Spring ligament A03.6.10.203 **31**
Squamomastoid suture A03.1.02.012 **26**
Squamosal
– border of parietal bone A02.1.02.012 **9**
– margin of sphenoid A02.1.05.034 **11**
Squamous
– part
– – of frontal bone A02.1.03.002 **10**
– – of occipital bone A02.1.04.010 **10**
– – of temporal bone A02.1.06.061 **13**
– suture A03.0.00.010 **25**, A03.1.02.010 **26**
Stalk of epiglottis A06.2.07.003 **58**
Stapedial
– branch of posterior tympanic artery A12.2.05.041 **80**
– membrane A15.3.02.059 **150**
Stapedius A15.3.02.062 **150**
Stapes A15.3.02.033 **149**
Stellate
– ganglion A14.3.01.020 **141**
– veins of kidney A08.1.04.006 **63**
Sternal
– angle A02.3.03.005 **18**
– branches of internal thoracic artery A12.2.08.035 **85**
– end of clavicle A02.4.02.002 **19**
– facet of clavicle A02.4.02.003 **19**
– line A01.2.00.013 **3**
– membrane A03.3.05.004 **28**
– part of diaphragm A04.4.02.009 **38**
– synchondroses A03.3.02.004 **28**
Sternalis A04.4.01.001 **37**
Sternoclavicular joint A03.5.04.001 **29**
Sternocleidomastoid A04.2.01.008 **35**
– branch of superior thyroid artery A12.2.05.004 **80**
– branches of occipital artery A12.2.05.033 **80**
– region A01.2.02.007 **3**
– vein A12.3.05.016 **93**
Sternocostal
– head of pectoralis major A04.4.01.004 **37**
– joints A03.3.05.001 **28**
– surface of heart A12.1.00.003 **75**
– triangle A04.4.02.015 **38**
Sternohyoid A04.2.04.002 **35**
Sternopericardial ligaments A12.1.08.003 **78**
Sternothyroid A04.2.04.006 **35**
Sternum A02.3.03.001 **18**
Stomach A05.5.01.001 **51**
Straight
– arterioles of kidney A08.1.03.008 **63**
– conjugate A02.5.02.016 **22**
– gyrus A14.1.09.218 **126**
– head of rectus femoris A04.7.02.019 **42**
– muscle A04.0.00.008 **33**
– part of cricothyroid A06.2.08.002 **59**
– seminiferous tubules A09.3.01.023 **68**
– sinus A12.3.05.112 **94**
– tubules A09.3.01.023 **68**
– venules of kidney A08.1.04.005 **63**
Stria A14.1.00.020 **104**
– medullaris of thalamus A14.1.08.106 **120, 121**
– of external granular layer A14.1.09.316 **128**
– – of isocortex A14.1.09.316 **128**
– of internal
– – granular layer of isocortex A14.1.09.317 **128**
– – pyramidal layer of isocortex A14.1.09.319 **128**
– of molecular layer of isocortex A14.1.09.315 **128**
– terminalis A14.1.09.275 **127**
– vascularis of cochlear duct A15.3.03.096 **152**

Striatum A14.1.09.516 **130**
Striola A15.3.03.087 **152**
Stroma A11.3.00.007 **74**
– of ganglion A14.2.00.004 **132**
– of iris A15.2.03.031 **145**
– of thyroid gland A11.3.00.007 **74**
Styloglossus A05.1.04.105 **49**
Stylohyoid A04.2.03.005 **35**
– branch of facial nerve A14.2.01.106 **135**
– ligament A03.1.01.003 **26**
Styloid
– process
– – of radius A02.4.05.015 **20**
– – of temporal A02.1.06.047 **13**
– – of third metacarpal [III] A02.4.09.005 **20**
– – of ulna A02.4.06.017 **20**
– prominence A15.3.02.007 **149**
Stylomandibular ligament A03.1.07.008 **27**
Stylomastoid
– artery A12.2.05.038 **80**
– foramen A02.1.06.048 **13**
– vein A12.3.05.044 **93**
Stylopharyngeal branch of glossopharyngeal nerve A14.2.01.145 **136**
Stylopharyngeus A05.3.01.114 **51**
Subacromial bursa A04.8.03.004 **44**
Subaortic lymph nodes A13.3.04.007 **103**
Subarachnoid
– cisterns A14.1.01.207 **105**
– space A14.1.01.202 **104**
– – of optic nerve A15.2.04.034 **146**
Subarcuate fossa A02.1.06.034 **12**
Subbrachial nucleus A14.1.06.329 **117**
Subcaerulean nucleus A14.1.05.437 **114**
Subcallosal
– area A14.1.09.211 **126**
– fasciculus A14.1.09.562 **131**
– gyrus A14.1.09.211 **126**
Subclavian
– artery A12.2.08.001 **84**
– groove A02.4.02.006 **19**
– lymphatic trunk A12.4.01.003 **99**
– nerve A14.2.03.013 **138**
– – plexus A14.3.03.008 **143**
– triangle A01.2.02.010 **3**
– trunk A12.4.01.003 **99**
– vein A12.3.08.002 **96**
Subclavius A04.4.01.007 **37**
Subcommissural organ A14.1.08.511 **121**
Subcostal
– angle A02.3.04.008 **18**
– artery A12.2.11.020 **87**
– nerve A14.2.04.016 **139**
– plane A01.2.00.008 **3**
– vein A12.3.07.013 **96**
Subcostales A04.4.01.015 **37**
Subcuneiform nucleus A14.1.06.335 **117, 118**
Subcutaneous
– abdominal veins A12.3.04.020 **92**
– bursa A04.8.01.001 **44**
– – of acromion A04.8.03.003 **44**
– – of laryngeal prominence A04.8.02.003 **44**
– – of lateral malleolus A04.8.05.028 **45**
– – of medial malleolus A04.8.05.029 **45**
– – of tuberosity of tibia A04.8.05.020 **45**
– calcaneal bursa A04.8.05.031 **45**
– infrapatellar bursa A04.8.05.018 **45**
– olecranon bursa A04.8.03.011 **44**
– part of external anal sphincter A04.5.04.013 **40, 54**
– perineal pouch A09.5.01.001 **71**
– prepatellar bursa A04.8.05.014 **45**
– tissue A16.0.03.001 **155**
– – of abdomen A04.5.02.021 **39**
– – of penis A09.4.01.027 **70**
– – of perineum A09.5.00.006 **71**
– trochanteric bursa A04.8.05.002 **45**
Subdeltoid bursa A04.8.03.005 **44**
Subdural space A14.1.01.109 **104**
Subendocardial branches of atrioventricular bundle A12.1.06.008 **77**
Subfascial
– bursa A04.8.01.003 **44**
– prepatellar bursa A04.8.05.015 **45**
Subfornical organ A14.1.08.412 **121, 127**, A14.1.09.449 **129**
Subhepatic space A10.1.02.426 **73**
Subhypoglossal nucleus A14.1.04.263 **111**
Subiculum
– of hippocampus A14.1.09.326 **128**
– of promontory of tympanic cavity A15.3.02.013 **149**
Sublenticular
– extended amygdala A14.1.09.420 **129**
– limb of internal capsule A14.1.09.544 **131**
Sublentiform limb of internal capsule A14.1.09.544 **131**
Sublingual
– artery A12.2.05.018 **80**
– caruncle A05.1.01.112 **47**
– fold A05.1.01.113 **47**
– fossa A02.1.15.014 **15**
– ganglion A14.3.02.011 **142**
– gland A05.1.02.008 **47**
– nerve A14.2.01.085 **135**
– vein A12.3.05.012 **93**
Submandibular
– duct A05.1.02.012 **47**
– fossa A02.1.15.015 **15**
– ganglion A14.3.02.009 **142**
– gland A05.1.02.011 **47**
– lymph nodes A13.3.00.016 **101**
– triangle A01.2.02.003 **3**
Submedial nucleus of thalamus A14.1.08.647 **122**
Submental
– artery A12.2.05.023 **80**
– lymph nodes A13.3.00.015 **101**
– triangle A01.2.02.006 **3**
– vein A12.3.05.030 **93**
Submucosa
– of bladder A08.3.01.022 **64**
– of bronchus A06.4.02.028 **60**
– of large intestine A05.7.01.005 **53**
– of oesophagus A05.4.01.014 **51**
– of pharynx A05.3.01.028 **51**
– of small intestine A05.6.01.008 **52**
– of stomach A05.5.01.026 **52**
Submucous nerve plexus A14.3.03.042 **143**
Submuscular bursa A04.8.01.002 **44**
Suboccipital
– muscles A04.2.02.001 **35**
– nerve A14.2.02.007 **137**
– venous plexus A12.3.04.016 **92**
Subparabrachial nucleus A14.1.05.440 **114**
Subparietal sulcus A14.1.09.205 **126**
Subphrenic space A10.1.02.425 **73**
Subpopliteal recess A04.8.05.024 **45**
Subpubic angle A02.5.02.004 **22**
Subpyloric lymph nodes A13.3.03.021 **102**
Subsartorial fascia A04.7.03.007 **43**
Subscapular
– artery A12.2.09.013 **85**
– branches of axillary artery A12.2.09.003 **85**
– fossa A02.4.01.003 **18**
– lymph nodes A13.3.01.005 **101**
– nerves A14.2.03.015 **138**
– vein A12.3.08.006 **96**
Subscapularis A04.6.02.012 **40**
Subserosa/Subserous layer
– of bladder A08.3.01.009 **64**
– of gallbladder A05.8.02.007 **56**
– of large intestine A05.7.01.003 **53**
– of liver A05.8.01.053 **55**
– of oesophagus A05.4.01.008 **51**
– of parietal pleura A07.1.02.011 **62**
– of pericardium A12.1.08.009 **78**
– of peritoneum A10.1.02.004 **72**
– of small intestine A05.6.01.003 **52**
– of stomach A05.5.01.020 **52**
– of testis A09.3.01.015 **67**
– of uterine tube A09.1.02.011 **65**
– of uterus A09.1.03.024 **66**
– of visceral pleura A07.1.02.004 **62**
Subserous nerve plexus A14.3.03.040 **143**

Substantia
– nigra A14.1.06.111 **116**
– propria
– – of cornea A15.2.02.020 **144**
– – sclerae A15.2.02.009 **144**
Subtalar joint A03.6.10.101 **31**
Subtendinous
– bursa A04.8.01.004 **44**
– – of iliacus A04.8.05.012 **45**
– – of infraspinatus A04.8.03.007 **44**
– – of latissimus dorsi A04.8.03.010 **44**
– – of obturator internus A04.8.05.008 **45**
– – of sartorius A04.8.05.021 **45**
– – of subscapularis A04.8.03.008 **44**
– – of teres major A04.8.03.009 **44**
– – of tibialis anterior A04.8.05.030 **45**
– – of trapezius A04.8.03.002 **44**
– – of triceps brachii A04.8.03.013 **44**
– prepatellar bursa A04.8.05.016 **45**
Subthalamic
– fasciculus A14.1.08.677 **122**, A14.1.09.522 **130**
– nucleus A14.1.08.702 **123**
Subthalamus A14.1.08.201 **120**, A14.1.08.701 **123**
Subtrigeminal part of lateral reticular nucleus A14.1.04.311 **112**
Sulcomarginal fasciculus A14.1.02.204 **107**
Sulcus
– limitans A14.1.05.724 **115**
– of auditory tube A02.1.05.041 **12**
– of corpus callosum A14.1.09.202 **126**
– sclerae A15.2.02.003 **144**
– tali A02.5.10.009 **24**
– terminalis cordis A12.1.01.013 **76**
Superciliary arch A02.1.03.005 **10**
Superficial A01.0.00.033 **1**
– anterior cervical lymph nodes A13.3.00.018 **101**
– brachial artery A12.2.09.019 **86**
– branch
– – of lateral plantar nerve A14.2.07.070 **141**
– – of medial
– – – circumflex femoral artery A12.2.16.022 **90**
– – – plantar artery A12.2.16.063 **91**
– – of radial nerve A14.2.03.056 **138**
– – of superior gluteal artery A12.2.15.014 **89**
– – of ulnar nerve A14.2.03.045 **138**
– cerebral veins A12.3.06.002 **94**
– cervical artery of transverse cervical artery A12.2.08.054 **85**
– circumflex iliac
– – artery A12.2.16.012 **90**
– – vein A12.3.11.005 **98**
– dorsal veins
– – of clitoris ♀ A12.3.11.008 **98**
– – of penis ♂ A12.3.11.008 **98**
– epigastric
– – artery A12.2.16.011 **90**
– – vein A12.3.11.006 **98**
– external pudendal artery A12.2.16.013 **90**
– fascia of scrotum A09.4.03.003 **70**
– fatty layer of subcutaneous tissue A16.0.03.002 **155**
– fibular nerve A14.2.07.050 **140**
– grey layer of superior colliculus A14.1.06.607 **118**
– head of flexor pollicis brevis A04.6.02.056 **41**
– inguinal
– – lymph nodes A13.3.05.003 **103**
– – ring A04.5.01.013 **38**
– investing fascia
– – of abdomen A04.5.02.018 **39**
– – of perineum A09.5.02.002 **71**
– lateral cervical lymph nodes A13.3.00.027 **101**
– layer
– – of cervical fascia A04.2.05.002 **35**
– – of levator palpebrae superioris A15.2.07.021 **147**
– – of temporal fascia A04.1.04.014 **35**
– lymph
– – nodes
– – – of front of neck A13.3.00.018 **101**
– – – of side of neck A13.3.00.027 **101**
– – – of popliteal fossa A13.3.05.012 **103**
– – – of upper limb A13.3.01.013 **102**
– – vessel A12.0.00.039 **75**
– middle cerebral vein A12.3.06.009 **94**
– palmar
– – arch A12.2.09.056 **86**
– – branch of radial artery A12.2.09.031 **86**
– parotid lymph nodes A13.3.00.004 **101**
– part
– – of anterior compartment of forearm A04.6.01.005 **40**
– – of external anal sphincter A04.5.04.014 **40, 54**
– – of masseter A04.1.04.003 **35**
– – of parotid gland A05.1.02.004 **47**
– – of posterior compartment of leg A04.7.01.007 **42**
– perineal
– – compartment A09.5.02.001 **71**
– – pouch A09.5.02.001 **71**
– – space A09.5.02.001 **71**
– peroneal nerve A14.2.07.050 **140**
– plantar arch A12.2.16.070 **91**
– popliteal lymph nodes A13.3.05.012 **103**
– posterior sacrococcygeal ligament A03.2.08.002 **27**
– temporal
– – artery A12.2.05.045 **80**
– – branches of auriculotemporal nerve A14.2.01.080 **135**
– – veins A12.3.05.032 **93**
– transverse
– – metacarpal ligament A04.6.03.011 **41**
– – metatarsal ligament A04.7.03.033 **44**
– – perineal muscle A09.5.02.003 **71**
– trigone A08.3.01.012 **64**
– vein/s A12.0.00.036 **75**
– – of lower limb A12.3.11.002 **98**
– – of upper limb A12.3.08.014 **96**
– venous palmar arch A12.3.08.026 **96**
Superior A01.0.00.017 **1**
– aberrant ductule A09.3.02.008 **68**
– – of epididymis A09.3.02.008 **68**
– alveolar nerves A14.2.01.049 **134**
– anal nerves A14.3.03.051 **143**
– anastomotic vein A12.3.06.012 **94**
– angle of scapula A02.4.01.018 **19**
– articular
– – facet of vertebra A02.2.01.015 **16**
– – process
– – – of sacrum A02.2.05.005 **17**
– – – of vertebra A02.2.01.014 **16**
– – surface
– – – of atlas A02.2.02.103 **16**
– – – of tibia A02.5.06.002 **23**
– aspect A02.1.00.003 **8**
– basal vein of lower lobe
– – of left lung A12.3.02.406 **92**
– – of right lung A12.3.02.206 **92**
– belly of omohyoid A04.2.04.004 **35**
– border
– – of body of pancreas A05.9.01.010 **56**
– – of petrous part A02.1.06.029 **12**
– – – of temporal bone A02.1.06.029 **12**
– – of scapula A02.4.01.014 **19**
– – of spleen A13.2.01.016 **100**
– – of suprarenal gland A11.5.00.005 **74**
– branch/es
– – of left inferior pulmonary vein A12.3.02.402 **92**
– – of oculomotor nerve A14.2.01.008 **133**
– – of right inferior pulmonary vein A12.3.02.202 **92**
– – of superior gluteal artery A12.2.15.016 **89**
– – of transverse cervical nerve A14.2.02.022 **137**
– bulb of jugular vein A12.3.05.002 **93**

– bursa of biceps femoris A04.8.05.013 **45**
– calyx of kidney A08.1.05.004 **64**
– central nucleus A14.1.05.603 **115**
– cerebellar
– – artery A12.2.08.025 **84**
– – peduncle A14.1.05.006 **112**, A14.1.06.009 **115**, A14.1.06.216 **116**, A14.1.07.417 **120**, A14.1.08.678 **122**
– cerebral veins A12.3.06.003 **94**
– cervical
– – cardiac
– – – branches of vagus A14.2.01.164 **136**
– – – nerve A14.3.01.015 **141**
– – ganglion A14.3.01.009 **141**
– choroid vein A12.3.06.029 **94**
– clunial nerves A14.2.05.006 **139**
– colliculus A14.1.06.015 **115, 118**
– conjunctival fornix A15.2.07.052 **147**
– constrictor A05.3.01.103 **51**
– cortical branches of middle cerebral artery A12.2.07.061 **83**
– costal facet A02.2.03.002 **17**
– costotransverse ligament A03.3.04.007 **28**
– deep
– – branch of superior gluteal artery A12.2.15.016 **89**
– – lateral cervical lymph nodes A13.3.00.028 **101**
– dental
– – branches A14.2.01.054 **134**
– – nerve plexus A14.2.01.053 **134**
– – nerves A14.2.01.054 **134**
– diaphragmatic lymph nodes A13.3.02.005 **102**
– duodenal
– – flexure A05.6.02.004 **52**
– – fold A10.1.02.410 **72**
– – fossa A10.1.02.411 **73**
– epigastric
– – artery A12.2.08.041 **85**
– – veins A12.3.04.019 **92**
– extensor retinaculum of foot A04.7.03.025 **43**
– extremity of kidney A08.1.01.008 **63**
– eyelid A15.2.07.025 **147**
– facet of talus A02.5.10.012 **24**
– fascia of pelvic diaphragm A04.5.03.012 **39**
– fibular retinaculum A04.7.03.028 **44**
– fovea of sulcus limitans A14.1.05.725 **115**
– frontal
– – gyrus A14.1.09.121 **125**
– – sulcus A14.1.09.122 **125**
– ganglion
– – of glossopharyngeal nerve A14.2.01.136 **136**
– – of vagus A14.2.01.154 **136**
– gemellus A04.7.02.013 **42**
– genial spine A02.1.15.010 **15**
– gingival
– – branches A14.2.01.055 **134**
– – nerves A14.2.01.055 **134**
– gluteal
– – artery A12.2.15.013 **89**
– – lymph nodes A13.3.04.020 **103**
– – nerve A14.2.07.031 **140**
– – veins A12.3.10.005 **97**
– head of lateral pterygoid A04.1.04.007 **35**
– hemi-azygos vein A12.3.07.005 **95**
– horn
– – of falciform margin of saphenous opening A04.7.03.018 **43**
– – of thyroid cartilage A06.2.02.010 **58**
– hypogastric nerve plexus A14.3.03.046 **143**
– hypophysial artery A12.2.06.017 **81**
– ileocaecal recess A10.1.02.418 **73**
– labial
– – branch/es
– – – of facial artery A12.2.05.026 **80**
– – – of infra-orbital nerve A14.2.01.063 **134**
– – vein A12.3.05.025 **93**
– laryngeal
– – artery A12.2.05.005 **80**
– – nerve A14.2.01.160 **136**
– – vein A12.3.05.017 **93**
– lateral
– – brachial cutaneous nerve A14.2.03.061 **139**
– – cutaneous nerve of arm A14.2.03.061 **139**
– – flexure of rectum A05.7.04.004 **54**
– – genicular artery A12.2.16.034 **90**
– ligament
– – of auricle A15.3.01.034 **148**
– – of epididymis A09.3.01.011 **67**
– – of incus A15.3.02.057 **150**
– – of malleus A15.3.02.055 **150**
– limb of ansa cervicalis A14.2.02.014 **137**
– linear nucleus A14.1.06.404 **118**
– lingular
– – artery A12.2.01.213 **79**
– – bronchus [B IV] A06.4.02.018 **60**
– – segment of left lung [S IV] A06.5.02.018 **61**
– lip A05.7.02.005 **53**
– lobar arteries
– – of left lung A12.2.01.203 **78**
– – of right lung A12.2.01.102 **78**
– lobe
– – of left lung A06.5.02.015 **61**
– – of lung A06.5.01.017 **60**
– – of right lung, A06.5.02.002 **60**
– longitudinal
– – fasciculus A14.1.09.557 **131**
– – muscle of tongue A05.1.04.106 **49**
– lumbar triangle A01.2.05.010 **4**
– lymph nodes of pancreas A13.3.03.024 **102**
– macular
– – arteriole A15.2.04.041 **146**
– – venule A15.2.04.048 **146**
– margin of cerebral hemisphere A14.1.09.010 **124**
– medial genicular artery A12.2.16.035 **90**
– mediastinum A07.1.02.102 **62**
– medullary velum A14.1.05.007 **112**, A14.1.05.719 **115**
– mental spine A02.1.15.010 **15**
– mesenteric
– – artery A12.2.12.053 **88**
– – ganglion A14.3.03.030 **143**
– – lymph nodes A13.3.03.033 **102**
– – nerve plexus A14.3.03.029 **143**
– – vein A12.3.12.018 **98**
– nasal
– – concha A02.1.07.013 **13**, A06.1.02.013 **57**
– – meatus A02.1.00.089 **9**, A06.1.02.023 **57**
– – retinal
– – – arteriole A15.2.04.039 **146**
– – – venule A15.2.04.046 **146**
– nuchal line A02.1.04.025 **11**
– oblique A15.2.07.016 **147**
– occipitofrontal fasciculus A14.1.09.562 **131**
– olivary
– – complex A14.1.05.415 **114**
– – nucleus A14.1.05.415 **114**
– ophthalmic vein A12.3.06.102 **95**
– orbital fissure A02.1.00.083 **9**, A02.1.05.023 **11**
– palpebral
– – arch A12.2.06.047 **82**
– – veins A12.3.05.022 **93**
– pancreatic lymph nodes A13.3.03.024 **102**
– pancreaticoduodenal lymph nodes A13.3.03.028 **102**
– parathyroid gland A11.4.00.002 **74**
– parietal lobule A14.1.09.130 **125**
– part
– – of diaphragmatic surface of liver A05.8.01.003 **54**
– – of duodenum A05.6.02.002 **52**
– – of lingular vein A12.3.02.309 **92**
– – of trapezius A04.3.01.002 **36**
– – of vestibular ganglion A14.2.01.125 **135**
– – of wing of central lobule of cerebellum A14.1.07.110 **119**
– peroneal retinaculum A04.7.03.028 **44**
– petrosal sinus A12.3.05.115 **94**
– phrenic
– – arteries A12.2.11.006 **86**
– – veins A12.3.07.010 **96**
– pole
– – of kidney A08.1.01.008 **63**
– – of testis A09.3.01.002 **67**

– posterior pancreaticoduodenal vein A12.3.12.014 **98**
– pubic
– – ligament A03.6.02.003 **30**
– – ramus A02.5.01.306 **21**
– recess
– – of omental bursa A10.1.02.405 **72**
– – of tympanic membrane A15.3.02.069 **150**
– rectal
– – artery A12.2.12.073 **88**
– – lymph nodes A13.3.03.045 **103**
– – nerve plexus A14.3.03.038 **143**
– – vein A12.3.12.035 **99**
– rectus A15.2.07.010 **147**
– root of ansa cervicalis A14.2.02.014 **137**
– sagittal sinus A12.3.05.109 **93**
– salivatory nucleus A14.1.05.413 **114**
– segment
– – of kidney A08.1.02.002 **63**
– – of left lung [S VI] A06.5.02.021 **61**
– – of right lung [S VI] A06.5.02.010 **61**
– segmental
– – artery
– – – of kidney A12.2.12.079 **88**
– – – of left lung A12.2.01.215 **79**
– – – of right lung A12.2.01.114 **78**
– – bronchus
– – – of left lung [B VI] A06.4.02.021 **60**
– – – of right lung [B VI] A06.4.02.010 **60**
– semilunar lobule of cerebellum A14.1.07.208 **119**
– sphincter A05.8.02.015 **56**
– – of bile duct A05.8.02.015 **56**
– suprarenal arteries A12.2.12.003 **87**
– synovial membrane A03.1.07.005 **27**
– – of temporomandibular joint A03.1.07.005 **27**
– tarsal muscle A15.2.07.045 **147**
– tarsus A15.2.07.038 **147, 154**
– temporal
– – gyrus A14.1.09.138 **125**
– – line of parietal bone A02.1.02.008 **9**
– – retinal
– – – arteriole A15.2.04.037 **146**
– – – venule A15.2.04.044 **146**
– – sulcus A14.1.09.145 **125**
– terminal branches A12.2.07.061 **83**
– – of middle cerebral artery A12.2.07.061 **83**
– thalamostriate vein A12.3.06.030 **94**
– thoracic
– – aperture A02.3.04.003 **18**
– – artery A12.2.09.004 **85**
– thyroid
– – artery A12.2.05.002 **79**
– – notch A06.2.02.005 **58**
– – tubercle A06.2.02.007 **58**
– – vein A12.3.05.014 **93**
– tibiofibular joint A03.6.09.001 **31**
– tracheobronchial lymph nodes A13.3.02.013 **102**
– transverse scapular ligament A03.5.01.003 **28**
– trunk of brachial plexus A14.2.03.004 **137**
– tympanic artery A12.2.05.067 **81**
– ulnar collateral artery A12.2.09.025 **86**
– vein
– – of lower lobe
– – – of left lung A12.3.02.402 **92**
– – – of right lung A12.3.02.202 **92**
– – of vermis A12.3.06.057 **95**
– veins of cerebellar hemisphere A12.3.06.059 **95**
– vena cava A12.3.03.001 **92**
– vermian branch A12.2.08.027 **85**
– vertebral notch A02.2.01.009 **16**
– vesical arteries A12.2.15.024 **89**
– vestibular
– – area of internal acoustic meatus A15.3.03.050 **151**
– – nucleus A14.1.05.429 **114**
Superodextral lateral flexure of rectum A05.7.04.004 **54**
Superolateral
– face of cerebral hemisphere A14.1.09.101 **124**
– superficial inguinal lymph nodes A13.3.05.005 **103**
Superomedial
– lobule of prostate A09.3.08.013 **69**
– superficial inguinal lymph nodes A13.3.05.004 **103**
Supination A03.0.00.061 **26**
Supinator A04.6.02.048 **41**
– crest A02.4.06.014 **20**
– muscle A04.0.00.026 **33**
Supra-acetabular groove A02.5.01.103 **21**
Supra-optic
– fibres A14.1.08.952 **124**
– nucleus A14.1.08.912 **123**
– recess A14.1.08.423 **121**
Supra-opticohypophysial tract A14.1.08.958 **124**
Supra-orbital
– artery A12.2.06.037 **82**
– margin A02.1.00.071 **9**, A02.1.03.008 **10**
– nerve A14.2.01.021 **133**
– notch/foramen A02.1.03.009 **10**
– vein A12.3.05.021 **93**
Suprachiasmatic
– artery A12.2.07.030 **82**
– nucleus A14.1.08.911 **123**
Suprachoroid lamina of sclera A15.2.03.003 **144**, A15.2.02.010 **144**
Supraclavicular
– lymph nodes A13.3.00.036 **101**
– nerves A14.2.02.024 **137**
– part of brachial plexus A14.2.03.010 **138**
Supracollicular sphincter A09.4.02.013 **70**
Supracondylar process A02.4.04.017 **19**
Supracristal plane A01.2.00.009 **3**
Supraduodenal artery A12.2.12.017 **87**
Suprageniculate nucleus A14.1.08.637 **122**
Supraglenoid tubercle A02.4.01.020 **19**
Suprahyoid
– branch of lingual artery A12.2.05.016 **80**
– muscles A04.2.03.001 **35**
Supralemniscal nucleus A14.1.05.450 **114**
Supramammillary nucleus A14.1.08.937 **124**
Supramarginal gyrus A14.1.09.131 **125**
Supramastoid crest A02.1.06.068 **13**
Suprameatal
– spine A02.1.06.070 **13**
– triangle A02.1.06.069 **13**
Supraoptic artery A12.2.07.026 **82**
Suprapalpebral sulcus A01.2.01.009 **3**
Suprapatellar bursa A04.8.05.017 **45**
Suprapineal recess A14.1.08.413 **121**
Suprapleural membrane A07.1.02.018 **62**
Suprapyloric lymph node A13.3.03.020 **102**
Suprarenal
– gland A11.5.00.001 **74**
– impression on liver A05.8.01.023 **55**
– nerve plexus A14.3.03.026 **143**
Suprascapular
– artery A12.2.08.051 **85**
– nerve A14.2.03.014 **138**
– notch A02.4.01.015 **19**
– vein A12.3.05.049 **93**
Supraspinal nucleus A14.1.04.268 **111**
Supraspinatus A04.6.02.006 **40**
Supraspinous
– fascia A04.6.02.007 **40**
– fossa A02.4.01.007 **18**
– ligament A03.2.01.005 **27**
Suprasternal
– bones A02.3.03.009 **18**
– notch A02.3.03.004 **18**
– space A04.2.05.003 **35**
Suprastyloid crest A02.4.05.016 **20**
Supratonsillar fossa A05.2.01.010 **50**
Supratragic tubercle A15.3.01.023 **148**
Supratrochlear
– artery A12.2.06.048 **82**

– lymph nodes A13.3.01.012 **101**
– nerve A14.2.01.024 **133**
– veins A12.3.05.020 **93**
Supravaginal part of cervix A09.1.03.011 **65**
Supravalvular ridge A12.2.01.003 **78**, A12.2.03.003 **79**
Supraventricular crest A12.1.02.007 **76**
Supravesical fossa A10.1.02.430 **73**
Supreme
– intercostal
– – artery A12.2.08.061 **85**
– – vein A12.3.04.023 **92**
– nasal concha A02.1.07.012 **13**
Sural
– arteries A12.2.16.037 **90**
– communicating branch/nerve A14.2.07.049 **140**
– nerve A14.2.07.062 **141**
– region A01.2.08.017 **5**
– veins A12.3.11.029 **98**
Surgical neck of humerus A02.4.04.004 **19**
Suspensory
– ligament
– – of axilla A04.6.03.003 **41**
– – of clitoris ♀ A04.5.02.019 **39, 67, 69**
– – of duodenum A05.6.02.011 **52**
– – of eyeball A15.2.07.005 **147**
– – of ovary A09.1.01.018 **65, 73**
– – of penis ♂ A04.5.02.019 **39, 67, 69**
– – of thyroid gland A04.2.05.005 **36**
– ligaments of breast A16.0.02.015 **155**
– muscle of duodenum A05.6.02.011 **52**
– retinaculum of breast A16.0.02.015 **155**
Sustentaculum tali A02.5.11.006 **24**
Sutural bone A02.1.00.043 **8**
Suture A03.0.00.008 **25**
Sweat gland A16.0.00.029 **154**
Sympathetic
– ganglion A14.2.00.011 **132**
– paraganglia A14.3.01.078 **142**
– part of autonomic division of nervous system A14.3.01.001 **141**
– root A14.3.02.010 **142**
– – of ciliary ganglion A14.3.02.004 **142**
– – of otic ganglion A14.3.02.015 **142**
– – of pelvic ganglia A14.3.02.019 **142**
– – of pterygopalatine ganglion A14.3.02.008 **142**
– – of sublingual ganglion A14.3.02.013 **142**, A14.3.03.005 **142**
– – of submandibular ganglion A14.3.02.010 **142**
– trunk A14.3.01.002 **141**
Symphysial surface A02.5.01.304 **21**
Symphysis A03.0.00.017 **25**
Synapse A14.0.00.004 **104**
Synarthrosis A03.0.00.003 **25**
Synchondrosis/es A03.0.00.016 **25**
– of first rib A03.3.02.003 **28**
– of thorax A03.3.02.001 **28**
– of vertebral column A03.2.02.001 **27**
Syndesmosis/es A03.0.00.005 **25**
– of pectoral girdle A03.5.01.001 **28**
– of pelvic girdle A03.6.01.001 **30**
– of shoulder girdle A03.5.01.001 **28**
– of thorax A03.3.01.001 **28**
– of vertebral column A03.2.01.001 **27**
Synostosis A03.0.00.019 **25**
Synovial
– bursa A03.0.00.039 **25, 34**
– fluid A03.0.00.031 **25**
– folds A03.0.00.029 **25**
– joint/s A03.0.00.020 **25**
– – of free
– – – lower limb A03.6.06.001 **30**
– – – upper limb A03.5.07.001 **29**
– – of pectoral girdle A03.5.02.001 **28**
– – of shoulder girdle A03.5.02.001 **28**
– – of thorax A03.3.03.001 **28**
– layer/membrane A03.0.00.028 **25**
– sheath/s A03.0.00.040 **25, 34**, A04.8.01.007 **44**
– – of digits of hand A04.8.04.018 **45**
– – of toes A04.8.06.017 **46**
– villi A03.0.00.030 **25**

T

Tactile elevations A16.0.00.007 **154**
Taenia/e A14.1.09.261 **127**
– cinerea A14.1.05.712 **115**
– coli A05.7.03.013 **53**
– of fornix A14.1.09.261 **127**
– thalami A14.1.08.105 **120, 121**
Tail A14.1.09.505 **130**
– of caudate nucleus A14.1.09.505 **130**
– of epididymis A09.3.02.005 **68**
– of helix A15.3.01.008 **148**
– of pancreas A05.9.01.014 **56**
Talar shelf A02.5.11.006 **24**
Talocalcaneal
– interosseous ligament A03.6.10.503 **31**
– joint A03.6.10.101 **31**
Talocalcaneonavicular joint A03.6.10.202 **31**
Talonavicular ligament A03.6.10.507 **31**
Talus A02.5.10.001 **23**
Tangential fibres of isocortex A14.1.09.320 **128**
Tapetum A14.1.09.252 **127**
Tarsal
– bones A02.5.09.001 **23**
– glands A15.2.07.042 **147**
– interosseous ligaments A03.6.10.502 **31**
– ligaments A03.6.10.501 **31**
– sinus A02.5.11.009 **24**
Tarsometatarsal joints A03.6.10.601 **31**
Taste
– bud A15.4.00.002 **153**
– pore A15.4.00.003 **153**
Tectal plate A14.1.06.011 **115, 118**
Tecto-olivary fibres A14.1.05.307 **113, 117**
Tectobulbar tract A14.1.04.147 **110**, A14.1.05.333 **113**, A14.1.06.218 **116**
Tectopontine
– fibres A14.1.05.108 **112**
– tract A14.1.05.334 **113**, A14.1.06.205 **116**, A14.1.06.219 **116**
Tectoreticular fibres A14.1.05.308 **113**
Tectorial membrane
– of atlanto-axial joint A03.2.04.007 **27**
– of cochlear duct A15.3.03.108 **153**
Tectospinal tract A14.1.02.211 **107**, A14.1.04.112 **109, 113, 116**
Tectum of midbrain A14.1.06.601 **118**
Teeth A05.1.03.001 **48**
Tegmen tympani A02.1.06.022 **12**
Tegmental
– decussations A14.1.06.220 **117**
– roof/wall A15.3.02.003 **149**
– – of tympanic cavity A15.3.02.003 **149**
Tegmentum
– of midbrain A14.1.06.007 **115–116**
– of pons A14.1.05.301 **112**
Tela choroidea
– of fourth ventricle A14.1.01.303 **105**
– of third ventricle A14.1.01.305 **105, 121**
Telencephalon A14.1.03.008 **108**, A14.1.09.001 **124**
Temple A01.1.00.004 **2**
Temporal
– bone A02.1.06.001 **12**
– branches of facial nerve A14.2.01.109 **135**
– crest of mandible A02.1.15.033 **15**
– fascia A04.1.04.013 **35**
– fossa A02.1.00.022 **8**
– horn of lateral ventricle A14.1.09.287 **128**
– line of frontal bone A02.1.03.013 **10**
– lobe A14.1.09.136 **125–126**
– muscle A04.1.04.005 **35**
– operculum A14.1.09.139 **125**
– plane A14.1.09.143 **125**
– pole A14.1.09.137 **125**

– process of zygomatic A02.1.14.005 **15**
– region A01.2.01.005 **3**
– surface
– – of frontal bone A02.1.03.011 **10**
– – of sphenoid A02.1.05.026 **11**
– – of temporal bone A02.1.06.065 **13**
– – of zygomatic A02.1.14.003 **15**
– veins A12.3.06.007 **94**, A12.3.06.016 **94**
Temporalis A04.1.04.005 **35**
Temporo-occipital branch of middle cerebral artery A12.2.07.059 **83**
Temporomandibular joint A03.1.07.001 **27**
Temporoparietalis A04.1.03.006 **34**
Temporopontine fibres A14.1.06.109 **116**, A14.1.09.548 **131**
Temporozygomatic suture A03.1.02.024 **26**
Tendinous
– arch A04.0.00.048 **34**
– – of levator ani A04.5.04.009 **40**
– – of pelvic fascia A04.5.03.010 **39**
– – of soleus A04.7.03.024 **43**
– chiasm of digits of hand A04.6.03.014 **41**
– cords of heart A12.1.00.023 **76**
– intersection/s A04.0.00.046 **34**
– – of rectus abdominis A04.5.01.002 **38**
– sheath
– – of abductor longus and extensor pollicis brevis A04.8.04.009 **44**
– – of extensor/es
– – – carpi
– – – – radiales A04.8.04.010 **44**
– – – – ulnaris A04.8.04.014 **45**
– – – digiti minimi brevis A04.8.04.013 **45**
– – – digitorum
– – – – and extensor indicis A04.8.04.012 **44**
– – – – longus A04.8.06.005 **45**
– – – hallucis longus A04.8.06.004 **45**
– – – pollicis longus A04.8.04.011 **44**
– – of flexor
– – – carpi radialis A04.8.04.006 **44**
– – – digitorum longus A04.8.06.007 **45**
– – – hallucis longus A04.8.06.009 **46**
– – – pollicis longus A04.8.04.005 **44**
– – of superior oblique A15.2.07.018 **147**
– – of tibialis
– – – anterior A04.8.06.003 **45**
– – – posterior A04.8.06.008 **45**
– sheaths
– – of lower limb A04.8.06.001 **45**
– – of toes A04.8.06.013 **46**
– – of upper limb A04.8.04.001 **44**
Tendon A04.0.00.044 **34**
– of infundibulum A12.1.00.028 **76**
– of valve of inferior vena cava A12.1.00.029 **76**
– sheath A04.8.01.005 **44**
– sheaths and bursae A04.8.00.001 **44**
Tension lines A16.0.00.008 **154**
Tensor
– fasciae latae A04.7.02.010 **42**
– of fascia lata A04.7.02.010 **42**
– tympani A15.3.02.061 **150**
– veli palatini A05.2.01.103 **50**
Tentorial
– basal branch of cavernous part of internal carotid artery A12.2.06.008 **81**
– marginal branch of cavernous part of internal carotid artery A12.2.06.009 **81**
– nerve A14.2.01.017 **133**
– notch A14.1.01.105 **104**
Tentorium cerebelli A14.1.01.104 **104**
Teres
– major A04.6.02.011 **40**
– minor A04.6.02.010 **40**
Terminal
– filum A14.1.01.401 **105**
– ganglion A14.2.01.003 **133**
– ileum A05.6.04.002 **53**
– nerve [0] A14.2.01.002 **133**
– notch of auricle A15.3.01.025 **148**
– nucleus A14.1.00.006 **104**
– sulcus of tongue A05.1.04.019 **49**
– ventricle A14.1.02.006 **105**
Testicular
– artery ♂ A12.2.12.086 **88**
– nerve plexus ♂ A14.3.03.035 **143**
– plexus ♂ A14.3.03.035 **143**
– serosa A09.3.01.014 **67**
– subserosa A09.3.01.015 **67**
Testis A09.3.01.001 **67**
Thalamic fasciculus [H1] A14.1.09.523 **130**, A14.1.08.679 **123**
Thalamogeniculate artery A12.2.07.090 **84**
Thalamoparietal fibres A14.1.09.538 **130**
Thalamoperforating artery A12.2.07.086 **84**
Thalamotuberal artery A12.2.07.076 **83**
Thalamus A14.1.08.101 **120**, A14.1.08.601 **121**
Thenar eminence A01.2.07.023 **5**
Thigh A01.1.00.035 **2**
– bone A02.5.04.001 **22**
Third
– molar tooth A05.1.03.008 **48**
– occipital nerve A14.2.02.009 **137**
– toe [III] A01.2.08.038 **6**
– trochanter A02.5.04.008 **22**
– ventricle A14.1.08.410 **120**
Thoracic
– aorta A12.2.11.001 **86**
– aortic nerve plexus A14.3.03.012 **143**
– cage A02.3.04.001 **18**
– cardiac branches
– – of thoracic ganglia A14.3.01.025 **141**
– – of vagus A14.2.01.170 **136**
– cavity A01.1.00.049 **2**, A02.3.04.002 **18, 62**
– constriction of oesophagus A05.4.01.004 **51**
– duct A12.4.01.007 **99**
– fascia A04.4.01.019 **37**
– ganglia A14.3.01.024 **141**
– inlet A02.3.04.003 **18**
– intertransversarii A04.3.02.403 **37**
– joints A03.3.00.001 **28**
– kyphosis A02.2.00.003 **16**
– lymph nodes A13.3.02.001 **102**
– nerves [T1–T12] A14.2.04.001 **139**
– outlet A02.3.04.004 **18**
– part
– – of iliocostalis lumborum A04.3.02.008 **36**
– – of oesophagus A05.4.01.003 **51**
– – of peripheral autonomic plexuses and ganglia A14.3.03.010 **143**
– – of spinal cord A14.1.02.015 **105**
– – of thoracic duct A12.4.01.010 **99**
– – of trachea A06.3.01.003 **59**
– pulmonary branches A14.3.01.026 **141**
– segments [1–12] A14.1.02.015 **105**
– skeleton A02.3.00.001 **17**
– splanchnic ganglion A14.3.01.029 **141**
– vertebrae [T I – T XII] A02.2.03.001 **17–18**
– vertebrae [T I – T XII] A02.2.03.001 **17–18**
Thoraco-acromial
– artery A12.2.09.005 **85**
– vein A12.3.08.016 **96**
Thoraco-epigastric veins A12.3.08.012 **96**
Thoracodorsal
– artery A12.2.09.014 **85**
– nerve A14.2.03.016 **138**
– vein A12.3.08.008 **96**
Thoracolumbar fascia A04.3.02.501 **37**
Thorax A01.1.00.014 **2**
Three-headed muscle A04.0.00.013 **33**
Thumb A01.2.07.027 **5**
Thymic
– branches of internal thoracic artery A12.2.08.031 **85**
– veins A12.3.04.005 **92**
Thymus A13.1.02.001 **100**
Thyro-arytenoid A06.2.08.008 **59**
Thyro-epiglottic

– ligament A06.2.07.005 **59**
– part of thyro-arytenoid A06.2.08.009 **59**
Thyrocervical trunk A12.2.08.042 **85**
Thyroglossal duct A05.1.04.021 **49**
Thyrohyoid A04.2.04.007 **35**
– branch of ansa cervicalis A14.2.02.016 **137**
– membrane A06.2.02.013 **58**
Thyroid
– articular surface on cricoid A06.2.03.005 **58**
– cartilage A06.2.02.002 **58**
– foramen A06.2.02.012 **58**
– gland A11.3.00.001 **74**
– ima artery A12.2.04.005 **79**
– lymph nodes A13.3.00.022 **101**
Thyropharyngeal part of inferior constrictor A05.3.01.112 **51**
Thyropharyngeus A05.3.01.112 **51**
Tibia A02.5.06.001 **23**
Tibial A01.0.00.042 **1**
– border of foot A01.2.08.027 **5**
– collateral ligament A03.6.08.012 **31**
– nerve A14.2.07.058 **141**
– nutrient artery A12.2.16.060 **91**
– tarsal tendinous sheaths A04.8.06.006 **45**
– tuberosity A02.5.06.012 **23**
Tibialis
– anterior A04.7.02.037 **42**
– posterior A04.7.02.051 **43**
Tibiocalcaneal part of medial ligament of ankle joint A03.6.10.005 **31**
Tibiofibular
– joint A03.6.09.001 **31**
– syndesmosis A03.6.05.001 **30**
Tibionavicular part of medial ligament of ankle joint A03.6.10.004 **31**
Tip
– of ear A15.3.01.021 **148**
– of nose A06.1.01.004 **57**
– of tongue A05.1.04.010 **49**
Toes A01.1.00.046 **2**, A01.2.08.035 **6**
Tongue A05.1.04.001 **49**
Tonsil of cerebellum A14.1.07.222 **119**
Tonsillar
– bed A05.2.01.009 **50**
– branch/es
– – of facial artery A12.2.05.022 **80**
– – of glossopharyngeal nerve A14.2.01.147 **136**
– – of lesser palatine nerves A14.2.01.048 **134**
– capsule A05.2.01.012 **50, 100**
– cleft A05.2.01.013 **50**
– crypts A05.2.01.015 **50, 100**, A05.3.01.008 **50, 100**, A13.2.02.002 **100**, A13.2.02.003 **100**
– fossa A05.2.01.009 **50**
– pits A05.2.01.014 **50, 100**, A05.3.01.007 **50, 100**
– sinus A05.2.01.009 **50**
Tooth/Teeth A05.1.03.001 **48**
– socket A05.1.03.074 **49**
Torus
– levatorius A05.3.01.015 **50**
– tubarius A05.3.01.012 **50**
Trabeculae A13.2.03.003 **100**
– carneae A12.1.00.020 **76**
– – of left ventricle A12.1.04.011 **77**
– – of right ventricle A12.1.02.021 **77**
– of corpora cavernosa A09.4.01.020 **69**
– of corpus spongiosum A09.4.01.021 **69**
– of lymph node A13.2.03.003 **100**
Trabecular
– bone A02.0.00.004 **7**
– tissue of sclera A15.2.02.004 **144**
Trachea A06.3.01.001 **59**
Tracheal
– bifurcation A06.3.01.008 **59**
– branches
– – of inferior thyroid artery A12.2.08.048 **85**
– – of internal thoracic artery A12.2.08.033 **85**
– – of recurrent laryngeal nerve A14.2.01.167 **136**
– cartilages A06.3.01.004 **59**
– glands A06.3.01.011 **59**
– mucosa A06.3.01.010 **59**
– veins A12.3.04.010 **92**
Trachealis A06.3.01.005 **59**
Tracheobronchial lymph nodes A13.3.02.012 **102**
Tract A14.1.00.011 **104**
Tractus spiralis foraminosus A15.3.03.054 **152**
Tragal lamina A15.3.01.051 **149**
Tragicus A15.3.01.039 **148**
Tragus A15.3.01.017 **148**
Transcapsular grey bridges A14.1.09.525 **130**
Transpyloric plane A01.2.00.007 **3**
Transversalis fascia A04.5.02.011 **39**
Transverse A01.0.00.026 **1**, A01.0.00.027 **1**
– abdominal A04.5.01.019 **38**
– acetabular ligament A03.6.07.009 **30**
– arytenoid A06.2.08.012 **59**
– branch of lateral circumflex femoral artery A12.2.16.030 **90**
– cerebral fissure A14.1.09.008 **124**
– cervical
– – artery A12.2.08.053 **85**
– – ligament A09.1.03.031 **66**
– – nerve A14.2.02.021 **137**
– – veins A12.3.05.050 **93**
– colon A05.7.03.004 **53**
– costal facet A02.2.03.004 **17**
– crest of internal acoustic meatus A15.3.03.047 **151**
– diameter of pelvis A02.5.02.011 **22**
– ductules of epoophoron A09.1.05.003 **66**
– facial
– – artery A12.2.05.047 **80**
– – vein A12.3.05.034 **93**
– fascicles of plantar aponeurosis A04.7.03.032 **44**
– folds of rectum A05.7.04.007 **54**
– head
– – of adductor
– – – hallucis A04.7.02.062 **43**
– – – pollicis A04.6.02.061 **41**
– humeral ligament A03.5.08.005 **29**
– ligament
– – of atlas A03.2.04.006 **27**
– – of knee A03.6.08.006 **30**
– ligaments of vertebral column A03.2.01.009 **27**
– medullary veins A12.3.06.051 **95**
– mesocolon A10.1.02.010 **72**
– muscle A05.1.04.108 **49**
– – of auricle A15.3.01.043 **149**
– – of tongue A05.1.04.108 **49**
– occipital
– – fasciculi A14.1.09.566 **131**
– – sulcus A14.1.09.135 **125**
– palatine
– – folds A05.1.01.106 **47**
– – suture A03.1.02.033 **26**
– part
– – of duodenum A05.6.02.007 **52**
– – of iliofemoral ligament A03.6.07.004 **30**
– – of left branch of portal vein A12.3.12.006 **98**
– – of nasalis A04.1.03.010 **34**
– – of trapezius A04.3.01.003 **36**
– pericardial sinus A12.1.07.001 **77**
– perineal ligament ♂ A09.5.03.003 **71**
– planes A01.2.00.006 **3**
– pontine
– – fibres A14.1.05.109 **112**
– – veins A12.3.06.046 **95**
– process of vertebra A02.2.01.013 **16**
– ridge/s
– – of sacrum A02.2.05.010 **17**
– – of tooth A05.1.03.014 **48**
– sinus A12.3.05.102 **93**
– tarsal joint A03.6.10.201 **31**
– temporal
– – gyri A14.1.09.140 **125**
– – sulcus A14.1.09.144 **125**
– vesical fold A10.1.02.503 **73**
Transversospinales A04.3.02.201 **37**
Transversus
– abdominis A04.5.01.019 **38**
– menti A04.1.03.027 **34**
– nuchae A04.3.01.005 **36**
– thoracis A04.4.01.016 **37**
Trapezium A02.4.08.008 **20**
Trapezius A04.3.01.001 **36**
Trapezoid A02.4.08.010 **20**

– area below prostate A09.3.08.021 **69**
– body A14.1.05.315 **113**
– ligament A03.5.03.005 **28**
– line A02.4.02.011 **19**
Triangle
– of auscultation A01.2.05.006 **4**
– of sinu-atrial node A12.1.00.030 **76**
Triangular
– fold A05.2.01.006 **50**
– fossa of auricle A15.3.01.010 **148**
– fovea of arytenoid A06.2.04.009 **58**
– muscle A04.0.00.009 **33**
– nucleus of septum A14.1.09.271 **127**, A14.1.09.448 **129**
– part of inferior frontal gyrus A14.1.09.115 **125**
– ridge of tooth A05.1.03.015 **48**
Triceps
– brachii A04.6.02.019 **40**
– surae A04.7.02.043 **43**
Tricuspid valve A12.1.02.003 **76**
Trigeminal
– cave A14.1.01.108 **104**
– cavity A14.1.01.108 **104**
– ganglion A14.2.01.014 **133**
– impression A02.1.06.028 **12**
– lemniscus A14.1.05.310 **113**, A14.1.06.208 **116**, A14.1.08.680 **123**
– nerve [V] A14.2.01.012 **133**
– tubercle A14.1.04.015 **109**
Trigeminospinal tract A14.1.02.238 **107**
Trigeminothalamic tract A14.1.05.310 **113**
Trigonal muscles A08.3.01.011 **64**
Trigone
– of bladder A08.3.01.024 **64**
– of hypoglossal nerve A14.1.05.708 **115**
– of lateral lemniscus A14.1.06.008 **115**
– of vagus nerve A14.1.05.709 **115**
Triquetrum A02.4.08.006 **20**
Triticeal cartilage A06.2.02.018 **58**
Trochanteric
– bursa/e of gluteus
– – maximus A04.8.05.003 **45**
– – medius A04.8.05.004 **45**
– – minimus A04.8.05.005 **45**
– fossa A02.5.04.006 **22**
Trochlea A02.4.04.023 **19**, A15.2.07.017 **147**
– of humerus A02.4.04.023 **19**
– of phalanx A02.4.10.009 **21**, A02.5.18.009 **24**
– – of foot A02.5.18.009 **24**
– – of hand A02.4.10.009 **21**
– of superior oblique A15.2.07.017 **147**
– of talus A02.5.10.011 **24**
Trochlear
– fovea A02.1.03.025 **10**
– nerve [IV] A14.2.01.011 **133**
– notch A02.4.06.006 **20**
– spine A02.1.03.024 **10**
True
– conjugate A02.5.02.014 **22**
– pelvis A02.5.02.006 **22**
– ribs [I–VII] A02.3.01.002 **17**
Trunk/s A01.1.00.013 **2**
– of accessory nerve A14.2.01.187 **137**
– of brachial plexus A14.2.03.003 **137**
– of corpus callosum A14.1.09.244 **127**
– of spinal nerve A14.2.00.031 **133**
Tubal
– air cells A15.3.02.077 **150**
– branch/es
– – of ovarian artery ♀ A12.2.12.088 **88**
– – of tympanic plexus A14.2.01.141 **136**
– – of uterine artery ♀ A12.2.15.034 **89**
– extremity of ovary A09.1.01.007 **65**
– glands A15.3.02.084 **151**
– tonsil A05.3.01.016 **50, 100**
Tuber A02.0.00.024 **7**
– cinereum A14.1.08.408 **120**
– of vermis [VII B] A14.1.07.212 **119**
Tubercle A02.0.00.025 **7**
– of rib A02.3.02.008 **18**
– of scaphoid A02.4.08.004 **20**
– of tooth A05.1.03.013 **48**
– of trapezium A02.4.08.009 **20**
– of upper lip A05.1.01.008 **47**
Tuberculum
– of iliac crest A02.5.01.108 **21**
– sellae A02.1.05.007 **11**
Tuberomammillary nucleus A14.1.08.932 **124**
Tuberosity A02.0.00.024 **7**, A02.0.00.026 **7**
– for coracoclavicular ligament A02.4.02.009 **19**
– for serratus anterior A02.3.02.019 **18**
– of cuboid A02.5.16.003 **24**
– of distal phalanx A02.4.10.005 **21**, A02.5.18.005 **24**
– – of foot A02.5.18.005 **24**
– – of hand A02.4.10.005 **21**
– of fifth metatarsal bone [V] A02.5.17.006 **24**
– of first metatarsal bone [I] A02.5.17.005 **24**
– of navicular A02.5.12.002 **24**
– of ulna A02.4.06.004 **20**
Tunica
– albuginea
– – of corpora cavernosa A09.4.01.017 **69**
– – of corpus spongiosum A09.4.01.018 **69**
– – of ovary A09.1.01.009 **65**
– – of testis A09.3.01.016 **67**
– externa A12.0.00.017 **75**
– intima A12.0.00.018 **75**
– media A12.0.00.019 **75**
– vaginalis testis A09.3.01.008 **67**
Two-bellied muscle A04.0.00.011 **33**
Two-headed muscle A04.0.00.012 **33**
Tympanic
– aperture of canaliculus for chorda tympani A15.3.02.027 **149**
– body A12.3.05.003 **93**
– canaliculus A02.1.06.049 **13**
– cavity A02.1.06.051 **13**, A15.3.02.002 **149**
– cells A15.3.02.030 **149**
– enlargement A14.2.01.139 **136**
– ganglion A14.2.01.139 **136**
– lamella A15.3.03.032 **151**
– lip of limbus of osseous spiral lamina A15.3.03.105 **152**
– membrane A15.3.01.052 **149**
– nerve A14.2.01.138 **136**
– notch A02.1.06.059 **13**, A15.3.01.047 **149**
– opening of pharyngotympanic tube A15.3.02.074 **150**
– part of temporal bone A02.1.06.052 **13**
– plexus A14.2.01.140 **136**
– ring A02.1.06.053 **13**
– sulcus A02.1.06.058 **13**
– surface of cochlear duct A15.3.03.100 **152**
– veins A12.3.05.043 **93**
Tympanomastoid fissure A02.1.06.077 **13**
Tympanosquamous fissure A02.1.06.076 **13**
Tympanostapedial syndesmosis A15.3.02.052 **150**

U

Ulna A02.4.06.001 **20**
Ulnar A01.0.00.040 **1**
– artery A12.2.09.041 **86**
– border A01.2.07.016 **5**
– canal A03.5.11.202 **29**
– collateral ligament
– – of elbow joint A03.5.09.005 **29**
– – of wrist joint A03.5.11.007 **29**
– head
– – of extensor carpi ulnaris A04.6.02.047 **41**
– – of flexor carpi ulnaris A04.6.02.032 **41**
– – of pronator teres A04.6.02.027 **41**
– nerve A14.2.03.040 **138**
– notch A02.4.05.019 **20**
– recurrent artery A12.2.09.042 **86**
– styloid process A02.4.06.017 **20**
– veins A12.3.08.030 **96**
Umbilical
– artery A12.2.15.020 **89**
– fascia A04.5.02.014 **39**
– fissure A05.8.01.034 **55**
– part of left branch of portal vein A12.3.12.008 **98**

– region A01.2.04.005 **4**
– ring A04.5.01.023 **38**
– vein A12.3.12.010 **98**
Umbo of tympanic membrane A15.3.01.059 **149**
Uncal artery A12.2.06.020 **81, 83**
Uncinate
– fasciculus A14.1.09.560 **131**
– – of cerebellum A14.1.07.420 **120**
– process
– – of cervical vertebra A02.2.02.002 **16**
– – of ethmoid A02.1.07.016 **13**
– – of first thoracic vertebra A02.2.03.005 **17**
– – of pancreas A05.9.01.003 **56**
Uncus A14.1.09.235 **126**
– of body
– – of cervical vertebra A02.2.02.002 **16**
– – of first thoracic vertebra A02.2.03.005 **17**
Unipennate muscle A04.0.00.015 **33**
Unpaired thyroid venous plexus A12.3.04.003 **92**
Unstratified part of detrusor A08.3.01.015 **64**
Upper
– dental arcade A05.1.03.002 **48**
– eyelid A15.2.07.025 **147**
– head of lateral pterygoid A04.1.04.007 **35**
– limb A01.1.00.019 **2**
– lip A05.1.01.006 **47**
– lobe of lung A06.5.01.017 **60**
– pole of testis A09.3.01.002 **67**
– trunk of brachial plexus A14.2.03.004 **137**
Ureter A08.2.01.001 **64**
Ureteric
– branches
– – of testicular artery ♂ A12.2.12.087 **88**
– – of inferior suprarenal artery A12.2.12.085 **88**
– – of ovarian artery ♀ A12.2.12.087 **88**
– – of umbilical artery A12.2.15.023 **89**
– mucosa A08.2.01.007 **64**
– nerve plexus A14.3.03.034 **143**
– orifice A08.3.01.026 **64**
Urethral
– artery A12.2.15.042 **89**
– carina of vagina A09.1.04.016 **66**
– crest A09.2.03.004 **67**, A09.4.02.007 **70**
– glands A09.2.03.013 **67**, A09.4.02.025 **70**
– lacunae A09.2.03.014 **67**, A09.4.02.024 **70**
– mucosa A09.2.03.012 **67**
– surface A09.4.01.006 **69**
Urinary
– bladder A08.3.01.001 **64**
– system A08.0.00.000 **63**
Urogenital
– hiatus A04.5.04.010 **40**
– peritoneum A10.1.02.501 **73**
– triangle A01.2.06.003 **4**
Uterine
– artery ♀ A12.2.15.029 **89**
– cavity A09.1.03.007 **65**
– extremity of ovary A09.1.01.008 **65**
– glands A09.1.03.028 **66**
– horn A09.1.03.004 **65**
– ostium of tube A09.1.02.009 **65**
– part of tube A09.1.02.008 **65**
– subserosa A09.1.03.024 **66**
– tube A09.1.02.001 **65**
– veins ♀ A12.3.10.015 **97**
– venous plexus ♀ A12.3.10.016 **97**
Uterosacral ligament A09.1.03.032 **66**
Uterovaginal
– nerve plexus ♀ A14.3.03.052 **143**
Uterus A09.1.03.001 **65**
Utricle A15.3.03.063 **152**
Utricular
– duct A15.3.03.077 **152**
– nerve A14.2.01.127 **135**
– recess A15.3.03.005 **151**, A15.3.03.064 **152**
Utriculo-ampullary nerve A14.2.01.126 **135**
Utriculosaccular duct A15.3.03.076 **152**
Uveal part of sclera A15.2.02.006 **144**
Uvula
– of bladder A08.3.01.006 **64**
– of palate A05.2.01.004 **50**
– of vermis [IX] A14.1.07.221 **119**

V

Vagal
– part of accessory nerve A14.2.01.185 **137**
– trigone A14.1.05.709 **115**
Vagina A09.1.04.001 **66**
Vaginal
– artery ♀ A12.2.15.035 **89**
– branches
– – of middle rectal artery ♀ A12.2.15.037 **89**
– – of uterine artery ♀ A12.2.15.031 **89**
– columns A09.1.04.013 **66**
– fornix A09.1.04.002 **66**
– mucosa A09.1.04.011 **66**
– nerves ♀ A14.3.03.053 **143**
– orifice A09.2.01.015 **67**
– part of cervix A09.1.03.014 **66**
– process of sphenoid A02.1.05.048 **12**
– rugae A09.1.04.012 **66**
– venous plexus ♀ A12.3.10.017 **97**
Vagus nerve [X] A14.2.01.153 **136**
Vallate papillae A05.1.04.016 **49**
Vallecula of cerebellum A14.1.07.005 **118**
Valve A12.0.00.020 **75**
– of coronary sinus A12.1.01.016 **76**
– of foramen ovale A12.1.03.005 **77**
– of inferior vena cava A12.1.01.015 **76**
– of navicular fossa A09.4.02.023 **70**
Vas
– deferens A09.3.05.001 **68**
– prominens of cochlear duct A15.3.03.098 **152**
– spirale A15.3.03.103 **152**
Vasa
– recta A08.1.03.008 **63**
– vasorum A12.0.00.028 **75**
Vascular
– bundles of renal medulla A08.1.01.024 **63**
– circle A12.0.00.007 **75**
– – of optic nerve A15.2.04.036 **146**
– fold of caecum A10.1.02.419 **73**
– lamina of choroid A15.2.03.005 **144**
– layer
– – of eyeball A15.2.03.001 **144**
– – of testis A09.3.01.017 **67**
– nerve plexus A14.2.00.043 **133**
– nerves A14.2.00.045 **133**
– organ of lamina terminalis A14.1.08.940 **124, 127**
– plexus A12.0.00.010 **75**, A14.2.00.043 **133**
– space A04.7.03.011 **43**
Vastus
– intermedius A04.7.02.022 **42**
– lateralis A04.7.02.021 **42**
– medialis A04.7.02.023 **42**
Vault of pharynx A05.3.01.004 **50**
Vein/s A12.0.00.030 **75**, A12.3.00.001 **91**
– of brainstem A12.3.06.038 **95**
– of bulb
– – of penis ♂ A12.3.10.023 **97**
– – of vestibule ♀ A12.3.10.023 **97**
– of caudate nucleus A12.3.06.035 **95**
– of cerebellomedullary cistern A12.3.06.055 **95**
– of cochlear
– – aqueduct A12.3.05.004 **93**, A15.3.03.136 **153**
– – window A15.3.03.143 **153**
– of heart A12.3.01.001 **91**
– of lateral recess of fourth ventricle A12.3.06.054 **95**
– of lower limb A12.3.11.001 **98**
– of medulla oblongata A12.3.06.048 **95**
– of olfactory gyrus A12.3.06.023 **94**
– of pterygoid canal A12.3.05.039 **93**
– of scala
– – tympani A15.3.03.139 **153**
– – vestibuli A15.3.03.138 **153**

– of semicircular ducts A15.3.03.135 **153**
– of spinal cord A12.3.07.023 **96**
– of uncus A12.3.06.014 **94**
– of upper limb A12.3.08.001 **96**
– of vertebral column A12.3.07.018 **96**
– of vestibular aqueduct A15.3.03.134 **153**
Vena comitans A12.0.00.031 **75**
– of hypoglossal nerve A12.3.05.011 **93**
Venous
– grooves A02.1.00.041 **8**
– plexus A12.0.00.011 **75**, A12.0.00.015 **75**
– – of foramen ovale A12.3.05.307 **94**
– – of hypoglossal canal A12.3.05.306 **94**
– valve A12.0.00.023 **75**
Ventral A01.0.00.013 **1**
– acoustic stria A14.1.05.319 **113**
– anterior nucleus of thalamus A14.1.08.652 **122**
– cochlear nucleus A14.1.04.249 **111**
– column A14.1.02.102 **106**
– corticospinal tract A14.1.02.205 **107**
– external arcuate fibres of medulla A14.1.04.009 **108, 109**
– fasciculus proprius A14.1.02.203 **107**
– funiculus of of spinal cord A14.1.02.202 **107**
– gigantocellular reticular nucleus A14.1.04.304 **111**
– grey
– – column of spinal cord A14.1.02.102 **106**
– – commissure of spinal cord A14.1.02.303 **108**
– horn of spinal cord A14.1.02.021 **106**, A14.1.02.103 **106**
– intermediate nucleus of thalamus A14.1.08.655 **122**
– lamella of principal olivary nucleus A14.1.04.222 **110**
– lateral
– – complex of thalamus A14.1.08.649 **122**
– – geniculate nucleus A14.1.08.806 **123**
– medial
– – complex of thalamus A14.1.08.644 **122**
– – nucleus of spinal cord A14.1.02.141 **106**
– – visceral nucleus A14.1.06.305 **117**
– median fissure
– – of medulla A14.1.04.001 **108**
– – of spinal cord A14.1.02.007 **105**
– nuclei of thalamus A14.1.08.639 **122**
– nucleus
– – of lateral lemniscus A14.1.05.434 **114**
– – of pons A14.1.05.203 **112**
– – of trapezoid body A14.1.05.422 **114**
– pallidum A14.1.09.438 **129, 130**
– paraflocculus [H IX] A14.1.07.222 **119**
– part/s
– – of anterior quadrangular lobule of cerebellum [H IV] A14.1.07.117 **119**
– – of central
– – – lobule of cerebellum [II] A14.1.07.106 **119**
– – – reticular nucleus A14.1.04.316 **112**
– – of culmen [IV] A14.1.07.113 **119**
– – of intertransversarii laterales lumborum A04.3.01.016 **36**
– – of lateral parabrachial nucleus A14.1.05.445 **114**
– – of wing of central lobule of cerebellum [H II] A14.1.07.109 **119**
– pontoreticulospinal tract A14.1.05.322 **113**
– posterior
– – inferior nucleus of thalamus A14.1.08.648 **122**
– – internal nucleus of thalamus A14.1.08.657 **122**
– – parvocellular nucleus of thalamus A14.1.08.658 **122**
– posterolateral nucleus of thalamus A14.1.08.641 **122**, A14.1.08.656 **122**
– posteromedial nucleus of thalamus A14.1.08.642 **122**
– premammillary nucleus A14.1.08.938 **124**
– principal nucleus of medial geniculate body A14.1.08.809 **123**
– rami
– of cervical nerves A14.2.02.011 **137**
– – of lumbar nerves A14.2.05.008 **139**
– – of sacral nerves and coccygeal nerve A14.2.06.007 **139**
– – of thoracic nerves A14.2.04.006 **139**
– raphespinal tract A14.1.02.212 **107**
– reticulospinal tract A14.1.04.124 **109**
– root of spinal nerve A14.2.00.029 **133**
– solitary nucleus A14.1.04.240 **111**
– spinocerebellar tract A14.1.02.226 **107**, A14.1.04.125 **109**, A14.1.05.323 **113**
– spinothalamic tract A14.1.02.214 **107**
– striatum A14.1.09.439 **129, 130**
– subdivision of nucleus of posterior commissure A14.1.06.310 **117**
– subnucleus of lateral parabrachial nucleus A14.1.05.445 **114**
– supra-optic commissure A14.1.08.959 **124**
– tegmental
– – decussation A14.1.06.222 **117**
– – nuclei of midbrain A14.1.06.330 **117**
– – nucleus of pons A14.1.05.435 **114**
– thalamus A14.1.08.201 **120**
– trigeminothalamic tract A14.1.05.311 **113**
– white commissure of spinal cord A14.1.02.305 **108**
Ventrobasal nuclear complex of thalamus A14.1.08.640 **122**
Ventrolateral
– nucleus
– – of principal sensory nucleus of trigeminal nerve A14.1.05.408 **114**
– – of spinal cord A14.1.02.105 **106**
– solitary nucleus A14.1.04.241 **111**
– sulcus
– – of medulla A14.1.04.005 **108**
– – of spinal cord A14.1.02.010 **105**
Ventromedial
– nucleus
– – of hypothalamus A14.1.08.928 **124**
– – of spinal cord A14.1.02.107 **106**
– part of supra-optic nucleus A14.1.08.915 **123**
Venulae rectae of kidney A08.1.04.005 **63**
Venule A12.0.00.037 **75**
Vermiform appendix A05.7.02.007 **53**
Vermis of cerebellum [I–X] A14.1.07.006 **118**
Vertebra/e A02.2.01.001 **16**
– prominens [C VII] A02.2.02.301 **17**
Vertebral
– arch A02.2.01.005 **16**
– artery A12.2.08.002 **84**
– body A02.2.01.002 **16**
– canal A02.2.00.009 **16**
– column A02.2.00.001 **16**
– foramen A02.2.01.011 **16**
– ganglion A14.3.01.017 **141**
– joints A03.2.00.001 **27**
– nerve A14.3.01.023 **141**
– – plexus A14.3.03.010 **143**
– part of costal surface of lung A06.5.01.007 **60**
– region A01.2.05.002 **4**
– synovial joints A03.2.03.001 **27**
– vein A12.3.04.012 **92**
Vertebromediastinal recess A07.1.02.016 **62**
Vertex A02.1.00.033 **8**
Vertical A01.0.00.001 **1**
– aspect A02.1.00.003 **8**

– crest of internal acoustic meatus A15.3.03.049 **151**
– limb of diagonal band A14.1.09.424 **129**
– muscle of tongue A05.1.04.109 **49**
– occipital fasciculi A14.1.09.563 **131**
Vesical
– nerve plexus A14.3.03.055 **143**
– surface of uterus A09.1.03.008 **65**
– veins A12.3.10.011 **97**
– venous plexus A12.3.10.012 **97**
Vesico-uterine pouch ♀ A10.1.02.504 **73**
Vesicoprostaticus ♂ A08.3.01.021 **64, 69**
Vesicovaginalis ♀ A08.3.01.021 **64, 69**
Vesicular
– appendices of epoophoron A09.1.05.004 **66**
– ovarian follicle A09.1.01.013 **65**
Vessels
– of internal ear A15.3.03.126 **153**
– of nerves A12.0.00.029 **75**
Vestibular
– aqueduct A15.3.03.057 **152**
– area A14.1.05.710 **115**
– caecum A15.3.03.109 **153**
– canaliculus A02.1.06.035 **12**
– crest A15.3.03.007 **151**
– fold A06.2.09.008 **59**
– fossa of vagina A09.2.01.012 **66**
– ganglion A14.2.01.123 **135**
– labyrinth A15.3.03.062 **152**
– lamella A15.3.03.031 **151**
– ligament A06.2.09.023 **59**
– lip of limbus of osseous spiral lamina A15.3.03.106 **153**
– membrane A15.3.03.094 **152**
– nerve A14.2.01.122 **135**
– nuclei
– – in medulla oblongata A14.1.04.242 **111**
– – in pontile tegmentum A14.1.05.425 **114**
– surface
– – of cochlear duct A15.3.03.094 **152**
– – of tooth A05.1.03.035 **48**
Vestibule A15.3.03.004 **151**
– of omental bursa A10.1.02.404 **72**
– of vagina A09.2.01.012 **66**
Vestibulocerebellum A14.1.07.007 **118**
Vestibulocochlear
– artery A15.3.03.129 **153**
– nerve [VIII] A14.2.01.121 **135**
– organ A15.3.03.002 **151**
– vein A15.3.03.140 **153**
Vestige
– of ductus deferens A09.1.06.002 **66**
– of processus vaginalis A09.3.04.006 **68**
Villous folds of stomach A05.5.01.031 **52**
Vincula tendinum
– of digits of hand A04.8.04.019 **45**
– of toes A04.8.06.018 **46**
Vinculum
– breve of digits of hand A04.8.04.021 **45**
– longum of digits of hand A04.8.04.020 **45**
Visceral
– abdominal
– – fascia A04.5.02.002 **38**
– – lymph nodes A13.3.03.014 **102**
– fascia A04.0.00.036 **33**
– layer
– – of serous pericardium A12.1.08.007 **78**
– – of tunica vaginalis testis A09.3.01.010 **67**
– lymph nodes A13.3.03.014 **102**, A13.3.04.023 **103**
– nerve plexus A14.2.00.042 **133**
– nuclei A14.1.06.304 **117**
– pelvic
– – fascia A04.5.03.002 **39**
– – lymph nodes A13.3.04.023 **103**
– peritoneum A10.1.02.006 **72**
– pleura A07.1.02.002 **62**
– serosa A07.1.02.003 **62**
– subserosa A07.1.02.004 **62**
– surface
– – of liver A05.8.01.012 **54**
– – of spleen A13.2.01.008 **100**
Viscerocranium A02.1.00.008 **8**
Vitreous
– body A15.2.06.008 **146**
– chamber of eyeball A15.2.06.006 **146**
– humor A15.2.06.014 **146**
– membrane A15.2.06.012 **146**
– stroma A15.2.06.013 **146**
Vocal
– fold A06.2.09.013 **59**
– ligament A06.2.09.025 **59**
– process of arytenoid A06.2.04.005 **58**
Vocalis A06.2.08.007 **59**
Voiding internal urethral orifice A09.2.03.002 **67**
Volar A01.0.00.043 **1**
Vomer A02.1.11.001 **14**
Vomerine
– crest of choana A02.1.11.004 **14**
– groove A02.1.11.003 **14**
Vomeronasal
– cartilage A06.1.01.016 **57**
– organ A06.1.02.008 **57**
Vomerorostral canal A02.1.00.066 **9**
Vomerovaginal
– canal A02.1.00.065 **9**
– groove A02.1.05.050 **12**
Vortex of heart A12.1.00.021 **76**
Vorticose veins A12.3.06.106 **95**
Vulva A09.2.01.001 **66**

W

White
– matter/substance A14.1.00.009 **104**
– – of basilar part of pons A14.1.05.102 **112**
– – of cerebellum A14.1.07.418 **120**
– – of hypothalamus A14.1.08.945 **124**
– – of medulla A14.1.04.101 **109**
– – of midbrain tegmentum A14.1.06.201 **116**
– – of pontile tegmentum A14.1.05.302 **112**
– – of spinal cord A14.1.02.024 **106**, A14.1.02.201 **107**
– – of thalamus A14.1.08.659 **122**
– pulp A13.2.01.006 **100**
– ramus communicans A14.3.01.007 **141**
Wing A02.2.05.004 **17**
– of central lobule of cerebellum A14.1.07.108 **119**
– of ilium A02.5.01.104 **21**
– of sacrum A02.2.05.004 **17**
Wisdom tooth A05.1.03.008 **48**
Wrist A01.1.00.026 **2**
– joint A03.5.11.002 **29**

X

Xiphisternal joint A03.3.02.005 **28**
Xiphoid process A02.3.03.007 **18**

Y

Yellow bone marrow A02.0.00.039 **7**

Z

Zona
– incerta A14.1.08.707 **123**
– orbicularis of hip joint A03.6.07.002 **30**
Zonal
– layer of superior colliculus A14.1.06.606 **118**
– subnucleus of spinal nucleus of trigeminal nerve A14.1.04.213 **110**
Zones of hypothalamus A14.1.08.941 **124**
Zonular
– fibres A15.2.05.016 **146**
– spaces A15.2.05.017 **146**
Zygapophysial joints A03.2.06.001 **27**
Zygomatic
– arch A02.1.00.023 **8**
– bone A02.1.14.001 **15**
– branches of facial nerve A14.2.01.110 **135**
– margin of sphenoid A02.1.05.031 **11**
– nerve A14.2.01.056 **134**
– process

– – of frontal bone A02.1.03.014 **10**
– – of maxilla A02.1.12.028 **14**
– – of temporal bone
A02.1.06.067 **13**
– region A01.2.01.015 **3**
Zygomatico-orbital
– artery A12.2.05.049 **80**
– foramen A02.1.14.009 **15**
Zygomaticofacial
– branch of zygomatic nerve
A14.2.01.058 **134**
– foramen A02.1.14.010 **15**
Zygomaticomaxillary suture
A02.1.12.012 **14**, A03.1.02.018 **26**
Zygomaticotemporal
– branch of zygomatic nerve
A14.2.01.057 **134**
– foramen A02.1.14.011 **15**
Zygomaticus
– major A04.1.03.029 **34**
– minor A04.1.03.030 **34**